D1591545

Chest Physiotherapy in the Intensive Care Unit

SECOND EDITION

Chest Physiotherapy in the Intensive Care Unit

SECOND EDITION

Colin F. Mackenzie, M.B., Ch.B., Editor

Associate Professor
Department of Anesthesiology
University of Maryland School of Medicine
Baltimore, Maryland

P. Cristina Imle, M.S., P.T.

Physical Therapist
Maryland Institute for Emergency Medical Services Systems
Clinical Instructor, Department of Physical Therapy
University of Maryland School of Medicine
Baltimore, Maryland

Nancy Ciesla, B.S., P.T.

Chief Physical Therapist
Maryland Institute for Emergency Medical Services Systems
and Montebello Rehabilitation Hospital
Clinical Instructor, Department of Physical Therapy
University of Maryland School of Medicine
Baltimore, Maryland

*With a contribution in the 1st Edition to Chapters 5 and
6 from **Nancy Klemic, B.S., P.T.**
Formerly, Senior Physical Therapist
Maryland Institute for Emergency Medical Services Systems
Baltimore, Maryland*

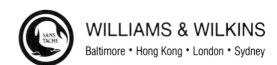

WILLIAMS & WILKINS
Baltimore • Hong Kong • London • Sydney

Editor: Timothy H. Grayson
Associate Editor: Carol Eckhart
Copy Editor: Arline Keithe, Amy Redmon
Design: JoAnne Janowiak
Illustration Planning: Lorraine Wrzosek
Production: Raymond E. Reter

Copyright © 1989
Williams & Wilkins
428 East Preston Street
Baltimore, Maryland 21202, USA

All rights reserved. This book is protected by copyright. No part of this book may
be reproduced in any form or by any means, including photocopying, or utilized
by any information storage and retrieval system without written permission from
the copyright owner.

Accurate indications, adverse reactions, and dosage schedules for drugs are
provided in this book, but it is possible that they may change. The reader is urged
to review the package information data of the manufacturers of the medications
mentioned.

Printed in the United States of America

First Edition 1981

Library of Congress Cataloging-in-Publication Data

Chest physiotherapy in the intensive care unit/Colin F. Mackenzie,
    editor; P. Cristina Imle, Nancy Ciesla, Nancy Klemic.—2nd ed.
        p. cm.
    Includes bibliographies and index.
    ISBN 0-683-05329-9
        1. Lungs—Diseases—Physical therapy.   2. Respiratory therapy.
    3. Critical care medicine.   I. Mackenzie, Colin F.   II. Imle, P.
    Christina.   III. Ciesla, Nancy.   IV. Klemic, Nancy.
        [DNLM: 1. Intensive Care Units.   2. Lung Diseases—therapy.
    3. Physical Therapy.   WF 145 C526]
    RC735.P58C48   1988
    617′.5406—dc 19
    DNLM/DLC
    for Library of Congress   88-37426
                                                                          CIP

                                                              89 90 91 92
                              1   2   3   4   5   6   7   8   9   10

Preface to the Second Edition

The second edition of *Chest Physiotherapy in the Intensive Care Unit* follows 8 years after the first. The object remains to provide a comprehensive reference source for all professionals involved in respiratory intensive care. Over 900 references are provided. A new section summarizes respiratory physiology and there are comprehensive reviews of respiratory mucus, cough, and suctioning techniques. Every chapter is extensively updated. This new edition adds over 300 references from material published since 1980.

The second edition addresses controversies about use of postural drainage, percussion, vibration, breathing exercises, cough, suctioning, and mobilization. Current theories and conflicts about indications and contraindications for chest physiotherapy are described and discussed. The authors' 15 years of experience of managing chest physiotherapy for critically ill patients is presented. The format of the second edition remains unchanged because the first edition had three printings, was published in Spanish and Portuguese and was favorably reviewed.

In Chapter 1 of the second edition, critical summaries of literature since 1981 describe pathophysiology of respiratory complications and techniques including chest physiotherapy, bronchoscopy and positive pressure, all of which are used to change pulmonary pressures and assist in the clearance of retained secretions. Chapter 2 provides new sections on respiratory physiology and respiratory mucus. Scientific data to justify postural drainage, positioning and breathing exercises, and percussion and vibration are updated in Chapters 3 and 4. Chapter 5 compares the effects of coughing and forced expiration and reviews the current techniques recommended for airway suctioning. Chapter 6 summarizes the important new aspects of patient mobilization used to minimize the need for chest physiotherapy. Chapter 7 includes more information on collateral airways and synthesizes some postulated mechanisms of action of chest physiotherapy. Treatment of patients with brain and spine injuries is comprehensively updated in Chapter 8. Chapter 9 covers some newer adjuncts to chest physiotherapy, most notably positive pressure techniques. Pain management techniques in the ICU are expanded in the revised Chapter 10. Statistics of patients treated since 1974 are now consolidated in Appendix I. Abbreviations and symbols are defined in Appendix II. An updated summary of chest physiotherapy treatment and evaluation is presented in Appendix III, and Appendix IV details the interventions in four critically ill patients. The index is now more comprehensive.

Preface to the First Edition

It is quite apparent, from even a casual conversation with physicians or other personnel involved in respiratory care management, that there is a large spectrum of differing treatments termed by their users as "chest physiotherapy." The literature is not helpful in specifying what chest physiotherapy is intended to include. Is the inhalation of bronchodilating or mucolytic agents part of chest physiotherapy? In tracheally intubated patients, is manual hyperinflation of the lung an inclusive part of chest physiotherapy? Many centers would use these therapies, others would not. All would claim to be treating the patient with chest physiotherapy. It is not surprising, therefore, that there are many contradictory opinions concerning the effects of chest physiotherapy. Because of these variations, if an improvement does occur, it is likely to be difficult to determine the beneficial component.

A homogeneous patient population treated in a similar manner by the same personnel over a number of years gives a useful clinical experience that frequently cannot be duplicated. At the Maryland Institute for Emergency Medical Services Systems (MIEMSS) in Baltimore, Maryland, there is a unique and homogeneous population of traumatized patients. Year after year, the admission statistics confirm the similarities in the patients, and their injuries, and in morbidity and mortality. The population is unique because about 60% of the 1,200 or more patients admitted each year come directly from the scene of their accident and about 75% of these patients come to the Institute by helicopter.

For the first 7 years, chest physiotherapy has been used in the critical care and intensive care units to treat patients with lung secretion retention. The physical therapists providing the therapy have a remarkable record of service. The three physical therapists who have contributed to this book have had between them 18 years of work at MIEMSS since 1973. The therapy they have provided encompasses five maneuvers: 1) postural drainage, 2) chest wall percussion and vibration, 3) coughing, 4) suctioning of the loosened secretions, and 5) breathing exercises in the spontaneously breathing patient. In addition, mobilization is used whenever possible.

Besides the similarities in patient population, personnel, and therapy, the mechanical ventilatory support was standardized at the Institute between 1973 and 1978 with the use of only one type of volume-present ventilator. Controlled mechanical ventilatory support was employed for resuscitation, for anesthesia and throughout recovery, providing humidification at all times. From October 1978 on, intermittent mandatory ventilation was occasionally used instead of controlled mechanical ventilation. No intermittent positive pressure breathing (IPPB) machines were used to deliver bronchodilator or mucolytic agents. No inhaled drugs, other than water vapor, were given in the critical or intensive care units. Tracheal lavage was rarely employed. The "bag squeezing" technique of chest physiotherapy, in which the lung is hyperinflated and the chest vibrated during expiration, was not used. No spontaneously breathing patients were treated with the aid of blow bottles or incentive inspiratory spirometers. Nasotracheal suctioning was seldom used or attempted. Tracheal suctioning was only carried out in intubated patients. Because these other respiratory maneuvers were excluded, the effect of chest physiotherapy alone was determined.

As with any book directed at diverse groups, such as critical care specialists, anesthesiologists, surgeons, internists, chest physiotherapists, nurse intensivists, and respiratory therapists, some areas of the text are more relevant than others to each group. For the physician, the changes that take place with therapy and the aggressive approach taken at MIEMSS are complemented by a considerable quantity of data and many case histories. To the physical therapist working in the intensive care unit, this book provides complete coverage of the specialty of chest physiotherapy. For the nurse intensivist and respiratory therapist, a practical approach to the respiratory management of the multiply-monitored intensive care unit patient is combined with a reference guide to the literature on chest physiotherapy. This book presents our experience with chest physiotherapy in the management of acute lung pathology in patients with previously normal and abnormal lungs. Over the 7 years (1973–80), a homogeneous patient population of over 3,000 intensive care unit patients was treated. The mechanical ventilation and physiotherapy techniques were standardized, and the medical and physical therapy personnel managing the respiratory care were constant. It is hoped that this book will provide others with a well-tested, practical approach to chest physiotherapy for intensive care patients.

C.F.M.
February 1981

Acknowledgments

First Edition. The majority of this book was written from knowledge acquired at the Maryland Institute for Emergency Medicine under the direction of R. Adams Cowley, M.D. We are greatly indebted to our mentors and colleagues, who have worked at the Institute with us during these years, for their teaching and assistance. Particular acknowledgment must be made to T. Crawford McAslan, M.D., who was Clinical Associate Director of MIEMSS. Under his guidance, chest physiotherapy was introduced to MIEMSS in 1973. He and Baekhyo Shin, M.D., provided a stimulating intellectual environment in which to study clinical respiratory physiology and the effects of chest physiotherapy. Our debt to Drs. McAslan, Shin, and Cowley is very great. We thank our colleagues, physicians and nurses, for their help and cooperation with the production of this book, and Gareth Green, M.D., Editor of the *American Review of Respiratory Diseases*, who kindly supplied drafts of the November 1980 supplement. We also owe thanks to Mark Moody, Ph.D., Director of Clinic and Field Evaluation at MIEMSS, for data concerning admissions appearing in Tables 1.1–1.6, and to T. Crawford McAslan, M.D., for the traces appearing in Figures 1.2–1.4.

For the photographs, we thank Colin Mackenzie, M.B., Ch.B., F.F.A.R.C.S., and Dick Register for taking them; and Frank Ciesla, MIEMSS and University of Maryland Hospital Illustrative Services, for printing them. For illustrations, we thank Chris McCullough-Green; and for proofreading, Barbara Eerligh and Beverley Sopp. Jeremy Hallisey, M.B., B.S., and David Clark helped with data analysis, proofreading and reference checking. Our thanks go to Marlene Wheeler and Kate McWilliams, who typed the final drafts, and to Sandy Bond-Lillicropp, who organized the typing of the earlier drafts.

Finally, we thank experts in the field of chest physiotherapy on both sides of the Atlantic who have read and criticized the manuscript at various stages. However, the final result should not be blamed on them. Rather, the end product is the result of our determination to keep some parts, such as the patient population data and the sections on special patients and mobilization which do not relate strictly to "chest therapy" or intensive care." The reviewers included Margaret Branthwaite, M.R.C.P., F.F.A.R.C.S., and Barbara Webber of the Brompton Hospital, London, England; Anthony Clement, M.B., B.S., F.F.A.R.C.S., of St. Thomas' Hospital, London; John Hedley-Whyte, M.D., and Cynthia Zadai of Beth Israel Hospital and Harvard Medical School, Boston, Massachusetts; T. Crawford McAslan, M.D., of Baltimore City Hospitals and The Johns Hopkins Medical School; Iain L. Mackenzie, M.D., of York Hospital, York, Pennsylvania, and Baekhyo Shin, M.D., Lucille Ann Mostello, M.D., and Martin Helrich, M.D., all of the University of Maryland Hospital and Medical School, Baltimore. Particular thanks are due Martin Helrich, M.D., Chairman, Department of Anesthesiology for his support and encouragement.

Second Edition. We gratefully acknowledge help from John New, B.A., with preparation of statistical data and we are grateful to Beverly Sopp and her staff (Lynn Kesselring and Eina Segal) for editorial assistance. Marlene Wheeler and Ruth Allan were unflagging typists. Justina Smith prepared the graphs in Appendix I and Appendix IV and assisted in many ways in the completion of this second edition. We are grateful to all of the reviewers of the first edition and hope to have answered their criticisms with the second edition. We are especially thankful to Nancy Klemic who, while not involved as an author in the second edition because of other commitments, skillfully reviewed each chapter with thoughtful criticism. In addition, George Barnas, Ph.D. provided excellent comments on Chapter 7. Finally, we thank our editor at Williams & Wilkins, Carol Eckhart, who cajoled and persuaded us sufficiently frequently to get the revision finished.

Contents

CHAPTER 1

History and Literature Review of Chest Physiotherapy, ICU Chest Physiotherapy, and Respiratory Care: Controversies and Questions

Colin F. Mackenzie, M.B., Ch.B., F.F.A.R.C.S.

As an introduction to this book, Chapter 1 is intended to put chest physiotherapy into historical perspective and provide a review of the literature. A brief description of the authors' understanding of chest physiotherapy and its objectives is followed by some comments on the variations found in the literature concerning indications, type, usage, and duration of chest physiotherapy. A chest physiotherapy program and techniques for respiratory management and assessment are discussed together with some controversial aspects of respiratory care that relate to secretion clearance. Finally the chapter summarizes conflicting data and points of contention concerning chest physiotherapy.

HISTORICAL SUMMARY AND LITERATURE REVIEW

1901   William Ewart described the beneficial effects of postural drainage in the treatment of bronchiectasis.

1908   Pasteur delivered the Bradshaw Lecture on massive collapse of the lung.

1910   Pasteur reported on the finding of acute lobar collapse as a complication of abdominal surgery.

1915   MacMahon described the use of breathing and physical exercises in patients with lung, diaphragm, and pleural injuries sustained in World War I.

1918   Bushnell used postural drainage for patients with pulmonary tuberculosis.

1919   MacMahon used breathing exercises for patients recovering from gunshot wounds of the chest.

1924   Featherstone described the causation of postoperative pneumonia, summarized the pertinent literature since 1895, analyzed the results of 1000 consecutive medical and surgical autopsies, compared the incidence of pneumonia after upper and lower abdominal surgery, and discussed his observations as an anesthetist on the causes of postoperative pneumonia. His pertinent findings are summarized in Table 1.1.
Dr. Featherstone's masterly work is impressive because its conclusions are almost all still valid, and because of the low incidence of pneumonia, which is little changed today from 1924.

1933   Jackson and Jackson wrote on the benefits of pulmonary drainage and coughing.

1934   Winifred Linton, a physiotherapist at the Brompton Hospital, London, England, introduced "localized breathing exercises" for the thoracic surgical patient (Gaskell and Webber, 1973).

1934   Nelson recommended bronchial drainage for management of bronchiectasis in children. He emphasized the use of physical and radiological examination to locate the specific position of the lung lesion and to determine patient positioning for drainage.

1938   Knies recommended bronchial drainage following thoracic surgery.

1950   Temple and Evans defined bronchopulmonary segments to identify areas of the lung needing resection.

1950   Felson and Felson used the silhouette sign to localize intrathoracic lesions radiographically.

1952–1953   Kane described pulmonary segmental localization on posteroanterior chest x-rays. He also noted that the more accurately gravity was applied to the draining bronchus, the more effective was the postural drainage.

Many reports of symptomatic and physiological benefits from breathing exercises and postural drainage appeared up to 1945 (Heckscher). However, until the 1950s there was little change in the incidence of atelectasis from that reported by Pasteur and no change in the incidence of pneumonia reported by Featherstone (1924), despite the ad-

Table 1.1
Summary of the Causes of Postoperative Pneumonia[a]

1. Postoperative pneumonia occurs with grave frequency (incidence in 1924 varied from 2.7 to 8.5%).
2. Often pneumonia is not recognized and figures that purport to give its incidence are unreliable.
3. The anesthetic agent and the method of administration, except in special cases, are seldom decisive factors.
4. Age and sex are not of importance.
5. General health and local disease of the lungs may play a considerable part.
6. At operation, every care should be taken to prevent loss of heat, of fluid, and of blood and especially exhaustion from trauma to nerve tissue and to highly vascular parts.
7. Infection of the lung is often by means of aspiration in the presence of certain other factors.
8. Severe sepsis in the other regions affects the lung via the blood stream.
9. There is evidence that lymphatic infection through the right half of the diaphragm leads first to pleurisy and then to pneumonia.
10. In the absence of severe sepsis, operations on the abdomen, and especially the upper abdomen, provide the start of the chain of events which leads to pneumonia.
11. Pain in the abdomen from operative trauma, or from inflammation, gives rise to rigidity of the anterior abdominal wall and to reflex inhibition of the diaphragm, together with some spasm of the lower intercostal muscles. The lower lobes of the lungs, then, do not freely expand and contract, so that congestion of the blood with edema sets in.

[a]From Featherstone (1924).

vances in surgery, anesthesia, and antibiotic usage. Pioneering work on the effects of chest physiotherapy was published by Palmer and Sellick in 1953. They described the use of breathing exercises, postural drainage with vibratory and clapping percussion, and inhalation of isoprenaline before and after surgery. This regime was significantly more effective than breathing exercises alone in reducing pulmonary atelectasis in 180 patients operated upon for hernia repair or partial gastrectomy. They also found that isoprenaline combined with postural drainage and vibratory and clapping percussion prevented atelectasis, but that neither intervention alone prevented it. These studies included controls but were based on the somewhat subjective data of atelectasis, as judged by clinical examination and chest x-ray. Thoren (1954), using diaphragmatic breathing and deep breathing while side-lying, postural drainage, and coughing, showed that without the use of inhalation therapy it was also possible to produce a significant reduction in pulmonary complications after cholecystectomy. Atelectasis developed in 11 of 101 patients treated before and after cholecystectomy, in 18 of 70 patients (25.7%) treated with chest physiotherapy only after cholecystectomy, and in 68 of the 172 patients (35.9%) who were not given chest physiotherapy after surgery.

Therefore, over 25 years ago, there appeared to be a specific indication for chest physiotherapy in the prevention of pulmonary complications after surgery. Since then, there has been an explosion in the apparent indications for chest physiotherapy. It is the application of chest physiotherapy with lack of specific indications that has rightly promoted adverse commentary. The original popularity of chest physiotherapy arose because of the benefits produced in patients with retained lung secretions. However, to our knowledge, no one has shown that treatment with chest physiotherapy has altered the morbidity or mortality of patients with chronic lung disease, whereas chest physiotherapy for acute lung pathology in a previously normal lung may produce a more favorable outcome.

The advent of controlled mechanical ventilation in 1953 (Crampton Smith et al., 1954) as a means of treating acute respiratory insufficiency also gave rise to the realization that during artificial respiration there is a special liability to pulmonary complications. Opie and Spalding (1958) produced a review of some of the physiological changes that occurred during chest physiotherapy and controlled mechanical ventilation, using intermittent positive pressure with a negative expiratory phase. The negative phase was then popular because this improved venous return to the heart. Advocates of intermittent mandatory ventilation make a similar claim about the spontaneous breath with this mode of ventilation.

Opie and Spalding noted that the rate of air flow in and out of the lungs was dependent upon the esophagotracheal pressure gradient, and that a rise in esophageal pressure with chest compression accelerated expiration (Fig. 1.1). Application of chest compression late in expiration caused only a very slight alteration in air flow. Two mechanisms for the action of chest physiotherapy were postulated. (1) By raising intrathoracic pressure as a whole, air was rapidly expelled from the lungs, carrying secretions with it, as in a cough. The paper, however, argues quite successfully against this mechanism. (2) By local compression of the lung underneath the physiotherapist's hands, secretions were pushed from the more peripheral airways into the main bronchi. This has since been disputed as the mode of action (Laws and McIntyre, 1969).

Wiklander and Norlin (1957) compared 100 patients who, following laparotomy, received chest physiotherapy, with 100 who did not. Chest physiotherapy was given before and after surgery, for usually 3 days, or as long as sputum was obtained. The incidence of atelectasis was 13% in those who received chest physiotherapy, and 24% in those who were asked to turn from side to side in bed and given instruction and help in coughing.

In a frequently quoted study on the value of lung physiotherapy in treatment of acute exacerbations in chronic bronchitis, Anthonisen and his colleagues (1964) compared conventional treatment and chest physiotherapy to conventional

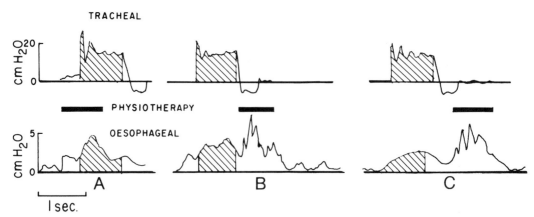

Figure 1.1. The effect of chest physiotherapy on tracheal and esophageal pressure in a patient ventilated with intermittent positive/negative pressure ventilation. *Hatched area,* inspiratory period. **(A)** Chest vibration during inspiration. **(B)** Chest vibration during the inspiratory–expiratory junction. **(C)** Chest vibration during the middle of the expiratory period. Note the greatest tracheoesophageal pressure differences occur with **B** and **C** which are normally used methods of applying chest vibration. (Tracing from Opie LH, Spalding JMK: *Lancet 2:*671–674, 1958.)

treatment alone. No differences in outcome were found between the groups randomly treated with and without chest physiotherapy. During an acute flare-up of chronic bronchitis, chest physiotherapy did not seem beneficial, but they did not exclude the possibility of benefit in lobar atelectasis.

In 1966, Holloway and his colleagues reported that chest physiotherapy appeared to cause a fall in arterial oxygenation when applied to neonates with tetanus. This preliminary observation was followed by the publication of a study on 22 patients with tetanus who received chest physiotherapy (Holloway et al., 1969). These patients were compared to a matched group of 14 spontaneously breathing patients and a group of 15 neonates receiving mechanical ventilation but not chest therapy. Chest physiotherapy, which took the form of clapping and compression, percussion and vibration, was followed by suctioning. A fall in PaO_2 occurred after chest physiotherapy, but it is doubtful if the changes of PaO_2 50.6 ± 6.4 to 47.0 ± 6.4 mm Hg (mean ± SD) were clinically significant, although it was apparently statistically so. The control group was ventilated but did not receive chest physiotherapy and was not turned to the same positions. Therefore, simple $\dot{V}/\dot{Q}$ changes cannot be excluded

as the cause for the fall in PaO_2 in the treated patients.

Further information about chest physiotherapy was published in 1969 when Laws and McIntyre described changes in gas exchange and cardiac output associated with chest physiotherapy in six patients in respiratory failure. All were ventilated with volume ventilators and a tidal volume (V_t) of 10–13 ml/kg. Cardiac output was measured with the dye dilution technique. Since this was before the era of flow-directed pulmonary artery catheters, neither pulmonary artery pressure nor mixed venous gases were monitored. However, mixed expired and inspired gases were analyzed. Alveolar-to-arterial tension gradients for both O_2 and CO_2 were derived and used to measure the efficiency of gas exchange before, during, and after chest physiotherapy. The procedures performed included postural drainage with percussion, shaking, and vibration. Artificial coughs were given in the supine position, and both lateral positions, and chest compression was performed during expiration. These procedures were followed by lung hyperinflation (V_t, 20–25 ml/kg). The patients were then suctioned; none had large amounts of sputum. This factor appeared to be crucial, as these authors were unable to show any improvement in gas exchange. They also cast doubt on the hypothesis that external chest compression squeezes secretions from completely occluded airways by direct lung compression. They suggest that the amount of compression required to do this would produce areas of collapse. As an alternative hypothesis, they put forward the idea that airway clearance requires some expansion of distal lung units. Indirect ventilation of these distal airways may be achieved by collateral channels. The more proximal airways are then cleared by increased expiratory flows, generated by the physiotherapists, from the distal airways. Our explanation of the mechanism of chest physiotherapy action is similar and is described in Chapter 7.

In the patients studied by Laws and McIntyre during physiotherapy, cardiac output varied up to 50% from the levels obtained before physiotherapy. These variations persisted for as long as 30 min. The greatest variation occurred during the artificial cough with inflation pressures of 60–100 cm H_2O. In some patients, cardiac output fell due to impaired venous return during this maneuver. In those who were conscious, the procedure was also found to be extremely unpleasant. During resistance to lung hyperinflation, and with patient apprehension, cardiac output rose. These hyperinflations, although causing such changes in the cardiovascular system, were not able to produce any lasting benefit to pulmonary gas exchange. These are some of the reasons for our omission of lung hyperinflation from physiotherapy treatment (see p. 225).

Lorin and Denning (1971) found that postural drainage produced more than twice the volume of sputum as an equal period of cough alone in 17 patients with cystic fibrosis. Postural drainage lasted 20 min and included positioning for the right middle lobe, lingula, and some basilar segments of the lower lobe. The patients received percussion and vibration in each position. The volume of sputum produced when compared with the volume produced by the same patient in the sitting position, coughing every 5 min for 20 min, averaged 3.4 ml and was significantly greater than that of the control of 1.6 ml (p < 0.0001).

Lord et al. (1972) showed anecdotal evidence for radiological and arterial blood gas improvement after chest physiotherapy in an infant and adults. Gormezano and Branthwaite (1972a) reported the effects of chest physiotherapy on 43 adults receiving intermittent positive pressure ventilation. The patients were considered in three groups: Group I included 18 patients with no cardiac disability; Group II, 13 patients with cardiovascular disability; and Group III, 11 patients with respiratory failure. Chest therapy included hyperinflation to 20 cm H_2O above previous ventilator settings, manual chest compression, and tracheal suctioning. Duration of treatment was was from 7 to 20 min, depending on whether copious secretions were mobilized. Arterial blood gases were sampled before and at 5, 15, and 30 min after cessation of therapy. Patients in Groups I and III did not show any change; Group II showed a maximum fall in PaO_2 of 14.9 ± 4.55 mm Hg (SE) 5 min after therapy. Within 30 min this had returned to the levels obtained before therapy. Hyperinflation caused a rise in PaO_2 in all groups. $PaCO_2$ increased in all groups, but a rebreathing circuit was used during manual chest compression. The authors postulated that during chest physiotherapy, (1) cardiac output fell; therefore, $P\bar{V}O_2$ fell; and, therefore, PaO_2 fell; (2) there was an increase in intrapulmonary shunt; and (3) there was increased oxygen consumption. Because no indications for chest physiotherapy were given, it is not known whether treatment was performed prophylactically or for a specific indication. Since the patients were turned on both left and right sides but were not apparently posturally drained with the affected lobe or segment uppermost, it is not certain whether chest physiotherapy produced these changes or whether they were due to changes in posture.

Gormezano and Branthwaite (1972b) also studied patients treated with chest physiotherapy and intermittent positive pressure breathing (IPPB). Thirty-two chronic bronchitic patients with airway obstruction and sputum production were divided into three groups: those with reversible airway obstruction (Group I), those with profuse secretions (Group II), and those with respiratory failure (Group III). Mean PaO_2 fell 4–6 mm Hg in all groups, but the fall was greatest in Group II. The fall was thought to be due to increased intrapulmonary shunt. However, no specific cause of the increased shunt was identified, although several were hypothesized, such as decreased pulmonary artery pressure with rest after therapy, increased pulmonary artery pressure due to increased cardiac output, and abolition of hypoxic pulmonary vasoconstriction.

In 1973, Clarke and his colleagues reported the effects of sputum on pulmonary function. Patients with copious sputum production and airway obstruction (forced expired volume in 1 sec (FEV_1)/ forced vital capacity (FVC) < 70% predicted) improved in all measured parameters, particulary specific airway conductance, following sputum removal. There was, however, no relationship between the volume of sputum produced and the improvement of pulmonary function. They concluded that although sputum volume production is important, its distribution within the bronchial tree and its viscoelastic properties may be of greater importance.

A report in which removal of inhaled radioactive tracers was used to measure pulmonary mucociliary clearance in cystic fibrosis appeared in 1973 (Sanchis et al.). Despite previous beliefs, mucociliary transport in 13 children with cystic fibrosis was found to take place at a similar rate to that found in normal adults. The theory that the viscid secretions found in cystic fibrosis (or mucoviscidosis) were inadequately cleared, resulting in blocked airways, stasis, and resultant infection, appeared to be considerably set back by this finding (Waring, 1973). However, one problem with the technique used was that the particle size of 3 μm was perhaps too large and, therefore, the radioactive particles did not penetrate the lung effectively. More central penetration occurred in children than in adults. Because mucociliary clearance is faster from larger airways than from smaller airways, the children may only

appear to have normal mucus clearance. The radioactive tracer clearance technique is now the accepted model for further investigation. However, peripheral deposition of radioaerosols is difficult in patients with chronic lung diseases because they often have impaired inhalation and they cough. Radioaerosols do not reach airways that are obstructed so that although airway clearance may occur, this is not demonstrated by the radioaerosol clearance technique. In 1974, the National Heart and Lung Institute, as it was then called, organized a conference, frequently referred to as the Sugarloaf Conference, on the scientific basis of respiratory therapy. This conference and a similar conference on in-hospital respiratory therapy published in 1980 are summarized in Chapter 7, pp. 245–248.

Campbell and his colleagues (1975) reported that bronchoconstriction, as measured by a fall in FEV_1, occurred in seven patients with exacerbation of chronic bronchitis following chest percussion or vibration. They found that bronchoconstriction was particularly noticeable in patients who did not have copious sputum production. The fall in FEV_1 was not confirmed by other studies of chest physiotherapy and chronic bronchitis (Cochrane et al., 1977; Newton and Stephenson, 1978; May and Munt, 1979).

Tecklin and Holsclaw (1975) found that following postural drainage, percussion, vibration and coughing in 26 patients with cystic fibrosis, significant increases occurred in peak expiratory flow rate, FVC, expiratory reserve volume and inspiratory reserve capacity. Larger airways appeared to be the sites of this beneficial action. There was no indication that these benefits lasted beyond 5 min after treatment had ceased. Cystic fibrosis is one of the few chronic lung diseases for which the benefits of chest physiotherapy are documented. A conference in Europe, published in 1977, summarized the state of the art (Baran and Van Bogaert, 1977).

Objective evidence of change in the lungs following sputum removal by chest physiotherapy in mechanically ventilated patients was reported by Winning and colleagues (1975). They estimated alveolar pressure by means of a retard mechanism applied to the lungs at end expiration. A significant fall in "alveolar pressure" was noted to occur after chest physiotherapy in 17 patients. Unfortunately the adjustment of the ventilator necessary to produce the "alveolar pressure" alters the characteristics of the lung under study. Therefore, it is difficult to determine whether the changes found were due to chest physiotherapy or ventilator manipulation.

The additional effect of only a mucolytic agent, or a bronchodilator and a mucolytic agent, on arterial oxygenation following chest physiotherapy was compared to the therapy alone. No differences were found (Brock-Utne et al., 1975). A similar finding was reported in which clearance of inhaled polystyrene particles tagged with technetium-99m was used to assess removal of lung secretions in a double-blind crossover trial in 16 patients with chronic bronchitis (Thomson et al., 1975). There was no significant difference in weight or radioactive content of sputum expectorated between the patients who were given S-carboxymethylcysteine, a mucolytic agent, and those who were not. Ventilatory capacity as assessed by dry spirometry was not changed, nor was there subjective improvement noted by the patients. Roper and colleagues (1976) found right upper lobe atelectasis occurred after tracheal extubation in 18 of 188 newborn infants. This was thought to result from the anatomical positions of the right upper lobe bronchus and damage from suction catheters. The atelectasis could usually be expanded by chest physiotherapy. If it was unresponsive, an orotracheal tube was inserted, and the lungs manually hyperinflated and suctioned until all secretions were mobilized. Following this the trachea was immediately extubated. This regime resulted in the elimination of recurrent atelectasis as a major problem after extubation. Tecklin and Holsclaw (1976) found that N-acetylcysteine (Mucomyst) and bronchial drainage and coughing produced the same changes in respiratory function in 20 patients with cystic fibrosis, that occurred without the use of the mucolytic agent. In fact, maximal

midexpiratory flow rate worsened, showing significant decrease with the inhalation. This was thought to be due to reflex small airway constriction and edema following N-acetylcysteine or due to coughing. Using technetium-99m, Pavia et al. (1976) found that a mechanically vibrating pad did not significantly alter clearance of sputum when compared in 10 patients who had histories of productive cough and difficulty expectorating phlegm; however, postural drainage was not used.

Martin et al. (1976) investigated the ability of unilateral breathing exercises to alter distribution of ventilation and blood flow in patients undergoing bronchospirometry. In no instance was the distribution of ventilation or blood flow altered to the side that was supposed to be limited. However, although these patients had active tuberculosis, there was no indication that the pathological lung was the target of the therapy, since both sides of the chest were treated. All patients had less than 15% involvement of the lung fields by chest x-ray, respiratory function tests were all normal, and only one subject was thought to have moderately advanced disease. Therefore, it is possible that in major lung pathology or in patients with chest splinting due to pain, breathing exercises may have a different effect, when large differences in lung/thorax compliance occur.

Removal of sputum by chest physiotherapy produced an improvement in specific airway conductance in 17 of 23 patients with chronic cough, airway obstruction, and at least a 30-ml sputum production per day (Cochrane et al., 1977). This improvement did not occur in 4 normal subjects, nor in 8 of the study patients who, on the following day, were given 150 mg isoprenaline base by inhalation instead of physiotherapy. Cochrane and his colleagues reiterated their belief that the distribution of sputum throughout the airways appeared to be more relevant than sputum volume, viscosity, or character. No correlation was found between changes in specific airway conductance and sputum volume produced by chest physiotherapy.

By using transcutaneous O_2 monitoring, the effect of chest physiotherapy on

PaO$_2$ in 45 patients who had undergone abdominal surgery was compared to three deep breaths using incentive spirometry, a mechanical lung insufflator, and the blowing up of a paper coil (Hedstrand et al., 1978). Chest physiotherapy produced a greater increase in PaO$_2$ than did the other maneuvers, though it is doubtful if a 7 mm Hg rise in PaO$_2$ is clinically any different from the 3 to 4.5 mm Hg obtained with the respiratory therapy devices. The reliability of transcutaneous O$_2$ monitoring, when used in adults, is also in question. This paper does not record why the patients needed therapy. The respiratory therapy devices may have been used in the recommended manner; however, chest physiotherapy, which apparently consisted of ten deep breaths and a minute of coughing followed by assisted costal breathing in the lateral position, at our institution would be considered inadequate to clear retained secretions.

Two abstracts (Finer et al., 1977; Fox et al., 1977) that described chest physiotherapy for the neonate were published as papers the following year. Finer and Boyd (1978) studied 20 neonates with a mean weight of 2.07 kg. Seven neonates were mechanically ventilated; all had respiratory failure and were receiving supplemental O$_2$. Respiratory failure was due to respiratory distress syndrome in 14 neonates, tachypnea in 2, pneumonia in 3, and apnea in 1. Arterial blood gases were analyzed before, and 15 min after, postural drainage and suction (10 infants) or postural drainage, percussion and suction (10 infants). The neonates showed a rise in PaO$_2$ when postural drainage, percussion and suction were used but no significant change with postural drainage and suction alone. The same findings, in a population of a different age and ventilated differently, were reported in the abstract. It is not clear why some patients, whose data appeared in the abstract, were omitted from the paper.

Fox and his colleagues (1978) studied 13 newborns to "determine the benefit/risk ratio of chest physiotherapy." All were intubated, breathing spontaneously with positive airway pressure, and were recovering from respiratory disease (respiratory distress, 10; aspiration, 2; apnea,

1). After a control period, 30 sec of anterior chest wall vibration was performed by using a mechanical vibrator. The infants were then suctioned and hyperventilated for ten breaths. Since neither postural drainage nor percussion was used, the treatment given was not strictly chest physiotherapy. However, there was a consistent trend in which compliance and functional residual capacity (FRC) increased in parallel throughout all the periods of study. Inspiratory airway resistance was noted to fall significantly following chest vibration and suctioning, but this had returned to control levels within 2 hr. Arterial oxygenation fell significantly following suctioning. This was reversed with hyperventilation. Two hours following therapy, PaO$_2$ levels did not differ from control. The fall in PaO$_2$, which was as high as 81 mm Hg in a patient breathing 55% oxygen, was not thought to be due to atelectasis because there was no change in FRC and no fall in lung compliance. It was, perhaps, due to the rise in pleural pressure accompanying coughing and suctioning which may have increased a right-to-left shunt.

Mackenzie et al. (1978) studied 47 patients with a variety of chest x-ray changes that included atelectasis, pneumonia, or lung contusion. Eight of the 47 patients were nontrauma and had multiple pathology; the remainder were trauma patients. All patients were mechanically ventilated with positive end-expiratory pressure (PEEP) (5–10 cm H$_2$O). Changes in arterial oxygenation were prospectively studied before and for 2 hr after chest physiotherapy. No significant changes in PaO$_2$ were found after chest physiotherapy. There were no differences between patients with or without trauma or between those treated with or without head-down postural drainage. The falls in arterial oxygenation reported by others to occur after chest physiotherapy may be reversed by the use of PEEP. Unilobar lung pathology showed radiological improvement in 74% (20/27) and multilobar pathology improvement in 60% (12/20). These radiological findings are similar to those obtained by fiberoptic bronchoscopy in patients resistant to routine respiratory therapy (Lindholm et al. 1974).

Chest physiotherapy produced a different effect on pulmonary function in patients with acute exacerbations of chronic bronchitis (Newton and Stephenson) than in patients with bronchiectasis and cystic fibrosis (Cochrane et al.). The 33 patients studied by Newton and Stephenson, within 4 days of admission for acute exacerbation of chronic bronchitis, had an FEV_1/FVC ratio of <50%, indicating considerable respiratory impairment and airway obstruction. They had less than 15% improvement after use of bronchodilators. Thoracic gas volumes and airway resistance were measured in a body plethysmograph, and specific conductance was derived. FEV_1, vital capacity, and inspiratory capacity were also measured before chest physiotherapy. All tests were repeated two times at half-hourly intervals after 15 min of physiotherapy. Positioning and chest physiotherapy maneuvers were not adequately described. No more than 5 ml of sputum was produced in any patient. An acute rise in lung volume, FRC and conductance occurred, but there was no change in arterial blood gases. No deterioration occurred in FEV_1. Most patients produced 2 ml of sputum or less; it is not surprising that the authors concluded that their patients did not show any obvious benefit from chest physiotherapy.

Graham and Bradley (1978) compared a randomized group of 27 patients, treated with chest physiotherapy and IPPB for 20 minutes, to a control group of 27 similar patients. Both groups had pneumonia, as judged by a compatible clinical history of fever and increased cough, radiological confirmation, and a positive gram stain of sputum and blood cultures (12% positive). They found no difference in duration of fever, extent of radiographic clearing, duration of hospital stay, or mortality between the control and treated groups. As was pointed out in the correspondence following this article, the authors excluded patients with bronchiectasis, lung abscess and cystic fibrosis who might have expected to benefit from chest physiotherapy. The establishment of a diagnosis of pneumonia in the intensive care unit (ICU) is not as simple as was cited by Graham and Bradley. As mentioned in Chapter 2, what appeared to be a pneumonic process was cleared in its early stages with treatment by chest physiotherapy (Case History 2.1). Restriction of chest physiotherapy to a predetermined time of 20 min may not provide sufficient duration to clear secretions, especially when IPPB is also given during the same 20 min. The conclusion by Murray (1979), that the use of chest physiotherapy for patients with otherwise uncomplicated pneumonia should stop, appears quite reasonable, especially if the patients are ambulatory or mobilized. For the mechanically ventilated patient in the ICU this may not be valid, since it is difficult to arrive at the diagnosis of pneumonia unless retained secretions are not cleared or radiological improvement fails to occur following chest physiotherapy. Recent data provide more objective evidence for diagnosis of pneumonia (Salata et al., 1987; Johanson et al., 1988a) and make some management suggestions for its prevention in the ICU (Driks et al., 1987; Johanson et al., 1988b).

An editorial in the *Lancet* (1978) scrutinized the use of chest physiotherapy and noted that surprisingly few studies showing objective assessment were published. Those that were published seemed to have concentrated on areas where physiotherapy is predictably ineffective. Chest physiotherapy was thought to be most useful when copious amounts of very sticky sputum were produced. It was also emphasized that by talking to, touching, and making the patient more comfortable, the physiotherapist provides an important link between the patient and other members of staff.

Newton and Bevans (1978) treated 39 patients with acute exacerbations of chronic bronchitis with antibiotics, bronchodilators and diuretics (standard treatment). These patients were compared with 40 patients treated with IPPB (3 times daily with nebulized saline) and chest physiotherapy for 10–15 min, in addition to the standard treatment. Arterial blood gases, sputum volume, FEV_1 and vital capacity were measured among other parameters. Only admission and discharge data were provided. Since discharge is frequently not a clinical but an administrative decision, it would be helpful if some daily data were included.

Chest physiotherapy was not adequately described and the results were at times confusing. However, no differences were found in PaO$_2$, PaCO$_2$, FEV$_1$, vital capacity, or duration of hospital stay between the two groups. The only difference was that men who received chest physiotherapy produced a greater sputum volume than those who did not.

The effects of chest percussion and postural drainage on respiratory function in 35 patients with stable chronic bronchitis were compared to sham treatment with an infrared lamp. (May and Munt, 1979). The conclusions were similar to the study of Newton and Stephenson on patients with acute exacerbations of chronic bronchitis and suggested that postural drainage and chest percussion did not benefit the patients. This study showed that although chest physiotherapy improved FVC and FEV$_1$, these also improved following the use of the infrared lamp (sham treatment). Sputum production was greater during percussion and postural drainage than during the infrared warming (5.5 vs. 1.4 ml average) or during coughing (9.0 vs. 3.5 ml average). Bateman and his colleagues (1979) did not use a sham treament but used a crossover control when they compared clearance of bronchial secretions labeled with technetium-99m from 10 patients with stable chronic airway obstruction and regular sputum production. They found that chest physiotherapy was highly effective in moving bronchial secretions from peripheral to more central lung regions and aided in expectoration.

Feldman et al. (1979) found that postural drainage with chest percussion, vibration and coughing resulted in significant improvement in expiratory flow at 50% and 25% of FVC. In the 19 patients studied who had chronic bronchitis or cystic fibrosis, there was no correlation between volume of sputum produced and changes in lung function.

Oldenburg et al. (1979) studied the effect of postural drainage, exercises and cough in 8 clinically stable patients with chronic bronchitis. They found that cough alone greatly accelerated bronchial clearance of a radioactive tracer deposited in the tracheobronchial tree. Postural drainage, with cough prohibited,

did not alter clearance. The differences in the findings of this study and that of Bateman et al. may be a function of study design and the properties of the radiolabeled aerosols used (Rochester and Goldberg, 1980). The site of deposition of radioactive aerosol showed considerable variation between the subjects in the study by Oldenburg and colleagues. Therefore, the conclusion that cough was effective in improving peripheral airway clearance may not be valid. These findings need confirmation in a larger patient population since they have not been confirmed by others (see Chapter 5). It is also doubtful if any clinician would use postural drainage and eliminate cough or huff. Bronchial clearance following postural drainage and coughing was not examined by these investigators. Camner et al. (1979) differentiated between healthy subjects and those with expectoration and lung disease on the basis of clearance of inhaled 6 μm radioactively tagged Teflon particles following coughing. Six of eight patients with lung disease reproducibly eliminated the tagged particles after 1–2 min of voluntary coughing. The rapid clearance suggests the particles were deposited in the central large airways.

Fiberoptic bronchoscopy is frequently used to clear acute lobar atelectasis (see Chapter 9). Marini et al. (1979) compared bronchoscopy to incentive spirometry, coughing, and tracheal suctioning in nonintubated patients. If they were intubated, they received IPPB with nebulized isoetharine (Bronkosol) and chest percussion and postural drainage. Neither bronchoscopy, nor the regime of respiratory therapy produced differences in resolution of the atelectasis at 24 or 48 hr. Patients who had air bronchograms seen on chest x-ray had slower resolution of the atelectasis. Marini et al. concluded that an air bronchogram is the result of satisfactory central clearance of secretions and, therefore, contraindicates fiberoptic bronchoscopy. However, bronchoscopy may be necessary when effective respiratory therapy cannot be accomplished or long-standing atelectasis and inspissated secretions remain unresponsive to respiratory therapy.

Murray (1979) likened the removal of

secretions from the respiratory tract to getting ketchup out of a bottle. He summarized the present debate about indications for chest physiotherapy in patients with chronic lung diseases. He did not discuss acute lung pathology in patients with otherwise normal lungs. What was considered of particular concern was the unnecessary use and cost of chest physiotherapy and other respiratory therapy procedures for patients with chronic obstructive pulmonary disease and other lung diseases in which no sputum was produced. The bottle must contain some ketchup before it can be emptied. No one would argue with this generality. Murray advocates that if chest physiotherapy does not produce in excess of 30 ml of sputum, it should be discontinued. This has not been found to be an appropriate guideline for patients with acute lung disease in the ICU, nor has it been substantiated as a guideline for patients with chronic lung disease.

Mackenzie et al. (1980), using calculation of lung/thorax compliance (C_T) described by Winning et al. (1975), but avoiding their adjustments of the ventilator that alter lung mechanics, found an increase in the C_T following chest physiotherapy. Forty-two patients who suffered trauma were studied. There appeared to be no difference in the C_T increase whether the patient had atelectasis, lung contusion, pneumonia, or respiratory distress syndrome. Nor did differences occur between patients ventilated with or without PEEP or between those treated for more or less than 1 hr. The greatest C_T increase occurred 2 hr after therapy had ceased, which suggested that changes continue to occur even after the completion of therapy.

Connors et al. (1980) found that acutely ill patients with lower lobe disease who produced little or no sputum showed a significant fall in PaO_2 during postural drainage and percussion. Those patients that produced more than 2 ml of sputum showed no change in PaO_2. The spectrum of intensive care and ward patients, diseases treated, and methods of ventilation are large in the study population. There are methodological variations in arterial blood gas sampling and oxygen delivery that detract from the data. They conclude that chest physiotherapy is not indicated in patients without sputum production.

The ability to perform chest physiotherapy and produce a favorable radiological outcome, when bronchoscopy was considered too hazardous, was reported in a case study by Ciesla and colleagues (1981). Despite severe trauma involving multiple body systems, intrapulmonary shunt was decreased and acute atelectasis reversed following chest physiotherapy. Hammond and Martin (1981) confirmed that advantages of chest physiotherapy over bronchoscopy and showed convincing radiological evidence of improvement when chest physiotherapy was used to treat acute atelectasis.

UPDATE OF LITERATURE SINCE 1980

In 1980, the first edition of *Chest Physiotherapy in the Intensive Care Unit* was completed and the most recent proceedings of the NHLBI Conference on the Scientific Basis of In-hospital Respiratory Therapy was published. For publications since 1980, added in this new edition, headings of broad interest are used to group critical summaries of similar topics.

Pathophysiology and Risk Factors for Postoperative Respiratory Complications

Andersen and Jespersen (1980) identified communications between neighboring lung segments in normal lungs using resin casts. They found collateral airways with a diameter of 80–150 μm (when fixed at 10 cm H_2O pressure) in all lobes, but especially in the lower lobes (Fig. 1.2A and B). These intersegmental respiratory bronchioles are probably of great importance in the reexpansion of atelectatic lung by chest physiotherapy. Macklem (1971) and Menkes and Traystman (1977) have previously suggested these alternative pathways, particularly the largest, the interbronchiolar channels of Martin, as a means of prevention and reexpansion of atelectasis beyond obstructed subsegmental or more peripheral airways. Resistance in collateral airways decreases with increased lung

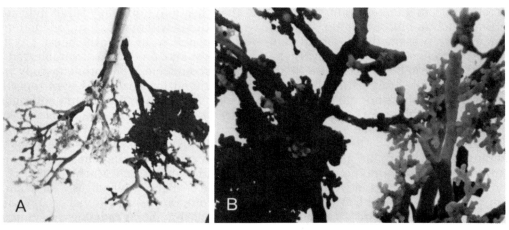

Figure 1.2. **(A)** Corrosion cast of two adjacent bronchopulmonary segments distal to 3 mm airways. The left segment is cast with light resin, the right with dark resin. Note that the light resin has crossed the segmental borders and occupies the distal part of the right segment. **(B)** A cast of a large intersegmental bronchiole from the lower lobe with a diameter of 110 μm. (From Andersen JB, Jespersen W: Demonstration of intersegmental respiratory bronchioles in normal human lung. *Eur J Respir Dis 61*:337–341, 1980.)

volume. The increased collateral ventilation that occurs with increased lung volume supports the use of deep breathing and positive airway pressure to reverse atelectasis found postoperatively (Craig, 1981).

The pathophysiology and management of atelectasis after anesthesia are discussed by Rigg (1981). He identifies many risk factors likely to increase alveolar collapse including low lung volume, high closing volume, oxygen therapy, rapid shallow ventilation, chronic lung disease, smoking, and obesity. Postoperative pain following abdominal or thoracic surgery and narcotic-induced ventilatory depression were additional factors together with neurological, neuromuscular, and musculosketetal diseases associated with impaired respiration. Management to prevent atelectasis includes chest physiotherapy, or delay in elective surgery. Improvement in respiratory function may be achieved with antibiotics, bronchodilators, and steroids, and by stopping smoking and weight loss. Elective postoperative ventilation may reduce atelectasis in selected patients. Whereas elective surgery may be delayed, emergency procedures and many of the identified risk factors are unavoidable or irreversible. Improvements in postoperative pain management can cer-

tainly avoid narcotic-induced ventilatory depression (see Chapter 10).

Vickers (1982) noted that the incidence of chest complications after surgery has not changed appreciably in 30 years, suggesting that the main determinants were largely unaffected by changes in medical and surgical practice. Although multiple etiologies are proposed for the cause of chest infection after surgery, none has produced unequivocally positive findings. Surveys of postoperative infections indicate upper abdominal or chest surgery as the most important causal determinant. Chronic respiratory disease tripled postoperative respiratory complications; obesity (over 120 kg), old age (above 70 years), and a history of smoking were also associated with a greater probability of postoperative pneumonia. Vickers discussed perioperative chest physiotherapy, IPPB, incentive spirometry, and bronchodilators, but stated that none made a difference in the development of pulmonary infection after upper abdominal surgery. Prophylactic antibiotics were viewed with disdain because resistant strains develop, and up to 80% of patients suffer no respiratory complications. Improvements in pain relief have not generally brought about a reduction in respiratory infections, though they may yet do so. Doxapram, a respiratory stimulant, may reduce the production of purulent sputum without influence on analgesia. However, when Doxapram was used in 20 postoperative patients greater than 126 kg in weight, there was no difference in the degree of hypoxemia or incidence of chest infections in the treated or untreated group (Holloway and Stanford, 1982). Garibaldi et al. (1981) found an association between obesity and postoperative pneumonia in patients weighing more than 100 kg. They also note that surgery lasting more than 4 hr, malnutrition (serum albumin less than 30 g/liter), and a preoperative stay of more than 7 days was associated with an increase in predisposition to pulmonary infection.

Natof (1980) described the postoperative complications in 13,433 patients having outpatient surgery. Only four patients (0.03%) had postoperative pulmonary infections, whereas Gracey at al. (1979) reported a 19% incidence of pulmonary complications after thoracic procedures and 25% after upper abdominal procedures in patients with chronic obstructive pulmonary disease (COPD). Garibaldi et al. found that the risk of developing postoperative pneumonia in patients with COPD is doubled by smoking. Bacterial filters on mechanical ventilators produced no reduction in the rate of postoperative pulmonary infections (Garibaldi et al.; Feeley et al., 1981).

The mechanism for postoperative hypoxia is not well understood. The early phase of hypoxia lasts only about 2 hr. The chest wall and diaphragm may be implicated (Craig, 1981; Schmid and Rehder, 1981) in addition to the ventilation/perfusion (V/Q) mismatch produced by some anesthetics. Hypoxia reduced the duration of breathing against resistance before diaphragmatic fatigue occurs (Macklem, 1980). The later phase of hypoxemia lasts up to a week after surgery, was more likely to occur after upper abdominal and thoracic surgery, and was characterized by a fall in FRC (Craig, 1981) and expiratory reserve volume (ERV) (Jones, 1982). The postoperative fall in lung volume was highly correlated with drop in PaO_2. Elderly patients were more likely to have low PaO_2 because of increased closing volume with increased

age (Jones, 1982). Catley et al. (1982) compared regional nerve block and continuous i.v. morphine infusion analgesia in patients following cholecystectomy and hip replacement. Comprehensive continuous monitoring of electroencephalogram (EEG), arterial O_2 saturation (SaO_2), ECG, and inductance pletysmography identified abnormal periods of apnea and paradoxical movement between rib cage and abdomen (Fig. 1.3), especially during sleep. The site of surgery had no influence on the abnormal respiratory patterns, but they occurred more frequently following morphine and with increased age. Paradoxical movements due to partial upper airway obstruction caused the greatest desaturation, to levels of 72%, on room air.

Whether respiratory infection in the postoperative period can be prevented by pre- or intraoperative measures was answered by many past studies that showed reduced complications for COPD patients with the preoperative use of bronchodilators and chest physiotherapy. Generally, prophylactic antibiotics are not recommended. However, Morran and McArdle (1980) found that trimethoprim and sulfamethoxazole (Bactrim) 1 hr before anesthesia reduced postoperative chest infections from 32% to 9% following cholecystectomy. For major elective procedures more likely to require postoperative ICU management, prophylactic antibiotics should be avoided because they are likely to cause overgrowth and development of resistant gram-negative organisms (Mackowiack, 1982). General anesthesia and surgery have an immunosuppressive effect (Serota et al., 1981) and nitrous oxide decreases neutrophil motility (Nunn and O'Morain, 1982), which may also predispose patients to chest infection after surgery. Shennib et al. (1984) showed in piglets that atelectasis predisposes the lung to infection due to impaired alveolar macrophage antibacterial function. There was progressive depression of phagocytic activity against *Pseudomonas aeruginosa* for up to 24 hr after atelectasis. Reexpansion of atelectasis with mechanical ventilation and 100% O_2 restored the impaired alveolar macrophage antibacterial activity.

Ventilatory failure, inadequate lung

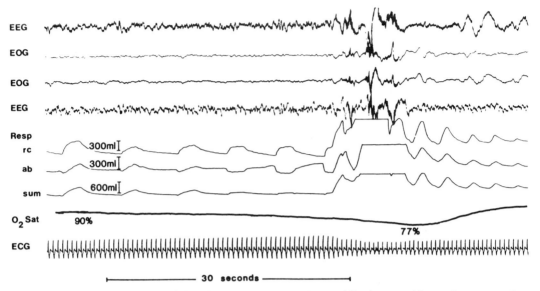

Figure 1.3. The movements of the rib cage (rc) and abdomen (diaphragm ab) are shown together with their sum, which is tidal volume. The trace shows obstructive apnea. rc and ab are first in phase for three breaths and then opposite in phase as upper airway obstruction becomes complete. The sum falls to zero as apnea occurs. The O_2 saturation (O_2 Sat) signal has a 10-sec delay so appears to go on falling after the patient shows arousal at the end of the period of obstructive apnea. EEG, electroencephalogram; EOG, electrooculogram; ECG, electrocardiogram. (From Jones JG: Pulmonary complications following general anesthesia. In *Anaesthesia Review,* edited by L Kaufman, 2nd Ed., Chapter 3, pp. 21–38. Churchill Livingstone, Edinburgh, 1984.)

expansion, and the postoperative fall in FRC and ERV may be due to respiratory muscle fatigue (Macklem, 1981; Craig, 1981; Jones, 1984). Fatigue of the diaphragm was predicted by the fall in force generated at low-frequency compared to high-frequency stimulation (Moxham et al., 1981). Respiratory muscle fatigue was relieved for long periods by a single unloaded breath (Lawler et al., 1979), and this may be the physiological basis for the beneficial effects sometime seen with intermittent mandatory ventilation (IMV). Phosphate depletion was associated with muscle weakness and hypoventilation, and may particularly be a cause of respiratory complications in alcoholics who receive dextrose intravenously and gastric antacids containing aluminum or magnesium (Newman, 1977). The mechanism determined by Aubier et al. (1985) was that hypophosphatemia impairs the contractile properties of the diaphragm during acute respiratory failure.

Enjeti et al. (1982) compared the effects of lung inflation of lobar and sublobar at-

electasis on vascular pressure-flow relationships in pigs with closed chests. With lobar atelectasis the atelectatic lobe behaved as a vascular resistor in parallel with the surrounding lung. When normal lung surrounding lobar atelectasis was inflated, its vascular resistance was increased and pulmonary blood flow was redistributed to the atelectatic lobe, causing a significant increase in intrapulmonary shunt. However, with sublobar atelectasis, lung inflation did not cause redistribution of blood flow. The explanation of these differences was that regional volume inhomogenicity occurs, which distorted the sublobar vessels and prevented redistribution of pulmonary blood flow. Enjet et al. suggested that their findings supported the use of selectively applied PEEP to diseased lung units in unilateral lung or lobar disease. There was, however, no discussion of the anatomic differences between pig and human lung. Collateral airways provide a means of ventilation to atelectatic sublobar units in humans but collateral airways are lacking in pigs.

Ford et al. (1983) studied diaphragmatic function in 15 patients before and after cholecystectomy. Diaphragmatic function was assessed by changes in transdiaphragmatic pressure swings during quiet tidal breathing, the ratio of changes in gastric to esophageal pressure swings, and the ratio of changes in abnormal rib cage diameters. There were significant falls in transdiaphragmatic and gastric-to-esophageal pressure changes after surgery, which reverted toward normal within 24 hr. Ford et al. suggest this reduction in diaphragm function may be responsible for the atelectasis, reduced vital capacity, and hypoxemia seen in patients after surgery. Different anesthetic techniques were used but not described. No assessment of neuromuscular function was made to confirm that complete reversal of muscle relaxants was present.

Because the role of pain in the etiology of postoperative respiratory dysfunction was still not fully established, Simonneau et al. (1983) examined diaphragm function after upper abdominal surgery. Opiate epidural analgesia on the first postoperative day did not modify diaphragmatic dysfunction, and measures of diaphragmatic function took until the seventh postoperative day to return to normal. They were able to demonstrate that the postoperative dysfunction was due to the upper abdominal surgery, not general anesthesia. Simonneau and associates implicated neuromuscular dysfunction or impairment of diaphragmatic mechanics induced by surgery as a possible mechanism of diaphragm dysfunction. Pain relief alone did not result in recovery of postoperative respiratory muscle abnormalities. Schur et al. (1984) measured pulmonary function in children before and after scoliosis surgery and compared them to a similar group of patients undergoing elective peripheral surgery. The peripheral surgery group had no postoperative change in lung volumes, whereas the scoliosis patients had 44% of their preoperative VC, 81% of FRC, 124% of preoperative residual volume, and 61% of total lung capacity. Schur et al. concluded that postoperative lung volume abnormalities were related

to the site and magnitude of surgery and associated abnormalities such as pain and preoperative respiratory dysfunction.

The mechanism of reduced vital capacity, hypoxemia and atelectasis that occurs after upper abdominal surgery remains unknown. However, Ford and Guenter (1984) quote Pasteur (1908, 1910) that a deficiency of inspiratory power is important and suggest that respiratory muscle activity may be reflexly modified by intraabdominal afferent nerves. Postoperative diaphragm function is impaired after cholecystectomy and breathing is predominantly thoracic. The return to normal thoracoabdominal breathing takes 24–48 hr. Animal studies suggest that when diaphragm function is impaired, expiratory muscles are activated and cause lung volumes to cycle below FRC. Therefore, despite loss of diaphragmatic contractility, there is still passive movement of the diaphragm. Expiratory muscle activation may cause atelectasis and hypoxemia because of small airway closure. Ford and Guenter (1984) suggest that the reduced tidal excursions of the lung adjacent to the diaphragm lead to the retained secretions, atelectasis, and infection seen in the lower lung fields. Intervention to block the reflex pathways responsible for decreased diaphragm activity may be possible when the afferent limb is established. Because diaphragm activity spontaneously reverts to normal, this definitive therapy will probably only be required for 24–48 hr.

Fletcher and Larsson (1985), in an interesting case report, monitored expired CO_2 curves and sulfahexafluoride SF6 washout (used to measure FRC) in an 11-month-old child who developed atelectasis. They found that alveolar dead space and intrapulmonary shunt were increased, but the blood shunt through the atelectatic lung was too small to account for the large increase in alveolar dead space. They suggest that atelectasis in the infant is associated with a more widespread disturbance in gas exchange due to the effects of interdependence on adjacent lung regions.

Celli et al. (1986) found that in patients with severe airway obstruction, arm exercises increased dyspnea and lead to dyssynchronous movements of the abdomen and chest wall. Celli et al. and the editorial that accompanied their article, concluded that breathing and simultaneously exercising of the shoulder girdle muscles, which are also accessory muscles of respiration, increased the demands on the other respiratory muscles, resulting in an increased load on the diaphragm. The diaphragm works inefficiently in chronic lung diseases; hyperinflation and loss of elastic recoil of the lungs cause diaphragm flattening. The dyssynchronous breathing noted in the study may be due to increased diaphragm flattening, and diminished expiratory ability of the abdominal muscles when the breathing rate increases and expiratory time decreases during exercise.

Durenil et al. (1986), after excluding neuromuscular dysfunction, concluded that postoperative diaphragm dysfunction was secondary to mechanisms such as a decrease in central nervous output. There may be inhibited phrenic nerve output due to reflexes from the chest or peritoneum. Local anesthetic nerve blockage of the sympathetic splanchnic, vagal abdominal, or afferent pathways from the esophagus or gallbladder may be therapeutic and relieve inhibition of central neural drive to the diaphragm.

Craven et al. (1986) identified risk factors for pneumonia and fatality in mechanically ventilated patients as univariately associated with the presence of intracranial pressure monitors ($p < 0.002$), cimetidine treatment ($p < 0.001$), fall–winter hospitalization ($p < 0.04$), and ventilator tubing changes every 24 hr rather than 48 hr ($p < 0.02$). The overall fatality rate for 49 of 233 patients who developed pneumonia was 55%, confirming the severity of illness of these patients. The diagnostic criteria used for pneumonia in this study are too nonspecific and do not provide a certain diagnosis of pneumonia. However, this study shows that there is a greater incidence of a pneumonia-like disease in patients who receive steroids (as in head injury) have increased gastric pH and get more frequent ventilator tubing manipulation.

The difficulties in diagnosis of nosocomial pneumonia in intubated intensive care unit patients were addressed by Salata et al. (1987). They noted that patients with tracheal tubes were at particularly high risk for colonization and subsequent pneumonia because of disrupted local clearance mechanisms, underlying immunosuppression, frequency of invasive procedures, use of respiratory therapy equipment, and location in an intensive care environment where exposure to numerous nosocomial pathogens was likely. Noninfectious pulmonary infiltrates may occur in the presence of colonization and this condition is difficult to distinguish from nosocomial pneumonia. Salata et al. studied 51 patients prospectively using three times weekly tracheal aspirates obtained by a sterile suction catheter. Suction catheter sampling almost certainly increases the false positives by contamination from tracheal tube to tracheobronchial tree, yet such sampling is frequently used in the ICU. Graded gram stains, quantitative bacterial cultures, and examination of aspirates for elastin fibers were used together with clinical and radiological observation. Grading of the gram stain for neutrophils, bacteria, and intracellular organisms correlated with quantitative tracheal aspirate culture. The presence of elastin fibers preceded pulmonary infiltrates by a mean of 1.8 ± 1.3 (SD) days and had a sensitivity of 52% and predictive value of 100%. Examination of serial tracheal aspirates for elastin fibers and by graded gram stain may improve differentiation of colonization from nosocomial pneumonia. Of the 51 patients, 34 developed pulmonary infiltrates on an average of 11 ± 13 days (range 1–60 days) after study entry and 21 of 34 were infected. Gram-negative bacilli were the most common isolates and were found most frequently in infected patients. Faling (1988) questions how the predictive value of elastin fibers might change in patients with adult respiratory distress syndrome (ARDS). Elastin fibers are produced by lung necrosis and this also occurs in ARDS, making differentiation from pneumonia difficult.

Driks et al. (1987) hypothesized that gram-negative nosocomial pneumonia may result from retrograde colonization of the pharynx from the stomach. The incidence of pneumonia in 132 mechanically ventilated patients in an ICU was twice as high in the patients given antacids or histamine type 2 (H2) blockers for stress ulcer prophylaxis compared to sucralfate. Sucralfate produced significantly lower gastric aspirate pH. Gram-negative bacilli were isolated more frequently and mortality rates were 1.6 times higher in the group of patients receiving antacids or H2 blockers. Driks et al. suggest that sucralfate may reduce the risk of nosocomial pneumonia in mechanically ventilated patients because it preserves the natural gastric acid barrier against bacterial overgrowth and prevents gastric colonization of the airway. Johanson and colleagues (1988a) examined diagnostic accuracy of bronchoalveolar lavage (BAL) in mechanically ventilated baboons compared to culture of tracheal secretions, protected specimen brush samples, and direct lung aspirates. The cultures of the three specimens obtained were compared with culture of lung homogenates. BAL produced the best reflection of lung infections both qualitatively and quantitatively. BAL recovered 74% of all microbes isolated and there were 15% false-positive specimens. Tracheal aspirates found 78% of the organisms in the lung tissue but 40% (14/30) of bacterial species isolated were not present in lung tissue. In a second paper, Johanson et al. (1988b) compared the occurrence of pneumonia after topical antibiotics, applied to the oropharynx and trachea, with and without the addition of intravenous antibiotics. Thirty-five baboons were studied for 7–10 days. Thirty animals had acute lung injury induced by oleic acid or hyperoxia. In 12 animals, no antibiotics or topical or intravenous antibiotics alone were given. Of the postmortem lung lobes 81% had severe pneumonia and none was sterile. Combinations of topical polymyxin and intravenous penicillin and gentamycin were efficacious in preventing pneumonia in 23 animals. Only 15% of lobes from these animals contained moderate to severe pneumonia and 52% of the lobes were sterile. Further studies are required in humans to assess the efficacy of these regimens in human subjects who may have

microbes with resistance to significant numbers of antibiotics.

Lack of mucociliary clearance occurs in subjects with Kartageners syndrome. Vevaina et al. (1987) examined radioisotopic mucociliary clearance and the ultrastructure of respiratory cilia in such a patient. They confirmed total absence of clearance of inhaled technetium-labeled sulfur colloid after 1 hr. Transmission electron microscopy of bronchial mucosal biopsy tissue showed that in virtually all cilia inner dynein arms were absent. The outer and inner dynein arms on the cilia are microtubule-associated proteins that are thought to be the transducers of mechanical forces necessary for ciliary motion. Inner dynein arms are of high molecular weight and have six electrophoretically distinct heavy chains. These proteins have unique and high adenosine triphosphatase activity in the presence of magnesium and calcium ions. Other causes for human ciliary immotility include abnormalities of the length and basal apparatus of cilia, radial spoke defects, outer or inner dynein arm deficiency, absence of microtubules within the cilia, and ciliary immotility induced by infection and injury (Eliasson et al., 1977; Suppl 127, *Eur J Resp Dis* 1983; Vevaina et al., 1987). All these recognized ultrastructural defects have the same clinical effect of causing impaired ciliary clearance from the tracheobronchial tree.

Tokis et al. (1987) examined whether spontaneous breathing, compared to controlled mechanical ventilation, muscle paralysis, and PEEP, was an etiology in the development of atelectasis and impaired gas exchange during general anesthesia. They used computerized axial tomographic (CT) scans and the multiple inert gas elimination technique (Wagner et al., 1974) for assessment of the distribution of V/Q ratios in 13 supine adult patients. Seven patients were smokers and two had obstructive airways disease. Ventilation of poorly perfused areas occurred in nine patients ranging from 9% to 19% of total ventilation. CT scans after 15 min of halothane anesthesia and mechanical ventilation showed densities in dependent lung regions in 11 of 19 patients (Figs. 1.4 and 1.5). There was close correlation (r=0.84) between the area of

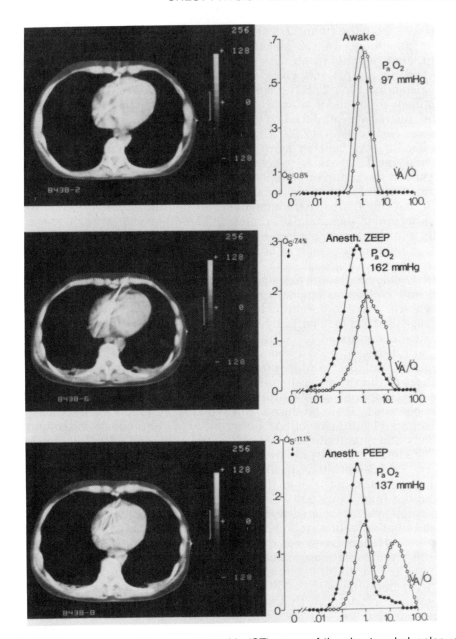

Figure 1.4. Transverse computerized tomographic (CT) scans of the chest and alveolar ventilation (V_A)/blood flow (Q) distribution (0 = V_A = Q liters/min), awake, during anesthesia, with conventional mechanical ventilation, and after the addition of 10 cm H_2O PEEP. There is a unimodal V_A/Q distribution awake with shunt (Q_s) of 0.8%. After induction of anesthesia, densities appear in the dependent lung and Q_s is 7.4%. PEEP reduces the densities but not the shunt and causes a high V_A/Q mode. PaO$_2$ is shown at each time. (From Tokis L, Hedenstierna G, Stranberg A, Brismar B, Lundquist H: Lung collapse and gas exchange during general anesthesia: Effects of spontaneous breathing, muscle paralysis and positive end-expiratory pressure. *Anesthesiology 66:*157–167, 1987.)

atelectasis on CT scan and the magnitude of shunt. Both CT density area and shunt increased after muscle paralysis. PEEP reduced the CT density area but did not consistently alter the shunt. During spontaneous breathing, shunt and density area were decreased compared to patients managed with muscle paralysis and mechanical ventilation. Tokis et al. suggested that anesthesia reduced or al-

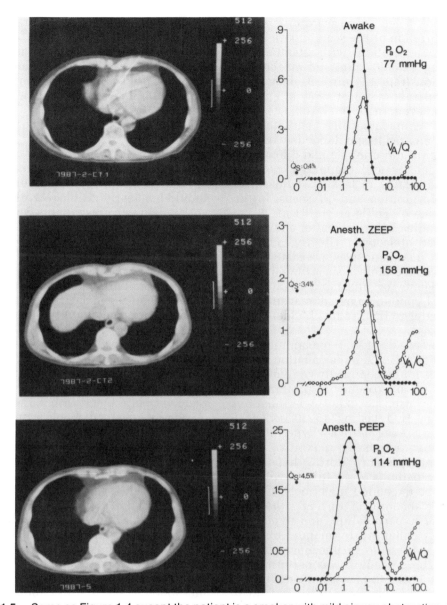

Figure 1.5.   Same as Figure 1.4 except the patient is a smoker with mild airway obstruction. During anesthesia (middle panel), the diaphragm moves cranially and appears as the white area, especially in the left lung. There is, however, only a small atelectatic area and low shunt (3.4%) although there are many low V_A/Q areas. PEEP reduced the atelectatic area but had minimal effects on V_A/Q. (From Tokis L, Hedenstierna G, Stranberg A, Brismar B, Lundquist H: Lung collapse and gas exchange during general anesthesia: Effects of spontaneous breathing, muscle paralysis and positive end-expiratory pressure. *Anesthesiology 66:*157–167, 1987.)

tered the tone of the diaphragm and caused development of atelectasis. The reason atelectasis increased after muscle paralysis was not explained.

FRC was reduced during anesthesia, and there was a cranial shift of the diaphragm. During positive pressure venti- lation, diaphragmatic movement occurs probably in a piston-like manner (K. Rehder, personal communication). Tokis et al. found no further cranial movement of the diaphragm (Fig. 1.5) after muscle paralysis, compared to spontaneous breathing during anesthesia. Because the CT scans took 5 sec, there were differences in the duration of the scan exposed during end expiration with spontaneous breathing (rate 20/min) and mechanical ventilation (rate 12/min). Atelectasis is more apparent on chest x-ray at end expiration, even in normal subjects. The changes in mechanically ventilated patients compared to spontaneously breathing patients and unexplained differences in CT density and diaphragm position could be related to lack of standardization of respiration and CT scans. In the experience of Tokis et al., 73 of 78 patients studied before and after anesthesia developed atelectasis. Clearly, anesthesia with halothane was associated with intraoperative atelectasis. Other inhalational agents or anesthetic techniques such as hypnotic or narcotic agents may not produce the same incidence of atelectasis.

Novak et al. (1987) reexamined the benefits of periodic hyperinflation on gas exchange for mechanically ventilated patients with hypoxemic respiratory failure. They used periodic hyperinflations of 40 cm H_2O lasting 15–30 sec as a sustained, exaggerated, hyperinflation rather than a sigh. To maximize transpulmonary pressure during hyperinflation, the patients were turned with the area to be expanded uppermost. Coughing was encouraged during exhalation from the hyperinflation, and expiratory flow was enhanced by manual external chest compression in uncooperative patients. The procedure was performed 10 times at 30-sec intervals between hyperinflations, five times with the patient in each of the right and left lateral positions, and was compared to standard bag-sigh suctioning. Neither technique, alone or in sequence, resulted in changes in gas exchange or lung/thorax compliance 5 or 30 min after treatment.

In view of the attempts made to increase transpulmonary pressures by use of incentive spirometry and inspiratory resistive breathing devices these findings are important. The reason that 40 cm H_2O was not able to recruit collapsed lung or improve oxygenation in patients with hypoxemic respiratory failure of more than 24 hr duration could be that end-expiratory pressure returned to baseline

levels, and collapse reoccurred, after each maneuver. Alternatively, either alveolar collapse was not the cause of hypoxemia, or viscid secretions blocking the airway caused overexpansion of the ventilated lung that further compressed the collapsed segments. Segmental bronchi blockage could be the mechanism, as blockage at a subsegmental or more peripheral airway would allow expansion through collateral airways and a cut off in the chest x-ray air bronchogram should be clearly visible. Novak et al. do not explain why the patients were turned on both left and right sides. Respiratory mechanics and gas exchange for unilateral lung lesions may improve in one lateral position and deteriorate in the other. For either hyperinflation or bag-sigh suctioning to be beneficial, secretions should be removed. The quantity of sputum removed was not described.

Mankikian et al. (1988) measured the effects of thoracic epidural block on diaphragm function in 13 patients after upper abdominal surgery. Fourth thoracic vertebral block with 0.5% plain bupivacaine reversed diaphragm dysfunction that occurred consistently after upper abdominal surgery. They suggested that inhibitory reflexes of phrenic motor activity arising from the abdominal wall and viscera may be involved in diaphragm dysfunction. They were unable to discriminate between potential inhibitory afferents from intraabdominal structure afferents and mechanical antagonism between abdominal muscles and the diaphragm. Using the same methodology as in this study, Simmoneau et al. (1983) showed that postoperative diaphragm dysfunction was unchanged with epidural opiates. Clergue et al. (1984) showed that shallow and rapid breathing that occurs after upper abdominal surgery was not modified by spinal morphine despite complete pain relief. It appears that pain is not the mechanism underlying respiratory dysfunction after upper abdominal surgery. Epidural block with 0.5% bupivacaine is the only technique to improve respiratory dysfunction after upper abdominal surgery. Clearly, studies examining the effects of continuous epidural anesthesia with lower concentration of bupivacaine are warranted to determine whether the incidence of postoperative respiratory complications can be reduced.

Therapy for Respiratory Complications

Since 1980, the reports on therapeutic interventions that may reverse respiratory complications or improve prognosis and reduce hospital stay for patients with respiratory complications have magnified. In this section, papers on chest physiotherapy and cough, techniques to change pulmonary pressure, and use of bronchoscopy, are critically summarized. Papers published since 1980 are compared to similar previous publications.

Chest Physiotherapy

Weller et al. (1980) found that chest physiotherapy resulted in significantly improved peak flow rates in 20 children with cystic fibrosis. No patients received aerosol therapy. On average, about 8 ml of sputum was produced. In 12 patients sputum grew *Pseudomonas aeruginosa*. Pulmonary function was assessed for 24 hr and compared to no chest physiotherapy. The authors suggest that central but not peripheral airway clearance occurred with chest physiotherapy. Bronchodilators had no added effects. Tecklin and Holsclaw (1975) also reported increased peak flow rates but did not follow up their 26 patients with cystic fibrosis and had no control group.

In a study designed to eliminate discrepancies in arterial blood gases due to changes in position, Holody and Goldberg (1981) examined the effect of mechanical vibrations over the anatomic area of acute lung disease during therapy for atelectasis or pneumonia. Patients were seated upright or in a high semi-Fowler position. Ten patients were studied, at least nine of whom had lower lobe lung pathology. Mechanical vibration lasted 30 min and the patients were suctioned only after completion of chest vibration therapy. Blood gases at 30 min and 1 hr after therapy showed average increases ($p < 0.05$) in PaO_2 of 10 and 15 mm Hg, respectively, when compared to baseline. In these acutely ill patients, 70% of whom were mechanically venti-

lated, the authors suggested that vibration therapy may be applied when patients were intolerant of postural drainage and percussion. There was no indication of how much sputum was produced with suctioning, no details of use of PEEP, and no information on the duration of improved PaO_2 beyond 1 hr. If the data from the three spontaneously breathing patients are extracted, there are probably no significant differences in PaO_2.

No difference was found between chest physiotherapy and IPPB in preventing postoperative pulmonary complications among patients who underwent upper abdominal surgery (Schuppisser et al., 1980). Because of the potential hazards with IPBB of cross-infection, gastric dilatation, ileus, tension pneumothorax, decrease in FRC and PaO_2, and increased airway resistance, hypotension, and gastrointestinal perforation, the authors recommended chest physiotherapy (see Chapter 9). Kigin (1981) published a comprehensive review of chest physical therapy for the postoperative or traumatic injury patient. She suggests that controlled studies of secretion removal techniques are a priority for this group of patients. She identifies the lack of studies determining the beneficial components of chest physiotherapy and states that clarification of contraindications and complications is required.

Kerrebijn et al. (1982) were unable to show clearance of mucus from peripheral airways in 25 clinically quiescent, sputum-producing children with cystic fibrosis. Chest physiotherapy or no therapy with or without aerosolized N-acetylcysteine was randomly compared on consecutive days. No effects on respiratory flows (maxium expiratory, FEV_1, or VC) and volumes (total lung capacity) were found. One of the points discussed by these authors was that the optimum frequency and strength of chest percussion were not the same at different ages because of changes in chest wall compliance and amounts of lung tissue. Patients with cystic fibrosis may respond differently to chest physiotherapy when in a quiescent, compared to an active phase. The papers in which beneficial effects occurred in patients with cystic fibrosis

(Tecklin and Holsclaw; Weller et al.) do not identify whether their patients were experiencing exacerbations at the time of therapy. The differences in techniques (frequency of percussion and force and frequency of chest vibration) may also influence the response of individual patients to chest physiotherapy. These techniques are discussed in Chapter 4. The conclusion of Kerrebijn et al. that no clearance of mucus from peripheral airways occurred in patients with cystic fibrosis confirmed the findings of Weller et al.

Rossman and colleagues (1982) compared the effectiveness of spontaneous cough (control), postural drainage (PD) with and without mechanical percussion, PD deep breathing with vibration and percussion administered by a physiotherapist, and directed vigorous cough. They found PD was not as effective as physiotherapy or cough and frequent self-directed vigorous cough was most effective. This was in contrast to the findings of Sutton et al. (1983) who report that the addition of PD nearly tripled the sputum yield achieved by cough alone. Rossman et al. did not differentiate between the use of a forced expiratory technique (FET) and cough. Sutton et al. (1983) found that cough alone did not enhance mucus clearance, but FET and PD did. The forced expiratory technique consisted of one or two forced expirations from mid- to low-lung volume, followed by a period of relaxation and diaphragmatic breathing. No glottic closure occurred and the airway compressive phase that characterizes coughing was avoided so that worsening of bronchospasm may be prevented by this forced expiratory maneuver (Sutton et al., 1983). (See Chapter 3, p. 121.) In 10 patients with copious sputum (mean 63 ml/24 hr) FET alone and with PD increased the clearance of sputum compared to control. Directed coughing without FET and PD was not different from control. Sutton et al. (1984) suggest that protracted coughing was fruitless and exhausting, leading to poor compliance.

Newhouse (1984) argued that the differences between the findings of the two studies investigating clearance of mucus probably related to secretion volume and rheology. Newhouse suggested that cough is more effective in clearing boluses of secretions rather than thin, watery, copious secretions, which were more likely to be cleared by PD. The conflicting results of Oldenberg et al. (1979), Bateman et al. (1981), and Rossman et al. (1982) concerning the role of cough independent of the other maneuvers used in chest physiotherapy stimulated De-Boeck and Zinman (1984) to assess conventional pulmonary function tests after cough alone or chest physiotherapy for patients with cystic fibrosis. Chest physiotherapy was standardized, consisting of 2 min of percussion and vibration in 11 postural drainage positions that proceeded sequentially from lower to upper lobes. The patient then performed three slow vital capacity maneuvers, during which exhalation was assisted by the physiotherapist. This was compared with a directed vigorous cough session repeated 11 times over 10 min in the seated position. The amount of sputum produced and the pattern and magnitude of changes in PFTs 1 hr after treatment on consecutive mornings were the same after cough or chest physiotherapy. De-Boeck and Zinman confirmed the lack of correlation between sputum produced and improvement in PFT. They suggested that vigorous coughing and FET should be further investigated for long-term effectiveness in cystic fibrosis.

The studies on patients with acute and chronic lung diseases comparing the effectiveness of the independent components of chest physiotherapy are confusing, because combinations of components may be more effective than a single variable under study. The multitude of possible permutations of chest vibration, percussion, cough, FET, PD, or tracheal suctioning in patients with different chronic or acute lung pathology makes clinically relevant studies difficult to find. The clinician wishes to know if lung reexpansion is achieved more efficiently when all the techniques are used or whether one or two of them may be omitted without loss of effectiveness. To date, this dilemma is unresolved.

Zapletal et al. (1983) found that chest physiotherapy that included manual chest percussion and vibration in various postural drainage positions and stimulation of cough produced adverse effects in 24 patients with cystic fibrosis. Despite production of 2–10 ml of sputum, flow at 25% vital capacity decreased significantly. The authors suggest that the flow limitation may result from adverse effects of prolonged coughing. Narrowing of bronchi was demonstrated on contrast cinebronchiographic studies (Fig. 1.6A and B).

For postoperative patients, Morran et al. (1983) showed in a prospective randomized controlled trial of 102 patients

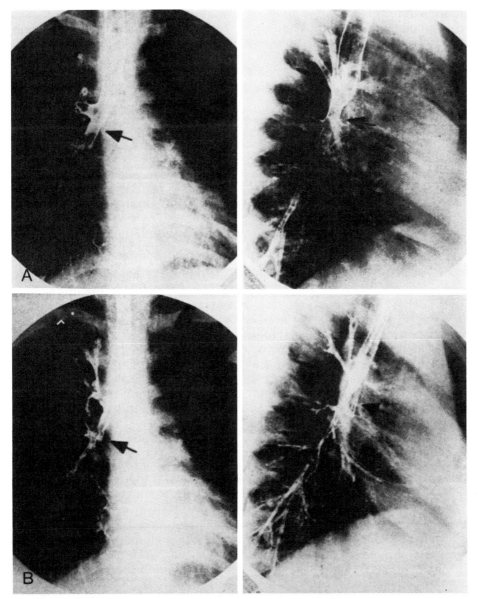

Figure 1.6. (**A**) Contrast bronchograms of the right lung of a 17-year-old female with cystic fibrosis. Arrow denotes significant narrowing of the right medial basal bronchus. On left is anteroposterior view and on right a lateral view during normal breathing. (**B**) Same as **A** during coughing. Note that there is marked narrowing of the airways during coughing and a lack of evacuation of the contrast material from peripheral airways. (From Zapletal A, Stefanova J, Horak J, Vavrova V, Somanek M: Chest physiotherapy and airway obstruction in patients with cystic fibrosis—a negative report. *Eur J Respir Dis 64*:426–433, 1983.)

that routine prophylactic chest physiotherapy significantly reduced the frequency of chest infection after elective cholecystectomy. The authors differentiated between routine and intensive chest physiotherapy. Postural drainage and bronchodilator therapy was referred to as intensive chest physiotherapy and breathing exercises, assisted coughing, and vibration of the chest wall were used as routine prophylactic chest physiotherapy. The control group in their study received only encouragement to breathe deeply and cough from nursing and medical staff. The authors specifically distinguished between atelectasis and infection. Although 18 patients receiving routine chest physiotherapy developed atelectasis, only 7 developed chest infection, whereas of patients not receiving chest physiotherapy, 11 had atelectasis and 19 developed chest infection ($p <$ 0.02). There were weaknesses in this clinical study because previous respiratory disease was not adequately defined and the means for confirming infection and use of antibiotics were vague. The authors suggested that routine chest physiotherapy prevented progression of atelectasis to chest infection.

Flower et al. (1979) showed that maximum peak vibration of the bronchial tree in adults occurred at about 16 Hz using an external chest pressure of about 2.5 kg. Hand clapping reaches only about 8 Hz. King et al. (1983), however, found that external chest wall compression at frequencies above 3 Hz and up to 17 Hz increased tracheal mucus clearance. Peak enhancement of clearance reached 340% of control at 13 Hz. King et al. suggested that the high-frequency chest wall compression may cause a reduction in cross-linking of mucus glycoproteins, resulting in improved mucus clearance. They did not consider other factors besides frequency when comparing manual and mechanical techniques of chest physiotherapy. The clinical advantages of manual percussion over mechanical devices are in our opinion, significant, and are fully discussed in Chapter 4.

Kigin (1984) comprehensively reviewed indications for chest physiotherapy and the effects of the individual components such as positioning, suctioning,

manual vibration, percussion, shaking, and cough. The use of chest physiotherapy in acute and chronically ill patients was described. Carswell et al. (1984) examined deoxyribonucleic acid (DNA) output in the sputum of patients with cystic fibrosis to determine if it was a useful indicator of pulmonary cellular damage. Aggressive therapeutic intervention may be more efficiently timed to coincide with increased rate of lung damage if DNA was such an indicator. However, sputum DNA showed similar variations to sputum weight and was not well correlated with lung damage. Sputum was obtained by physiotherapy using percussion and postural drainage, breathing exercises and chest shaking, assisted panting, huffing, and coughing. Physiotherapy sessions lasted 25 min. Patients carried out this therapy at home two times per day for 3 weeks, followed by 3 weeks parental use of a mechanical percussor. For the next 3 weeks a professional physiotherapist visited the home 5 days a week and provided a third session in addition to parental chest physiotherapy. In two of the three subjects in which data were gathered, the professional and parental regimen produced significantly greater quantities of DNA than the percussor or parental therapy alone. Sputum weight correlated well ($p = 0.90$) with DNA (Fig. 1.7). This suggests that the professional physical therapists treatment was more effective than the parental or percussor therapy in removing secretions.

Buscaglia and St. Marie (1983) found no dangerous hypoxemia using continuous oximetry monitoring of arterial O_2 saturation during chest percussion and vibration with postural drainage. Ten spontaneously breathing patients with acute exacerbation of severe COPD were studied. Although most patients had elevated PCO_2 and required O_2 to maintain PaO_2 above 60 mm Hg, the largest decrease in saturation was 2%, and the lowest absolute value was 91%. These findings are surprising, considering the variability of FiO_2 in spontaneously breathing patients receiving O_2. In addition, even in normal individuals, arterial saturation frequently falls below 91% during coughing and breathholding.

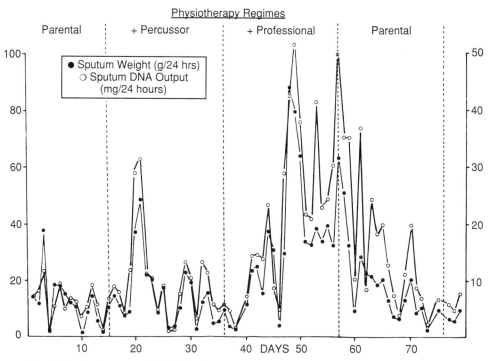

Figure 1.7.   Weight of sputum (solid circles) and DNA (open circles) is compared ($p = 0.9$) in the course of parental chest physiotherapy twice a day (parental), mechanical percussor twice a day (percussor), and parental and physiotherapist treatment for a total of three treatments per day (professional). Sputum production was greater but peak expiratory flow less with the professional than percussor regimen. (From Carswell F, Robinson DW, Ward CCL, Waterfield MR: Deoxyribonucleic acid output in the sputum from cystic fibrosis patients. *Eur J Respir Dis 65*:53–57, 1984.)

Sutton et al. (1985) examined the value of percussion, vibratory shaking, and breathing exercises with and without postural drainage and FET in eight patients with copious sputum production. Using inhaled aerosols, bronchial secretions were labeled and their clearance monitored by gamma camera. Randomized treatments included vibratory shaking during relaxed expiration followed by maximum inspiration, percussion during tidal breathing compared to a control period of 30 min postural drainage, and voluntary cough. Vibration (12–16 Hz), shaking (2 Hz), and percussion (approximately 5 Hz) were used to enhance mucus clearance. No differences in clearance of radioisotope were found between any of the treatments, although the wet weight of sputum was increased by vibration and percussion with deep breathing. Why radioisotope clearance was no different when sputum clearance was increased with vibration and percussion was not explained, but may be due to

particle penetration of the peripheral airways. The techniques of labeling and scanning of the three regions are open to criticism because of the inability to adequately visualize the isotope in three dimensions. The requirement that the patients are in exactly the same position with the same lung volume to make valid comparisons before and after each of the therapies that were as many as 1–4 days apart is not addressed. Although the eight patients did have copious sputum, the range varied by over 100%. The eight patients had three different causative pathologies, which suggests that they might have responded differently to the therapies under study. Some of the variations found in studies using radioisotopes may be due to different techniques for aerosol deposition and measurement of clearance.

Chest percussion was found to be of little value as an adjunct to postural drainage and instructed coughing in the treatment of 10 patients with chronic bronchitis (Wollmer et al., 1985). Percussion was associated with a small decrease in FEV_1 after therapy; however, this was not associated with any changes in O_2 saturation. Radioisotope penetration was higher following chest physiotherapy with percussion. The two patients who produced 100 ml and 130 ml of sputum had substantially higher clearance of inhaled radioisotope particles when percussion was included, compared to when it was omitted. The findings were not, therefore, clear-cut. Mazzocco et al. (1985) found that chest percussion and postural drainage were helpful, safe, and effective in assisting 13 patients with stable bronchiectasis to clear secretions. There were no adverse effects on heart rate or rhythm, pulmonary function or O_2 saturation.

Mackenzie and Shin (1985) measured cardiorespiratory function before, immediately after, and 2 hr after chest physiotherapy in 19 patients with posttraumatic respiratory failure. Cardiac index was unchanged and intrapulmonary shunt fell, followed at 2 hr by an increase in lung/thorax compliance. The reduced cardiac output after chest physiotherapy reported by Laws and McIntyre (1969) was not found, but cardiac output was not measured during chest physiotherapy. In addition, the patient population was young and did not have preexisting cardiac disease. None of the detrimental cardiopulmonary changes associated with bronchoscopy occurred in these critically ill patients, yet beneficial effects on gas exchange and lung mechanics were documented.

Klein et al. (1988) found that heart rate, systolic and mean blood pressure, and cardiac output were increased during chest physiotherapy. Metabolic rate determined by measurement of O_2 consumption and CO_2 production was increased. In no patient was PaO_2 changed but in some groups $PaCO_2$ increased with chest physiotherapy. The increases in blood pressure and heart rate were attenuated by continuous infusion of 3 μg/kg fentanyl but not 1.5 μg/kg fentanyl. Fentanyl did not alter the increased metabolic response with chest physiotherapy. Cardiac output increased up to 50%

above baseline values in two patients who did not receive fentanyl only placebo infusion. Cardiac output was measured in 6/10 patients in the groups that received 3.0 and 1.5 μg/kg fentanyl. Neither dose prevented elevation of baseline cardiac output by about 20–25% during chest physiotherapy. In all instances within 15 min of the finish of chest physiotherapy cardiac output was not different to baseline whether the patients received fentanyl or placebo. The unchanged cardiac output and PaO_2 immediately after therapy confirms the findings of Mackenzie et al. (1987b) and Mackenzie and Shin (1985). The issue is whether elevation of cardiac output and metabolic rate during chest physiotherapy is clinically significant. Is this a reason to withhold chest physiotherapy in critically ill patients with cardiovascular dysfunction? These are the very patients who can least tolerate pulmonary deterioration. In our opinion chest physiotherapy should not be withheld because cardiac output and metabolic rate increase. Instead sedation and analgesia are used before and during therapy.

Van der Schans et al. (1986) examined percussion in nine patients with stable chronic airflow obstruction and excessive tracheobronchial secretions. Manual percussion was no different when applied in combination with PD coughing and breathing exercises for 20 min, compared to the same regimen without percussion. The addition of PD and coughing with or without percussion improved mucociliary clearance. The authors suggested that because manual percussion as a single procedure was found to improve tracheobronchial clearance, it may be useful when a patient was not able to cough or cannot tolerate postural drainage.

An editorial on management of acute bronchiolitis in infancy (Milner and Murray, 1988) suggests that chest physiotherapy, although a popular therapy, may not be beneficial. In a controlled study of 96 children with bronchiolitis chest physiotherapy was not found to be beneficial (Webb et al., 1985). The criteria for assessment of benefit were clinical and, therefore, subjective. The authors do not recommend chest physiotherapy in the management of acute bronchiolitis as the babies require considerable disturbance and many children were noted to become more distressed during and immediately after chest physiotherapy. Directed, supervised coughing was found to be equally effective as chest physiotherapy in management of 39 patients hositalized for treatment of an exacerbation of pulmonary symptoms from cystic fibrosis (Bain et al., 1988). Directed coughing consisted of five quick small huffs or pants followed by expiratory huffs and coughing until all loosened sputum was cleared from the airways. The sequence was then repeated twice every 5 min for 35 min. No differences were found in pulmonary function tests and sputum characteristics.

Cardiac output, oxygen consumption, and arterial and mixed venous saturation ($S\overline{V}O_2$) were measured during suctioning in 10 acutely ill mechanically ventilated patients (Walsh et al., 1989). Suctioning produced significant decreases in $S\overline{V}O_2$ predominantly due to increased O_2 consumption but also due to an inadequate rise or even a fall in cardiac output. Arterial saturation was virtually unchanged partly because the patients were preoxygenated with 100% O_2 before suctioning. The authors comment that arterial saturation was not a sensitive indicator of changes in $S\overline{V}O_2$. The mechanism postulated for fall in $S\overline{V}O_2$ was decreased cardiac output occurring from decreased intrathoracic pressure with suctioning. If this is indeed the mechanism, closed sheath suction catheters which prevent entrainment of atmospheric air during suctioning may potentiate this effect. The solution is to sedate agitated patients before suctioning so that O_2 consumption is reduced and to restrict suctioning if no secretions are obtained.

Techniques to Change Transpulmonary Pressures

By producing either subatmospheric pleural pressure or positive airway pressure, bilateral lung expansion is achieved because both maneuvers increase transpulmonary pressure. Mechanical means that generate a subatmospheric pleural pressure greater than the normal 5–10 cm H_2O include inspiratory incentive spirometry, inspiratory resistive breathing, and, in patients with diaphragmatic paralysis, electrical pacing. Positive airway pressure is obtained by mechanical ventilation with or without PEEP, continuous positive airway pressure (CPAP) during spontaneous respiration, or IPPB. Pressure support and changing inspiratory/expiratory ratios may alter the length of time during the respiratory cycle that transpulmonary pressure is increased. Inspiratory resistive breathing may also increase respiratory muscle endurance and strength. Mechanical means of altering local lung expansion include selective positive pressure inflation of an atelectatic lung segment, recruitment by collateral ventilation, and interdependence.

Anderson et al. (1979) showed that atelectatic lung can be recruited through collateral airways by positive pressure ventilatory techniques. They suggested that time constants (product of compliance and resistance) for collateral airways during exhalation were longer than during inspiration, so more air entered the lung at the periphery of an atelectatic area than left during exhalation. As a result, pressure rose distal to the obstruction and became greater than the pressure in the surrounding lung. Collateral airway reinflation, therefore, potentially forced secretions centrally to larger bronchi where they may be more easily removed. Andersen et al. (1980) suggested the use of periodic applications of continuous positive airway pressure (CPAP) by face mask to increase collateral ventilation of obstructed lung regions. Twenty-four patients with postoperative atelectasis were studied in a prospective randomized controlled clinical trial. CPAP with 15 cm H_2O once per hour and conventional therapy was compared to conventional therapy alone. Conventional therapy included humidification, oxygen, intensive chest physical therapy with three times daily postural drainage, tracheal suctioning, and instruction in deep breathing. The comparison was made over 24 hr and successful therapy was considered to be an increase in PaO_2 of at least 15% or decrease in area of radiological atelectasis by 50%. Significantly more patients were treated successfully with the addition of CPAP.

Chest wall strapping, such as occurs with dressings around chest tubes or after thoracotomy, reduces respiratory excursion and the ability to generate subatmospheric intrapleural pressures and increases the elastic work of breathing. After strapping the chest of four healthy young men, DeTroyer (1980) found that both FRC and chest wall compliance were decreased. FRC decreased about 1 liter and compliance of the chest wall fell from 22.9 to 10.6 ml/cm H_2O (Fig. 1.8). Whenever possible, chest wall restriction should be minimized as it reduces subatmospheric pleural pressure causing lung volume to fall below FRC.

Belman and Mittman, in an editorial (1981), raised the issue of the unproven efficacy and widespread use of incentive spirometry. They found the evidence against the efficacy of incentive spirometry convincing, yet they concede that the theoretical basis for expecting this approach to be effective was also convincing. Lung hyperinflation by whatever means reverses low lung compliance caused by quiet breathing. They suggest that when multiple measures in addition to lung hyperinflation were used, encouraging results were obtained. Lung hyperinflation affects the high compliance lung units and needs to be supplemented with other measures that direct ventilation to the low compliance compartments in the lung, particularly in the high-risk patients with obesity or obstructive lung disease.

Falk et al. (1984) suggest that periodic application of face mask positive expiratory pressure (PEP) with forced expiratory technique (FET) improved sputum production and was better tolerated by 74 patients with cystic fibrosis than postural drainage, percussion and chest vibration, or PD and periodic application of PEP or FET. They thought that PEP may be beneficial to other patients with excessive secretions.

Celli et al. (1984) showed that IPPB, incentive spirometry (IS), and deep breathing exercises (DBE) were superior to no treatment at all in preventing pulmonary complications in a controlled trial among 172 patients after abdominal surgery. Hospital stay for 21 of 81 patients who underwent upper abdominal surgery and received incentive spirometry was

Figure 1.8. Effects of chest strapping on the pressure–volume curve of the relaxed chest wall in four subjects. Control data are shown as solid circles data after strapping as open circles. Transthoracic pressure shown on the abscissa is the difference between esophageal and barometric pressures. (From DeTroyer A: Mechanics of the chest wall during restrictive thoracic strapping. *Respiration* *39:*241–250, 1980.)

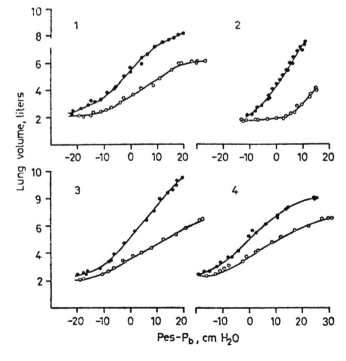

shorter than the control group who received no therapy. The authors acknowledge that the optimal treatment schedule for these techniques remains unknown and they recommend further study of IS and DBE in patients at high risk of pulmonary complications. Many of the arguments they use to support DBE would equally apply to chest physiotherapy. This was not considered. An editorial (Ford and Guenter) referring to Celli's paper stressed that the most important factor predicting the development of postoperative pulmonary complications was the upper abdominal site of surgery. It may also be important to know which organs were involved in the upper abdominal surgery.

Dull and Dull (1983) found that 49 adult patients who underwent cardiopulmonary bypass and were assigned to either mobilization, incentive spirometry, or maximal inspiratory breathing exercises all experienced decreases in lung volume. No advantage was shown with incentive spirometry or breathing exercises in addition to mobilization, compared to mobilization alone. Stock et al. (1985) demonstrated that the use of incentive spirometry with documented maximal volume inhalations was not superior to deep breathing exercises in preventing postoperative pulmonary complications after upper abdominal surgery. Respiratory function tests including FRC, FeV_1, and FVC were not different. CPAP produced a more rapid increase in FRC than incentive spirometry or deep breathing.

The effect of continuous positive airway pressure (CPAP) and blow bottles on FRC was examined by Heitz et al. (1985) in two groups of comparable patients undergoing elective abdominal surgery. Both blow bottles and CPAP increased FRC by 50% both preoperatively and postoperatively. The significant reduction in FRC seen postoperatively returned within 10 min of stopping either therapy. CPAP had a lower resistive work of breathing and was better tolerated by patients. The average postoperative reduction in FRC in the 20 patients who underwent upper abdominal surgery was 20–30%. Both CPAP and blow bottles increased FRC, but most authori-

ties suggest CPAP is superior to achieve the increase. The rapid reversal of benefit on cessation suggests that CPAP should be used continuously for the therapy to alter outcome and reduce postoperative complications.

Incentive spirometry was not found to be beneficial in producing differences in chest x-ray, PaO_2, spirometric evaluation, or clinical evaluation 2 and 4 days after elective cholecystectomy, compared to a group of similar patients who had no specialized respiratory care (Schweiger et al., 1986). Both groups of 20 patients had 12–16% pulmonary complications. The low-risk patients with subcostal cholecystectomy incisions did not benefit from incentive spirometry. IPPB is reported to improve lung compliance in subjects with kyphoscoliosis (Sinha and Begofsky, 1972). IPPB was examined to see if it conferred benefit on patients with respiratory muscle weakness. However, in 14 subjects with either quadriplegia or muscular dystrophy, no immediate improvements were derived in ventilatory mechanics (McCool et al., 1986).

The study by Zibrak et al. (1986) strongly suggested that a concerted effort to set priorities for the use of respiratory therapy techniques (bronchodilator aerosols, ultrasonic mist aerosols, IPPB, incentive spirometry, and oxygen therapy) for patients in at least seven common diagnostic categories can be successful. Implementation of these priorities did not change overall mortality, although patients stayed a shorter time in the hospital after coronary artery bypass surgery and the staffing of respiratory therapists was reduced. In an editorial commenting on rational respiratory therapy stimulated by the study of Zibrak et al., Petty (1986) identified the core of a major problem. He states that the prescribing physician's lack of firm grounding in the rational ordering of respiratory therapy is one of the factors that created the uncontrolled and excessive use of respiratory therapy. A large difference in usage of IS and chest physiotherapy after coronary artery surgery exists in the United States and Great Britain. Only 44% of 39 hospitals used IS in Britain, whereas O'Donohue (1985) reported 95% used IS in the

United States. Chest physiotherapy was only used in 41% of U.S. hospitals after cardiac surgery, whereas in Britian all hospitals surveyed used CPT (Jenkins and Soutar, 1986).

Strohl et al. (1984) reported on the effects of bilateral phrenic nerve pacing in a C_2 quadriplegic. The results are summarized in Figure 1.9. Both upper and lower rib cage showed paradoxical motion during paced breaths in the supine and 85° upright position. Abdominal compression decreased supine tidal volume 10–20%, whereas in the upright posture it increased tidal volume 200%. Abdominal compression changed only the movement of the lower ribs. These observations suggested that the diaphragm can move the lower ribs independently of the upper ribs. Tidal volume during diaphragmatic pacing is determined both by the resting length and diaphragm load. Lisboa et al. (1986) showed that unilateral diaphragm paralysis resulted in use of intercostal and accessory inspiratory muscle or compensatory use of abdominal expiratory muscles. Vital capacity was reduced in all cases of unilateral diaphragmatic paralysis. There is a decrease in inspiratory muscle efficiency that may contribute to regional V/Q mismatch, diminished lung volumes, and decreased endurance during inspiratory resistive loading at lung volumes higher than FRC (such as occur in emphysema). The mechanisms for the increase in O_2 cost of breathing that results include changes in mechanical coupling, the pattern of re-

cruitment of respiratory muscles, or the intrinsic properties of the inspiratory muscles at shorter length (Collett and Engel, 1986).

High-frequency ventilation produces positive airway pressure and changes transpulmonary pressures like PEEP. George et al. (1985) found that high-frequency oscillation (HFO) at 8–12 Hz by means of a bass loudspeaker applied through a mouthpiece in seven normal subjects increased clearance of radioisotope compared to a control group with no HFO. HFO may alter the viscoelastic properties of the mucus either by increased vagal discharge or an effect on the cross-linking altering mucociliary coupling and viscoelasticity. Further studies are clearly required to confirm these findings and examine the effects on patients with excessive sputum production and purulent sputum because there is conflicting evidence of the benefits of HFO on mucus clearance. Purulent sputum contains copious white blood cells, bacteria, and their products. Neutrophil elastase and bacterial products damage human ciliated epithelium and reduce ciliary beat frequency in vitro (Wilson et al., 1985, 1986).

Ricksten et al. (1986) studied 43 consecutively randomized patients who had elective upper abdominal surgery. They compared CPAP, PEP, and a control group using a deep breathing device (Triflo). One of the three therapies was administered for 30 consecutive breaths every waking hour for 3 days postopera-

Figure 1.9. Upper and lower rib cage motion and tidal volume are shown during a postural shift from full recumbency to 85° upright posture and subsequent application of abdominal compression. The diaphragm is paced by phrenic nerve stimulation. (From Strohl KP, Mead JM, Banzett RB, Lehr J, Loring SH, O'Cain CF: Effect of posture on upper and lower rib cage motion and tidal volume during diaphragm pacing. *Am Rev Respir Dis* *130*:320–321, 1984.)

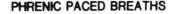
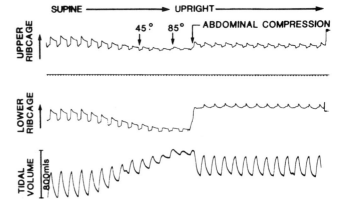

PHRENIC PACED BREATHS

tively. Postoperative pain was controlled using lumbar epidural morphine for at least 2 days postoperatively. Pulmonary function tests and chest x-ray were measured regularly before and after surgery. Alveolar arterial PO_2 difference increased in all groups but was significantly lower in the PEP group after 2 days and after 3 days with CPAP and PEP compared to control. Peak expiratory flow was not different, but FRC was higher in the PEP and CPAP groups by the third day after surgery. Atelectasis occurred in 6 of 15 control patients, no PEP, and 1 of 13 CPAP patients. Ricksten et al. concluded that the simple PEP mask was equally effective as the CPAP system in preservation of lung volumes and prevention of atelectasis after upper abdominal surgery.

Hofmeyer et al. (1986) compared three treatment regimens for assisting clearance of secretions in patients with cystic fibrosis to determine if PEP with or without postural drainage increased sputum yield. Postural drainage without PEP produced more sputum than PEP and postural drainage. Both the postural drainage regimens produced more sputum

than PEP therapy in the sitting position. Sputum clearance was less effective when PEP was included in the treatment regimen.

Albert et al. (1987) examined the effects of the prone position in oleic acid-induced acute lung injury in dogs. The prone position produced an immediate and persistent increase in PaO_2 and decrease in $\dot{Q}_s/\dot{Q}_t$, which was reversed on turning the animals supine (Fig. 1.10). The improvement in gas exchange was not related to changes in FRC, regional diaphragmatic motion, cardiac output, or pulmonary vascular pressures. The authors were unable to explain the mechanism. The prone position is also beneficial in improving oxygenation in patients with acute respiratory failure (Douglas et al., 1977). Jones et al. (1986), however, using two gases of markedly different diffusivities in nine normal subjects, found that the effect of posture on gas mixing represents a convective and diffusive-dependent change in the distribution of ventilation. The effect of posture was not solely due to lung volume changes. However, this report and the two previously published human studies suggest that pa-

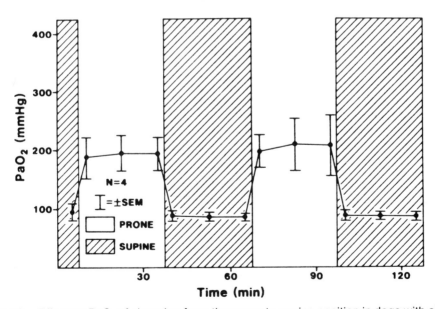

Figure 1.10. Effect on PaO_2 of changing from the prone to supine position in dogs with oleic acid-induced acute lung injury. Animals were kept prone for 15–45 min after oleic acid injection before the first measurement. (From Albert RK, Leasa D, Sanderson M, Robertson HT, Hlastala MP: The prone position improves arterial oxygenation and reduces shunt in oleic-acid-induced acute lung injury. *Am Rev Respir Dis 135*:628–633, 1987.)

tient positioning should be used as a means of reducing the requirements for oxygen and PEEP during mechanical ventilation. The prone position is the postural drainage postion for drainage of the superior segments of the lower lobes. Quadriplegic patients nursed on Stryker frames may spend considerable time prone. The lack of information provided about positioning of patients during chest physiotherapy, in many publications, makes interpretation of pulmonary function changes due to the therapy alone difficult.

Use of Bronchoscopy

Perruchoud et al. (1980) found that bronchoscopic lavage and aspiration with saline and acetylcysteine, followed by positive pressure inflation of the atelectatic lung through the bronchoscope, was successful in reexpanding atelectasis in 37 of 51 patients. Rigid bronchoscopy was used in the 11 spontaneously breathing patients and fiberoptic bronchoscopy in the 40 mechanically ventilated patients. Eleven patients had partial reexpansion of the atelectasis and three showed no change. Atelectasis recurred in three patients on the first day and five on the second, and seven patients developed pneumonia. Lobar atelectasis was more successfully cleared (85%) than segmental atelectasis (47%) using these techniques. Segmental atelectasis also occurred more frequently. All the patients described had recent radiological evidence of mucoid impaction. Some of the patients were apparently given physiotherapy, but no information is provided about the success rate of reexpansion with physiotherapy alone. Bronchoscopy may be indicated if chest physiotherapy fails to reexpand an atelectasis.

Bronchoscopy may be more efficacious in the nonintubated patient with atelectasis than in the intubated patient (Friedman, 1982). There are a few indications for fiberoptic bronchoscopy after an initial aggressive regimen of respiratory therapy. Bronschoscopy may be necessary when a symptomatic patient is unable to tolerate vigorous respiratory therapy, an important diagnostic question coexists, massive collapse is unrespon-

sive to respiratory therapy, or when patients do not show improvement after 24 hr of respiratory therapy (Marini et al., 1982). Selective positive pressure ventilation through the suction port of a cuffed fiberoptic bronchoscope was found effective in the expansion of refractory atelectasis (Harada et al., 1983). Fourteen of 15 patients wre successfully managed; however, in six patients atelectasis recurred.

Bronchoscopy produces marked hemodynamic changes when performed under topical anesthesia. Lundgren et al. (1982) found mean arterial pressure increased by 30%, heart rate by 43%, cardiac index by 28%, and pulmonary wedge pressure by 86% compared to prebronchoscopic control values in 10 patients. The patients were premedicated with morphine and scopolamine and the pharynx, larynx, trachea, and bronchi were anesthetized with 250 mg of lidocaine. Flexible fiberoptic bronchoscopy was performed without supplemental oxygen and PaO_2 decreased significantly from 75 ± 3 mm Hg before bronchoscopy to 67 ± 3 mm Hg during bronchoscopy.

Jaworski et al. (1988) found that fiberoptic bronchoscopy was no better than routine physical therapy in prevention of atelectasis after lobectomy for lung tumor. Twenty postoperative patients were studied. Five of six patients who produced more than 30 ml sputum per day developed atelectasis. One patient who received only physiotherapy required therapeutic bronchoscopy. In the group who received routine bronchoscopy in the postanesthesia recovery room, one patient also required repeated bronchoscopy. There was no difference in ICU or hospital stay or duration of chest tube placement postoperatively. These findings make fiberoptic bronchoscopy undesirable in most critically ill patients. The majority of critically ill ICU patients can tolerate the position changes necessary for chest physiotherapy (see Chapter 3). In our experience (Mackenzie et al., 1980; Mackenzie and Shin, 1986) and others (Friedman, 1982; Marini et al., 1979, 1982) bronchoscopy is only used when atelectasis persists longer than 48 hr or a realistic diagnostic dilemma exists.

Summary of Literature Update Since 1980

The importance of diaphragmatic malfunction as an etiology in development of respiratory complications has been established since 1980. The interaction of the chest wall and abdomen in the relationship that leads to reduced lung volume and atelectasis has not been as well investigated. Pain is now considered less of a causative factor in the postoperative fall in FRC than was thought before 1980. Certainly epidural and intrathecal opiates have revolutionized pain relief after surgery so that in many studies this is no longer a confounding variable (Ricksten et al.). However, epidural and intrathecal opiates have not reduced the incidence of postoperative respiratory complications or resulted in improved diaphragm function. Epidural bupivacaine does improve diaphragmatic function after upper abdominal surgery (Mankikian et al., 1988) but as yet has not been shown to reduce respiratory complications.

A major confusion that has developed since 1980 is in the effects of posture on gas exchange in patients with unilateral lung disease. Prone positioning, dependent positioning of the good lung, and the effects of chest wall compliance are factors that may improve gas exchange irrespective of the therapeutic modality under study. The effects of increases in transpulmonary pressures on lung and cardiac function are numerous. The data are confusing in many of the reported studies that employ small numbers of patients. It seems physiologically unlikely that PEP is greatly different from CPAP or PEEP if they are all applied intermittently. None of these means of increasing transpulmonary pressure may be different from deep breathing. As shown so dramatically by Driks et al., PEEP may reduce atelectasis but increase VA/Q mismatch. The mechanics of what occurs during surgery requires more investigation to find the causes of loss of lung volume and impaired diaphragmatic function after surgery. All the relatively noninvasive techniques for removal of secretions are generally preferred over bronchoscopy, which produces major cardiorespiratory disturbance in the critically ill patient and requires physician participation. Bronchoscopy is more costly and no more effective than chest physiotherapy maneuvers for secretion removal.

WHAT IS CHEST PHYSIOTHERAPY?

Encompassed in the use of the term chest physiotherapy are five maneuvers: (1)postural drainage, (2) chest wall percussion and vibration, (3) coughing, (4) suctioning, and (5) breathing exercises in the spontaneously breathing patient. Breathing exercises include the forced expiration technique or huffing, diaphragmatic costal excursion, and lateral costal excursion exercises. In addition, patient mobilization is used whenever possible. These maneuvers are discussed in detail in subsequent chapters. Postural drainage, manual percussion, and chest vibration are applied until specific endpoints indicate therapy should cease. The end-points include increased air entry, reduced adventitial breath sounds, increased lung/thorax compliance, cessation of sputum production, or patient intolerance. Duration of therapy may, therefore, vary from 15 to 90 min and reflects the extent of pulmonary dysfunction. Chest physiotherapy, including instructions on turning, frequency of application, methods of performance, things to avoid, and evaluation of effectiveness, is described in abbreviated form in Appendix III.

WHAT ARE THE OBJECTIVES OF CHEST PHYSIOTHERAPY

The objectives of chest physiotherapy include clearance of secretions from large and small airways and reexpansion of nonventilated lung. The goal of chest physiotherapy is to obtain this favorable outcome equally or more effectively than bronchoscopy without the invasiveness, trauma, risk of hypoxemia, complications, physician involvement, and cost that bronchoscopy requires (Mackenzie and Shin, 1986). A further objective of chest physiotherapy is to specifically improve ventilation to areas of local lung obstruction. In this respect it differs from blow bottles, incentive spirometry, bronchodilators, mucolytic agents, IPPB, pressure support, or application of positive pressure (CPAP) that are applied to both lungs indiscriminately. Chest physiotherapy aims to alter local lung expansion and is physically directed at the local lesion. Postural drainage places the local lesion in the ideal position for gravity to promote drainage of secretions. Percussion and vibration over the skin surface area of the local lesion assist postural drainage and are also directed at the lung with the local lesion. In addition, one of the objects of chest physiotherapy is to produce benefit when infiltrates are generalized.

If the objectives of the chest physiotherapy are achieved, an increase in local lung expansion should occur and a parallel increase in perfusion to the affected area would result. If secretions are cleared from larger airways, airway resistance and flow obstruction should decrease. Clearance of secretions and improved ventilation of small airways should increase lung compliance. If clearance of secretions from both large and small airways occurs, it is reasonable to assume that the work of breathing and oxygen consumption should decrease, and gas exchange improve. Furthermore, if these objectives are achieved, the incidence of postoperative respiratory infection, morbidity, and hospital stay for those with acute and chronic lung diseases should be reduced. The mechanisms by which chest physiotherapy attempts to achieve these objectives are discussed in Chapter 7, pp. 237–242.

CHEST PHYSIOTHERAPY ORGANIZATION

The number of patients treated with chest physiotherapy at our institution has risen annually. The statistics for the types and numbers of patients treated with chest physiotherapy appear in Appendix I. The patient population is summarized in Appendix I. There are 16 full-time physical therapists who provide not only chest, but also rehabilitation care. The physical therapists train the nurses by means of in-service tutorials. Audiovisual aids assist in this process (Mackenzie et al., 1978). The nursing staff, therefore, supplements chest physiotherapy treatments on evening and night shifts. Nurses can also help by providing a backup when the case load becomes too great for the number of physical therapists.

The essence of application of chest physiotherapy to these patients with acute lung problems lies in a cooperative approach that includes the critical care physician, radiologist, physical therapist, and nurse. Patients receive a daily portable anteroposterior chest x-ray that is reviewed in the morning critical care conference by the radiologist, following the patient case presentation. At least one physical therapist attends the daily morning rounds. An attempt is made by the radiologist to identify not just lobar involvement but, more particularly, segments within a lobe. This approach, even with potential sources of error, has a relatively high success rate (Ayella, 1978).

The chest physical therapist, therefore, approaches the patient with knowledge of the early morning chest x-ray and a verbal report that enables the patient to be positioned with the affected segment uppermost. After chest physiotherapy, a follow-up chest x-ray is requested on a patient with a complete lobar atelectasis. Treatment is given until clinical signs of improvement are noted and as long as sputum is obtained. Details of the exact procedures and the outcome are discussed in later chapters and are summarized in Appendix III.

RESPIRATORY MANAGEMENT

Physiotherapy should not be considered in isolation from overall respiratory care management. All the data in mechanically ventilated patients presented in this book before October 1978 refer to ventilation that was completely controlled by means of a time-cycled volume-preset mechanical ventilator, the Engström 300. Since 1978, intermittent mandatory ventilation, high-frequency ventilation, CPAP, pressure support ventilation, independent lung ventilation, continuous flow ventilation, and combinations of high-frequency and continuous flow ventilation and conventional positive pressure ventilation were used.

Indications for Intubation, Ventilation, Weaning, and PEEP

To prevent unnecessary complications, minimize confusion resulting from different techniques and ideas used by other training centers, and aid in collection of meaningful data, respiratory care may be standardized. The following suggestions for respiratory care are, therefore, dogmatic and certainly are not necessarily applicable in all situations.

Intubation

The indications for intubation include

1. Airway obstruction that cannot be simply relieved
2. PaO_2 of less than 80 mm Hg on supplemental O_2 or of less than 60 mm Hg on room air
3. Patient in shock with a systolic blood pressure of less than 80 mm Hg
4. Severe head injury or unconsciousness
5. Anticipated surgery.

In an emergency patients are preoxygenated, and cricoid pressure (Sellick, 1961) is applied to prevent regurgitation of gastric contents during rapid sequence intubation, with thiopental (when indicated) and succinylcholine. Intubation is initially carried out by the orotracheal route.

If the patients are incapable of protecting their own airway due to unconsciousness, incompetent laryngeal reflexes, or upper airway obstruction, then, after about 10–14 days a tracheostomy is usually performed, and a cuffed tracheostomy tube is placed. Patients with severe head injury and spasticity may have a tracheostomy much earlier, within 1–3 days of ICU admission. Since tracheal tubes promote secretion production and reduce the effectiveness of coughing, extubation is carried out once the tube is no longer indicated to protect the airway, and the patient meets weaning criteria. Therefore, patients would not normally breathe spontaneously for prolonged periods through orotracheal or nasotracheal tubes; instead, a tracheostomy is performed or the patient is extubated. Similarly when airway protection and me-chanical ventilation are no longer required in a patient with a tracheostomy, the patient is extubated. Use of fenestrated tracheostomy tubes and progressive reduction in tracheostomy tube size needlessly prolong tracheal intubation and efforts to decannulate. Both the fenestrated and small tracheostomy tube increase airway resistance and the work of breathing and decrease cough effectiveness and secretion clearance (Criner et al., 1987).

Mechanical Ventilation

Mechanical ventilation is used during tracheal intubation unless the patient is about to be extubated or spontaneous respiration with PEEP is employed. For completely controlled mechanical ventilation minute ventilation of the ventilator is adjusted to satisfy respiratory drive, so that the patient is kept in phase. This commonly means hyperventilation to a $PaCO_2$ of 30–35 mm Hg. Ventilation is most frequently kept at a rate of 12–20 breaths/min, and a tidal volume in the range of 10–15 ml/kg is used. Many centers use a high tidal volume and low respiratory rate (Bendixen et al., 1963). The patient with a head injury is routinely hyperventilated to a $PaCO_2$ of 25–30 mm Hg as one part of the therapeutic maneuvers to reduce intracranial pressure. Other maneuvers for this purpose may include steroids, diuretics, barbiturates, and monitoring of intracranial pressure.

If the patient is out of phase with the ventilator, pneumothorax, inadequate minute ventilation, retained secretions and inadequate sedation should be considered, investigated, and if present, corrected. Narcotics and benzodiazepines or both are used for sedation and pain relief. Muscle relaxants, such as vecuronium or pancuronium, are used only if the cause of asynchrony cannot be found and corrected. The two groups of patients in whom muscle relaxants are used most frequently are decorticate or decerebrate patients with head injury and those who develop generalized sepsis. Patients with severe head injury and elevated intracranial pressure may also receive high doses of barbiturates.

Weaning from Mechanical Ventilation

The weaning criteria that are used include

1. Partial pressure of arterial oxygen/fractional inspired oxygen (PaO_2/FIO_2) greater than 250
2. V_d/V_t less than 0.55 (by nomogram or direct measurement)
3. Maximum inspiratory force greater than -20 cm H_2O
4. Vital capacity 15 ml/kg body weight or greater than 1000 ml
5. Total lung/thorax compliance greater than 30 ml/cm H_2O
6. No muscular fatigue, neurological or nutritional indication for continued mechanical ventilation.

If all the weaning criteria are met, the patient may be placed on a T-piece or tracheostomy collar. A T-piece is normally used when the patient has an orotracheal or nasotracheal tube. Arterial blood gases are measured after 30 min and 1 hr of spontaneous breathing. If the patients maintain adequate arterial blood gases, extubation is indicated. Gradual weaning is not used. As an alternative to the T-piece, gradually decreasing rates of IMV, CPAP, and pressure support may be employed. This approach considerably increases the duration of weaning but has many advocates.

The indications for reinstitution of mechanical ventilation include

1. Fall in PaO_2 below 60 mm Hg when breathing 10 liters/min of 40% O_2 by an aerosol humidifier
2. Increase in $PaCO_2$ of 10 mm Hg/hr, or 5 mm Hg/hr for 3 consecutive hours
3. Respiratory rate consistently exceeding 50/min
4. Sudden deterioration of consciousness.

PEEP

PEEP may be applied if PaO_2/FIO_2 is less than 200. However, there are many critical care physicians who advocate use of PEEP of at least 5 cm H_2O in all mechanically ventilated patients. Initially, 5 cm H_2O is applied, and arterial blood gas analysis is repeated after about 15 min. If

PaO_2/FIO_2 is still not in excess of 200, chest physiotherapy may be indicated if there is retention of lung secretions. If, following chest physiotherapy, the ratio is still not in excess of 200, further increments of PEEP are added to a maximum of 10 cm H_2O. If, with 10 cm H_2O, PEEP, and chest physiotherapy, the PaO_2/FIO_2 is still not greater than 200, a Swan-Ganz flow-directed, thermistor-tipped, pulmonary artery catheter is inserted. Further increases of PEEP above 10 cm H_2O may be detrimental to cardiorespiratory function and should be monitored with arterial, mixed venous gas, and cardiac output determinations.

Normally PaO_2 is maintained at about 100 mm Hg by adjustment of FIO_2 and PEEP. FIO_2 is not normally increased above 0.6. Exceptions may occur with carbon monoxide poisoning, chest physiotherapy in an extremely unstable patient, hyperbaric oxygen therapy, and diffusion problems in the lung.

Alternative Modes of Mechanical Ventilation

Intermittent Mandatory Mechanical Ventilation

Intermittent mandatory ventilation (IMV) was introduced in 1973 by Downs et al. Compared to conventional intermittent positive pressure ventilation, the essential difference is provision of a parallel inspiratory gas circuit that allows the patient to breathe spontaneously between mechanical breaths. The advantages and disadvantages of intermittent mandatory ventilation are summarized by Benzer (1982) and Willatts (1985a,b). The advantages claimed for IMV include reduced sedation requirements, spontaneous breathing that may prevent respiratory muscle atrophy, improved autoregulation of acid–base balance, reduced mean intrathoracic pressure, reduced risk of barotrauma, and an improvement in renal excretory function. The claimed benefits of earlier weaning are not substantiated by clinical trials (Weisman et al., 1983). Modification of simple IMV circuits is necessary to reduce the work of breathing and respiratory muscle fatigue.

Airway pressures during IMV may be equally high as with conventional mechanical ventilation.

High-Frequency Ventilation. High-frequency ventilation (HFV) utilizing low tracheal pressures can maintain gas exchange while reducing the effects of pressure on the lung and circulation. HFV is indicated in bronchopleural fistula and necrotizing pneumonia. HFV may be beneficial in respiratory failure unresponsive to conventional techniques, although there is little agreement in the literature on benefits of HFV compared to conventional mechanical ventilation. High frequency jet ventilation at 60–300 breaths/min (bpm) produces gas exchange by modifications in gas mixing and streaming. Air trapping occurs at higher frequencies. High-frequency oscillation has the advantage of an active expiratory phase that prevents gas trapping and allows frequencies of 1000–3000 bpm to be achieved using small tidal volumes. It may be clinically valuable to combine HFV with conventional mechanical ventilation (Nunn, 1987).

Differential Lung Ventilation (DLV). In circumstances where disease or surgery result in pathological changes in one lung not found in the other, DLV may be beneficial. Use of two synchronized ventilators enables ventilation and PEEP to be adjusted independently. A double-lumen cuffed tube is used to separate ventilation to the right and left lung. DLV has limited long-term use because double-lumen tubes are large and traumatize the larynx, trachea, and particularly the mainstem bronchi.

Continuous Flow Ventilation (CFV)

Apneic oxygenation (AO) and tracheal insufflation of oxygen (TRIO) were described by Hirsch (1905) and Meltzer and Auer (1909). More recently Lenhert et al. (1982) described a technique of endobronchial insufflation (EI) of flows of 1 liter/kg/min. AO, TRIO, and EI are all CFV techniques and they produce gas exchange without any chest movements. EI differs from the others in producing normal oxygenation and CO_2 excretion for up to 5 hr with room air insufflation. Both AO and TRIO require O_2 and do not excrete adequate amounts of CO_2 for prolonged use without development of respiratory acidosis. CFV techniques may be used as adjuncts to conventional and DLV techniques. The main clinical use of CFV occurs during extracorporeal membrane CO_2 removal. CFV may be a useful adjunct to augment oxygenation (Gattinoni et al., 1980).

Inverse Ratio Ventilation

This technique aims to increase the relative duration of inspiration but may cause gas trapping and elevated intrathoracic pressure. Depending on the respiratory pathology, reversal of the normal I:E ratio of 1:2 to 3:1 may decrease intrapulmonary shunt, dead space, and $PaCO_2$ (Perez-Chada et al., 1983). If decreased lung compliance occurs with normal airway resistance, time constants for inspiration are reduced. In those patients, prolongation of inspiration by inverse ratio ventilation may improve gas exchange by increasing the time that otherwise closed alveoli are held open (Willatts, 1985b).

Exclusions in Respiratory Care

No assist modes or sigh mechanisms were used during mechanical ventilation of any of the patients treated at our institution. No IPPB machines were used for delivery of bronchodilators or mucolytic agents to assist secretion clearance and no inhaled drugs, other than water vapor, were used in any of the patients treated before 1980. All patients received humidification from the moment of intubation, through anesthesia, and during any subsequent mechanical ventilation. No spontaneously breathing patients were treated with blow bottles. Tracheal lavage was rarely part of routine patient care.

Secretions were removed in intubated patients by means of postural drainage, percussion, vibration or shaking therapy, and tracheal suctioning. Mobilization was encouraged in all patients, and coughing, in those who were spontaneously breathing. Lung hyperinflation or "bagging" was not employed when chest physiotherapy was given to mechanically ventilated patients. Breathing exercises were used in spontaneously breathing patients. Rarely was bronchoscopy used. Chest physiotherapy replaced bronchoscopy as the first treatment of choice for removal of retained secretions at our institution in 1974. The number of therapeutic bronchoscopies between 1972 and 1979 is shown in Table 1.2. Bronchoscopy is not used when an air bronchogram is visible on chest x-ray to peripheral lung. Bronchoscopy is employed for therapeutic effect when 24 hr of chest physiotherapy has failed to reexpand atelectatic lung and a diagnostic dilemma exists. Details of procedures followed in application of chest physiotherapy are discussed in subsequent chapters and summarized in Appendix III.

MISCONCEPTIONS ABOUT EFFECTS OF CHEST PHYSIOTHERAPY

Misconceptions exist about the use of chest physiotherapy in patients with acute lung pathology. Many reports in the literature discuss the use of chest physiotherapy in patients with chronic lung diseases, such as bronchiectasis, cystic fibrosis, or bronchitis. These patients may not be hospitalized and often receive treatment at a clinic or on an outpatient basis. They have chronically abnormal lungs. Therefore, it may not be justified to extrapolate what occurs following chest physiotherapy in these patients to those who have acute lung disease in otherwise normal lungs.

The patient population studied also influences the likely outcome of maneuvers designed to remove retained lung secretions. For example, the response following chest physiotherapy of a patient with atelectasis secondary to pain from a stab wound in the chest is more likely to be favorable than is the response to chest physiotherapy of a patient with adult respiratory distress syndrome and multisystem blunt trauma. When comparisons are made between two forms of therapy designed to remove secretions from the tracheobronchial tree, a single use of the therapy should be compared on similar patient populations with similar lung pathology. Confounding variables such as differences in position during therapy may produce changes in oxygenation that are unrelated to the therapy. Apples must not be compared to oranges. When chest physiotherapy is compared to any other therapy, both therapies must be performed on a similar patient population. This is not always done. Therefore, confusion may exist concerning effectiveness of the therapy in improving the patient. This, of course, brings up a most important point. What is meant by improvement?

There is difficulty in adequately quantitating the effectiveness of chest physiotherapy. Subjective claims that the patient feels better, that clinical signs

Table 1.2
The Number of Patients Receiving Therapeutic Bronchoscopy for Retention of Lung Secretions for 1972–1980 Is Compared to the Total Number of Admissions[a]

Year	Total Admissions	Number of Bronchoscopies	Number of Patients Requiring Bronchoscopy	Comments
1972	615	31	19	One patient had 7 Six patients had 2
1973	982	21	17	Four patients had 2
1974	872	7	7	
1975	920	9	9	
1976	1,105	14	12	Two patients had 2
1977	1,023	9	7	Two patients had 2
1978	1,053	8	6	Two patients had 2
1979	1,249	18	14	One patient had 3 Two patients had 2

[a]The data for 1972–1975 were kindly supplied by J. Hankins, M.D., Thoracic Surgical Consultant to MIEMSS.

improve, or that the chest x-ray appearance is more favorable are very difficult to interpret. Objective evidence is sparse, and it was agreed, in the excellent conferences sponsored by the American Thoracic Society in 1974 (National Heart and Lung Institute) (NHLI) and in the similar conference (National Heart, Lung and Blood Institute) (NHLBI) in 1979 (see pp. 245–248 for summary), that there are very few, adequate, and acceptable ways reported that provide evidence of the effectiveness of chest physiotherapy in chronic lung diseases. Lung function tests would appear to be the best parameter for comparison. However, even they may be prejudiced either by requiring invasive and sophisticated techniques for measurements, such as xenon inhalation, or by the tests themselves altering the parameter that they purport to measure. For example, the maneuver of forced expiration is known to cause small airway closure and may induce bronchospasm in some patients (Nunn et al., 1965). FEV_1 measurement may, therefore, not accurately reflect the effect of chest physiotherapy, as some authors have suggested (Campbell et al.). Another important reason why confusion may exist about the use of chest physiotherapy is the wide range of therapies that are described. Claims that chest vibration did not produce a statistically significant difference in clearance of sputum when compared to coughing alone must be questioned when it is learned that the therapy was performed in the sitting position with a mechanical vibrating pad (Pavia et al.). In our experience, upper lobe secretion retention is uncommon (see Appendix I). Far more frequently, lower lobe collapse is seen, especially left lower lobe collapse. Therefore, the sitting position is inappropriate for drainage of lower lobe secretions. If chest vibration was performed by a physiotherapist, with the patient in the appropriate postural drainage position, until there was clinical evidence of secretion clearance, the outcome may be different.

In other reports, "chest physiotherapy" includes suctioning but no percussion, manual vibration or postural drainage (Fox et al., 1978). Some physiotherapy techniques include bagging (where the lungs are hyperinflated), and vibration or chest shaking is applied during expiration (Gormezano and Branthwaite, 1972a). The duration of therapy also shows an amazingly wide variation. This reasonably may be expected to produce different results. In some centers, therapy lasts only a few minutes (Hedstrand et al.). In other centers, it may be applied for 7–20 min (Gormezano and Branthwaite, 1972a), or in others the therapy is restricted to a predetermined duration of 10–15 min (Newton and Bevans, 1978). Some reports also include the administration of nebulized solutions by IPPB as part of chest physiotherapy (Graham and Bradley, 1978). Therefore, a reported 20 min of chest physiotherapy may actually consist of 15 min of IPPB and only a short period of postural drainage percussion and coughing. All these variables must be appreciated before drawing conclusions from the literature.

It seems reasonable to assume that unless sputum is produced by chest physiotherapy, the treatment is not likely to be beneficial. It is, however, doubtful that the more sputum produced, the greater the benefit. Sputum removal may cause a fall in PaO_2 and an increase in intrapulmonary shunt because of alteration in ventilation perfusion relationships. This was suggested as the probable cause for the falls in PaO_2 noted by Gormezano and Branthwaite (1972b) following chest physiotherapy in chronic lung disease patients. Partial reexpansion of a lobar atelectasis may reverse the vascular compensating mechanisms that previously reduced intrapulmonary shunt.

Most clinicians agree with Murray that sputum production is essential if chest physiotherapy is to be effective for the treatment of chronic lung disease. However, the removal of 30 ml, that he states as the minimum necessary to produce benefit, is excessive in the patient with normal lungs and acute secretion retention. If sputum is removed from the smallest airways, less should produce beneficial effects (see p. 220).

Sputum volume measurement is notoriously unreliable (Bateman et al.). The expectorated measurement has considerable sources of error, as the patient can swallow sputum, so reducing the volume collected, and equally, the patient can add saliva apparently increasing the quantity. The effectiveness of humidification and patient hydration may also affect sputum volume. Except for our data presented in Chapter 7, few studies measure volume of sputum production in tracheally intubated patients. The cuffed tracheal tube removes two of the major sources of error in sputum collection mentioned above. Volume of sputum may not be the primary consideration for assessing chest physiotherapy effectiveness for the ICU patient. In our experience treating acute lung pathology, there is little relationship between the volume of sputum produced in excess of 5 ml and the benefits in terms of improved physiological parameters. In acute processes, as in chronic lung disease, different lung problems produce different volumes and types of sputum. The lung contusion produces mostly blood, not sputum, yet chest physiotherapy may improve ventilation/perfusion relationships (Mackenzie and Shin, 1979a). Lobar and segmental atelectasis may clear when only a small volume of sputum is removed, yet dramatic improvement in intrapulmonary shunt and total lung/thorax compliance may occur on reexpansion. In patients with established pneumonia, little improvement may be apparent whether a large or a negligible amount of sputum is produced. The long-term benefits of removal of retained sputum are unknown. It is thought that it does not alter the course of chronic lung diseases (NHLI, 1974), but in acute lung diseases, especially in an ICU environment, it seems likely that it would reduce the incidence of respiratory tract infection and, therefore, morbidity (and possibily mortality). Areas of dispute concerning the components, alternatives and disease processes treated by chest physiotherapy are summarized in Table 1.3. This table also provides our opinion on some controversial points.

SUMMARY

Objective studies of chest physiotherapy are few and the techniques employed are not standardized or adequately described. The patient population studied are variable, sometimes inappropriately excluding those patients likely to or including those least likely to benefit.

Chest physiotherapy is used frequently in pediatric ICUs, surgical ICUs for respiratory problems occurring after surgery, and for treatment of chronic lung disease. In the acute setting, physiotherapy appears equally as good as bronchoscopy for reexpansion of atelectasis. For patients with chronic lung disease it seems effective when production of secretions is great.

Some common misconceptions about chest physiotherapy that occur because of the lack of standardization were emphasized. Chest physiotherapy techniques were briefly described.

Controlled mechanical ventilation was considered the treatment of choice for the acute management of the severely injured and pathological lung. Removal from mechanical ventilatory support does not need to be gradual in patients recovering from acute lung pathology. Changes in lung/thorax compliance were thought to be a good indicator of the benefits and end point of chest physiotherapy.

Assist modes of ventilation, sighs and hyperinflation, bronchodilator and mucolytic agent inhalations, and use of blow bottles and incentive spirometers have clouded the interpretation of the results of chest physiotherapy. Therapeutic bronchoscopy is rarely required for sputum removal when chest physiotherapy is employed. It is clear from the literature since 1980 that posoperative pain is not the major factor in development of respiratory complications. Diaphragmatic dysfunction after upper abdominal surgery appears to be an important etiology for respiratory complications that is reversed by epidural bupivacaine but not by spinal or epidural opiates. Despite a multitude of mechanical aids to lung expansion such as PEEP, CPAP, PEP, pressure support, and inverse ratio ventilation none is convincingly superior to chest physiotherapy, deep breathing, and position changes in prevention of respiratory complications in the ICU. For mechanically ventilated patients, the recently described techniques to improve

Table 1.3
Conflicting Data and Points of Contention Concerning Chest Physiotherapy

Component	For	Against	Authors Opinion and Practice
Percussion and vibration	Assists secretion clearance[1-3]	May not add to the effect of cough and suction[4,5]	Assists secretion clearance; mode of action postulated in Chapter 4 and on p. 240–242
Postural drainage (PD)	Peripheral clearance of secretions is enhanced with PD.[6] Significantly more sputum is produced with PD and the forced expiratory technique.[7] PD without positive expiratory pressure (PEP) produced more sputum than PEP therapy in the sitting position.[8] The addition of PD and coughing improves mucociliary clearance[9]	Both cough and exercise are superior to PD at clearance of secretions.[10] Sputum production is reduced with CPT including PD compared to FET or PEP without PD.[11] PD is no better than cough alone[12,13]	Identification of the involved lung segment is essential to determine which of 11 different positions is correct for gravity assisted segmental drainage.[14] PD has an additive effect to percussion, vibration, coughing, and FET. PD improves central airway clearance when cough is impaired
Cough	CPT does not add benefits to cough alone.[12] Both clear central and peripheral airways[6]	CPT but not cough produces peripheral clearance of secretions.[6] Cough effects are limited to the central airways, proximal to the fifth generation.[15] Repetitive coughing may cause fatigue[16] and bronchospasm[17]	It is inappropriate to separate cough from other CPT techniques. Cough occurs spontaneously and concurrently when secretions are loosened or suctioned. Cough is important for removal of secretions advanced to the central airways. Protracted coughing should be avoided
Forced expiratory technique (FET) and PEP	FET is more effective than cough alone. FET with PD produced more sputum than CPT.[6] PEP prevents atelectasis after upper abdominal surgery.[18] FET is better tolerated than CPT[19]	Sputum clearance was less effective when PEP is included in treatment. PEP clears less secretions than PD alone[8]	FET is not shown to improve mucus clearance in peripheral airways. May be helpful to clear central airways. Physiological basis unknown.[19] PEP produces only short-lived benefits

Table 1.3
Conflicting Data and Points of Contention Concerning Chest Physiotherapy—Continued

Component	For	Against	Authors Opinion and Practice
Component			
Tracheal suctioning in nonintubated patients	Is safe since it is widely used and advocated	Is dangerous and may cause cardiac dysrhythmia[20] or arrest[21]; it may stimulate vomiting and cause aspiration (p. 179–180)	It is dangerous; if the patient cannot cough up secretions by using other techniques to stimulate cough, tracheal intubation with a cuffed tube is required
Mechanical chest vibrators/percussors	Manufacturers claim that they provide percussive directional stroking for postural drainage.[22] Hand clapping frequency of up to 8 Hz is too low for sputum clearance[23]	Manufacturers claims not substantiated in clinical practice.[24] Percussion frequencies of 3–17 Hz is adequate for secretion clearance.[26]	No mechanical devices used; hands on care provides better, safer, more adaptable, and cheaper therapy. Manual techniques can be varied to suit patient tolerance
Sputum volume	If less than 30 ml is produced, chest physiotherapy should be discontinued[26]	Sputum measurement is not accurate; importance is not the volume, but where it comes from	Sputum must be obtained, but removal of 5 ml may frequently result in impressive physiological and radiological changes
Short duration of therapy	Widely practiced; it ranges from a few minutes,[27] 7–20 min,[28] or is restricted to predetermined time[29]	Treatment times less than 20 min have not been sufficient to clear atelectasis or produce radiographic or physiological improvement	Treatment may last 1 hr; if there is improvement in lung/thorax compliance and clinical signs, it may be stopped earlier
Adjuncts			
Mucolytic agents	Reduced sputum viscosity, increased pourability, subjective and objective clinical improvement following use[30]	Using radioactive tracer techniques has not been shown to increase sputum clearance[31]	Not used
Bronchodilators	Improvement in arterial O_2 following chest physiotherapy may be more obvious if therapeutic levels of aminophylline are obtained[32]	Not better than placebo when given by IPPB[33]	If patient is a known asthmatic taking regular bronchodilator therapy, drugs by continuous i.v. infusion are appropriate during mechanical ventilation; otherwise, they are not routinely used

Tracheobronchial lavage or instillation	Promotes cough and helps humidify and loosen secretions; lavage volume of up to 200 ml is used with bronchoscopy[34]	No amount of lavage will loosen viscid tenacious sputum from small airways; large volumes may cause deterioration of chest x-ray and accumulate in the lungs[35]	Provided there is adequate systemic and local hydration (humidity), bronchial lavage is not used

Alternatives

Bronchoscopy	Highly successful at clearing atelectasis; performed under visual control; can identify obstruction if present.[36] Selective positive pressure ventilation through suction port may expand refractory atelectasis[37]	Traumatic, expensive, and not more effective at secretion clearance[38]; it cannot reach peripheral airways; fiberoptic bronchoscopy cannot suction large quantities of tenancious secretions[39], needs a physician's participation, causes rises in systemic and pulmonary artery pressure in the critically ill patient[40]	If an atelectasis cannot be cleared after 36 hr of physiotherapy, bronchoscopy is appropriate to exclude other pathology; bronchoscopy is not the first treatment for lobar segmental collapse
Incentive spirometry (IS)	Cheap, prevents atelectasis, and reduces hospital stay compared to IPPB, and patients like it.[41,42] Superior to no treatment at all[43]	Did not increase PaO_2 as significantly as physiotherapy[27] and has not been shown to be better than deep breathing.[44] No benefit compared to specialized respiratory care[45]	Incentive spirometry may be used; mobilization and verbal encouragement to cough are cheaper and probably equally effective
IPPB	IPPB modifies lung compliance[46] and lung mechanics[47]; maximum volume IPPB treats atelectasis[48]	In controlled studies in postoperative patients, IPPB did not reduce the incidence of pulmonary complications[49–51]; it may harm the patient.[52] It does not help patients with quadriplegia[53]	IPPB is not used and is not thought to help clearance of retained secretions; IPPB has no ability to alter local lung expansion; chest physiotherapy increases lung compliance and may alter local lung expansion
CPAP	Increases PaO_2 and reduces radiological density when used with CPT.[54] Increases FRC more rapidly than IS or breathing exercises[55]	No advantage over mobilization.[56] Increases in FRC found with CPAP ceases within 10 min of stopping therapy.[57] PEP mask is equally effective and simpler[18]	CPAP is useful during spontaneous respiration in the intubated patient. Mask CPAP is not practical in the critically ill. CPAP lacks the regional specificity necessary for effective expansion of segmental or lobar collapse

Table 1.3
Conflicting Data and Points of Contention Concerning Chest Physiotherapy—Continued

	For	Against	Authors Opinion and Practice
Transtracheal catheters and minitracheostomy	Lavage fluid instillation precipitates coughing in the otherwise uncooperative patient; this may clear secretions; apparently frequently used in the ICU[58]	May cause death, uncontrollable tracheal hemorrhage, pneumomediastinum, local infection, etc.[59] Catheter may be aspirated[60]	Transtracheal catheters are dangerous. Alternative techniques to stimulate cough and clear secretions are clearly preferable
Disease Processes Treated by Chest Physiotherapy			
Pneumonia	Pneumonia may be aborted by chest physiotherapy preventing retention of secretions. Pneumonia in the ICU is difficult to distinguish from atelectasis or ARDS[61]	Chest physiotherapy and IPPB do not hasten the resolution of pneumonia[29]	The diagnosis of pneumonia in the ICU is very subjective; more recent diagnostic aids are helpful[61–63]; reversal of a pneumonia-like process is possible with chest physiotherapy (see Case History 2.1)
Chronic bronchitis	Subjective improvement in dyspnea and reduced obstruction and increased clearance of sputum after chest physiotherapy	Chest physiotherapy had no effect on acute exacerbations of the disease[64,65]	In the ICU, infection is present; it is, therefore, mandatory that all patients with preexisting chronic sputum producing respiratory disease should obtain prophylactic therapy to reduce the retention of secretions, until the patient is mobilized

Condition			
Cystic fibrosis (CF)	CPT improves mucous clearance and pulmonary function[66,67]	CPT does not clear peripheral secretions in patients with CF.[68,69] Vital capacity decreases[70]	CPT is beneficial. Efficacy may vary when disease is quiescent and active. See Chapters 2–5
Acute atelectasis	Radiological and clinical benefit from CPT.[67,71,72] Oxygenation[27] and lung/thorax compliance[14] increased	No better than encouragement of deep breathing and mobilization.[73] CPT is not effective and causes a fall in PaO_2[74]	
Lung contusion	CPT decreases intrapulmonary shunt[75] and increases lung/thorax compliance[14]	May cause transbronchial aspiration of blood. CPT is contraindicated[76]	See Chapters 2 and 10

1 Bateman et al., 1979.
2 Cochrane et al., 1977.
3 Opie and Spalding, 1958.
4 Murray, 1979b.
5 Mellins, 1974.
6 Bateman et al., 1981.
7 Sutton et al., 1983.
8 Hofmeyer, 1986.
9 Van der Schans et al., 1986
10 Oldenberg et al., 1979.
11 Falk et al., 1984.
12 Rossman et al., 1982.
13 DeBoek and Zinman, 1984.
14 Mackenzie et al., 1980.
15 Smaldone and Smith, 1985.
16 Sutton et al., 1984.
17 Zapletal et al., 1983.
18 Ricksten et al., 1986.
19 Pryor and Webber, 1979.
20 Shim et al., 1969.
21 Welply et al., 1975.
22 General Physiotherapy, 1979.
23 Flower et al., 1979.
24 Pavia et al., 1976.
25 King et al., 1983.
26 Murray, 1979a.
27 Hedstrand et al., 1978.
28 Gormenzano and Branthwaite, 1972a.
29 Graham and Bradley, 1978.
30 Aylward, 1973.
31 Thomson et al., 1975.
32 Menkes and Britt, 1980.
33 Shim et al., 1978.
34 Barrett, 1978.
35 Sackner et al., 1972.
36 Sackner, 1975.
37 Harada et al., 1983.
38 Mackenzie and Shin, 1986.
39 Feldman and Huber, 1976.
40 Lundgren et al., 1982.
41 McConnell et al., 1974.
42 Dohi and Gold, 1978.
43 Celli et al., 1984.
44 Ingram, 1980.
45 Schweiger et al., 1986.
46 Murray, 1980.
47 Sinha and Bergofsky, 1972.
48 O'Donohue, 1979.
49 Sands et al., 1961.
50 Barach and Segal, 1975.
51 Petty, 1974a.
52 Gold, 1976.
53 McCool et al., 1986.
54 Andersen et al., 1986.
55 Stock et al., 1985.
56 Dull and Dull, 1983.
57 Heitz et al., 1983.
58 Matthews and Hopkinson, 1984.
59 Schmerber and Deltenre, 1978.
60 Charnley and Verma, 1986.
61 Faling, 1988.
62 Salata et al., 1987.
63 Johanson et al., 1988a.
64 Newton and Stephenson, 1978.
65 May and Munt, 1979.
66 Tecklin and Holsclaw, 1975.
67 Kirilloff et al., 1985.
68 Weller et al., 1980.
69 Kerrebijn et al., 1982.
70 Zapletal et al., 1983.
71 Hammond and Martin, 1981.
72 Mackenzie et al., 1978.
73 Fairley, 1980.
74 Connors et al., 1980.
75 Mackenzie and Shin, 1979a.
76 Tyler, 1982.

diagnosis, prevention, and management of pneumonia may reduce the incidence and fatality of nosocomial pneumonia. There are many conflicting opinions that confuse the interpretation of the effects of chest physiotherapy. Particularly the different combinations of chest physiotherapy maneuvers used by different investigators creates difficulty in determining efficacy.

References

Albert RK, Leasa D, Sanderson M, Robertson HT, Hlastala MP: The prone position improves arterial oxygenation and reduces shunt in oleic acid-induced acute lung injury. Am Rev Respir Dis 135:628–633, 1987

Andersen JB, Jespersen W: Demonstration of intersegmental respiratory bronchioles in normal human lung. Eur J Respir Dis 61:337–341, 1980

Andersen JB, Qvist J, Kahn T: Recruiting collapsed lung through collateral channels with positive end-expiratory pressure. Scand J of Resp Dis 60:260–266, 1979

Andersen JB, Olesen KP, Eikard B, Jansen E, Qvist J: Periodic continuous positive airway pressure, CPAP, by mask in the treatment of atelectasis. Eur J Respir Dis 61:20–25, 1980

Anthonisen P, Riis P, Sogaard-Andersen T: The value of lung physiotherapy in the treatment of acute exacerbations in chronic bronchitis. Acta Med Scand 175:715–719, 1964

Aubier M, Murciano D, LeCocgnic Y, Viires N, Jacquens Y, Squara P, Parienote R: Effect of hypophosphatemia on diaphragmatic contractility in patients with acute respiratory failure. N Eng J Med 313:420–424, 1985

Ayella RJ: Radiologic Management fo the Massively Traumatized Patient, pp 93–97. Williams & Wilkins , Baltimore, 1978

Bain J, Bishop J, Olinsky A: Evaluation of directed coughing in cystic fibrosis. Br J Dis Chest 82:138–148, 1988

Baran D, Van Bogaert E (eds): Chest Physical Therapy in Cystic Fibrosis and Chronic Obstructive Pulmonary Disease. European Press, Ghent, Belgium, 1977

Bateman JRM, Newman SP, Daunt KM, Pavia D, Clarke SW: Regional lung clearance of excessive bronchial secretions during chest physiotherapy in patients with stable chronic airways obstruction. Lancet 1:294–297, 1979

Bateman JRM, Newman SP, Daniel KM, Sheahan NF, Pavia D, Clarke SW: Is cough as effective as chest physiotherapy in removal of excessive tracheobronchial secretions? Thorax 36:683–687, 1981

Beecher HK, Todd DP: A study of the deaths associated with anesthesia and surgery. Ann Surg 140:2–34, 1954

Belman M, Mittman C: Incentive spirometry. The answer is blowing in the wind. Chest 79:254–255, 1981

Bendixen HH, Hedley-Whyte J, Laver MB: Impaired oxygenation in surgical patients during general anesthesia with controlled ventilation. N Engl J Med 260:991–996, 1963

Benzer H: The value of intermittent mandatory ventilation. Editorial. Intensive Care Med 8:267–268, 1982

Bergman NA: Effects of varying respiratory waveforms on gas exchange. Anesthesiology 28:390–395, 1967

Bone RC: Compliance and dynamic characteristic curves in acute respiratory failure. Crit Care Med 4:173–179, 1976

Brock-Utne JG, Winning TJ, Botha E, Goodwin NM: Chest physiotherapy during mechanical ventilation. Anaesth Intensive Care 3:234–236, 1975

Buscaglia AJ, St. Marie M: Oxygen saturation during chest physiotherapy for acute exacerbation of severe chronic obstructive pulmonary disease. Resp Care 28:1009–1013, 1983

Bushnell GE: The treatment of tuberculosis. Am Rev Tuberc 2:259–275, 1918

Campbell AH, O'Connell JM, Wilson F: The effect of chest physiotherapy upon the FEV$_1$ in chronic bronchitis. Med J Aust 1:33–35, 1975

Canner P, Mossberg B, Philipson K, Strandberg K: Elimination of test particles from the human tracheobronchial tract by voluntary coughing. Scand J Resp Dis 60:52–62, 1979

Carswell F, Robinson DW, Ward CCL, Waterfield MR: Deoxyribonucleic acid output in the sputum from cystic fibrosis patients. Eur J Respir Dis 65:53–57, 1984

Casaburi P, Wasserman K: Exercise training in pulmonary rehabilitation. Editorial. N Eng J Med 314:1509–1511, 1986

Catley DM, Thornton C, Jordan C, Royston D, Lehane JR, Jones JG: Postoperative respiratory depression associated with continuous morphine infusion. Br J Anaesth 54:235, 1982

Celli BR, Rodriguez KS, Snider GL: A controlled trial of intermittent positive pressure breathing, incentive spirometry and deep breathing exercises in preventing pulmonary complications after abdominal surgery. Am Rev Respir Dis 130:12–15, 1984

Celli BR, Rassulo J, Make BJ: Dyssynchronous breathing during arm but not leg exercise in patients with chronic airflow obstruction. N Engl J Med 314:1485–1490, 1986

Cherniack RM: Physical therapy. Am Rev Respir Dis 122(2):25–27, 1980

Ciesla N, Klemic N, Imle PC: Chest physical therapy to the patient with multiple trauma. Two case studies. Phys Ther 61:202–205, 1981

Clarke SW, Cochrane GM, Webber BA: Effects of sputum on pulmonary function (abstract). Thorax 28:262, 1973

Clergue F, Montembault C, Despierre O, Ghesquiere F, Harari A, Viars P: Respiratory effects of intrathecal morphine after upper abdominal surgery. Anesthesiology 61:677–685, 1984

Cochrane GM, Webber BA, Clarke SW: Effects of sputum on pulmonary function. Br Med J 2:1181–1183, 1977

Collett PW, Engel LA: Influence of lung volume on oxygen cost of resistive breathing. J Appl Physiol 61:16–24, 1986

Connors AF, Hammon WE, Martin RJ, Rogers RM: Chest physical therapy: The immediate effect on oxygenation in acutely ill patients. *Chest* 78:559–564, 1980

Craig DB: Postoperative recovery of pulmonary function. *Anesth Analg* 60:46–52, 1981

Crampton Smith A, Spalding JMK, Russell WR: Artificial respiration, by intermittent positive pressure in poliomyelitis and other diseases. *Lancet* 1:939–945, 1954

Craven DE, Kunches LM, Kilinsky V, Lichtenberg DA, Make BJ, McCabe WR: Risk factors for pneumonia and fatality in patients receiving continuous mechanical ventilation. *Am Rev Respir Dis* 133:792–796, 1986

Criner G, Make B, Celli B: Respiratory muscle dysfunction secondary to chronic tracheostomy tube placement. *Chest* 91:139–141, 1987

Dammann JF, McAslan TC: Optimal flow pattern for mechanical ventilation of the lungs: Evaluation with a model lung. *Crit Care Med* 5:128–136, 1977

Darrow G, Anthonisen NR: Physiotherapy in hospitalized medical patients. *Am Rev Respir Dis* 122(2):155–158, 1980

DeBoeck C, Zinman R: Cough versus chest physiotherapy. A comparison of the acute effects on pulmonary function in patients with cystic fibrosis. *Am Rev Respir Dis* 129:182–184, 1984

DeTroyer A: Mechanics of the chest wall during restrictive thoracic strapping. *Respiration* 39:241–250, 1980

Dohi S, Gold MI: Comparison of two methods of postoperative respiratory care. *Chest* 73:592–595, 1978

Douglas WW, Rehder K, Beynen FM, Sessler AD, Marsh HM: Improved oxygenation in patients with acute respiratory failure; the prone position. *Am Rev Respir Dis* 115:559–566, 1977

Downs JB, Klein ER, Desautels D, Modell JH, Kirby RR: Intermittent mandatory ventilation: new approach to weaning patients from mechanical ventilators. *Chest* 64:331–335, 1973

Driks MR, Craven DE, Celli BR, Manning M, Burke RA, Garvin GM, Kunches L, Farber HW, Wedel SA, McCabe WR: Nosocomial pneumonia in intubated patients given Sucralfate as compared with antacids or histamine Type 2 blockers. *N Engl J Med* 317:1376–1382, 1987

Dull JL, Dull WL: Are maximal inspiratory breathing exercises or incentive spirometry better than early mobilization after cardiopulmonary bypass? *Phys Ther* 63:655–659, 1983

Durenil B, Viires N, Cantineau JP, Aubier M, Desmonts JM: Diaphragmatic contractility after upper abdominal surgery. *J Appl Physiol* 61:1775–1780, 1986

Eliasson R, Mossberg B, Camner P, Afzelius BA: The immobile cilia syndrome. A congenital ciliary abnormality as an etiologic factor in chronic airway infections and male sterility. *N Engl J Med* 297:1–6, 1977

Engström Respiratory System ER 300 Instruction Manual VI. LKB Medical, Stockholm, Arne Tryckare, 1974

Enjeti S, O'Neill JT, Terry PB, Menkes HA, Traystman RJ: Effects of positive and expiratory pressure on shunt flow in atelectasis. *Respir Physiol* 48:243–254, 1982

Ewart W: The treatment of bronchiectasis and of chronic bronchial affections by posture and respiratory exercises. *Lancet* 2:70–72, 1901

Fairley HB: Oxygen therapy for surgical patients. *Am Rev Respir Dis* 122(2):37–44, 1980

Faling LJ. Editorial. New advances in diagnosing nosocomial pneumonia in intubated patients. Part 1. *Am Rev Respir Dis* 137:253–255, 1988

Falk M, Kelstrup M, Andersen JB, Kinoshita T, Falk P, Stoving S, Gothgen I: Improving the ketchup bottle method with positive expiratory pressure, PEP, in cystic fibrosis. *Eur J Resp Dis* 65:423–432, 1984

Featherstone H: An inquiry into the causation of postoperative pneumonia. *Br J Surg* 12:482–523, 1924

Feeley TW, Hamilton WK, Xavier B, Moyers J, Egar EI: Sterile anesthesia breathing circuits do not prevent postoperative pulmonary infection. *Anesthesiology* 54:369–372, 1981

Feldman J, Traver GA, Taussig LM: Maximal expiratory flows after postural drainage. *Am Rev Respir Dis* 119:239–245, 1979

Feldman NT, Huber GL: Fiberoptic bronchoscopy in the intensive care unit. *Int Anesthesiol Clin* 14:31–42, 1976

Felson B, Felson F: Localization of lesions by means of the postero-anterior roentgenogram. *Radiology* 55:363–373, 1950

Finer NN, Boyd J: Chest physiotherapy in the neonate. A controlled study. *Pediatrics* 61:282–285, 1978

Finer NN, Grace MG, Boyd J: Chest physiotherapy in the neonate with respiratory distress (abstract 1189). *Pediatr Res* 11:570, 1977

Fletcher R, Larsson A: Gas exchange in the partially atelectatic lung. *Anaesthesia* 40:1186–1188, 1985

Flower KA, Eden RI, Mann NM, Burges J: New mechanical aid to physiotherapy in cystic fibrosis. *Br Med J* II:630–631, 1979

Ford GT, Whitelaw WA, Rosenal TW, Cruse PJ, Guenter CA: Diaphragm function after upper abdominal surgery in humans. *Am Rev Respir Dis* 127:431–436, 1983

Ford GT, Guenter CA: Toward prevention of postoperative pulmonary complications (editorial). *Am Rev Respir Dis* 130:4–5, 1984

Fox WW, Schwartz JG, Shaffer TH: Alterations in neonatal respiratory function following chest physiotherapy (abstract 1192). *Pediatr Res* 11:570, 1977

Fox WW, Schwartz JG, Shaffer TH: Pulmonary physiotherapy in neonates: Physiologic changes and respiratory management. *J Pediatr* 92:977–981, 1978

Friedman SA (letter), Marini JJ, Pierson DJ, Hudson LD (reply): Comparison of fiberoptic bronchoscopy and respiratory therapy. *Am Rev Respir Dis* 126:367–368, 1984

Fuleihan SF, Wilson RS, Pontoppidan H: Effect of mechanical ventilation with end-inspiratory pause on blood gas exchange. *Anesth Analg (Cleve)* 55:122–130, 1976

Garibaldi RA, Britt MR, Coleman ML, Reading JC, Pace NL: Risk factors for postoperative pneumonia. *Am J Med* 70:677–680, 1981

Gaskell DV, Webber BA: *The Brompton Hospital Guide to Chest Physiotherapy* (preface), 2nd ed. Blackwell Scientific Publications, London, 1973

Gattinoni L, Pesenti A, Rossi GP et al: Treatment of acute respiratory failure by low frequency positive pressure ventilation and extracorporeal removal of CO_2. Lancet 2:292–294, 1980

General Physiotherapy: G5 Massage Apparatus. General Physiotherapy, St. Louis, 1979

George RJD, Johnson MA, Pavia D, Agnew JL, Clark SW, Geddes DM: Increase in mucociliary clearance in normal man induced by oral high frequency oscillation. Thorax 40:433–437, 1985

Gold MI: Is intermittent positive-pressure breathing therapy (IPPB Rx) treatment necessary in the surgical patient? Ann Surg 184:122–123, 1976

Gormezano J, Branthwaite MA: Effects of physiotherapy during intermittent positive pressure ventilation. Anaesthesia 27:258–263, 1972a

Gormezano J, Branthwaite MA: Pulmonary physiotherapy with assisted ventilation. Anaesthesia 27:249–257, 1972b

Gracey DR, Divertic MB, Didier EP: Preoperative pulmonary preparation of patients with chronic obstructive pulmonary disease. Chest 76:123–129, 1979

Graham WG, Bradley DA: Efficacy of chest physiotherapy and intermittent positive-pressure breathing in the resolution of pneumonia. N Engl J Med 299:624–627, 1978

Grimby G: Aspects of lung expansion in relation to pulmonary physiotherapy. Am Rev Respir Dis 110(2):145–153, 1974

Hammond WE, Martin RJ: Chest physical therapy for acute atelectasis. Phys Ther 61:217–220, 1981

Harada K, Mutsuda T, Saoyama N, Tainki T, Kimura H: Reexpansion of refractory atelectasis using a bronchofiberscope with a balloon cuff. Chest 84:725–728, 1983

Heckscher H: The emphysema of the lungs, its symptoms and relations to other diseases. Acta Med Scand 120:349–383, 1945

Hedstrand U, Liw M, Rooth G, Ogren CH: Effect of respiratory physiotherapy on arterial oxygen tension. Acta Anaesthesiol Scand 22:349–352, 1978

Heitz M, Holzach P, Dittman M: Comparison of the effects of continuous positive airway pressure and blowing bottles on functional residual capacity after abdominal surgery. Respiration 48:277–284, 1985

Herzog P: Advice and practical instruction for the use of the Engström respirator. Opusc Med Bd 9(8):17, 1964

Herzog P, Norlander DD: Distribution of alveolar volumes into different types of positive pressure gas flow patterns. Opusc Med Bd 13(11):1–45, 1968

Hirsch M: Uber Kunstliche aemung durch ventilation der trachea. Dissertation Gressen, 1905.

Hofmeyer JL, Webber BA, Hodson ME: Evaluation of positive expiratory pressure as an adjunct to chest physiotherapy in the treatment of cystic fibrosis. Thorax 41:951–954, 1986

Holloway R, DeSai SD, Kelly SD, Thambiran AK, Strydom SE, Adams EB: The effect of chest physiotherapy on the arterial oxygenation of neonates during treatment of tetanus by intermittent positive pressure respiration. S Afr Med J 40:445–447, 1966

Holloway R, Adams EB, Desai SD, Thambiran AK: Effect of chest physiotherapy on blood gases of neonates treated by intermittent positive pressure respiration. Thorax 24:421–426, 1969

Holloway TE, Stanford BJ: Effect of doxopram on postoperative oxygenation in obese patients. Anaesthesia 37:718–721, 1982

Holody B, Goldberg HS: The effect of mechanical vibration physiotherapy on arterial oxygenation in acutely ill patients with atelectasis or pneumonia. Am Rev Respir Dis 126:372–375, 1981

Ingram RH: Mechanical aids to lung expansion. Am Rev Respir Dis 122(2):23–24, 1980

Jackson C, Jackson CL: Peroral pulmonary drainage: Natural and therapeutic with special reference to the tussive squeeze. Am J Med Sci 186:849–854, 1933

Jaworski A, Goldberg SK, Walkenstein MD, Wilson B, Lippmann ML: Utility of immediate postlobectomy fiberoptic bronchoscopy in preventing atelectasis. Chest 94:38–43, 1988

Jenkins SC, Soutar SA: A survey into the use of incentive spirometry following coronary artery bypass graft surgery. Physiotherapy 72:492–493, 1986

Johanson WG, Seidenfeld JJ, Gomez P, De Los Santos R, Coalson JJ: Bacteriologic diagnosis of nosocomial pneumonia following prolonged mechanical ventilation. Am Rev Respir Dis 137:259–264, 1988a

Johanson WG, Seidenfeld JJ, De Los Santos R, Coalson JJ, Gomez P: Prevention of nosocomial pneumonia using topical and parenteral antimicrobial agents. Am Rev Respir Dis 137:265–272, 1988b

Jones HA, Davies EE, Hughes JMB: Modification of pulmonary gas mixing by postural changes. J Appl Physiol 61:75–80, 1986

Jones JG: Pulmonary complications following general anesthesia. Chapter 3 in Anesthesia Review 2, edited by L Kaufman, pp 21–37. Churchill Livingstone, Edinburgh, 1984

Jones JG, Minty BD, Royston D: The physiology of leaky lungs. Br J Anaesth 54:705–721, 1982

Jones NL: Physical therapy—present state of the art. Am Rev Respir Dis 110(2):132–136, 1974

Kane IJ: Segmental localization of pulmonary disease on the postero-anterior chest roentgenogram. Radiology 59:229–237, 1952

Kane IJ: Segmental postural drainage in pulmonary diseases. Dis Chest 23:418–427, 1953

Kerrebijn KF, Veentzer R, Bonzet E, Water VD: The immediate effect of physiotherapy and aerosol treatment on pulmonary function in children with cystic fibrosis. Eur J Resp Dis 63:35–42, 1982

Kigin CM: Chest physical therapy for the postoperative or traumatic injury patient. Phys Ther 61:1724–1736, 1981

Kigin CM: Advances in chest physical therapy. In Current Advances in Respiratory Care, edited by WJ O'Donohue, pp 37–71. American Coll. Chest Physicians, Park Ridge, IL, 1984

King M, Phillips DM, Gross D, Vartian V, Chang HK, Zidulka A: Enhanced tracheal mucus clearance with high frequency chest wall compression. Am Rev Respir Dis 128:511–515, 1983

Kirilloff LH, Owens HR, Rogers RM, Mazzocco MC: Does chest physical therapy work? Chest 88:436–444, 1985

Klein P, Kemper M, Weissman C, Rosenbaum SH,

Askanazi J, Hyman AI: Attenuation of the hemodynamic responses to chest physical therapy. Chest 93:38–42, 1988

Knies PT: Physical therapy in thoracic diseases. Phys Ther Rev 18:239–243, 1938

Lambert MW: Accessory bronchiole—alveolar communications. J Pathol Bacteriol 70:311–314, 1955

Lancet Editorial: Chest physiotherapy under scrutiny. Lancet 2:1241, 1978

Lawler P, Jones JG, Loh L, Lonn M: Inability to maintain ventilation against large inspiratory threshold loads: muscle fatigue or progressive failure of coordination. Br J Anaesth 51:994P, 1979

Laws AK, McIntyre RW: Chest physiotherapy: A physiological assessment during intermittent positive pressure ventilation in respiratory failure. Can Anaesth Soc J 16:487–493, 1969

Lenhert BE, Oberdorster G, Slutsky AS: Continuous flow ventilation of apneic dogs. J Appl Physiol 53:483–489, 1982

Lillehei RC: Surgery. Med World News 10:102, 1969

Lindholm CE, Ollman B, Snyder J. Mullen E, Grenvik A: Flexible fiberoptic bronchoscopy in critical car medicine. Crit Care Med 2:250–261, 1974

Lisboa C, Pare PD, Pertuze J, Contreras G, Moreno R, Guillemi S, Cruz E: Inspiratory muscle function in unilateral diaphragmatic paralysis. Am Rev Respir Dis 134:488–492, 1986

Lord GP, Herbert CA, Francis DT: A clinical, radiologic and physiologic evaluation of chest physiotherapy. J Maine Med Assoc 63:142–150, 1972

Lorin MI, Denning CR: Evaluation of postural drainage by measurement of sputum volume and consistency. Am J Phys Med 50:215–219, 1971

Lundgren R, Haggmark S, Reiz S: Hemodynamic effects of flexible fiberoptic bronchoscopy performed under topical anesthesia. Chest 82:295–299, 1982

Lyager S, Wernberg M, Rajani N, Boggild-Madsen B, Nielsen L, Nielsen HC, Andersen M, Moller J, Silberschmid M: Can postoperative pulmonary conditions be improved by treatment with the Bartlett-Edwards Incentive Spirometer after upper abdominal surgery? Acta Anaesthesiol Scand 23:312–319, 1979

Mackenzie CF, Ayella RJ, Imle PC: Chest Physiotherapy—An Alternative to Bronchoscopy. Department of Physical Therapy, University of Maryland Hospital, Audiovisual Services, 1978a

Mackenzie CF, Shin B, McAslan TC: Chest physiotherapy: The effect on arterial oxygenation. Anesth Analg 57:28–30, 1978b

Mackenzie CF, Shin B: Evaluation of respiratory physical therapy (letter). N Engl J Med 301:665–666, 1979a

Mackenzie CF, Shin B, Fisher R, Cowley RA: Two year mortality in 760 patients transported by helicopter direct from the road accident scene. Am Surg 45:101–108, 1979b

Mackenzie CF, Shin B, McAslan TC, Blanchard CL, Cowley RA: Severe stridor after prolonged endotracheal intubation using high volume cuffs. Anesthesiology 50:235–239, 1979c

Mackenzie CF, Shin B, Friedman S, Wai M: Evaluation of total lung/thorax vs static lung compliance. Anesthesiology 51:S381, 1979d

Mackenzie CF, Shin B, Hadi F, Imle PC: Changes in total lung/thorax compliance following chest physiotherapy. Anesth Analg 59:207–210, 1980

Mackenzie CF, Shin B: Cardiorespiratory function before and after chest physiotherapy in mechanically ventilated patients with post-traumatic respiratory failure. Crit Care Med 13:483–486, 1985

Mackenzie CF, Shin B: Chest physiotherapy vs bronchoscopy. Crit Care Med 14:78–79, 1986

Macklem PT: Airway obstruction and collateral ventilation. Physiol Rev 51:368–436, 1971

Macklem PT: Respiratory muscles: The vital pump. Chest 78:753–758, 1980

Macklem PT: Normal and abnormal function of the diaphragm. Thorax 36:161–163, 1981

Mackowiack PA: The normal microbial flora. N Engl J Med 307:83–93, 1982

MacMahon C: Breathing and physical exercises for use in cases of wounds in the pleura and lung and diaphragm. Lancet 2:769–770, 1915

MacMahon C: Some cases of gunshot wounds and other affectations of the chest treated by breathing and physical exercises. Lancet 1:697–699, 1919

Mankikian B, Cantineau JP, Bertrand M, Kieffer E, Sartene R, Viars P: Improvement of diaphragmatic function by a thoracic extradural block after upper abdominal surgery. Anesthesiology 68:379–386, 1988

Marini JJ, Pierson DJ, Hudson LD: Acute lobar atelectasis: A prospective comparison of fiberoptic bronchoscopy and respiratory therapy. Am Rev Respir Dis 119:971–978, 1979

Marini JJ, Pierson DJ, Hudson LD: Comparison of fiberoptic bronchoscopy and respiratory therapy (letter). Am Rev Respir Dis 126:368, 1982

Martin CJ, Ripley H, Reynolds J, Best F: Chest physiotherapy and the distribution of ventilation. Chest 69:174–178, 1976

Martin HB: Respiratory bronchioles as the pathway for collateral ventilation. J Appl Physiol 21:1443–1447, 1966

May DB, Munt PW: Physiologic effects of chest percussion and postural drainage in patients with stable chronic bronchitis. Chest 75:29–32, 1979

Mazzocco MC, Owens GR, Kirilloff LH, Rogers RM: Chest percussion and postural drainage in patients with bronchiectasis. Chest 88:360–363, 1985

McAslan TC: Automated respiratory gas monitoring of critically ill patients. Crit Care Med 4:255–260, 1976

McConnell DH, Maloney JV, Buckberg GD: Postoperative intermittent positive-pressure breathing treatments. J Thorac Cardiovasc Surg 68:944–952, 1974

McCool FD, Mayewski RF, Shayne DS, Gibson CJ, Griggs RC, Hyde RW: Intermittent positive pressure breathing in patients with respiratory muscle weakness. Chest 90:546–552, 1986

McIntyre RW, Laws AK, Ramanchandran PR: Positive expiratory pressure plateau: Improved gas exchange during mechanical ventilation. Can Anaesth Soc J 16:477–486, 1969

Mellins RB: Pulmonary physiotherapy in the pediatric age group. Am Rev Respir Dis 110(2):137–142, 1974

Meltzer SJ, Auer J: Continuous respiration without respiratory movements. *J Exp Med* 11:622–625, 1909

Menkes HA, Traystman RJ: State of the art: collateral ventilation. *Am Rev Respir Dis* 116:287–309, 1977

Milner AD, Murray M: Acute bronchiolitis in infancy: Treatment and prognosis. Editorial. *Thorax* 44:1–5, 1989

Morran C, McArdle CS: The reduction of postoperative chest infection by prophylactic co-trimoxazole. *Br J Surg* 67:464, 1980

Morran CG, Finlay IG, Matheson M, McKay AJ, Wilson N, McArdle CS: Randomized controlled trial of physiotherapy for postoperative pulmonary complications. *Br J Anaesth* 55:1113–1116, 1983

Mossberg B, Camner P: Mucociliary transport and cough as tracheobronchial clearance mechanims in pathological conditions. *Eur J Respir Dis* 61:Suppl 110, 47–55, 1980

Moxham J, Morris AJR, Spiro SG, Edwards RHT, Green M: Contractile properties and fatigue of the diaphragm in man. *Thorax* 36:164–168, 1981

Murray JF: Editorial: The ketchup-bottle method. *N Engl J Med* 300:1155–1157, 1979a

Murray JF: Reply to correspondence on evaluation of respiratory physical therapy. *N Eng J Med* 301:666, 1979b

Murray JF: Indication for mechanical aids to assist lung inflation in medical patients. *Am Rev Respir Dis* 122(2):121–125, 1980

National Heart, Lung and Blood Institute (NHLBI): Proceedings of the 1979 conference on the scientific basis of in-hospital respiratory therapy. *Am Rev Respir Dis* 122(2):161, 1980

National Heart and Lung Institute (NHLI): Proceedings of the conference on the scientific basis of respiratory therapy. *Am Rev Respir Dis* 110(2):1–204, 1974

Natof HE: Complications associated with ambulatory surgery. *JAMA* 244:1116–1118, 1980

Nelson P: Postural drainage of the lungs. *Br Med J* 2:251–255, 1932

Newhouse MT, Rossman CM: Response to Sutton PP et al, 1984 letter. *Am Rev Respir Dis* 127:391, 1984

Newman JH, Neff TA, Ziporin P: Acute respiratory failure associated with hypophosphatemia. *N Engl J Med* 296:1101–1103, 1977

Newton DAG, Bevans HG: Physiotherapy and intermittent positive-pressure ventilation of chronic bronchitis. *Br Med J* 2:1525–1528, 1978

Newton DAG, Stephenson A: Effect of physiotherapy on pulmonary function. *Lancet* 2:228–230, 1978

Novak RA, Shumaker L, Snyder JV, Pinsky MR: Do periodic hyperinflations improve gas exchange in patients with hypoxemic respiratory failure? *Crit Care Med* 15:1081–1085, 1987

Nunn JF, Coleman AJ, Sachithanandan J, Bergman NA, Laws JW: Hypoxaemia and atelectasis produced by forced expiration. *Br J Anaesth* 37:3–11, 1965

Nunn JF: Artificial ventilation. Chapter 21 In *Applied Respiratory Physiology*, 3rd ed., pp 392–422. Butterworth, London, 1987

Nunn JF, O'Morain C: Nitrous oxide decreases motility of human neutrophils in vitro. *Anesthesiology* 56:45–48, 1982

O'Donohue WJ: Maximum volume IPPB for the management of pulmonary atelectasis. *Chest* 76:683–687, 1979

O'Donohue WJ: National survey of the usage of lung expansion modalities for the prevention and treatment of postoperative atelectasis following abdominal and thoracic surgery. *Chest* 87:76–80, 1985

Oldenburg FA, Dolovich MB, Montgomery JM, Newhouse MT: Effect of postural drainage, exercise and cough on mucus clearance in chronic bronchitis. *Am Rev Respir Dis* 120:739–745, 1979

Opie LH, Spalding JMK: Chest physiotherapy during intermittent positive pressure respiration. *Lancet* 2:671–674, 1958

Pardy RL, Rivington RN, Despas PJ, Macklem PT: Inspiratory muscle training compared with physiotherapy in patients with chronic airflow limitation. *Am Rev Respir Dis* 123:421–425, 1981

Palmer KNV, Sellick BA: The prevention of postoperative pulmonary atelectasis. *Lancet* 1:164–168, 1953

Pasteur W: The Bradshaw Lecture on massive collapse of the lung. *Lancet* 2:1351–1355, 1908

Pasteur W: Active lobar collapse of the lung after abdominal operations. A contribution to the study of post operative lung complications. *Lancet* 2:1080–1083, 1910

Pavia D, Thomson ML, Phillipakos D: A preliminary study of the effect of a vibrating pad on bronchial clearance. *Am Rev Respir Dis* 113:92–96, 1976

Perez-Chada RD, Gardez J-P, Madgewick P, Sykes MK: Cardiorespiratory effects of an inspiratory hold and continuous positive pressure ventilation in goats. *Intensive Care Med* 9:263–269, 1983

Perruchoud A, Ehrsam R, Heitz M, Kopp C, Tschan M, Herzog H: Atelectasis of the lung: Bronchoscopic lavage with acetylcysteine. Experience in 51 patients. *Eur J Resp Dis* 61:Suppl III, 163–168, 1980

Peters RM, Turnier E: Physical therapy: Indications for and effects in surgical patients. *Am Rev Respir Dis* 122(2):147–154, 1980

Petty TL: A critical look at IPPB (editorial). *Chest* 66:1–3, 1974a

Petty TL: Physical therapy. *Am Rev Respir Dis* 110(2):129–130, 1974b

Petty TL: Rational respiratory therapy, Editorial. *N Engl J Med* 315:317–318, 1986

Piehl MA, Brown RS: Use of extreme position changes in acute respiratory failure. *Crit Care Med* 4:13–14, 1976

Pontoppidan H: Mechanical aids to lung expansion in nonintubated surgical patients. *Am Rev Respir Dis* 122(22):109–119, 1980

Pryor JA, Webber BA: An evaluation of the forced expiratory technique as an adjunct to postural drainage. *Physiotherapy* 65:304–307, 1979

Ricker JB, Haberman B: Expired gas monitoring by mass spectrometry in a respiratory intensive care unit. *Crit Care Med* 4:223–229, 1976

Ricksten SE, Benglsson A, Soderberg C, Thordeu M, Kwist H: Effects of periodic positive airway pressure by mask on postoperative pulmonary function. *Chest* 89:774–781, 1986

Rigg JRA: Pulmonary atelectasis after anaesthesia: Pathophysiology and management. *Can Anaesth Soc J* 28:305–313, 1981

Rochester DF, Goldberg SK: Techniques of respiratory physical therapy. *Am Rev Respir Dis* 122(2):133–146, 1980

Roper PC, Vonwiller JB, Fisk GC, Gupta JM: Lobar atelectasis after nasotracheal intubation in newborn infants. *Aust Paediat J* 12:272–275, 1976

Rossman CM, Waldes R, Sampson D, Newhouse MT: Effect of chest physiotherapy on the removal of mucus in patients with cystic fibrosis. *Am Rev Respir Dis* 126:131–135, 1982

Rubi JAG, Sanartin A, Diaz GG, Apezteguia C, Martinez GT, Rubi JCM: Assessment of total pulmonary airway resistance under mechanical ventilation. *Crit Care Med* 8:633–636, 1980

Sackner MA: State of the art bronchofiberscopy. *Am Rev Respir Dis* 111:62–88, 1975

Sackner MA: State of the art bronchofiberoscopy. *Am Rev Respir Dis* 111:62–88, 1975

Salata RA, Lederman MM, Shlaes DM, Jacobs MR, Eckstein E, Tweardy D, Toossi Z, Chmielewski R, Marino J, King CK, Graham RC, Ellner JJ: Diagnosis of nososomial pneumonia in intubated intensive care unit patients. *Am Rev Respir Dis* 135:426–437, 1987

Sanchis J, Dolovich M, Rossman C, Wilson W, Newhouse M: Pulmonary mucociliary clearance in cystic fibrosis. *N Engl J Med* 288:651–654, 1973

Sands JH, Cypert C, Armstrong R, Ching S, Trainer D, Quinn W, Stewart D: A controlled study using routine intermittent positive-pressure breathing in the post-surgical patient. *Dis Chest* 40:128–133, 1961

Schmerber J, Deltenre M: A new fatal complication of transtracheal aspiration. *Scand J Resp Dis* 59:232–235, 1978

Schmid ER,Rehder K: General anesthesia and the chest wall. *Anesthesiology* 55:668–675, 1981

Schuppisser JP, Brandi O, Meili U: Postoperative intermittent positive pressure breathing versus physiotherapy. *Am J Surg* 140:682–686, 1980

Schur MS, Brown JT, Kafer ER, Strope GL, Greene WB, Mandell J: Postoperative pulmonary function in children. *Am Rev Respir Dis* 130:46–51, 1984

Schweiger I, Garnlin Z, Foster A, Meyer P, Gemperle M, Suter PM: Absence of benefit of incentive spirometry in low risk patients undergoing elective cholecystectomy. *Chest* 89:652–656, 1986

Sellick BA: Cricoid pressure to control regurgitation of stomach contents during induction of anaesthesia. *Lancet* 2:404–406, 1961

Serota AI, Meyer RD, Wilson SE, Edestein PH, Finegold SM: Legionnaire's disease in the postoperative patient. *J Surg Res* 30:417–427, 1981

Shennib H, Mulder DS, Chiu RCJ: The effects of pulmonary atelectasis and re-expansion on lung cellular immune defenses. *Arch Surg* 119:274–277, 1984

Shim C, Fine N, Fernandez R, Williams MH: Cardiac arrhythmias resulting from tracheal suctioning. *Ann Intern Med* 71:1149–1153, 1969

Shim C, Bajwa S, Williams MH: The effect of inhalation therapy on ventilatory function and expectoration. *Chest* 73:798–801, 1978

Simonneau G, Vivien A, Sartene R, Kunstlinger F,

Sania K, Noviant Y, Duroux P: Diaphragm dysfunction induced by upper abdominal surgery. Role of postoperative pain. *Am Rev Respir Dis* 128:899–903, 1983

Sinha R, Bergofsky EH: Prolonged alteration of lung mechanics in kyphoscoliosis by positive pressure hyperinflation. *Am Rev Respir Dis* 106:47–57, 1972

Stock CM, Downs JB, Ganer PK, Alster JM, Purrey PB: Prevention of postoperative pulmonary complications with CPAP incentive spirometry and conservative therapy. *Chest* 87:151–157, 1985

Strohl KP, Mead J, Banzett RB, Lehr J, Loring SH, O'Cain CF: Effect of posture on upper and lower rib cage motion and tidal volume during diaphragm pacing. *Am Rev Respir Dis* 130:320–321, 1984

Sutton PP, Parker RA, Webber BA, Newman SP, Garland N, Lopez-Vidriero MT, Pavia D, Clarke SW: Assessment of the forced expiration technique, postural drainage and directed coughing in chest physiotherapy. *Eur J Resp Dis* 64:62–68, 1983

Sutton PP, Lopez-Vidriero MT, Pavia D, Newman SP, Clarke SW: Effect of chest physiotherapy on the removal of mucus in patients with cystic fibrosis (letter). *Am Rev Respir Dis* 127:390–391, 1984

Sutton PP, Lopez-Vidriero MT, Pavia D, Newman SP, Clay MM, Webber B, Parker RA, Clarke SW: Assessment of percussion vibratory-shaking and breathing exercises in chest physiotherapy. *Eur J Respir Dis* 66:147–152, 1985

Tecklin JS, Holsclaw DS: Evaluation of bronchial drainage in patients with cystic fibrosis. *Phys Ther* 55:1081–1084, 1975

Tecklin JS, Holsclaw DS: Bronchial drainage with aerosol medication in cystic fibrosis. *Phys Ther* 56:999–1003, 1976

Temple HL, Evans JA: The bronchopulmonary segments. *Am J Roentgenol Rad Ther* 63:26–46, 1950

Terry PB, Traystman RJ, Newball HH, Batra G, Menkes HA: Collateral ventilation in man. *N Eng J Med* 298:10–15, 1978

Thomson ML, Pavia D, Jones CJ, McQuiston TAC: No demonstrable effect of S-carboxymethylcysteine on clearance of secretions from the human lung. *Thorax* 30:669–673, 1975

Thoren L: Post-operative pulmonary complications. Observations on their prevention by means of physiotherapy. *Acta Chir Scand* 107:193–204, 1954

Tokis L, Hedenstierna G, Stranberg A, Brismar B, Lundquist H: Lung collapse and gas exchange during general anesthesia: effects of spontaneous breathing, muscle paralysis and positive end-expiratory pressure. *Anesthesiology* 66:157–167, 1987

Tyler ML: Complications of positioning and chest physiotherapy. *Resp Care* 27:458–466, 1982

Van der Schans CP, Piers PA, Postma DS: Effect of manual percussion on tracheobronchial clearance in patients with chronic airflow obstruction and excessive tracheobronchial secretion. *Thorax* 41:448–452, 1986

Veviana JR, Teichberg S, Buschman D, Kirapatrick CH: Correlation of absent inner dynein arms and mucociliary clearance in a patient with Kartageners syndrome. *Chest* 91:91–95, 1987

Vickers MD: Postoperative pneumonias, Editorial. *Br Med J* 284:292–293, 1982

Vraciu JK, Vraciu RA: Effectiveness of breathing exercises in preventing pulmonary complications following open heart surgery. *Phys Ther* 57:1367–1371, 1977

Wagner PD, Naumann PF, Laravuso RB: Simultaneous measurement of eight foreign gases in blood by gas chromatography. *J Appl Physiol* 36:600–605, 1974

Wahba WB: Influence of aging on lung function—Clinical significance of changes from age twenty. *Anesth Analg* 62:764–776, 1983

Walker J, Cooney M: Improved respiratory function in quadriplegics after pulmonary therapy and arm ergometry (letter). *N Engl J Med* 316:486–487, 1987

Waring WW: Editorial. Cilia and cystic fibrosis. *N Engl J Med* 288:681–682, 1973

Webb MSC, Martin JA, Cartlidge PHT, Ng YK, Wright NA: Chest physiotheapy in acute bronchiolitis. *Arch Dis Child* 60:1078–1079, 1985

Weil MH, Shubin H: The "VIP" approach to the bedside management of shock. *JAMA* 207:337–340, 1969

Weisman IM, Rinaldo JE, Rogers RM, Sanders MH: Intermittent mandatory ventilation. *Am Rev Respir Dis* 127:641–647, 1983

Weller PH, Bush E, Preece MA, Mathew DJ: Short-term effects of chest physiotherapy on pulmonary function in children with cystic fibrosis. *Respiration* 40:53–56, 1980

Welply NC, Mathias CJ, Frankel HL: Circulatory reflexes in tetraplegics during artificial ventilation and general anaesthesia. *Paraplegia* 13:172–182, 1975

Wiklander O, Norlin U: Effect of physiotherapy on post operative pulmonary complications. A clinical and roentgenographic study of 200 cases. *Acta Chir Scand* 112:246–254, 1957

Willats SM: Alternative modes of ventilation. Part I. Disadvantages of controlled mechanical ventilation: intermittent mandatory ventilation. *Intensive Care Med* 11:51–55, 1985a

Willats SM: Alternative modes of ventilation. Part II. High and low frequency positive pressure ventilation, PEEP, CPAP, reversed ratio ventilation. *Intensive Care Med* 11:115–122, 1985b

Wilson R, Roberts D, Cole P: Effects of bacterial products on human ciliary function in vitro. *Thorax* 40:125–131, 1985

Wilson R, Sykes D, Currie DC, Cole PJ: Beat frequency of cilia from sites of purulent infection. *Thorax* 41:453–458, 1986

Winning TJ, Brock-Utne JG, Goodwin NM: A simple clinical method of quantitating the effects of chest physiotherapy in mechanically ventilated patients. *Anaesth Intensive Care* 3:237–238, 1975

Wollmer P, Ursing K, Midgren B, Eriksson L: Inefficiency of chest percussion in the physical therapy of chronic bronchitis. *Eur J Respir Dis* 66:233–239, 1985

Zapletal A, Stefanova J, Horak J, Vavrova V, Samanek M: Chest physiotherapy and airway obstruction in patients with cystic fibrosis—a negative report. *Eur J Respir Dis* 64:426–433, 1983

Zibrak JD, Dosetti P, Wood E: Effect of reductions in respiratory therapy on patient outcome. *N Eng J Med* 315:292–295, 1986

CHAPTER 2

Clinical Indications and Usage of Chest Physiotherapy: Anatomy, Physiology, Physical Examination, and Radiology of the Airways and Chest

Colin F. Mackenzie, M.B., Ch.B., F.F.A.R.C.S.

Prophylactic Use of Chest Physiotherapy
Chronic Sputum-Producing Lung Disease
Acute Quadriplegia
Smoke Inhalation and Aspiration
Depressed Level of Consciousness
Obesity

The intention of this chapter is primarily to assist the clinician in determining the need for chest physiotherapy. A brief review of airway and lung anatomy is included so that clinical examination and the chest x-ray may be most usefully interpreted. Respiratory physiology is reviewed with the purpose of assisting understanding of the research reported in the literature and the objectives of chest physiotherapy. Research on human respiratory mucus and mucus properties is described. A section covers examination of the chest in mechanically ventilated patients together with a summary of some commonly found acute lung lesions. An approach to chest x-ray interpretation is described, and finally, the acute and prophylactic uses of chest physiotherapy are discussed.

Initially, the indication for chest physiotherapy for the intensive care unit (ICU) patient with acute lung disease is based on bedside examination, the chest x-ray, and blood gas analysis. A knowledge of the anatomy of the tracheobronchial tree and lung lobes and segments is essential to allow the maximum amount of information to be obtained from clinical and radiological examination of the chest, since this enables correct patient positioning for postural drainage.

ANATOMY OF THE AIRWAY AND LUNG SEGMENTS AND LOBES

Surface Anatomy of the Lung Lobes

The lungs rise cranially to above the first rib. During full inspiration the lower lobes descend to the tenth thoracic vertebra posteriorly and to the xiphoid process anteriorly. Parts of all lung lobes (right upper, middle, and lower; left upper and lower) are adjacent to the anterior chest wall, while only parts of the

upper and lower lobes are found posteriorly. Both oblique fissures (separating upper and middle from lower lobes) run from the spine of the third thoracic vertebra to the sixth costochondral junction. The horizontal fissure (found only on the right and separating the upper from the middle lobe) runs from the oblique fissure in the midaxillary line to the level of the fourth costal cartilage anteriorly. Consequently, both upper lobes (excluding the lingula) are located above the spinous process of T3 or the spine of the scapula posteriorly and above the fourth and the sixth costal cartilage anteriorly. The lingula and right middle lobe are predominantly anterior to the midaxillary line and are found between the fourth costal cartilages. The lower lobes of the lungs are located between the levels of thoracic vertebra 3 and 10 posteriorly (or as low as 1 hand breadth below the inferior angle of the scapula posteriorly in the adult) and lateral to the xiphisternum anteriorly. It should be noted that these surface markings are described in reference to a full inspiration. Breathing, however, is not static; therefore, landmarks may vary with the phases of ventilation, lung disease, surgical intervention, and changes in ventilatory patterns (Lockhart et al., 1959; Downie, 1979). There are 11 segmental postural drainage positions used when performing chest physiotherapy (see Fig. 3.1A–T). The corresponding surface markings of these lung segments and the overlying anatomic landmarks are shown in Figure 2.1A–C.

Upper Airway

The pharynx extends from the base of the skull to the esophagus and communicates with the nose, mouth, and larynx (Fig. 2.2). The pharynx serves as a com-

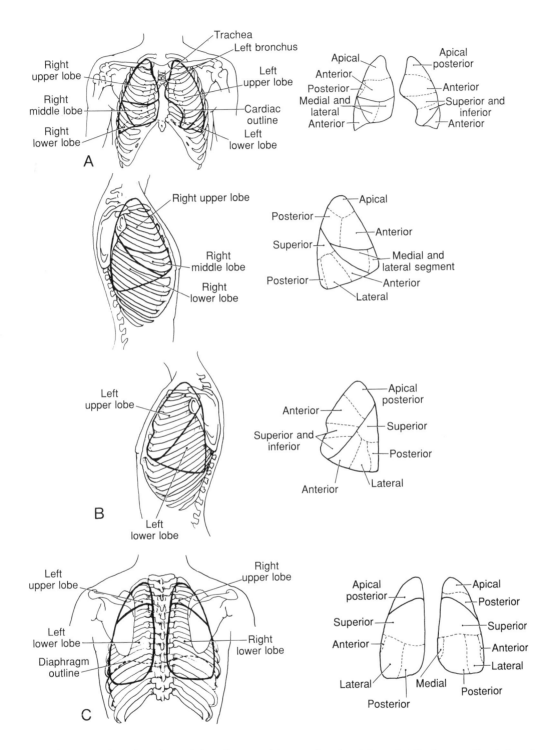

Figure 2.1. (**A**) Anterior view of the chest and lungs showing lobar distribution on the *left* and bronchopulmonary segments on the *right*. (**B**) Lateral views of the right chest and lungs *(upper)* and left chest and lungs *(lower)*. The lobar distribution is shown on the *left* and the bronchopulmonary segments are shown on the *right*. (**C**) Posterior view of the chest and lungs showing lobar distribution on the *left* and bronchopulmonary segments on the *right*.

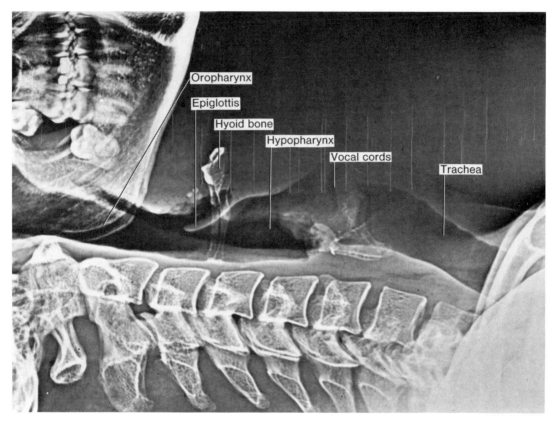

Figure 2.2. Xeroradiograph of a normal lateral cervical spine showing the pharynx and its communications. (Kindly supplied by E. McCrea, M.D., Department of Radiology, University of Maryland Hospital, Baltimore, MD.)

mon passage for air and food; breathing and swallowing cannot take place simultaneously in the adult.

Phonation and prevention of aspiration into the tracheobronchial tree are the important functions of the larynx. Aspiration protection is achieved by the sphincteric action of the aryepiglottic and vestibular folds. The infant larynx is funnel-shaped, with its narrowest point 1 cm below the vocal cords, and is situated higher in the neck than is the adult larynx. A neonate can elevate the larynx so that the epiglottis touches the soft palate. Breathing can, therefore, continue even when liquids are swallowed. This ability is lost after 6 months. The larynx contains the vocal cords which vibrate to produce phonation on expiration. The larynx is composed mostly of the thyroid and cricoid cartilages and the hyoid bone. The thyroid is made up of two plates of cartilage joined anteriorly, form-

ing the laryngeal prominence or Adam's apple. This is greater in the male (where the apple is said to have stuck). The upper border of the thyroid cartilage is attached to the hyoid bone by the thyrohyoid membrane (Fig. 2.3). The angle of

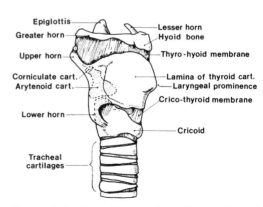

Figure 2.3. The laryngeal cartilages viewed from the anterolateral aspect.

the thyroid laminae within the larynx is the attachment for the epiglottic cartilage. The epiglottis projects up behind the tongue as a flap and fuses with the aryepiglottic folds that are the boundaries of the laryngeal inlet. The cricoid cartilage is attached to the lower border of the thyroid cartilage by the cricothyroid membrane which can be palpated anteriorly as the notch just beneath the Adam's apple. Two arytenoid cartilages articulate with the upper body of the cricoid cartilage. The arytenoid cartilages have two processes at their bases. Anteriorly, the vocal process gives attachment to the vocal cords; laterally, the muscular process is the insertion site for the posterior and lateral cricoarytenoid muscles. These muscles abduct and adduct the vocal cords. The pair of vocal cords and the arytenoid elevations comprise the glottis. The intervening sagittal slit, known as the rima glottidis, is the narrowest part of the larynx at rest (Lockhart et al. (Fig. 2.4). The width of the rima glottidis is altered by the cricoarytenoid muscles, and air flow is controlled.

Trachea

The adult trachea extends from the lower border of the cricoid cartilage (which lies opposite the sixth cervical vertebra) to the carina. This is found over the fifth thoracic vertebra and under the sternal angle of Louis. The trachea is composed of many flexible interlacing cartilages with a posterior membrane (Fig. 2.5A–C). The unstretched adult autopsy specimen varies in length from 8 to 12 cm. Stretching the trachea with a 500-gm weight increases the length approximately 30%. During extension of the neck and inspiration the trachea is stretched. The cartilage of the trachea

may have six cross-sectional shapes: C, U, D, elliptical, triangular, and circular (Fig. 2.6). The shape varies throughout the length of the trachea and changes with inspiration, expiration, coughing, mechanical ventilation, and posture. The trachea enlarges with inspiration and contracts with expiration. The most common cross-sectional autopsy tracheal shapes are C and U (Mackenzie et al., 1978a). There is no correlation between adult tracheal shape, size, or circumference and height, or weight (Mackenzie et al., 1979, 1980b). Because the posterior membranous portion has a higher compliance than the anterior cartilage, it is more readily deformed during changes in intratracheal pressure. Tracheal compliance decreases progressively with age, and calcification of the cartilages may be seen after age 35 years and is almost always seen to some degree in those patients older than 60 years of age. The infant trachea differs from the adult trachea in several respects; these are summarized in Table 2.1.

Bronchi to Alveoli

At the carina the trachea bifurcates into right and left main stem bronchi (Fig. 2.5). The right main stem bronchus differs in several ways from the left. The right is usually shorter and wider and comes off the trachea at an angle of about 15°, whereas the left branches at about 35° to a midline sagittal plane. This does not necessarily always occur, however (Fig. 2.5A). Also, the right main bronchus branches into three lobar bronchi; the left, only two. Lobar bronchi supply different lobes of the lung, and they branch within the lung to give rise to the segmental bronchi. The segmental or third generation bronchi supply a portion of

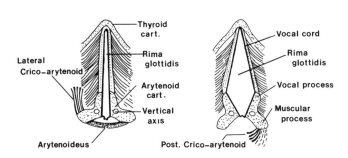

Figure 2.4. The glottis—on the *left* shown at rest; on the *right* shown during forced expiration. The lateral cricoarytenoid muscle and the arytenoideus adduct. The posterior cricoarytenoid muscle is the only abductor of the vocal cords and is, therefore, vital for respiration.

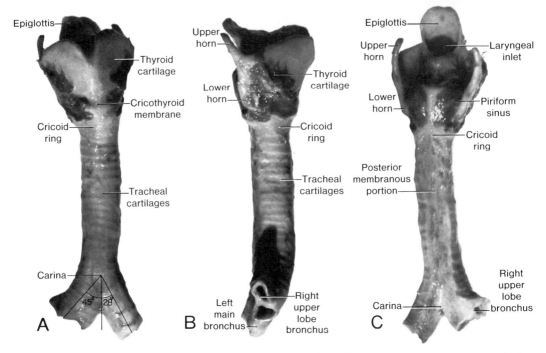

Figure 2.5. (**A**) Anterior view of a normal larynx and trachea. The trachea is shown as interlacing cartilages. In this specimen the right main stem bronchus is shorter and wider than the left and makes a 45° angle with the sagittal plane; the left main stem bronchus makes a 28° angle. These anatomical differences from the normal may account for some success in cannulation of the left bronchus with a straight catheter. (**B**) Right lateral view of a normal larynx and trachea. The right upper lobe bronchus is seen coming off the right main stem bronchus 3 mm below the tracheal bifurcation. Compare the laryngeal structures shown in this photograph with those in Figure 2.3. The hyoid bone has been removed in the photographs. (**C**) Posterior view of the normal larynx showing the compliant posterior membrane, the epiglottis, and other laryngeal structures.

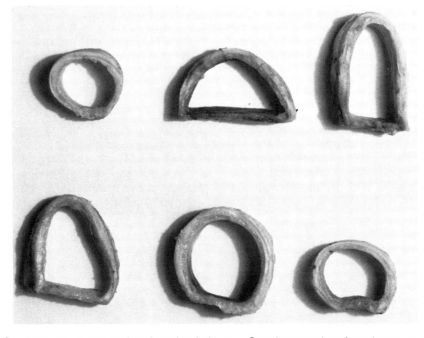

Figure 2.6. Autopsy cross-sectional tracheal shapes. Specimens taken from between the fourth and seventh tracheal cartilages. From *top left,* clockwise, these are circular D-Shaped, U-shaped, elliptical, C-shaped, and triangular. C and U shapes are the most common. (From Mackenzie CF, et al: The shape of the human adult trachea. *Anesthesiology* 49:48–50, 1978a.)

Table 2.1
Major Anatomical Differences Between the Adult and Infant Trachea[a]

	Unstretched Length (cm)	Number of Tracheal Cartilages	Cross-sectional Shape	Lumen Circumference (cm)	Posterior Membrane Length (cm)	Level of Carina	Narrowest Portion of Upper Airway
Adult	8–12	12–19	See Fig. 2.6	6.0–7.6	0.7–2.3	T5	Vocal cords
Infant (birth to 6 months)	3.5–4.5	Same but closer together	Nearly circular	1.4–1.7[b]	0.05–0.1	T3–T4	Cricoid

[a]Data are from Mackenzie et al. (1978a, 1979, and 1980b; and Unpublished data).
[b]Specimens preserved in a dilute formalin solution.

lung known as the bronchopulmonary segment. The distribution of these bronchopulmonary segments is shown in Figure 2.7. The main, lobar and segmental bronchi normally remain patent during inspiration and expiration and coughing, but they are susceptible to collapse with changes in intrathoracic pressure. When intrathoracic pressure exceeds intraluminal pressure by about 50 cm H_2O, as may occur during forced expiration, the larger bronchi collapse and limit peak expiratory flow (Nunn, 1977).

Small bronchi branch from the segmental bronchi, and their diameters, progressively decrease from 3.5 to 1 mm until, at the twelfth generation, the airway divisions cease to have cartilage in their walls and become known as bronchioles. The caliber of the bronchioles is influenced by lung volume. Each bronchiole enters a lobule of the lung and gives off five to seven terminal bronchioles (generations 12–16). The lung lobule served by terminal bronchioles is termed an acinus. The terminal bronchioles are the last of the conducting air passages and derive blood supply from the bronchial circulation. Distal to this, the air passages take on the function of gas exchange and are supplied by the pulmonary circulation.

Beyond the terminal bronchioles (generations 17–23) the acinus is composed of respiratory bronchioles, alveolar ducts, alveolar sacs, and alveoli. As many as 20 alveoli communicate with the central chamber of the alveolar sac. Small openings (5–10 μm in diameter) found in the alveoli, termed pores of Kohn, permit air to pass from one alveolus to another (Menkes and Traystman, 1977).

Interbronchiolar channels were de-scribed by Martin (1966), and bronchiolar-alveolar communications were reported by Lambert (1955) (Fig. 2.8). The communicating lobules are sometimes bifid and connected with the adjacent alveoli. When found in generations 12–14, they may connect with their own subdivided alveoli, but in generations 14–16 (terminal bronchioles) they may connect with other alveoli (interacinar connections). These connections are much bigger (about 30 μm in diameter) than the pores of Kohn and can remain open despite bronchiolar smooth muscle contraction (Krahl, 1964). They are, therefore, important avenues of collateral ventilation and may be highly significant in the reexpansion of collapsed airways by such maneuvers as deep inspiration and chest physiotherapy (see p. 237-242).

PHYSIOLOGY OF RESPIRATION

Respiratory Mechanics

Airways and Lung Volumes

The conducting airways include the trachea and all branches of the airway down to the terminal bronchioles that are supplied with blood from the bronchial artery. The conducting airways contain no alveoli, do not take part in gas exchange, and, therefore, constitute what is known as the anatomic dead space (often referred to as the Fowler dead space). Distal to the terminal bronchioles, the respiratory bronchioles, which contain alveoli, take on the function of gas exchange and derive their blood supply from the pulmonary artery. There is so much branching of the airways in the respiratory gas exchange zone that the

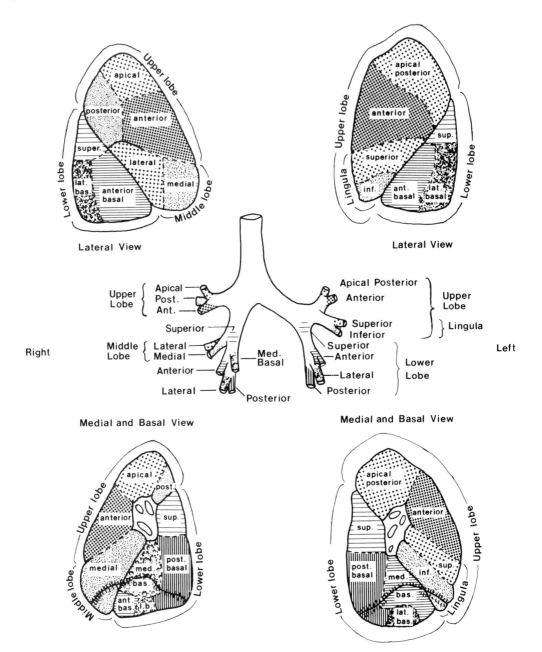

Figure 2.7. The distribution of the bronchopulmonary segments. (Redrawn from Krahl V: The anatomy of the mammalian lung. In *Handbook of Physiology,* vol 1, *Respiration,* p 248, Fig. 23, American Physiological Society, Washington, DC, 1964.)

sum of the cross-sectional area of the airways increases (Fig. 2.9). As a result, respiratory gas flow over the last 5 mm before reaching the alveolus is slowed markedly. Oxygen diffusion occurs into the adjacent pulmonary capillaries, and CO_2 diffuses out of the blood along partial

pressure gradients between the blood and the respiratory zone airways.

The volume of gas in the lung at the end of a quiet exhalation is the functional residual capacity (FRC). The normal values for subjects in different positions are shown in Table 2.2. FRC is a

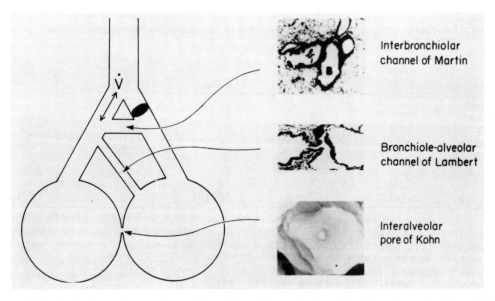

Figure 2.8. Potential pathways for collateral flow. (From Menkes HA, Traystman RJ, Terry P: Collateral ventilation. *Fed Proc* 38:22–26, 1979.)

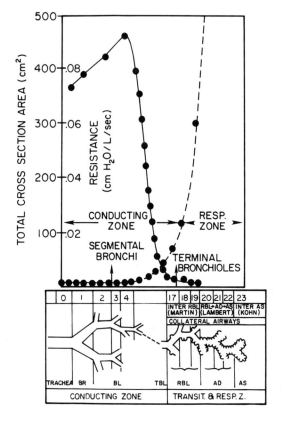

Figure 2.9. A comparison of human airway generation [according to Weibel's (1963) idealization] airway resistance and cross-sectional area (from West, 1985), showing the extremely rapid increase in total cross-sectional area of the airways in the respiratory zone and the location of the chief site of airway resistance in the intermediate-sized bronchi. Little resistance is located in the very small airways where cross-sectional area is greatest and airflow low. L, liter(s); transit and resp. z., transitional and respiratory zones; BR, bronchus; BL, bronchiole; TBL, terminal bronchiole; RBL, respiratory bronchiole; AD, alveolar duct; and AS, alveolar sac. (Adapted from Weibel ER: *Morphometry of the Human Lung,* p 111, Springer-Verlag, Berlin, 1963; and West JB: *Respiratory Physiology—The Essentials,* ed 3, pp 7 and 104. Williams & Wilkins, Baltimore, 1985.)

Table 2.2
Physical Characteristics and FRC Measurements in 100 Subjects Sitting and Supine[a]

Sex	Age (yr)	Height (m)	Weight (kg)	FRC Sitting (liters)	FRC Supine (liters)
Women					
Mean	33	1.6	56	2.45	1.80
SD	12.6	0.07	48	0.43	0.34
Range	20–63	1.45–1.77	48–83	1.52–3.49	1.08–2.43
Men					
Mean	36	1.69	71	2.99	0.61
SD	13.3	0.06	9	0.66	
Range	22–65	1.57–1.81	52–101	1.72–4.54	1.27–2.63

[a]FRC was measured by the helium dilution closed circuit method. Twenty-five women and 30 men were smokers, but no differences were found in FRC between smokers and nonsmokers. FRC always decreased when the subject changed from sitting to supine. Correlation coefficients between FRC and height were significant for both sexes. Age and weight had negligible effect on FRC. (From Ibanez J, Raurich JM: Normal values of functional residual capacity in sitting and supine positions. *Intensive Care Med* 8:173–177, 1982.)

commonly used starting point for considering lung volumes, as it is the resting place of normal lung for the majority of its working life. FRC is the volume of gas left in the lungs after passive exhalation and allows gas mixing and exchange to take place during the expiratory pause. Other lung volumes of clinical importance are vital capacity and residual volume (RV). All lung volumes except FRC and RV are measured by spirometry (Fig. 2.10). FRC is determined by washout of

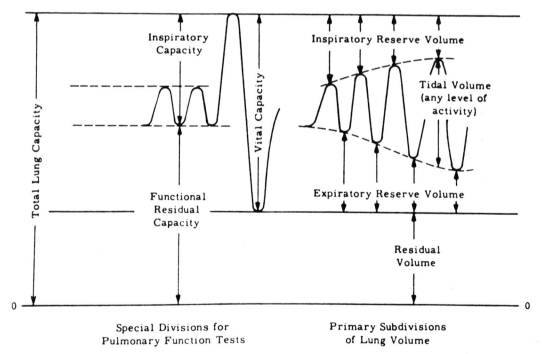

Figure 2.10. Spirometric subdivision of the lung showing four volumes and four capacities. Each capacity is made up of the combination of two or more volumes. (From Pappenheimer JR, Comroe JH, Cournand A, Ferguson JWK, Filley GF, Fowler WS, Gray JS, Helmholz HF, Obis AB, Rahn H, Riley RL: Standardization of definitions and symbols in respiratory physiology. *Fed Proc* 9:602–615, 1950.)

N_2 or other tracer gas or by measurement of volume changes in a body box.

Respiratory Pressures and Flow

At FRC the elastic recoil forces of the chest wall tending to expand outward are exactly matched by the elastic recoil forces of the lung collapsing inward. The traction between the two pleural surfaces covering the lung and lining the chest wall generates a subatmospheric pleural pressure of 5 cm H_2O at FRC. Because there is no airflow at FRC, alveolar pressure is atmospheric. The pressure difference between the pleura and alveolus at FRC, of 5 cm H_2O, is known as the transpulmonary pressure. With inspiration of a tidal volume breath (usually 8–10 ml/kg), a greater subatmospheric pressure is generated. The amount of increased subatmospheric pressure that is generated to produce a tidal volume change is a measure of compliance.

Compliance is defined as volume change per unit pressure change. Pleural pressure may be estimated from an esophageal balloon placed in the lower third of the esophagus. If pressure is measured during inspiration of the tidal volume, a subatmospheric alveolar pressure develops. If inspiratory flow is also determined, airway resistance may be calculated by dividing alveolar pressure by flow. Normal values for airway resistance and compliance as well as causes of abnormality are shown in Table 2.3. Airway conductance is the reciprocal of airway resistance. There is a linear relationship between airway conductance and lung volume: as the lungs increase in size, the diameter and length of the airways increase proportionately (Fig. 2.11).

Respiratory Muscles and Rib Cage

Because of the shape of the ribs and the way in which the intercostal muscles are attached in parallel to the chest circumference, anteroposterior and lateral expansion of the chest takes place by contraction of intercostal muscles. During inspiration the anteroposterior and lateral diameters increase, and the ribs are raised. The movement of the ribs about their axis of rotation is analogous to the arc described by a bucket handle. The point at which the radial distance from the axis of rotation is greatest (where a bucket handle would be held) is anterior in the upper chest and more lateral in the lower ribs. The movement of the sternum during inspiration has the action of a pump handle moving up and out.

The diaphragm is the most important muscle of inspiration. In quiet breathing it normally contributes 70–80% of the tidal volume. Contraction of the diaphragm causes descent of its dome, expansion of the base of the thorax, increase in intraabdominal pressure, and decrease in intrathoracic pressure. In normal tidal breathing the diaphragm moves about 1 cm; with exercise and forced inspiration and expiration it may move 10 times that amount. The diaphragm is not essential for respiration, as there are other accessory muscles of respiration. When the diaphragm is paralyzed, it moves up rather than down with inspiration, because the intrathoracic

Table 2.3
Definitions, Measurement Requirements, Typical Values, and Causes of Abnormality for Compliance and Resistance

	Definition	Measurement	Typical Values
Compliance[a]	Volume change produced by a unit of pressure change	Static pressure and volume	Lung/thorax = 50–100 ml/ cm H_2O
Resistance[b]	Pressure difference required for a unit flow change	Dynamic pressure and flow	0.5–1.5 cm H_2O (liters/sec)

[a]Low compliance occurs with pulmonary edema, pneumonia, lung contusion, interstitial fibrosis, and respiratory distress syndrome.
[b]High resistance occurs with asthma, emphysema, bronchitis, bronchospasm, sputum retention in large airways, airway compression, and narrowing or stenosis.

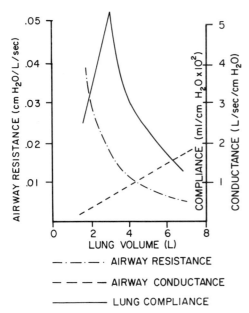

- — · — · — AIRWAY RESISTANCE

- — — — — AIRWAY CONDUCTANCE

——————— LUNG COMPLIANCE

Figure 2.11. Airway resistance, airway conductance, and specific lung compliance are plotted against lung volume in liters (L). Airway resistance falls in an exponential manner with increasing lung volume, while airway conductance increases linearly. Compliance is at its greatest at about a FRC of 2.5–3 liters and then falls progressively as lung volume rises above FRC.

pressure falls. The most important muscles of expiration are the abdominal muscles. The external, internal oblique, and transversus abdominis muscles compress the abdomen. The rectus abdominis muscle draws the anterior ribs to the symphysis pubis and compresses the abdomen during expiration. Expiratory muscles are active at high rates of ventilation when movement of air out of the lungs is impeded, such as in respiratory failure. The expiratory muscles also regulate breathing, as is required during talking, singing, coughing, defecation, and parturition. In addition to the three major muscles of respiration, the diaphragm, the intercostals, and the abdominal muscles, there are secondary muscles. The scaleni muscles elevate and fix ribs 1 and 2; the sternocleidomastoids elevate the sternum and may be an important means of ventilation for quadriplegic patients, as they are innervated by the spinal accessory nerve and C1–C3. The

alae nasi flare the nostrils, and the suprahyoid elevates and stabilizes the larynx.

Gas Exchange

The major mechanism by which gas passes through the conducting airways during spontaneous respiration or conventional mechanical ventilation is bulk convection. Bulk convection is the physical mass transport of gas from one part of the airway to another. Once in the respiratory zone airways, gas exchange takes place by passive diffusion, first in the gaseous medium of the alveolus and then across the blood–gas barrier between the alveoli and pulmonary capillaries.

The relative rates of diffusion of gases in a gaseous medium are inversely proportional to the square root of their densities. Because O_2 has a smaller molecular weight than CO_2 ($O_2 = 32$, $CO_2 = 44$), O_2 diffuses more rapidly in alveolar gas than does CO_2. A normal human alveolus is 100 μm in diameter; diffusion of gas is 80% complete in 0.002 sec if the diffusion distance is 0.5 mm. In emphysema, groups of alveoli may become one air sac, however, the distances for diffusion are much greater. If the diffusion distance in an air sac is 7 mm, 0.38 sec would be required for 80% completion. The area of the blood–gas barrier is 50–100 m^2, and the alveolar-mixed venous partial pressure difference for O_2 is $100 - 40 = 60$ mm Hg (breathing room air) and is $46 - 40$ (alveolar CO_2) $= 6$ mm Hg for CO_2. The alveolar-capillary membrane is normally less than 0.5 μm thick. The amount of gas transferred across the alveolar-capillary membrane is proportional to the area, a diffusion constant, and the difference in partial pressure and is inversely proportional to the thickness of the membrane. The diffusion constant is proportional to gas solubility and inversely proportional to molecular weight.

Gas diffusion occurs between a gaseous phase (the alveolus) and a liquid phase (the pulmonary capillary blood). Because CO_2 is 24 times more soluble than O_2 in water at atmospheric pressure, there is far more rapid diffusion of CO_2 from the capillary blood than entry of O_2, even though O_2 has a more rapid diffusion in the gas phase of the alveolus.

In disease states, the path for diffusion may become longer. The alveolar wall may be thickened as in fibrosis or edema, the capillary membrane may be thickened or the capillaries may be dilated, and edema may occur between the alveoli or in the alveolus. These causes of alveolar capillary block all result in a decreased pulmonary diffusing capacity. To test the ability of alveolar capillary membranes to transfer or conduct gases, the diffusing capacity for carbon monoxide (DCO) is frequently employed. DCO is specific for impaired diffusion. Decreased DCO occurs in pulmonary edema, fibrosis, and emphysema. DCO is decreased in pulmonary embolus or when blood flow to the lung is decreased as in shock. DCO may be normal in uncomplicated bronchial asthma but may be increased in high blood flow or pressure states such as pulmonary hypertension. DCO is measured because CO has an affinity for hemoglobin (Hb) 210 times that of O_2. So very low CO concentrations suffice to saturate Hb. The diffusion capacity for O_2 can be obtained by multiplying DCO by 1.23 (Comroe, 1975).

Gas Mixing

The majority of gas volume in the lungs is contained within the acini in airways and air spaces distal to terminal bronchioles. Most gas mixing takes place in acinar units with volumes less than 0.2 ml. An airway 2–3 mm in diameter may subtend about 35 terminal bronchioles and their acini. During inspiration of fresh gas the separation of fresh from "alveolar" gas occurs within the acinus, where the magnitude of bulk convection and diffusion gas transport mechanisms are similar. The volume contained in the airways more central to the point of separation of alveolar and fresh gas defines the Fowler (anatomical) dead space. Because of the asymmetrical branching of airways within the acinus, there are inequalities of gas concentrations within alveolar gas despite equal volume expansion. Mixing between lung units with different time constants results in a to-and-fro motion between adjacent areas. This phenomena is often called pendelluft. Incomplete alveolar gas mixing constitutes a measurable limitation to gas exchange in the normal lung.

The major gas transport mechanisms during spontaneous respiration and conventional positive pressure mechanical ventilation are bulk convection and molecular diffusion. Bulk convection occurs when lung expansion increases the total number of gas molecules in the lung. There is a random dispersion of these molecules, so that differences in gas concentrations are evened out. Mixing by molecular diffusion is enhanced by oscillations in acinar gas (cardiogenic oscillations) produced by cardiac activity. During high-frequency oscillation, bulk convection becomes a less important means of gas exchange than during conventional mechanical ventilation. High-frequency jet ventilation or high-frequency flow interrupter techniques, however, still rely heavily on bulk convection for gas transport. Cardiogenic oscillations and to-and-fro gas mixing become more important mechanisms of gas mixing in peripheral airways during high-frequency oscillation and continuous-flow ventilation techniques of gas exchange.

Pulmonary Blood Flow

The lungs and heart are the only two organs in the body through which the entire circulation flows. Normal blood flow measured as cardiac output per minute ranges from 5 to 15 liters/min at rest and during exercise, respectively. The right heart moves venous blood and pumps it into the pulmonary artery (Pa). The Pa progressively branches into successively smaller vessels adjacent to the branching airways. Beyond the terminal bronchioles the capillary branches of the Pa contain mixed venous blood. The pulmonary capillaries form an almost continuous thin sheet of blood flowing in the alveolar walls of the airways in the respiratory zone. The pulmonary vein leaves the capillary bed and is composed by addition of all the oxygenated blood flowing in progressively larger vessels, which empty into the left heart. A diagrammatic representation of partial pressures of O_2 and CO_2 and of the intravascular pressures is shown in Figure 2.12.

Resistance in the pulmonary circulation is normally about one tenth of the systemic vascular resistance (normal pulmonary = 50–150 dynes/sec/cm^{-5}; normal systemic = 900–1500 dynes/sec/cm^{-5}). The entire circulation flows through the pulmonary vasculature. Functionally, this requires less blood flow regulatory capability than the systemic circulation, which distributes portions of the circulation to organs and tissues above or distant from the heart. There are three major types of pulmonary vessels: the pulmonary capillaries, the alveolar vessels, and the major vessels around the mediastinum. The pulmonary capillaries are unusual in that they are surrounded by gas in the alveolus. When alveolar pressure rises above pulmonary capillary pressure, the capillary collapses and blood flow ceases. Extraalveolar vessels within the lung parenchyma respond in the same way as

airways and increase their dimensions with increasing lung volume. Due to radial traction of elastic lung parenchyma, pressure in these extraalveolar vessels is reduced as lung volume increases. The major vessels around the mediastinum respond to intrapleural pressure. Intrapleural pressure may be less subatmospheric than extraalveolar vessel pressures because of dynamic forces within lung parenchyma. The pulmonary vasculature is able to reduce acute rises in vascular resistance that might normally occur during the increased blood flow, e.g., during exercise. The two mechanisms that prevent marked rises in pulmonary pressures are the opening of previously closed vessels (recruitment) and the increase in caliber of already-open vessels (distension).

If the pressure difference between the alveolus and the pulmonary capillaries falls because of either an elevation in alveolar pressure or a fall in pulmonary capillary pressure, the resistance in pulmonary capillaries rises because of compression of the thin capillary walls. Re-

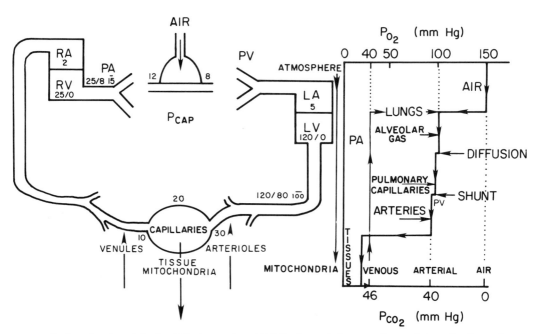

Figure 2.12. On the *right* the PO$_2$ *(upper)* and PCO$_2$ *(lower)* changes from air to mitochondria are shown. The depression in PO$_2$ caused by diffusion and shunt is illustrated. On the *left,* pressures (in mm Hg) in the pulmonary and systemic circulation including capillaries are compared. RA, right atrium; PA, pulmonary artery; RV, right ventricle; PV, pulmonary vein; LA, left atrium; LV, left ventricle. (Modified from West JB: *Respiratory Physiology—The Essentials,* ed 3, pp 32 and 53. Williams & Wilkins, Baltimore, 1985.)

sistance continues to rise as the transmural gradient between the alveolar and capillary pressure falls. At the point the alveolar pressure exceeds capillary pressure, transmural pressure becomes positive, pulmonary capillaries close, and blood flow through them ceases. There is an increase in pulmonary vascular pressures from apex to base. As a result of gradients in vascular transmural pressures, there are regional differences in perfusion ($\dot{Q}$). A model of distribution of ($\dot{Q}$) is shown in Figure 2.13 (West, 1964). In zone 1, alveolar pressure (PA) is greater than either pulmonary artery (Pa) or pulmonary vein (Pv) pressures. The pulmonary capillary is compressed, and no blood flow (shown on the right side of the diagram) occurs. In zone 2, Pa is greater than PA, but PA is greater than Pv. Blood flow in zone 2 is determined by the difference Pa − PA. Blood flow through the pulmonary capillaries progressively increases down zone 2 as Pa hydrostatic pressure increases and transpulmonary pressure falls. In zone 3, vascular pressures are greater than PA, and Pa is greater than Pv. Blood flow in zone 3 is determined by the usual arteriovenous pressure differences.

Regional differences also occur in ventilation ($\dot{V}$). At the base of the lungs, when a person is sitting or standing, pleural pressure becomes less subatmospheric because of the weight of the lungs. At FRC, PA is atmospheric throughout the lung. Therefore, the difference between PA and pleural pressure (known as transpulmonary pressure) becomes less from the apex to the base of the lung. The greater transpulmonary pressure at the apex of the lung results in open peripheral airways and alveoli, whereas at the bases, airways and alveoli are closed at low lung volumes. Normally, the apical alveoli remain open and have volume. They are higher up the pressure/volume curve of the lung at end expiration. Apical alveoli, therefore, have less potential for further volume increase with inspiration. The alveoli at the base of the lung are emptied at end expiration, and they are at the bottom of the pressure volume curve. With a tidal volume inspiration, the apical alveoli are ventilated initially because they are open. As lung volume increases, basal alveoli open and receive the majority of the tidal volume increase. Therefore, ventilation is greater in the base than in the apex. As was shown above, there is no perfusion of apical alveoli; the apical alveoli however, are open and do have some ventilation so that, relative to $\dot{Q}$; there is a large excess of $\dot{V}$. The $\dot{V}/\dot{Q}$ relationship is greater than 1 and tending toward infinity, since there is no blood flow in zone 1. In zone 2, there is better matching of $\dot{V}$ and $\dot{Q}$, and $\dot{V}/\dot{Q}$ is more nearly equal to 1. In zone 3, because blood flow ($\dot{Q}$) increases more than ventilation from the apex to the base of the lung, there is an excess of $\dot{Q}$ over $\dot{V}$. The $\dot{V}/\dot{Q}$ relationship in zone 3 is, therefore, less than 1.

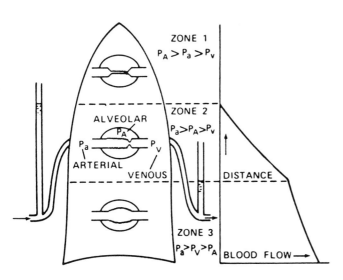

Figure 2.13. Model showing West's three zones and the uneven distribution of blood flow in the lung based on pressures affecting the capillaries. (From West JB, Colley CT, Naimak A: Distribution of blood flow in isolated lung: relation to vascular and alveolar pressures. *J Appl Physiol* 19:713, 1964.)

Dead Space and the Intrapulmonary Shunt

Considering the state in the zone 1 regions of the lung, there is an excess of ventilation over perfusion. The excess ventilation does not take part in gas exchange and is termed dead space. High $\dot{V}/\dot{Q}$ causes alveolar dead space. The combination of anatomical dead space and dead space occurring due to excess of ventilation over perfusion in the respiratory zone is called the physiological or Bohr dead space. Physiological dead space is always greater than anatomical dead space, since it is a combination of anatomical and alveolar dead space. When there is an excess of perfusion over ventilation, as in zone 3, some of the blood in the pulmonary capillaries is not in contact with alveolar gas across the alveolar-capillary membrane, and gas exchange does not take place. The nonoxygenated blood is referred to as intrapulmonary shunt or venous admixture. Both names are synonymous with blood that passes through the lungs and does not become oxygenated or remove CO_2. Anatomical intrapulmonary shunt is due to the bronchial blood supply that empties into the pulmonary vein and the thebesian veins that drain from the coronary sinus into the left ventricle. In congenital cardiac diseases such as atrial or ventricular septal defects, much greater anatomical right-to-left shunts may cause severe arterial hypoxemia. Hypoventilation causes hypoxemia if the rate of supply of O_2 to the alveolus is less than the rate of removal of O_2 by the blood. Although decreased diffusion of O_2 is a minor cause

of hypoxemia while breathing room air, when low inspired O_2 mixtures are breathed (such as occurs at high altitude), the alveolar end capillary blood O_2 content differences can become quite large.

By far, the most common and important cause of hypoxemia is ventilation/perfusion mismatch. When $\dot{V}/\dot{Q}$ is greater than 1, there is excess ventilated dead space. When $\dot{V}/\dot{Q}$ is less than 1, there is venous admixture. The possible relationships of $\dot{V}/\dot{Q}$ are summarized succinctly in the O_2–CO_2 diagram in Figure 2.14. In the extreme case where the airway is obstructed ($\dot{V} = O$) but blood flow ($\dot{Q}$) persists, there is intrapulmonary shunt (left side of diagram). The alveolar gas trapped behind the occluded airway would have the composition of mixed venous blood, namely, $PO_2 = 40$ mm Hg and $PCO_2 = 46$ mm Hg. In the opposite extreme, ventilation occurs and there is no blood flow (right side of diagram); the composition of alveolar gas would be the same as the inspired gas, namely, $PO_2 = 150$ mm Hg and $PCO_2 = 0$ mm Hg. Between these two extremes are gradations of $\dot{V}/\dot{Q}$ mismatch which are described by the solid line. Figure 2.13 shows how $\dot{V}/\dot{Q}$ decreases down the upright lung. Note that both blood flow and ventilation increase from the apex to the base of the lung, but blood flow increases more than ventilation. Opposite the third rib, ventilation and perfusion are matched and $\dot{V}/\dot{Q} = 1$ (West's zone 2). As a result of these regional differences in $\dot{V}/\dot{Q}$, O_2 is higher and CO_2 lower at the apex, and the reverse is true at the base of the upright lungs.

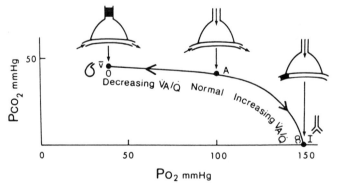

Figure 2.14. O_2–CO_2 diagram in which a single $\dot{V}/\dot{Q}$ ratio line is shown, representing the extremes of dead space and intrapulmonary shunt, with the PO_2 and PCO_2 at various $\dot{V}/\dot{Q}$ ratios. A, alveolar gas ($PO_2 = 100$, $PCO_2 = 40$); V, mixed venous point ($PO_2 = 40$, $PCO_2 = 45$); I, inspired point ($PO_2 = 150$, $PCO_2 = 0$ = room air). (From West JB: Ventilation/Blood Flow and Gas Exchange, ed 3. Blackwell Scientific Publications, Oxford, 1977.)

$\dot{V}/\dot{Q}$ mismatching occurs if a patient breathes at low lung volume because airways close. At low lung volumes, some airways are closed for part of each breath, and $\dot{V}/\dot{Q}$ is, therefore, reduced. With age, airways close at progressively larger lung volumes and gas exchange deteriorates. In pathological states such as atelectasis, lung contusion, or infection, a reduction in lung volume increases the amount of airway closure during tidal volume breathing, and gas exchange is impaired. Multiple inert gas tracer techniques are used to distinguish between intrapulmonary shunt and low $\dot{V}/\dot{Q}$ without altering their values (Wagner et al., 1974).

What are the clinical implications of $\dot{V}/\dot{Q}$ and shunt? Increasing the inspired oxygen concentration cannot directly increase the oxygenation of shunted blood but can improve O_2 content in the blood passing through low $\dot{V}/\dot{Q}$ units. In a patient with an early pneumonia, there is hypoxemia during room air breathing. $\dot{V}/\dot{Q}$ mismatch occurs as more lung regions become zone 3 (low $\dot{V}/\dot{Q}$). If oxygen is given, this compensates for $\dot{V}/\dot{Q}$ mismatch and allows more of the excessive blood perfusion to be oxygenated. As the pneumonia progresses and the inspired O_2 concentration is raised, more airways become obstructed and absorption atelectasis occurs. When atelectasis occurs $\dot{V}/\dot{Q}$ mismatch becomes intrapulmonary shunt. There is no gas exchange if blood flows past a collapsed alveolus. Increasing inspired oxygen does not improve arterial oxygenation if the cause of hypoxemia is intrapulmonary shunt. Raising the fraction of inspired O_2 (FIO_2) becomes progressively less and less effective as $\dot{V}/\dot{Q}$ mismatch converts to intrapulmonary shunt. Distinction between $\dot{V}/\dot{Q}$ mismatch and intrapulmonary shunt used to be made on the basis of measuring the partial pressure of oxygen (PaO_2) on 100% O_2. Hypoxemia due to the intrapulmonary shunt cannot be improved by increasing FiO_2, and PaO_2 remains low, whereas hypoxemia due to $\dot{V}/\dot{Q}$ mismatch can be improved. Two major errors, however, result from this technique: breathing 100% O_2 reverses hypoxic pulmonary vasoconstriction and

diverts blood to low $\dot{V}/\dot{Q}$ units, and 100% O_2 causes absorption atelectasis once nitrogen (from air) is washed out.

Gas Transport

Oxygen is carried attached to Hb and in solution. The oxygen capacity of arterial blood is determined by the product of Hb content, arterial saturation, and 1.39 ml/100 ml (the amount of O_2 carried by 1 gm of Hb; some authorities use 1.34 or even 1.36 ml/100 ml). Normal arterial oxygen content (CaO_2) is approximately 20 ml/100 ml of blood. Delivery of oxygen to the tissues is determined by the product of CaO_2 and cardiac output ($\dot{Q}_t$). Since $\dot{Q}_t$ at rest is approximately 5 liters/min, O_2 delivery is $5 \times 20 \times 10$ (to convert to ml/100 ml) or about 1000 ml/min. The only three variables that may be manipulated to improve O_2 delivery in a situation where there is evidence of inadequate tissue perfusion (evidence includes metabolic acidosis, low mixed venous O_2 tension, oliguria) are Hb, $\dot{Q}_t$, and arterial O_2 saturation. Cardiac failure in an anemic patient would require management to ensure that arterial desaturation was prevented. Chest physiotherapy, by removal of secretions, and mechanical ventilation, by decreasing O_2 consumption, may improve arterial saturation and O_2 delivery to the tissues.

Oxyhemoglobin Dissociation

The shape of the oxyhemoglobin (HbO_2) dissociation curve favors HbO_2 dissociation in capillary blood supplying metabolically active cells, and Hb gives up O_2 especially easily in the PO_2 range of 20–40 mm Hg where the curve is so steep (Fig. 2.15). The HbO_2 curve shifts to the right with decreasing pH, increasing PCO_2, increasing temperature, 2, 3-DPG and anemia. In low tissue perfusion states when acidosis occurs, the curve shifts to the right, and O_2 unloading at the tissues is facilitated, because at the same PO_2 the blood is less saturated. The difference between the amount of O_2 saturation at different pH and PCO_2 levels is

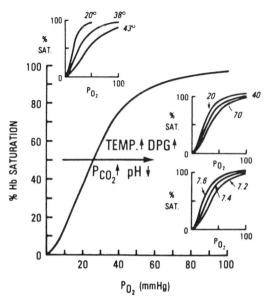

Figure 2.15. Oxyhemoglobin dissociation curve showing the right shift with changes in pH, PCO_2, temperature (TEMP.), and 2,3-diphosphoglycerate (DPG). Anemia also shifts the curve to the right. (From West JB: *Respiratory Physiology—The Essentials*, ed 3, p 71. Williams and Wilkins, Baltimore, 1985.)

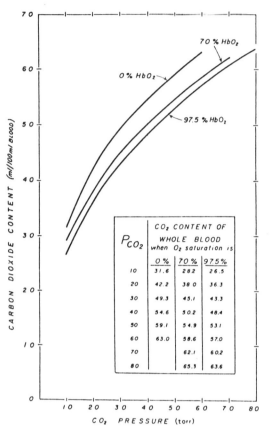

Figure 2.16. CO_2 dissociation curve. The relationship of CO_2 content of whole blood and PCO_2 varies with changes in saturation of Hb with O_2 (box insert). PCO_2 of the blood, therefore, influences O_2 saturation (Bohr effect), and O_2 saturation of the blood influences CO_2 content (Haldane effect). Note the CO_2 dissociation curve is almost linear between 40 and 60 mm Hg. (From Comroe JH: *Physiology of Respirations*, 2 ed, p 165. Year Book Medical Publishers, Chicago, 1965.)

known as the Bohr effect and results in extra O_2 availability for the tissues when pH falls and PCO_2 rises.

CO₂ Dissociation Curve

O_2 saturation of the blood also influences CO_2 carriage. Desaturated blood can carry more CO_2 than oxygenated blood. This effect of additional CO_2 carriage is called the Haldane effect. The CO_2 dissociation curve differs from the HbO_2 dissociation curve because in the physiological range it is essentially linear (Fig. 2.16). If alveolar ventilation is doubled, alveolar CO_2 is halved, and if alveolar ventilation is halved, alveolar CO_2 is doubled. This means that if atelectasis or other pulmonary pathology in one lung prevents adequate CO_2 removal in the diseased lung, hyperventilation of the good lung can compensate and prevent rises in arterial CO_2 above a normal value of 40 mm Hg. The end capillary CO_2, even in a totally nonventilated lung, does not exceed mixed venous CO_2, which is normally about 46 mm Hg.

O₂–CO₂ Diagrams

O_2 and CO_2 dissociation curves may be plotted together to show the O_2 saturation at any given PO_2 and PCO_2 (Fig. 2.17). The diagram allows arterial saturation to be determined when PCO_2 is either greater than or less than 40 mm Hg. A low arterial saturation may occur because of the effect of increased PCO_2.

Figure 2.14 shows another application of the information that can be obtained from the O_2–CO_2 diagram in which a single line represents the entire spectrum of possible $\dot{V}/\dot{Q}$ ratios. The result of analy-

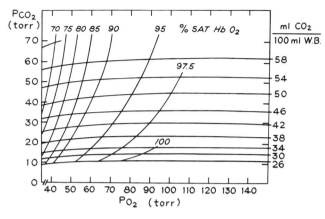

Figure 2.17. O_2–CO_2 diagram of Rahn and Fenn. PO_2 is plotted against PCO_2. There are seven lines of % saturation of HbO_2 called isopleths that represent equal volumes of O_2 combined with Hb at saturation between 70% and 100%. There are nine lines that are isopleths of CO_2 in vol %. The HbO_2 dissociation curve can be reconstructed from the HbO_2 saturation shown at each PO_2 when following the 40 mm Hg PCO_2 line from left to right. More specifically, this O_2–CO_2 diagram shows that with CO_2 retention, O_2 saturation falls, e.g., if PO_2 is 93 mm Hg and PCO_2 is 70 mm Hg, HbO_2 saturation is only 95% (when if PCO_2 was 40 mm Hg, HbO_2 saturation would be 97%). The lower saturation is not a function of diffusion impairment or other pulmonary disease. (From Comroe JH: *Physiology of Respiration,* 2 ed, p 166. Year Book Medical Publishers, Chicago, 1965.)

sis of alveolar PO_2 and PCO_2 at any point on the curve is obtained from the axis. At the extreme of dead space shown at *point I* (inspired point), alveolar gas is room air, contains no CO_2, and has a PO_2 of 150 mm Hg. This is quantitatively similar to the apex of the lung or West's zone 1. At the other end of the curve, which shows "true" intrapulmonary shunt, the alveolar gas tensions are the same as those found in mixed venous blood, namely, PO_2 = 40 mm Hg and PCO_2 = 46 mm Hg. The spectrum of increasing and decreasing $\dot{V}/\dot{Q}$ on either side of *point A* represents $\dot{V}/\dot{Q}$ mismatching, the most common cause of hypoxia. *Point A* (alveolar gas) describes the ideal alveolus where ventilation and perfusion are equal ($\dot{V} = \dot{Q} = 1$). This is similar to West's zone 2.

Human Respiratory Mucus

In a National Institutes of Health conference on human respiratory mucus published in the *American Review of Respiratory Diseases* (134:612–621, 1986) are summarized the present state of knowledge and approaches to management of bronchorrhea in adults. There was also a workshop to elucidate mechanisms of cough and the nature of bronchial expectoration which was published as a supplement to the *European Journal of Respiratory Disease* (61 (Supplement 110):

21–25, 1980). The following information is mostly abstracted from these sources.

The normal volume of tracheobronchial secretions is estimated to range from 10 to 100 ml/day. Mucus coats the airway from alveoli to the trachea and is 2–5 μm thick. The secretion is a heterogenous mixture derived from several sources. The four major constituents are mucus glycoprotein (MGP), lipids, proteins, and water. The cells producing the secretion include alveolar type II cells, Clara cells, goblet cells, and mucous and serous glandular cells of the surface epithelium. Duct cells from the submucous glands line the cartilage containing airways. Goblet cells occur throughout the respiratory tract down to the alveolar duct, where Clara cells are found.

Respiratory mucus has protective functions, which include lubrication, humidification, waterproofing, insulation, and provision of the environment for ciliary action (Kaliner et al., 1984). Mucus also acts as a selective macromolecular sieve to trap microorganisms and as an extracellular surface for immunoglobulin and enzyme action. Mucus neutralizes toxic gases, as in smoke inhalation, and, together with cilia, has a transport function in disposal of trapped materials. The defense mechanisms of mucus may be overwhelmed by excessive secretions or an increase in the proteins or cells. Noninfected tracheobronchial secretions are composed of 95% water, 0.5–1% protein, 0.5–0.8% lipid and 1–3% MGP (Potter et al., 1963, Lopez-Vidriero and Reid, 1980). With infection, more protein glycoprotein or deoxyribonucleic acid (DNA) from dead neutrophils is present in secretions. Increases in DNA decrease the flow of mucus. The viscosity and the elasticity of tracheobronchial secretions are due to the MGP. Patients with viral infections have impaired mucociliary clearance (Camner et al., 1973). *Mycoplasma pneumoniae* infection causes severely impaired mucociliary transport (Jarstand et al., 1974). Infections of the airway are probably unlikely unless mucociliary transport is depressed. Congenital nonfunctioning cilia cause chronic bronchitis, rhinitis, and sinusitis in early childhood (Camner et al., 1975; Eliasson, 1977; Mossberg and Camner, 1980).

Cholinergic nerves innervate and affect secretions from the airways; therefore, vagal stimulation and muscarinic agonists such as neostigmine cause increased secretion, and atropine, a muscarinic antagonist, reduces secretion. Adrenergic (α-agonist) drugs such as phenylephrine selectively stimulate secretion of lysozyme from serous cells of submucosal glands. Secretions after α-stimulation are of low viscosity and low elasticity. These sympathetically produced secretions could assist airway defenses, e.g., by diluting inhaled irritant materials. Circulating catecholamines, particularly epinephrine, with more adrenergic effects, however, produce more viscous secretions. Both α- and β-adrenergic mechanisms regulate the production of macromolecular secretions. Neuropeptides, such as substance P, and vasoactive intestinal peptides may also cause mucus secretion. The degradation of neuropeptides may regulate mucus secretion. Because there appears to be no motor nerve supply to surface submucosal glands and there is no response to cholinergic or adrenergic antagonists, secretory stimulation of surface cells is probably by neural mechanisms (Borson and Nadel, 1986). The effects of α-, β-, and muscarinic agonists on tracheal secretions in animals are shown in Table 2.4.

Using techniques to distinguish surface cells secretions from those of submucous glands, Varsano et al. (1986) have suggested that the macromolecules released by surface cells contribute to the viscoelastic properties of the mucous gel. Because of their location, surface cells probably play a role in airway inflammation (bacterial infections, bronchitis, asthma, cystic fibrosis). Surface cells also release arachidonic acid metabolites. In asthma, mucociliary clearance is delayed, and lipoxygenase products of arachidonic acid metabolism released from mast cells (located immediately outside vascular capillaries) appear to be the active mediators (Wanner et al., 1975). Inflammatory changes in asthma are responsible for many of the mucociliary changes in the disease, including status asthmaticus (Borson and Nadel, 1986). Mast cell degradation results from antigen interaction with immunoglobulin E and release of anaphylaxis mediators including prostaglandins, leukotrienes, lipoxygenase products, and bradykinin (Wasserman, 1983).

Products of the cyclooxygenase pathway of arachidonic acid metabolism (namely, prostaglandins A_2, D_2, E_1, and $F_{2\alpha}$) stimulate MGP secretion (Patow, 1986), as does histamine (Shelhamer et al., 1980). Cyclooxygenase inhibition,

Table 2.4
Effects of Adrenergic and Cholinergic Agonists on Properties of Tracheal Secretions on Animal Models[a]

Effect	α-Adrenergic Agonist	β-Adrenergic Agonist	Muscarinic Agonist
Fluid secretion from glands	↑↑↑	↑	↑↑↑
Macromolecular secretion	↑↑↑	↑↑	↑↑↑
Protein concentration	↓	↑	→
Mucus viscosity	↓	↑	→
Mucus elasticity	→	↓	→

[a]↑, increase; ↓, decrease; →, no change.

however, causes even greater secretion of MGP, implying that the lipoxygenase pathway is important in the regulation of MGP production. Leukotriene C_4 and D_4 are potent stimulants of MGP secretion (Marom, 1986).

The pulmonary macrophage functions as the first line of defense against inhaled particles, recruits other cell types to the inflamed lung, and participates in the mucous secretion process (Marom et al., 1984). Human macrophages and monocytes release a potent mucus secretagogue on surface activation. The secretagogue increases MGP secretion in pulmonary inflammatory states and infections and in smoking-related bronchitis. Complement may also be associated with increased mucous production. There is substantial data that C5a is generated during adult respiratory distress syndrome and that C5a is a potent mucus secretagogue (Marom, 1986).

Several therapies may reduce excessive mucus secretion: prostaglandin E_2, eicosatetraynoic acid and other lipoxygenase inhibitors (Table 2.5), atropine, cimetidine inhibition of histamine, vasoactive intestinal peptides, and glucocorticosteroids (Kaliner, 1986). As a clinical example of therapeutic application for asthmatic patients, systemic corticosteroids in bursts, inhaled corticosteroids and then atropine may be given when systemic steroids are tapered. Mucolytic agents and potassium iodide are not generally helpful. A single daily dose of tetracycline and inhaled β_2-adrenergic agonists, followed by postural drainage with chest percussion and vibration, may be a useful approach to mucous hypersecretion in the asthmatic (Kaliner, 1986).

EXAMINATION OF THE CHEST IN MECHANICALLY VENTILATED PATIENTS

Examination of the chest in mechanically ventilated patients is such a frequent necessity in the ICU that it is surprising how little is written about it. It differs from examination of the chest in nonintubated cooperative patients in several important respects. With controlled mechanical ventilation, there is loss of the patient's respiratory pattern and rate as indicators of disease. These may, however, still be usefully noted

Table 2.5
Human Respiratory Mucus Secretory Responses[a]

Agent	Airway Mucus	Nasal Turbinate Mucus
Methacholine	↑	↑
Atropine	NE	NE
Methacholine + atropine	NE	NE
α-Adrenergic agonists	↑	↑
β-Adrenergic agonists	NE	NE
Cyclic guanosine monophosphate	↑	—
Cyclic adenosine monophosphate	NE	—
Arachidonic acid	↑	NE
Prostaglandins E_1, $F_{2\alpha}$, D_2, I_2, A_2	↑	NE
Prostaglandin E_2	↓	—
Aspirin	↑	NE
Indomethacin	↑	NE
Eicosatetraynoic acid	↓	—
5-, 8-, 9-, 11-, or 15-Hydroxyeicosatetraenoic acid	↑	NE
5- and 9-Hydroperoxyeicosatetraenoic acid	↑	NE
Leukotriene C_4 or D_4	↑	NE
Anaphylaxis	↑	↑
Histamine	↑	↑
Prostaglandin-generating factor	↑	—
Macrophage or monocyte mucus secretagogue	↑	—
C3a	↑	—

[a] ↑, increased; NE, no net effect on mucus secretion; —, not studied.

when assisted or intermittent mandatory ventilation is used. The ventilated patient is unable to cooperate in such maneuvers as are required to elicit tactile vocal fremitus and vocal resonance because of tracheal intubation. There may be difficulties with percussion when dressings over chest tubes, incisions, or intravenous sites cover the chest. Frequently the patient cannot be positioned favorably for examination and is unable to clear adventitial sounds by coughing. Auscultatory sounds may, therefore, need interpretation in the light of mechanical ventilation and these possible restrictions.

Mechanical ventilation may, in some respects, make assessment of the respiratory system easier, but it requires adaption of other parts of the physical examination. Many of these problems have been overcome in the intensive care patient, and some of the compromises used are discussed. Examination, as is traditional, should be divided into inspection, palpation, percussion and auscultation.

Inspection

During controlled mechanical ventilation with the patient supine, discrepancies between movement of the two sides of the chest are easy to observe. The lungs are inflated with the same volume of gas at each breath, and the usual inspired volume variation seen in a spontaneously breathing patient is avoided. Diminished movement indicates disease of the lung, pleura, or chest wall of that side. The only exception to this may be caused by external restrictions. In the ICU, these include chest tubes and intravenous line dressings, arm slings, figure-of-eight bandages for clavicle fractures, and high abdominal binders. These all may cause diminished chest movement and almost certainly give rise to atelectasis if left in position (Fig. 2.18). The halo vest used in the management of cervical spine injuries may also prevent adequate inspection of the chest. If it is applied too tightly, it restricts chest movement, causing atelectasis in this particularly vulnerable patient population. Compared to the body cast, however, the halo vest has advantages, in that it may be loosened, allowing inspection, palpation, percussion, and auscultation. There is also less radiological interference from the vest than from the body cast. Unilateral application of external restrictions to the chest should, therefore, be considered as an

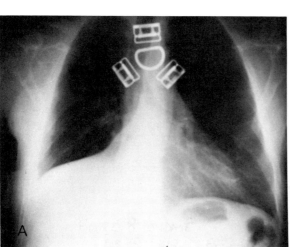 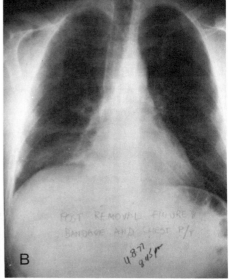

Figure 2.18 (**A**) A portable anteroposterior chest x-ray taken 36 hr after admission and application of a figure-of-eight bandage for the right fractured clavicle. (**B**) The right lower lobe atelectasis cleared completely after chest physiotherapy and removal of the bandage, as shown on the chest film taken 8 hr later.

important cause of diminished movement apart from disease of the underlying lung, pleura, or chest wall.

The first observation, therefore, is the equality of movement of either side of the chest. Notice should be taken of external evidence of trauma or previous operation. If chest tubes are present, these can be very helpful in determining the likely diagnosis on completion of the examination. Blood in a chest tube suggests a different respiratory problem from pus or serosanguineous drainage. The hourly rate of production of the drainage should also be noted. A chest tube may enable the diagnosis of bronchopleural fistula to be made, when air is seen bubbling through the water seal drainage bottle with inspiration of the ventilator. This is most easily observed when there is no suction applied to the water seal. Measurement of inspired and expired volume, which are separated by placing a shunt valve in the Y-piece of the ventilator tubing, enables this leak to be quantitated.

Lastly, the ventilator airway pressure gauge can give useful information concerning total lung/thorax compliance (C_t) and airway resistance. Details of the calculations are given in Chapter 7. Examination for cyanosis and finger clubbing, the observation of the anteroposterior (AP) diameter of the chest, and note of any kyphoscoliosis may provide additional information about a previous history of respiratory disease.

Palpation

Palpation may be restricted because of dressings covering incisions, chest tubes, and intravenous infusion sites, particularly those in the subclavian area. Rib fractures may be felt as crepitus during inspiration, expiration, and coughing. If the patient is conscious, tenderness may be elicited. The clinical diagnosis of rib fractures is helpful, since this finding may be missed on the initial chest radiograph of a patient with multiple trauma, if specific rib films are not taken. Subcutaneous emphysema may also be present and palpable, initially over the neck and chest wall. In mechanically ventilated patients this is frequently due to small

airway rupture. Air can be identified in the mediastinum on chest x-ray and may give rise to pneumothoraces (Macklin and Macklin, 1944). If coughing occurs and a pneumothorax is present, it may be further aggravated, giving rise to a tension pneumothorax. Observation of ventilator airway pressure may be diagnostic. A sudden rise in peak and end-inspiratory pressures is indicative of a rise in intrathoracic pressure that accompanies pneumothorax.

Tactile vocal fremitus may not be elicited in mechanically ventilated patients unless there are rhonchi present. Rhonchi are low pitched and usually associated with large airway pathology. They may, therefore, be palpable. Crackles are not palpable. Tracheal deviation may normally be a useful sign of upper lobe pathology or pneumothorax. In the intubated patient, this happens less frequently because the tracheal tube tends to prevent it. Despite the presence of a tracheal tube, deviation away from the side of a tension pneumothorax may commonly occur and should always be looked for when a pneumothorax is suspected.

Percussion

Percussion is useful in the diagnosis of pneumothorax. Besides the reduction in chest movement, a pneumothorax is hyperresonant to percussion and is, therefore, immediately differentiated from fluid, which gives a stony dullness to percussion. In a patient with fluid in the chest, turning may elicit a shift in the dullness to the dependent part of the lung. This does not occur if the fluid is loculated. Shifting dullness should differentiate free fluid from consolidation, collapse or fibrosis which also elicit dullness and cause diminished chest movement. Clinical examination of the patient who cannot sit up may be obtained by percussion bilaterally over the anterior chest. This should be followed by percussion in both midaxillary lines before turning the patient laterally for posterior chest examination. Examination of the chest by percussion in the lateral position of a multiply monitored patient may cause more problems than there is additional information gained. This is a useful way to confirm fluid, however, if there is more resonance in the axilla after turning. Percussion, palpation, and auscultation should be performed in relation to the underlying lung lobes. The surface anatomy of these is shown in Figure 2.1A–C.

Auscultation

The first questions the examiner should ask on placing a stethoscope on the chest of a mechanically ventilated patient are: "Do I hear breath sounds?"; and if so, "Are the breath sounds vesicular or bronchial?" A vesicular breath sound is louder during inspiration and has a longer expiration, and there is no pause between inspiration and expiration. It is normally heard over all peripheral lung fields. Bronchial breathing is louder than vesicular breathing and has a pause between inspiration and expiration. Expiration is louder and longer than inspiration. Bronchial breath sounds are harsh and abnormal except when heard over the trachea anteriorly and between the scapulae posteriorly. The usual plots of normal breath sounds are helpful in making the distinction between vesicular and bronchial breath sounds (Fig. 2.19).

Bronchial breathing occurs when there is loss of the normal air/alveolus interface. In other words, when the lung becomes solid due to consolidation, fluid, fibrosis, or collapse of peripheral bronchi, the sounds that are normally heard in the central region of the tracheobronchial tree are now transmitted peripherally by the physical means of the solid lung. Bronchial breathing is, therefore, likely to be heard in pneumonia, lung contusion, or segmental collapse. It is abnormal when heard in areas of the lungs where vesicular breathing occurs normally. The bronchial breath sounds are heard over the area where the disease process is taking place. The surface anatomy should, therefore, be noted and related to the underlying lung lobes and segments (Fig. 2.1A–C). In lung contusion, one of the characteristic clinical and radiological findings is that the contused area does not conform to, and is not restricted by, normal anatomical lung segmental distribution, as would be expected in other pathology. Maximum radiological change is commonly seen 12 or more hours after injury, and clinical and

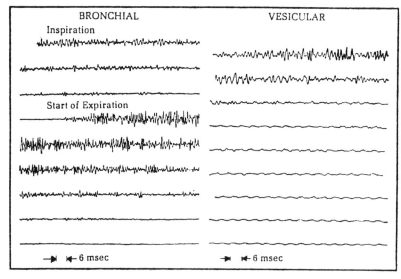

Figure 2.19. On the *left* is shown a time intensity plot of a normal bronchial breath sound. Inspiration is shorter than expiration. There is a well-marked pause between inspiration and expiration. Expiration is louder and longer than inspiration. On the *right* is shown a time intensity plot of a normal vesicular breath sound. The trace begins at inspiration. Inspiration is louder than expiration. There is no clear demarcation between inspiration and expiration. (From Murphy RLH: *A Simplified Introduction to Lung Sounds.*)

radiological examinations frequently underestimate the extent of the contusion (Shin et al., 1979).

If no breath sounds are heard when listening over the chest, this is indicative that there is no air entry to the underlying lung or that something is preventing the transmission of the breath sounds. A comparison should be made with the same area of lung on the other side of the chest. Absence of breath sounds indicates lung pathology. Diminution of breath sounds may be present in obesity or increased muscle mass but may also indicate underlying lung pathology. Breath sounds may be absent in the presence of a pneumothorax, pleural fluid, or a major lobar collapse. Atelectasis or fibrosis cause diminished breath sounds.

Next, the presence of any adventitial sounds should be noted. An adventitial sound is any sound not normally occurring. These can be described in many ways. Various names have been attached to adventitial sounds. A low-pitched sound may be referred to as a rhonchus (or a low-pitched wheeze), and a high-pitched sound, as a wheeze, rale, crackle, or crepitation. Since the latter sound may frequently be divided into fine or coarse, which may be synonymous with a particular lung pathology, considerable confusion exists as to their precise meaning. Therefore, only three terms are used: crackle, rhonchus, and wheeze. The crackle is high pitched, the rhonchus is low pitched, and the wheeze is high pitched and most common and loud in expiration which is also prolonged. Murphy et al., (1977), by means of time-expanded wave-form analysis, showed that crackles are discontinuous sounds and wheezes are continuous sounds. Visualization of these lung sounds by electronic means is extremely helpful and is shown in Figure 2.20 together with nomenclature. Crackles are associated with pulmonary edema, interstitial fibrosis, or pneumonia. Rhonchi are found with excess sputum production, in bronchitis, and in association with absorption atelectasis. They are produced by narrowing of the bronchial lumen due to spasm, swelling, or secretions. Bleeding from a severe lung contusion may give rise to rhonchi in other areas of lung not origi-nally affected by the contusion. Rhonchi may clear after coughing or tracheal suctioning. Wheezes are found with airway narrowing and obstruction. If the cause of wheezing is bronchoconstriction, this may be aggravated by coughing and suctioning. Wheezing due to retained secretions, however, may diminish after their removal. Some of these clinical signs may now be associated with commonly occurring acute lung pathology. This is conveniently done in Table 2.6.

Pitfalls of Clinical Examination in the Mechanically Ventilated Patient

There are several pitfalls in clinical examination of the chest of intubated and mechanically ventilated patients. These may be deceptive to even a most experienced clinician. For example, a right endobronchial intubation may give rise to signs resembling an atelectasis of the left lung. If allowed to persit, it commonly produces both left lung and right upper lobe atelectasis. Because the right upper lobe bonchus branches off the main stem bronchus about 2–3 mm below the carina, it is very susceptible to occlusion with endobronchial intubation (Fig. 2.5C). Unlike atelectasis, signs of decreased movement, dullness to percussion, and decreased air entry completely disappear on extubation of the right bronchus if this is recognized soon enough. A deceptive adventitial sound may be heard if air leaks around the cuff of a tracheal tube. Since airway pressure of mechanical ventilators is highest on inspiration, the leak is likely to be heard and felt at this time; if only slight, it can mimic a wheeze. If this is thought to be the cause, brief compression of the pilot balloon of the tracheal tube should raise cuff pressure sufficiently to occlude the trachea and prevent the air leak around the cuff. Auscultation over the neck should verify this finding.

Obstruction of the tracheal tube by inspissated secretions or partial kinking may produce elevated airway pressures, and the resulting turbulence may alter the character of the breath sounds. Water in the ventilator tubing that has spilled over from a humidifier or kinking of compliant ventilator tubing can give a se-

Lung Sounds' Classifications and Nomenclature

Acoustic Characteristics	Time-Expanded Waveform	Recommended Term	English	French	German	Japanese	Portuguese	Spanish	Some Common Clinical Associations
Discontinuous, interrupted, explosive sounds—loud, duration of about 10 ms; low in pitch: initial deflection, width averaging 1.5 ms.	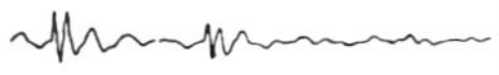	Coarse crackle	Coarse crackles	Râles bulleux ou Sous-crepitants	Grobes Rassein	強髪音	Estertores grossos	Estertores gruesos	Pulmonary edema resolving pneumonia
Discontinuous, interrupted, explosive sounds—less loud and of shorter duration; they average less than 5 ms in duration and are lower in pitch; initial deflection width averages about 0.7 ms	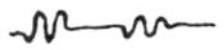	Fine crackle	Fine crackles	Râles crepitants	Feines Rassein	水泡音	Estertores finos	Estertores finos	Interstitial fibrosis (eg, asbestosis)
Continuous sounds—longer than 250 ms, high-pitched dominant frequency of 400 Hz or more; a hissing sound	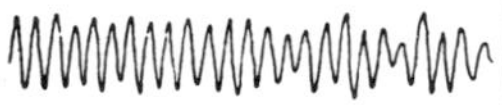	Wheeze	Wheezes	Râles sibilants	Pfeifen	ヒュー（笛）音	Sibilos	Sibilancias	Airway narrowing (eg, asthma)
Continuous sounds—longer than 250 ms, low-pitched, dominant frequency about 200 Hz or less; a snoring sound	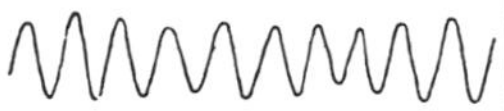	Rhonchus	Rhonchus	Râles ronflants	Brummen	いびき（様）音	Roncos	Roncus	Sputum production (eg, bronchitis)

Figure 2.20. Time-expanded wave forms of crackles, rhonchi, and wheezes together with International nomenclature. (From Andrews JL Jr, Badges IL: Lung sounds through the ages. *JAMA* 241:2629, 1979, and Cugell DW: Lung sound nomenclature. *Am Rev Respir Dis* 136:1016, 1987.)

Pathological Process	Inspection	Palpation	Percussion	Auscultation
Pneumothorax	↗ or ↓ movement; C_T ↓, P_{max} ↑, P_{IE} ↑ if tension; otherwise may be N	Possible subcutaneous emphysema; tracheal deviation away from pneumothorax if tension	Hyperresonance over pneumothorax	Breath sounds ↓ or absent
Pulmonary edema	Movement N; frothy sputum in tracheal tube; C_T ↓, P_{max} N or ↗, P_{IE} ↑	If florid, palpable fluid in airways	Dullness	Crackles and wheezes
Atelectasis	↓ movement; C_T ↓; P_{max} N or ↗; P_{EE} ↑	Tracheal deviation towards lesion if complete upper lobe atelectasis	Dullness over area of collapse	Breath sounds ↓ or absent with major collapse; maybe bronchial breathing and crackles
Contusion	Bruising may be present; movement N or ↓; C_T ↓; P_{max} N or ↗; P_{IE} ↑	May be tenderness and crepitus over fractured ribs	Dullness over contusion	Bronchial breathing; wheezes and rhonchi if excessive bleeding
Aspiration	Movement N or ↓; C_T N or ↓; P_{max} N or ↗; P_{IE} N or ↗	Rhonchi may be palpable	Dullness may be present	Vesicular breathing; rhonchi
Pleural fluid	Movement ↓; C_T N or ↓; P_{mzx} N or ↑; P_{IE} N or ↑ depending on quantity	No breath sounds palpable; tracheal deviation away from fluid if voluminous	Stony dullness may clear on turning patient if fluid not loculated	Breath sounds absent; may be bronchial breathing about fluid
Pneumonia	Movement ↓; C_T ↗; P_{max} ↗; P_{IE} ↗	Pleural rub may be palpable	Dullness over consolidation	Early breath sounds ↓; bronchial breathing crackles and pleural rub
Fibrosis	Movement ↓; C_T ↓; P_{max} ↑; P_{IE} ↑	Tracheal deviation toward fibrosis	Dullness over fibrosis	Breath sounds ↗; bronchial breathing and crackles

[a] ↘, slightly decreased; ↓, decreased; ↑, increased; ↗, slightly increased; P_{max}, maximum airway pressure; P_{IE}, end-inspiratory pressure; N, normal.

ries of apparently unexplainable sounds that may, at times, resemble mucus secretions in the larger airways. Sump drains in the subhepatic or splenic bed areas may considerably confuse auscultation of the chest when they are connected to vacuum suction. Equally, nasogastric tubes on continuous low suction drainage may cause additional sounds. The loudest and most easily recognizable additional sound occurs with chest tubes connected through drains to vacuum suction. This abruptly terminates if the chest tube is briefly clamped.

RADIOLOGICAL INDICATIONS FOR CHEST PHYSIOTHERAPY

Almost without exception in a critical care unit, the patient has a daily portable chest x-ray. The practice of clinical examination backed up by radiological confirmation ensures a high degree of success in establishing the area of pulmonary infiltrates. Although clinical examination is often correct, the chest x-ray offers an additional dimension that is frequently not possible with clinical examination alone. The additional dimension is the ability to pinpoint the lung infiltrate not just to a lobar distribution but to a specific segment within the lobe. This is of utmost importance to the chest physical therapist in determining the correct postural drainage position.

Patients in the ICU are unable to be transported to the radiology department for a chest x-ray if they are critically ill. Routinely, therefore, portable AP chest x-rays are taken of these patients. If these are taken with the patient in the erect position, there are several advantages. The erect chest x-ray allows better visualization of the superior mediastinum (Ayella, 1977) and comparative assessment of heart size on a daily basis if the film is exposed with the same degree of inspiration. The erect position accentuates the presence of free pleural fluid which gravitates, giving a characteristic blunting of the costophrenic angle seen with pleural effusion. In patients with spinal and pelvic injuries, the x-ray is normally taken with the patient in the supine position. The radiograph should be exposed on full inspiration; therefore, the radiology technician should be familiar with the association of ventilator airway pressure and full inspiration for mechanically ventilated patients.

Localization of Lung Segments

Based on anatomical bronchial segments, specific areas of the lung correspond to individual bronchi on a straight AP chest x-ray. There is, however, some overlapping of areas due to superimposition of the lobes in the AP projection. The localization of these segments is somewhat different from many other similar diagrams, but the designations shown in Figure 2.21A–C are based on the anatomy of the bronchial tree segments on bronchography and on nuclear scanning (Ayella, 1978a). The silhouette sign and air bronchogram together with the segmental anatomy are used to localize lung pathology, so that chest physiotherapy is directed at specific lung segments.

Silhouette Sign

The silhouette sign occurs when two separate structures adjacent to each other have the same densities. The border between the two is not identifiable on x-ray because of the lack of contrast in densities. In normal circumstances on chest x-ray the heart, diaphragm, and mediastinum have contrasting densities to the aerated lung. The borders of the heart, diaphragm, and upper mediastinum are, therefore, clearly visible on chest x-ray. When lung pathology occurs in segments adjacent to these structures and the lung becomes consolidated, atelectatic, edematous, or fibrotic, however, its density increases, and the contrast with the cardiac, mediastinal, and diaphragmatic borders is lost. The lung segments adjacent to various structures within the chest are shown in Figures 2.22, 2.24, 2.26, and 2.30. Loss of the definition of these borders infers pathological involvement of the adjacent lung segment. It appears to be quite specific. Figure 2.23A shows atelectasis of the right upper lobe which responded to a single treatment with chest physiotherapy (Fig. 2.23B). Silhouette of the left and right heart borders is shown diagrammatically in Figure 2.24 and in clinical practice in Figure 2.25A. The atelectasis of

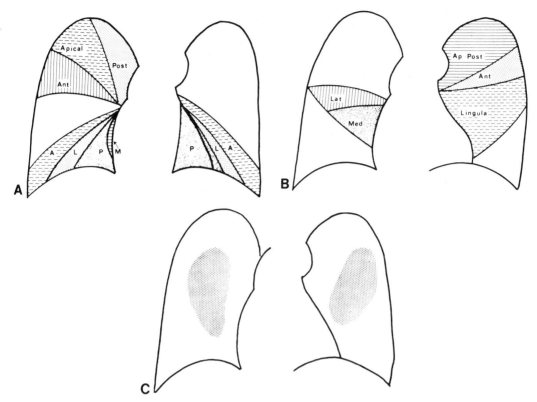

Figure 2.21. (A) Bronchopulmonary segments of the right upper lobe and basal segments of both lower lobes as seen on a straight AP chest x-ray. The mediastinum and diaphragm are outlined in this and in B and C. Note contact of lower lobes with diaphragm and right upper lobes with superior mediastinum. (B) Bronchopulmonary segments of the right middle and left upper lobe. Note contact with right heart border, left heart border, and superior mediastinum. (C) Superior segments of both lower lobes are large but make no contact with mediastinum or diaphragm. Compare the radiological bronchopulmonary segmental distribution shown here with the surface anatomy shown in Figure 2.1. (From Ayella RJ: *Radiologic Management of the Massively Traumatized Patient,* p 95, Figs. 8.25–8.27. (Williams & Wilkins, Baltimore, 1978.)

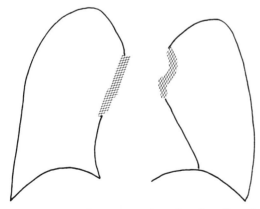

Figure 2.22. Silhouette sign showing "loss" of the superior mediastinum bilaterally. This indicates right posterior and left apical posterior segmental atelectasis of the upper lobes. (From Ayella RJ: *Radiologic Management of the Massively Traumatized Patient,* p 96, Williams & Wilkins, Baltimore, 1978a.)

the lingula is successfully cleared by physiotherapy, and the left heart border becomes visible (Fig. 2.25B). The silhouette sign of lower lobe atelectasis is shown in Figure 2.26. The diaphragm from the outer third, medially, silhouettes the anterior lateral and posterior segments of the lower lobe, respectively. The diaphragm appears to be "lost" opposite the anterior (Fig. 2.27) and the posterior segments (Fig. 2.28) in these AP erect portable chest x-rays. A complete atelectasis of the left lower lobe (Fig. 2.29A) partially reexpands with chest physiotherapay (Fig. 2.29B). To completely clear this atelectasis of the posterior basal segment of the left lower lobe, the patient required the correct, specific, postural drainage position. Each segment of the lower lobe has a different postural

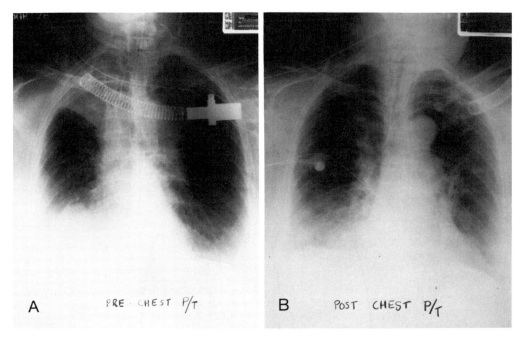

Figure 2.23. (A) Note "loss" of the right superior mediastinum and atelectasis of the right upper lobe. Also, there is "loss" of the right hemidiaphragm, indicating atelectasis of the right lower lobe. (B) After a single treatment with chest physiotherapy the right upper lobe is now reexpanded, and the right superior mediastinum outline is clearly visible. The right lower lobe atelectasis has also reexpanded, and the diaphragm outline is now visible.

drainage position, so that identification before therapy is of the utmost importance. In order to clear a total lower lobe atelectasis completely, five different postural drainage positions may be required.

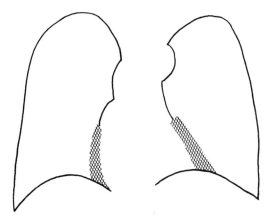

Figure 2.24. Silhouette sign showing "loss" of the right and left heart borders. This indicates middle lobe and lingula involvement. (From Ayella RJ: *Radiologic Management of the Acutely Traumatized Patient,* p 96, Fig 8.28B. Williams & Wilkins, Baltimore, 1978a.)

The importance of identification of segmental involvement to the chest physical therapist is, therefore, immense. If the involved segment can be identified, the patient can be positioned in the ideal drainage position, and percussion and vibration therapy can be carried out in this position. In our opinion this approach greatly increases the likelihood of clearance of the area of lung involvement. A complete atelectasis of the left upper lobe (including lingula) silhouettes the left heart and the superior mediastinum (Fig. 2.30). The chest x-ray shows haziness of the left heart border and superior mediastinum (Fig. 2.31A) which cleared with chest physiotherapy (Fig. 2.31B).

Air Bronchogram

The air bronchogram is the reverse of the phenomenon that causes the silhouette sign. Since air is less dense than consolidated, edematous, contused, or fibrosed lung, the differing densities result in a line of demarcation visible on chest x-ray. In normal circumstances there is

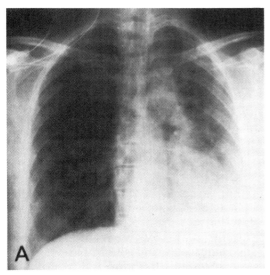 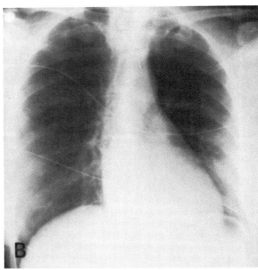

Figure 2.25 (**A**) Note loss of the left heart border in this chest x-ray showing atelectasis of the lingula. The diaphragm is visible. (**B**) After chest physiotherapy the heart has now moved to the right, and the lingula is reexpanded. The left heart border is now clearly visible.

no demarcation because the lungs, and the bronchi are both well aerated. With loss of air in the lung the density contrast is apparent between the air in the bronchi and the more dense lung. If a mucus plug is thought to be the cause of the atelectasis, this may be apparent, on the straight AP film, as a sharp cutoff of the

air bronchogram. If an air bronchogram is visible to the peripheral lung fields, the lesion is unlikely to be due to a mucus plug. Bronchoscopy is usually not helpful in patients who have an air bronchogram that can be traced to the peripheral lung field. This is because most fiberoptic

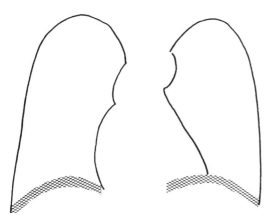

Figure 2.26. Silhouette sign showing "loss" of diaphragms. If the outer one third is missing, the anterior segment is indicated; if the middle one third is missing, the lateral segment is indicated; and if the inner one third is missing, the posterior segment of the lower lobes is indicated. (From Ayella RJ: *Radiologic Management of the Massively Traumatized Patient,* p 96, Fig 8.28C. Williams & Wilkins, Baltimore, 1978a.)

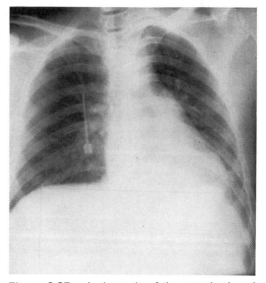

Figure 2.27. Atelectasis of the anterior basal segment of the left lower lobe. The lateral third of the diaphragm is "lost." (From Ayella RJ: *Radiologic Management of the Massively Traumatized Patient,* p 121, Fig 8.90. Williams & Wilkins, Baltimore, 1978a.)

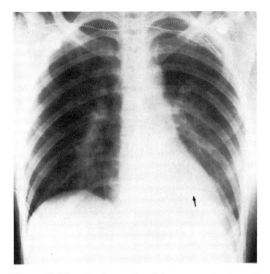

Figure 2.28. Atelectasis of the posterior basal segment of the left lower lobe. The medial third of the diaphragm, from the *arrow,* is missing. (From Ayella RJ: *Radiologic Management of the Massively Traumatized Patient,* p 120, Fig 8.89. Williams & Wilkins, Baltimore, 1978a.)

bronchoscopes are too large to be passed beyond the third generation of bronchial divisions and the secretion retention involves the 16–23 generations much more peripherally (see p. 308).

ACUTE INDICATIONS FOR CHEST PHYSIOTHERAPY

Blood Gas Changes

If a patient requires mechanical ventilation, a controlled readily determined FIO_2 is administered, and arterial blood gas analyses are necessary. Critically ill patients may have three arterial blood gas analyses during a 24-hr period. Other analyses are done if the clinical situation is believed to justify the requirement or after ventilator adjustment. With use of the pulse oximeter and the on-line end-tidal CO_2 monitor, blood gases may be less frequently analyzed.

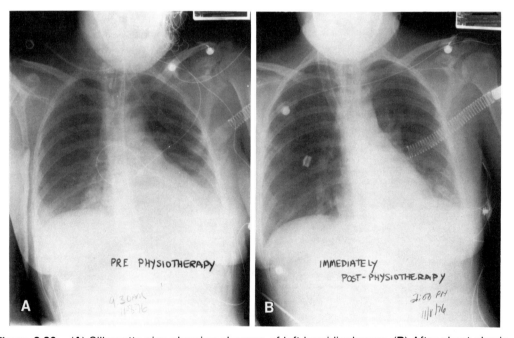

Figure 2.29. (**A**) Silhouette sign showing absence of left hemidiaphragm. (**B**) After chest physiotherapy the outer two thirds of the left hemidiaphragm is clearly visible. There is still an infiltrate in the posterior segment of the left lower lobe which silhouettes with the medial third of the diaphragm.

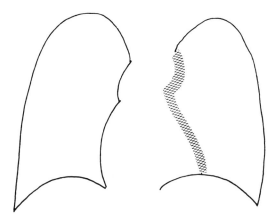

Figure 2.30. Complete loss of the left heart border and superior mediastinum indicates a complete left upper lobe atelectasis. (From Ayella RJ: *Radiologic Management of the Massively Traumatized Patient*, p 96, Fig. 8.28D. Williams & Wilkins, Baltimore, 1978a.)

Accurate knowledge of the PaO_2 and FIO_2 enables calculation of the PaO_2/FIO_2 ratio to approximate the degree of blood shunting occurring in the lungs. PaO_2/FIO_2 is a good approximation of intrapulmonary shunt (Q_s/Q_t) up to 20%

(Aye et al., 1978). If PaO_2/FIO_2 is less than 200, the patient, the ventilator, and the current chest x-ray should be examined to determine any clinical, mechanical, or radiological reason for the increased shunt. If there was clinical or radiological evidence of retained secretions, the most involved lung segments are identified, and chest physiotherapy is performed with the patient in the postural drainage position for the affected segments. After repeating the blood gas analysis, if PaO_2/FIO_2 is not greater than 200, positive end-expiratory pressure (PEEP) is added in increments to a maximum of 10 cm H_2O so that functional residual capacity may be increased and intrapulmonary shunt improved (McIntyre and Laws, 1969). Further increases in PEEP beyond 10 cm H_2O are monitored with a pulmonary artery catheter in order to exclude a cardiac cause of increased shunt. Patients with high shunts may benefit from chest physiotherapy alone, without the addition of further increments of PEEP. Causes of $\dot{V}/\dot{Q}$ mismatch that may be improved by chest physiotherapy include atelectasis and secretion retention.

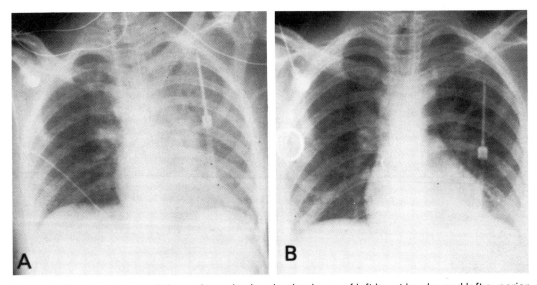

Figure 2.31.   A. Left upper lobe atelectasis showing haziness of left heart border and left superior mediastinum. **B.** After physiotherapy and reexpansion of the atelectasis these borders become clearly visible. (From Ayella RJ: *Radiologic Management of the Massively Traumatized Patient*, p 119, Fig. 8.85A and B. Williams & Wilkins, Baltimore, 1978a.)

Pneumonia

Pneumonia may be improved by chest physiotherapy, but this is controverisal and hinges on the definition of pneumonia. Graham and Bradley (1978) could show no improvement, using intermittent positive-pressure breathing and 20 min of chest physiotherapy, in the resolution of pneumonia. They have however, excluded many of the diseases associated with pneumonia, such as lung abscess, bronchitis, and bronchiectasis, that are thought to benefit from therapy. They also used the therapy for only 20 min at each treatment session. In our experience this duration may not be sufficient to clear retained secretions (Mackenzie et al., 1980a). The concept of a predetermined length of therapy is unacceptable; rather, the chest physical therapist should continue until there is clinical evidence of improvement in the area being treated or sputum production ceases. Evidence for the benefit of chest physiotherapy in a patient with pneumonia is presented in the case history below.

Case History 2.1. A 19-year old male was admitted by helicopter directly from the scene of an automobile accident. The patient was a passenger in a truck hit by a train. He arrived unconscious, with a right tension pneumothorax, absent bowel sounds, and hematuria. Chest x-ray showed fracture of the first right and second left ribs. Minilaparotomy was positive, and the patient went to the operating room for placement of an intracranial pressure monitor (intracranial pressure, 9 mm Hg) and for laparotomy, which revealed a ruptured spleen and renal contusion.

The patient remained unconscious due to cerebral contusion for 17 days. Starting 9 days after admission, *Pseudomonas aeruginosa* was grown for 3 successive days from tracheal cultures. Maximum daily temperature (T_{max}), white blood cell count, and chest x-ray findings from the time of positive tracheal cultures are shown in Table 2.7.

Eleven days after admission, there was no obvious source found for the leukocytosis and pyrexia, and the chest x-ray was not thought to be sufficient to account for these changes despite the positive tracheal cultures. On the twelfth day after admission, the morning chest x-ray showed development of fluffy infiltrates in the left lower lobe and right middle and lower lobes (Fig. 2.32). These, and clinical examination, were thought to be compatible with a left lower lobe pneumonia. Tobramycin and ticarcillin were suggested but not given, because, following 45 min of chest physiotherapy, arterial oxygenation (PaO_2), C_T, and temperature all improved significantly. A repeat chest x-ray also showed improvement. The PaO_2, C_T and temperature changes before and after chest physiotherapy are shown in Table 2.8.

The leukocytosis and pyrexia decreased (Table 2.7), and the chest x-ray showed marked improvement by the following day (Fig. 2.33). The patient had two further chest physiotherapy treatments, on days 14 (Fig. 2.34) and 15 (Fig. 2.35). Chest x-ray confirmed complete resolution, and he was extubated on the seventeenth day after admission. The laboratory, chest x-ray, and clinical data strongly suggested that chest physiotherapy had played a significant role in reversal of the patient's pneumonia.

Table 2.7
T_{max}, **White Blood Cell Count (WBC), and Chest X-ray Findings of Patient in Case History 2.1 for 1 Week after *P. aeruginosa* Cultures Showing Pyrexia, Leukocytosis, and Development of Pneumonia (Chest Physiotherapy Given on Days 12–15)**

Day from Admission	T_{max} (°F)	WBC	Chest X-ray
9	101.6	24,600	Clear
10	101.8	33,800	Clear
11	102.6	37,400	Slight infiltrate in left lower and right middle lobes
12	103	36,100	Fig. 2.31
		First Chest Physiotherapy Given	
13	100.4	27,600	Fig. 2.32
14	101.8	22,500	Fig. 2.33
15	100.8	24,200	Fig. 2.34

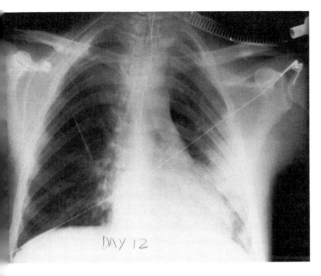

Figure 2.32. Fluffy infiltrates in the left lower lobe and lingula and right lower lobe developed on the twelfth day after admission.

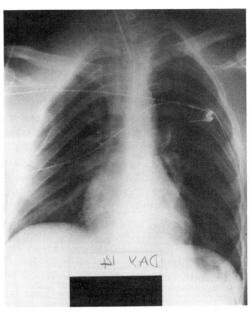

Figure 2.34. Morning chest x-ray on the fourteenth day after admission.

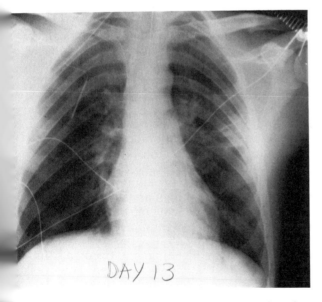

Figure 2.33. Marked clearing of pneumonitis the day after chest physiotherapy was given.

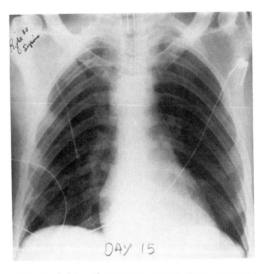

Figure 2.35. Complete resolution of pneumonia on the fifteenth day after admission.

In the ICU, pneumonia commonly occurs as the end product of secretion retention behind blocked airways. It is an extremely difficult diagnosis to make. Positive bacteriological cultures from the airway of tracheally intubated patients are commonplace. The difficulty occurs in identifying whether these are pathological. A method of increasing the likelihood of obtaining cultures of a pathological organism from tracheally intubated patients by peripheral sampling has been described. By using this method the pathological organism was successfully cultured at a peripheral airway despite polymicrobial colonization of the upper airways (Matthew et al., 1977). This method, however, has been disputed as an effective diagnostic aid (Boysen et al., 1980). Also, the ICU patient commonly has a temperature elevation and leukocytosis that may be related to a pneumonic process. Lastly, the presence of infiltrates within the lung does not necessarily signify pneumonia. Radiological infiltrates in 70% of cases that are unilateral and 60% that are bilateral may be improved by one treatment of chest physiotherapy (Mackenzie et al. 1978b). These are, therefore, unlikely to be pneumonia. The cardinal signs of pneumonia, positive sputum culture, temperature with a leukocytosis, and compatible radiological infiltrate have little meaning as criteria for making the diagnosis in the ICU. Were these circumstances allowed to persist without attempts at removal of the retained secretions, however, the accumulation would certainly give rise to pneumonia. More recent data (Salata et al., 1987) indicate that examination of serial tracheal aspirates for elastin fibers and by graded gram's strain may enable differentiation of colonization from nosocomial pneumonia. The presence of elastin fibers in sterile suction catheter aspirations occurred about 2 days before radiological pulmonary infiltrates. Sucralfate for stress ulcer prophylaxis rather than antacids or histamine type 2 blockers prevents gastric colonization of the airway and reduces the risk of nosocomial pneumonia in mechanically ventilated patients (Driks et al., 1987) Bronchioalveolar lavage and a combination of topical and intravenous antibiotics improve the diagnosis and prevent development of nosocomial pneumonia in animals (Johanson et al., 1988a,b).

In practice, if lung infiltrates that cannot be cleared within 36 hours of their appearance and the other criteria exist, a diagnosis of pneumonia is made. At this point Graham and Bradley's conclusions that pneumonia does not benefit from chest physiotherapy may be true. The treatment now includes appropriate antibiotics. Until this point, the removal of retained secretions and the opening up of blocked airways may prevent the propagation of pneumonia.

Lung Contusion

Lung contusion may also be improved after chest physiotherapy. Lung contusion is commonly the result of a high-speed automobile accident. In the early stages there may be no radiological evidence of lung damage (Ayella, 1978b), particularly when rapid evacuation from the scene of the accident by helicopter occurs. If increasing intrapulmonary shunt, a confirmed history of blunt trauma, bloody tracheal secretions, and crackles on auscultation of the chest are present, however, chest physiotherapy is indicated. When the contusion is caused by rapid deceleration creating an implosion effect within the lung (Zuckerman, 1940), there may be no fractured ribs or any external signs of injury. Improvement in intrapulmonary shunt after chest physiotherapy may be obtained by removal of bloody secretions from the areas of normal lung around the contused area into which bleeding has occurred. Improvement is not always seen, however. If the lung is severely contused and lacerated as a result of the injury, there may be copious bleeding. Deterioration after chest physiotherapy in this set of circumstances may be noted (see p. 222, Case History 7.1). Nevertheless, morbidity, as measured in terms of duration of mechanical ventilation, was reduced in our institution as a result of managing lung contusion with a combination of early initiation of mechanical ventilation, chest physiotherapy, and PEEP where indicated (Shin et al., 1979; Mackenzie and Shin, 1981). The reported mortality of lung contusion has varied between 20% and 50% (Roscher et al., 1974). By using the early approach to intubation outlined in Chapter 1 and the support of controlled mechanical ventilation and chest physiotherapy, this has been reduced to mortality of 10% in 132 patients (Shin et al.). If the bloody secretions occuring in lung contusion are allowed to remain within the lung, they act as a perfect culture medium. Therefore, infection may be a common sequela of lung contusion. Similarly, traumatic lung cysts at the focus of the contusion can also become infected, giving rise to lung abscesses if the area is not adequately drained (Ayella, 1978b). Chest physiotherapy may be highly successful at draining a lung abscess that communicates with the tracheobronchial tree.

PROPHYLACTIC USE OF CHEST PHYSIOTHERAPY

Chronic Sputum-Producing Lung Disease

In circumstances in which there are excessive secretions or the ability to clear secretions is impaired, the use of prophylactic chest physiotherapy may be indicated. Smokers who produce morning phlegm or patients with chronic lung disease and copious sputum production probably benefit from chest physiotherapy, especially after major surgical procedures or during prolonged tracheal intubation, ventilation, and immobilization. In an ideal situation, breathing exercises should be practiced by the patient before operation. When acute circumstances precipitate admission, this is not possible. Patients with normal lungs may also benefit from preventive measures aimed at reducing pulmonary complications when they are immobilized.

Acute Quadriplegia

The acutely quadriplegic patient is unable to clear secretions effectively be- cause of the loss of motor function below the spinal cord transection. The amount of respiratory impairment is generally related to the level of transection; C6–C8 function ensures competent diaphragmatic innervation and often allows patient involvement in secretion clearance. In the acutely quadriplegic patient, however, pulmonary complications are frequently fatal (McMichan et al., 1980). Aggressive tracheobronchial toilet on a prospective basis, in an attempt to prevent secretion retention, is indicated in this group of patients. It is reported to be highly successful in reducing mortality (McMichan et al.). The approach to chest physiotherapy for the quadriplegic patient is described further in Chapter 8.

Smoke Inhalation and Aspiration

Secretion and particulate matter retention should be prevented in the patient suffering from inhalation of smoke or gastric contents. Lung parenchymal damage may develop from inhaled irritants, such as soot and cyanide from burning plastics, or from acid aspiration. Smoke inhalation victims may also suffer from the effects of carbon monoxide inhalation, causing a reduced level of consciousness. The damaged lung, after smoke inhalation injury or aspiration, may become infected. To reduce this likelihood, drainage of lung secretions and particulate matter should be assisted by chest physiotherapy.

Depressed Level of Consciousness

The unconscious or semiconscious patient who breathes spontaneously requires prophylactic chest physiotherapy because coughing and deep breathing are depressed. The unconscious patient with head injury may frequently breathe spontaneously with spastic respiration, using an active expiration. The combination of low tidal volume (300 ml or less) and high frequency (30–50 breaths/min) is another variant of abnormal respiration found with depressed levels of consciouness. Both may cause small airway closure and secretion retention. The chest physical therapist may alter these respiratory patterns and induce deeper breathing and generate coughs in otherwise-unresponsive patients. The techniques employed are described in Chapters 3 and 5.

Obesity

The obese patient is well recognized as having a higher incidence of pulmonary complications after surgery than normal subjects. Obesity and immobilization in the supine position predispose to inadequate lung expansion and, therefore, small airway closure and secretion retention (Cherniack et al., 1986). In our experience the best chest therapy for the obese patient is deep breathing and coughing that can be induced with early and aggressive attention to mobilization. The sooner the patient is moved out of bed and is walking, the more quickly the respiratory problems resolve. In obese patients with a tracheostomy, early tube removal appears to greatly assist the process of lung reexpansion and secretion clearance. Mobilization is, therefore, used prophylactically for the obese patient.

SUMMARY

A knowledge of the anatomy of the airways, lung segments, and lobes is essential for clinical and radiological examination of the chest and the performance of effective chest physiotherapy. An outline of pulmonary physiology is useful, especially the concepts of dead space, shunt, and $\dot{V}/\dot{Q}$ mismatch, to understand how they may be changed by chest physiotherapy. Details of the production, function, and biochemistry of sputum may provide therapeutic strategies for increasing its removal. Some pitfalls of chest examination in mechanically ventilated patients were described. Identification of atelectatic lung segments or lobes on chest x-ray by means of the silhouette sign is the major radiological indication for chest physiotherapy. This technique enables correct patient posi-

tioning for postural drainage and ensures application of chest physiotherapy to the involved areas of lung.

Deterioration of arterial blood gas due to increased intrapulmonary shunt is an indication for chest physiotherapy when the cause of the shunt is acute atelectasis, secretion retention, or lung contusion. Pneumonia may be difficult to diagnose and may in the early stages respond favorably to chest physiotherapy. Patients with chronic sputum-producing lung disease, acute quadriplegia, smoke inhalation, aspiration, depressed levels of consciousness, and obesity who are admitted to the ICU, especially if they require tracheal intubation and mechanical ventilation, benefit from prophylactic chest physiotherapy.

References

Aye S, Shin B, Mackenzie CF, Milholland AV, Helrich M: Tracking of respiratory function: Evaluation of respiratory index and PaO_2/FIO_2 ratio (abstract). Am Soc Anesth 391–392, 1978

Ayella RJ: Radiologic Management of the Massively Traumatized Patient, pp 93–96. Williams & Wilkins, Baltimore, 1978a

Ayella RJ: Radiologic Management of the Massively Traumatized Patient, pp 129–140. Williams & Wilkins, Baltimore, 1978b

Ayella RJ, Hankins JR, Turney SZ, Cowley RA: Ruptured thoracic aorta due to blunt trauma. J Trauma 17:199–205, 1977

Borson B, Nadel J: Neurophysiologic control of airway secretions in experimental animals. Kaliner M, Moderator: Human respiratory mucus. Am Rev Respir Dis 134:614–617, 1986

Boysen PG, Jenkins RB, Murphy EJ: Prospective comparison of cultures of proximal and peripheral endotracheal aspirates in intubated patients (abstract). Crit Care Med 8:238, 1980

Camner P, Jarstrand C, Philipson K: Tracheobronchial clearance in patients with influenza. Am Rev Respir Dis 108:131–135, 1973

Camner P, Mossberg B, Afzelius BA: Evidence for congenitally non-functioning cilia in the tracheobronchial tract in two subjects. Am Rev Respir Dis 112:807–809, 1975

Cherniack RM, Zwillich CW, Maclem PT, Kryger MH, Olson GH: Obesity. Am Rev Respir Dis 134:827–828, 1986

Comroe JH: Physiology of respiration, ed 2, p 165. Yearbook Medical Publishers, Chicago, 1975

Downie PA: Cash's Textbook of Chest, Heart and Vascular Disorders for Physiotherapists, pp 17–34. Faber & Faber, London, 1979

Driks MR, Craven DE, Celli BR, Manning M, Burke RA, Garvin GM, Kunches L, Farber HW, Wedel SA, McCabe WR: Nosocomial pneumonia in intubated patients given sucralfate as compared with antacids or histamine type 2 blockers. N Engl J Med 317:1376–1382, 1987

Eliasson R, Mossberg B, Camner P, Afzelius BA: The immobile cilia syndrome. A congenital ciliary abnormality as an etiologic factor in chronic airway infections and male sterility. N Engl J Med 297:1–6, 1977

Fowler WS, Gray JS, Helmholz HF Jr, Otis AB, Rahn H, Riley RL: Standardization of definitions and symbols in respiratory physiology. Fed Proc 9:602–615, 1950

Graham WGB, Bradley DA: Efficacy of chest physiotherapy and intermittent positive-pressure breathing in the resolution of pneumonia. N Engl J Med 299:624–627, 1978

Jarstrand C, Camner P, Philipson K: Mycoplasma pneumoniae and tracheobronchial clearance. Am Rev Respir Dis 110:415–419, 1974

Johanson WG, Seidenfeld JJ, Gomez P, De Los Santos R, Coalson JJ: Bacteriologic diagnosis of nosocomial pneumonia following prolonged mechanical ventilation. Am Rev Respir Dis 137:259–264, 1988a

Johanson WG, Seidenfeld JJ, De Los Santos R, Coalson JJ, Gomez P: Prevention of nosocomial pneumonia using topical and parenteral antimicrobial agents. Am Rev Respir Dis 137:265–272, 1988b

Kaliner M: Pharmacologic approach to the treatment of mucus hypersecretion. Kaliner M, moderator: Human respiratory mucus. Am Rev Respir Dis 134:618–619, 1986

Kaliner M, Maroon J, Patow C, Shelhauser J: Human respiratory mucus. J Allerg Clin Immunol 73:318–323, 1984

Krahl V: Anatomy of the mammalian lung In Handbook of Physiology, vol 1, Respiration, edited by WO Fenn and H Rahn, American Physiological Society, Washington DC, 1964

Lambert MW: Accessory bronchiole-alveolar communications. J Pathol Bacteriol 70:311–314, 1955

Lockhart RD, Hamilton GF, Fyfe FW: Anatomy of the Human Body, pp 535–548. Faber & Faber, London, 1959

Lopez-Vidriero MI, Reid L: Respiratory tract fluid—chemical and physical properties of airway mucus. Eur J Respir Dis 61 (Suppl 110):21–25, 1980

Mackenzie CF, Shin B: Sequential respiratory function following human lung contusion (abstract). Crit Care Med 9:205, 1981

Mackenzie CF, McAslan TC, Shin B, Schellinger D, Helrich M: The shape of the human adult trachea. Anesthesiology 49:48–50, 1978a

Mackenzie CF, Shin B, McAslan TC: Chest physiotherapy: the effect on arterial oxygenation. Anesth Analg 57:28–30, 1978b

Mackenzie CF, Shin B, Whitley N, Schellinger D: The relationship of human tracheal size to body habitus. Anesthesiology 51:S378, 1979

Mackenzie CF, Shin B, Hadi F, Imle PC: Changes in total lung/thorax compliance following chest physiotherapy. Anesth Analg 59:207–210, 1980a

Mackenzie CF, Shin B, Whitley N, Helrich M: Human tracheal circumference as an indicator of correct cuff size. Anesthesiology 53:S414, 1980b

Macklin MT, Macklin CC: Malignant interstitial emphysema of the lungs and mediastinum as an important occult complication in many respiratory diseases and other conditions: An interpretation of the clinical literature in the light of laboratory experiment. Medicine 23:281–358, 1944

Marom Z: The effects of macrophage (monocyte) products on respiratory mucus secretion. In, Kaliner M, Moderator: Human respiratory mucus. Am Rev Respir Dis 134:618, 1986

Marom Z, Shelhamer JH, Kaliner M: Human pulmonary macrophage derived mucus secretagogue. J Exp Med 159:844–860, 1984

Martin HB: Respiratory bronchioles as the pathway for collateral ventilation. J Appl Physiol 21:1443–1447, 1966

Matthew EB, Holmstrom FMG, Kasper RL: A simple method for diagnosing pneumonia in intubated or tracheostomized patients. Crit Care Med 5:76–81, 1977

McIntyre RW, Laws AK, Ramanchandran PR: Positive expiratory pressure plateau: improved gas exchange during mechanical ventilation. Can Anaesth Soc J 16:477–486, 1969

McMichan JC, Michel L, Westbrook PR: Pulmonary dysfunction following traumatic quadriplegia. JAMA 243:528–531, 1980

Menkes HA, Traystman RJ: Collateral ventilation. Am Rev Respir Dis 116:287–309, 1977

Menkes HA, Traystman RJ, Terry P: Collateral ventilation. Fed Proc 38:22–26, 1979

Mossberg B, Camner P: Mucociliary transport and cough as tracheobronchial clearance mechanisms in pathological conditions. Eur J Respir Dis 61 (Suppl 110):47–55, 1980

Murphy RLH, Holford SK, Knowler WC: Visual lung-sound characterization by time-expanded waveform analysis. N Engl J Med 296:968–971, 1977

Nunn JF: Applied Respiratory Physiology, ed 2, p 9. Butterworth, London, 1977

Patow C: Studies on control of mucus secretion in human airways. Kaliner M, moderator: Human respiratory mucus. Am Rev Respir Dis 134:617–618, 1986

Potter JL, Matthews LW, Lemm J, Spector S: Human pulmonary secretions in health and disease. Ann NY Acad Sci 106:692–697, 1963

Roscher R, Bittner R, Stockmann U: Pulmonary contusion. Arch Surg 109:508–510, 1974

Salata RA, Lederman MM, Shloes DM, Jacobs MR, Eckstein E, Tweardy D, Toossi Z, Chmielewski R, Marino J, King CK, Graham RC, Ellner JJ: Diagnosis of nosocomial pneumonia in intubated intensive care unit patients. Am Rev Respir Dis 135:426–432, 1987

Shelhamer JH, Marvin Z, Kaliner M: Immunologic and neuropharmacologic stimulation of mucus glycoproteins release from human airways. J Clin Invest 66:1400–1408, 1980

Shin B, McAslan TC, Hankins JR, Ayella RJ, Cowley RA: Management of lung contusion. Am Surg 45:168–175, 1979

Varsano S, Borson DB, Gold M, Forsberg LS, Basbaum C, Nadel JA: Proteinases release $^{35}SO_4$-labeled macromolecules from cultured airway epithelial cells. Fed Proc 43:786, 1986

Wagner PD, Saltzman HA, West JB: Measurement of continuous distribution of ventilation perfusion ratios: Theory. J Appl Physiol 36:588–599, 1974

Wanner A, Zarzecki S, Hirsch J, Epstein S: Tracheal mucus transport in experimental canine asthma. J Appl Physiol 39:950–957, 1975

Wasserman SI: Mediators of immediate hypersensitivity. J Allerg Clin Immunol 72:101–115, 1983

Weibel ER: Morphometry of the Human Lung, 111. Springer-Verlag, Berlin, 1963

West JB: Respiratory Physiology—The Essentials, ed 3, pp 7 and 104. Williams & Wilkins, Baltimore, 1985

West JB, Dolley CT, Naimak A: Distribution of blood flow in isolated lung: Relation to vascular and alveolar pressures. J Appl Physiol 19:713–724, 1964

Zuckerman S: Experimental study of blast injuries to the lungs. Lancet 2:219–224, 1940

CHAPTER 3

Postural Drainage, Positioning, and Breathing Exercises

Nancy Ciesla, B.S., P.T.

Chest physiotherapy consists of (1) postural drainage, (2) percussion and vibration, (3) coughing, (4) suctioning, (5) breathing exercises if the patient is not mechanically ventilated, and (6) optimal patient mobilization as the medical condition allows. This chapter discusses positioning the patient for optimal postural drainage and the use of breathing exercises.

POSTURAL DRAINAGE

Postural drainage, often referred to as bronchial drainage, is achieved by positioning the patient to promote gravity-assisted drainage of retained secretions. The lung segments receiving drainage are positioned uppermost. Patients are therefore placed in the sitting, side-lying, supine, prone, and head-down positions. The side-lying head-down position is used most frequently. The majority of intensive care unit (ICU) treatments are given to the lower lobes (see Appendix A 1.3).

Studies evaluating the efficacy of postural drainage as a single component of chest physiotherapy are limited, although this is an accepted treatment component. The addition of postural drainage to cough instruction was shown by Bateman et al. (1981) to enhance peripheral lung clearance in patients with chronic obstructive pulmonary disease (COPD). Marini et al. (1984) documented that lung volumes and oxygenation were not significantly changed by using the head down position in 25 COPD patients, although 8 patients demonstrated an increased functional residual capacity (FRC). In a similar patient population, Buscaglia and St. Marie (1983) documented no change in oxygen saturation with the prone and supine head-down positions. Radioaerosol clearance of central lung regions, increased sputum expectoration (Sutton et al., 1983; Maloney et al., 1981), and accelerated mucus clearance (Wong, 1977) were also noted with postural drainage. Cardiorespiratory function was studied by Mackenzie and Shin (1985) in 19 trauma patients requiring controlled mechanical ventilation and positive end expiratory pressure (PEEP). Intrapulmonary shunt and lung thorax compliance were significantly improved without a decrease in arterial oxygenation during chest physical therapy that included postural drainage.

The effects of position changes in acutely ill patients following thoracic and abdominal surgery, or in patients with acute unilateral lung disease have been studied by several authors. Patients turned every 2 hr immediately after coronary artery bypass surgery had a decreased stay in the surgical ICU and a lower postoperative fever compared with a control group (Chulay et al., 1982). Clauss et al. (1968) and Douglas et al. (1977) also demonstrated improved oxygenation with the simple maneuver of turning side to side or prone. Spontaneously breathing patients with pneumonia, lung contusion, and pleural effusion and those mechanically ventilated with PEEP demonstrated improved arterial oxygenation when positioned laterally with the "good lung down" (Zack et al., 1974; Seaton, 1979; Dhainaut et al., 1980; Ibanez et al., 1981; Remolina et al., 1981; Sonnenblick et al., 1983; Rivara et al., 1984). Piehl and Brown (1976) compared PaO_2 in adults with acute respiratory failure positioned prone and supine. Oxygenation was improved by prone positioning. Improved perfusion of the dependent lung is also noted with positioning the "good lung down" (Arborelius et al., 1974).

Ventilation and perfusion are primarily gravity dependent (West, 1962; Glaister, 1967; Nye, 1968). Lung ventilation varies according to the amount of active diaphragmatic contraction. Froese and Bryan (1974) and Bryan (1974) found that the dependent lung volume was decreased with mechanical ventilation. Recent studies suggest the diaphragm moves with a piston-like motion with mechanical ventilation (Rheder, 1987, personal communication). Kaneko et al. (1966) noted that, in spontaneously breathing normal subjects, ventilation was greater in dependent lung zones at low lung volumes.

Studies evaluating the respiratory effects of changes in body position are not as conclusive in infants and patients with stable chronic lung disease. Wagamen et al. (1979) noted that lung compliance, tidal volume, and PaO_2 improved when changing the position of 14 mechanically ventilated infants from supine to prone, although Heaf et al. (1983) noted transcutaneous oxygen measurements to be better with the "good lung up." Improved distribution of ventilation was noted in the uppermost lung in four subjects with asymptomatic and stable COPD (Chang et al., 1986).

Available literature supports positioning adults with the "good lung down." This is the usual position for delivering chest physiotherapy to patients with unilateral lung disease. The positions into which clinicians are often reluctant to place critically ill patients (right or left lateral, prone, and one-quarter turn from prone) appear optimal for maximum matching of ventilation and perfusion. In these positions improved oxygenation may occur.

Patients with bilateral lung disease are assessed individually. In some patients it may be difficult to determine the most involved lung by clinical examination and chest x-ray. These patients should be closely monitored while turning, a marked deterioration in oxygenation may occur (Fig. 3.1). The side-lying position may provide better oxygenation than the sitting position (Table 3.1). Monitoring vital signs, lung volumes, and oxygen saturation may promote safe and effective treatment.

Response to chest physiotherapy treat-

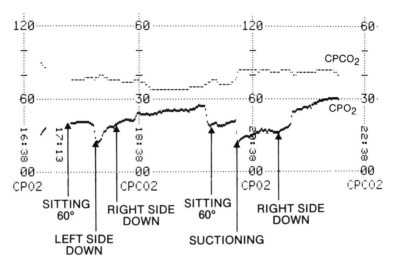

Figure 3.1. Transcutaneous oxygen (CPO_2) and carbon dioxide ($CPCO_2$) measurements for a patient with closed head injury, pulmonary contusion, and a fractured left femur. The patient was turned with the better lung (right) down after developing pneumonia and an ARDS pattern on chest x-ray. Data provided by Joan Stoklosa, B.S.

ment varies depending on the type of mechanical ventilation or whether the patient is spontaneously breathing. Prokocimer and associates (1983) found that the head-down position improved oxygenation in patients with bilateral lower lobe lung disease receiving mechanical ventilation with PEEP. Patients with severe posttraumatic ARDS unresponsive to conventional mechanical ventilation and therapeutic position change may require simultaneous independent lung ventilation (SILV) (Siegel, 1988). Chest physiotherapy may be performed, if indicated, for patients receiving (SILV) (Fig. 3.2). The tidal volume delivered to each lung may be increased when necessary with changes in position.

The findings of Oldenburg et al. (1979) that intermittent postural drainage is less effective without cough than with exercise or cough and Zinman's (1984) evaluation of stable cystic fibrosis children demonstrating cough to be equally as effective as postural drainage do not seem clinically relevant for the intensive care patient who cannot be mobilized. Newhouse (1984) states that postural drainage is likely to be most effective when secretions are thin and copious. Postural drainage may be especially beneficial in acutely ill patients who are often intubated, in pain, or have a decreased level of consciousness, because, spontaneous cough is less effective.

The following section discusses meth-

Table 3.1
Respiratory Effects of Changing Position for Patient in Figure 3.1[a]

	Position			
	SIT 60	RT LAT	SIT 60	RT LAT
Time	17:45	19:00	21:10	22:20
FIO_2 .65				
PEEP 20				
PaO_2 (mm Hg)	70	85	63	84
$PaCO_2$ (mm Hg)	34	29	41	37
$\dot{Q}_s/\dot{Q}_t$	29%			24%
CO (liters/min)	9.1			7.4

[a]Data provided by Joan Stoklosa, B.S.

Figure 3.2. Patient receiving SILV and chest physiotherapy to the left upper lobe, posterior segment. Therapist should closely monitor changes in respiratory parameters of each lung.

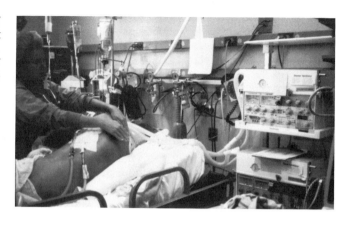

ods of achieving optimum segmental bronchial drainage for the ICU patient. Clinicians ordering or performing chest physiotherapy should encourage use of the optimum postural drainage positions to remove retained secretions and improve matching of ventilation and perfusion. This is most important for patients immobilized or with poor cough ability. Both lungs should be drained in patients with lung contusion or lung abscess when adventitial breath sounds occur during treatment and denote spillage of secretions to the dependent lung. Treatment of all involved lung segments minimizes spillage of secretions and bacterial contamination of the "good lung." The therapist should closely monitor the patient's vital signs during treatment. Arterial blood gas, SaO_2, and chest x-ray results allow the clinician to tailor treatment to the needs of the individual patient. Monitoring is particularly important following cardiac surgery, when cardiac output and mixed venous saturation may be decreased during treatment (Barrell and Abbas, 1978). It is important to note that a single measurement of arterial oxygenation is only temporal for a specific body position and may change dramatically with time and treatment. Some patients may have a decrease in PaO_2 during treatment that increases once secretions are removed from the peripheral airways. In the author's experience the majority of ICU patients tolerate position changes necessary for postural drainage quite well.

Illustrations showing the position and angle of tilt necessary to drain each segment (colored black) appear in Figure 3.3A–T. Zausmer (1968) suggests that cil-

iary action and consequently the movement of copious and viscous mucus toward the major bronchi are influenced by forces of gravity. By utilizing the following methods to turn critical multiply injured patients, improved ventilation and perfusion relationships and secretion removal may be obtained.

PROBLEMS ASSOCIATED WITH OBTAINING IDEAL POSTURAL DRAINAGE POSITIONS IN THE INTENSIVE CARE UNIT

Discussion and observation of treatment given by other physical therapists, nurses, and respiratory therapists confirm that chest physiotherapy is often not performed in the optimal bronchial drainage positions. This may be due to the apparent difficulty of positioning a patient who has multiple injuries or monitoring devices. Methods of obtaining optimum bronchial drainage by turning patients despite the presence of multiple injuries, lines, catheters, tubes and monitoring equipment are discussed in the following section.

Turning the Patient with Multiple Injuries

The following guidelines are helpful for turning the patient with multiple injuries:

1. Obtain the patient's history and diagnosis.
2. Observe the patient supine and identify the presence of fractures and soft-tissue injuries or placement of lines, tubes, catheters, and monitoring equipment.

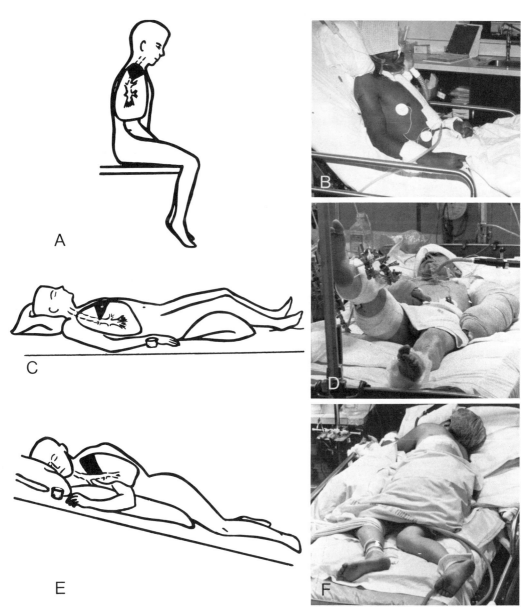

Figure 3.3. (**A**) The apical segments of both upper lobes are drained with the patient sitting upright. (**B**) This spontaneously breathing patient is receiving postural drainage of the apical segments of both upper lobes. (**C**) The anterior segments of both upper lobes are drained with the patient supine. (**D**) This patient, positioned for drainage of the anterior upper lobe segments, had a closed head injury and was unconscious. He also had multiple orthopedic injuries. (**E**) The left upper lobe apical posterior segment is drained with the thorax elevated approximately 30°. This can be achieved by raising the head of the bed or by placing the whole bed 30° up from horizontal. The patient is also positioned one-quarter turn from prone. (**F**) After a left thoracotomy and exploratory laparotomy, this patient received postural drainage to the apical posterior segment of the left upper lobe.

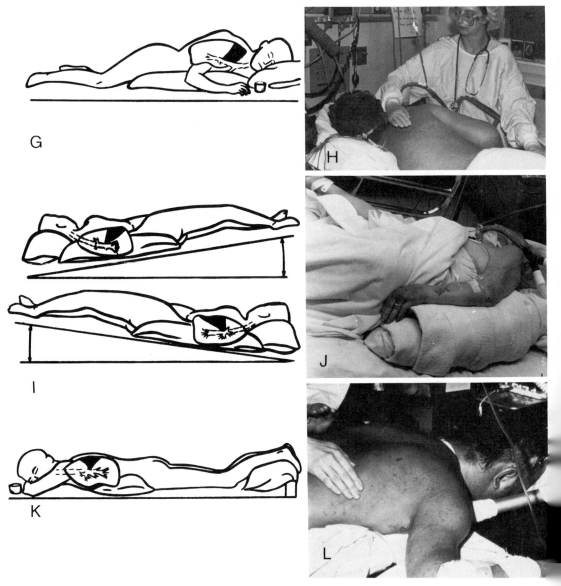

Figure 3.3. (Continued) (**G**) The posterior segment of the right upper lobe is drained with the patient positioned one-quarter turn from prone. The bed remains flat. (**H**) Postural drainage of the right upper lobe posterior segment in a patient with a head injury, left pulmonary contusion, fractured ribs, left pneumothorax, and pelvic and limb fractures. He received physiotherapy following splenorrhaphy and internal fixation of bilateral femur fractures. (**I**) *Upper:* right middle lobe position; *lower:* lingula position. The right middle lobe and lingula are drained with the patient one-quarter turn from supine. A 12-inch bed elevation is recommended. (**J**) A patient receiving postural drainage of the lingula. (**K**) The bed is flat and the patient is prone to drain the superior segments of both lower lobes. (**L**) A patient with multiple-system involvement, including cervical spinal cord, chest and abdominal injuries.

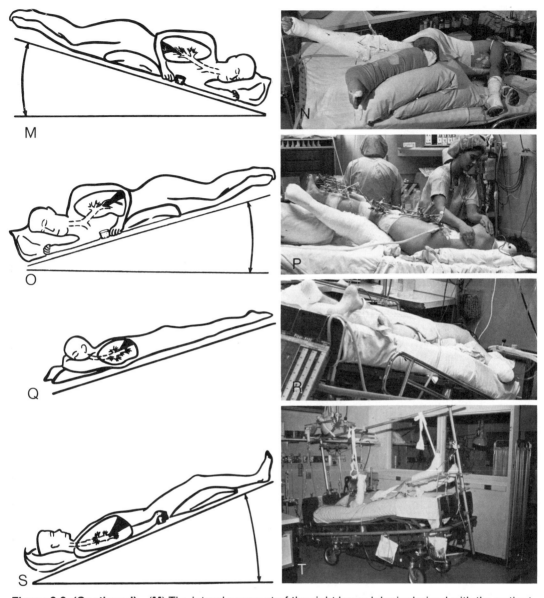

Figure 3.3. (Continued) (**M**) The lateral segment of the right lower lobe is drained with the patient lying on the left side. The foot of the bed is elevated. (**N**) Postural drainage of the lateral segment of the right lower lobe is shown in a patient who sustained a head injury, a fractured left femur, fractured right lateral malleolus and fibula, ruptured spleen, and liver lacerations. Pancuronium, a neuromuscular blocking agent, was used because the patient was agitated and out of phase with the ventilator. The patient has resting hand splints to preserve functional range of motion. Neufeld traction permits turning to the left side. (**O**) The right side-lying head-down position is used for postural drainage of the lateral segment of the left lower lobe and the medial segment of the right lower lobe. (**P**) The lateral segment of the left lower lobe is posturally drained in a patient with bilateral femoral fractures, a fractured left tibia, left lung contusion, and a chest tube draining a left hemothorax. Neufeld traction and exoskeletal fixation devices allow the patient to be turned. A Philadelphia collar is being worn since the seventh cervical vertebra could not be visualized on lateral cervical spine x-ray. (**Q**) The posterior segments of both lower lobes are drained in the prone head-down position. (**R**) This patient had a right pneumothorax, lung contusion and soft-tissue lacerations around the right elbow. He also had a laparotomy for repair of liver lacerations and mesenteric tears. (**S**) The supine head-down position is used to drain the anterior segments of both lower lobes. (**T**) This patient with multiple extremity fractures receives postural drainage of the anterior segments of the lower lobes.

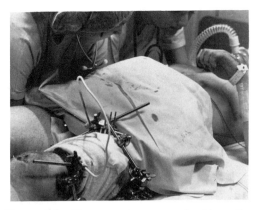

Figure 3.4. Two people are required to pull a patient with multiple injuries to the side of the bed.

3. Move the patient to the side of the bed before turning (Fig. 3.4). If the patient cannot assist, two people slide the patient to the side of the bed. One person lifts the thorax while the second moves the hips.
4. Move lines and electrocardiogram wires away from the side onto which the patient is turning.
5. While facing the patient, place one hand over the shoulder and the other over the hip to rotate the patient onto the side. A second person may be required to move the hip and shoulder back so that the patient remains correctly positioned (Fig. 3.5). A roll may be used to prevent the patient from rolling supine. Rolls, which can be made from folded sheets or blankets, are better than pillows because they are less easily compressed (Fig. 3.6).

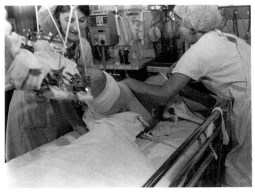

Figure 3.5. One therapist places a hand over the shoulder and hip; a second pulls the hips back to position the patient on his side.

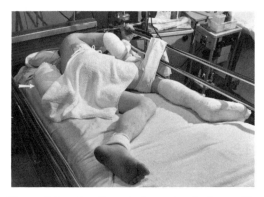

Figure 3.6. A roll made from sheets *(arrow)* is very practical and can be used to maintain the patient in a side-lying position.

Turning the Patient into the Prone Position

The following guidelines have been found useful for turning the patient into the prone position:

1. Flex the dependent shoulder 180° or position the dependent arm so that the patient can be rolled over it. One therapist raises the trunk while the second moves the arm and shoulder from under the patient. Patients with orotracheal or nasotracheal tubes can maintain the prone position as long as cervical rotation is not restricted (Fig. 3.7). Sometimes it may be necessary to prop the patient's head on a pillow or rolled towel to prevent kinking of the tracheal and/or ventilator tubes.

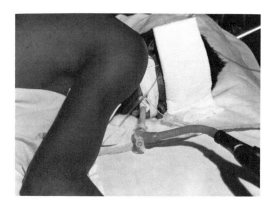

Figure 3.7. Three people are required to turn a patient with a tracheal tube prone. The dependent arm is moved under the patient's thorax and positioned comfortably. A roll is then placed under the chest to prevent the tracheal tube from becoming occluded.

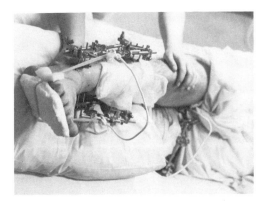

Figure 3.8. A massively fractured extremity requires careful positioning with turning.

2. Patients who have orthopedic injuries or pain that inhibits turning onto the dependent shoulder may be turned prone over the noninvolved upper extremity.
3. Patients with skeletal traction or external skeletal fixation on the lower extremity require a third person for prone positioning. The extra person is required to position the involved extremity carefully, avoiding motion that is detrimental to the injury (Fig. 3.8).
4. Mechanically ventilated patients with tracheostomies also require the assistance of three people for turning into the prone position. Two are required to raise the patient's upper thorax, while one places a roll under the chest to prevent occlusion or pressure on the tracheostomy tube (Fig. 3.9).

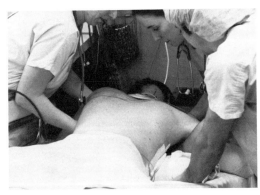

Figure 3.9. Placing a roll under the chest allows a patient with a tracheal tube to be turned three-quarters prone. There is then adequate space for the tracheal and ventilator tubes.

5. Once the patient is turned into the appropriate position, the ventilator tubing and monitoring equipment are checked and readjusted as necessary.

Turning the Patient with Intravascular Lines

Central Intravenous Subclavian Lines

Suturing of central intravenous subclavian lines so that the external tubing runs parallel to the patient's thorax allows full shoulder movement. The 90° side-lying position, the prone position, and full shoulder horizontal adduction can then be obtained without the line being pulled out or kinked (Fig. 3.10).

Peripheral Intravenous Lines

Peripheral intravenous lines usually do not interfer with turning. Preferably, in order to allow better mobilization, they should not cross a joint.

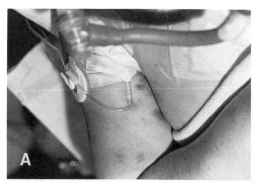
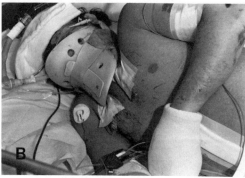

Figure 3.10. **(A)** Tubing of a subclavian line may become kinked when the patient lies on the same side. **(B)** Suturing subclavian lines parallel to the patient's chest allows adequate side-to-side turning and proper positioning for postural drainage.

Arterial Lines

Radial lines are maintained in good position with a secure dressing. In addition, an armboard or splint may help avoid displacement. Femoral lines function in all the required positions for postural drainage, including sitting. Occasionally, hip flexion affects line function. The hip is then further extended until the proper wave form is again observed on the monitor. The prone and supine positions are ideal for maintaining a good femoral arterial line wave form. The presence of umbilical catheters in neonates should not be a contraindication to prone positioning.

Turning the Patient with Chest, Tracheal, Feeding, and Sump Tubes

Chest Tubes

Chest tubes are placed for treatment of hemopneumothorax and to adeqately drain the pleural cavity in cases of patients with empyema. They are routinely connected to an underwater seal. Suction is often added for adequate expansion of pneumothorax or to increase drainage of the pleural cavity. Kinks or compresson of the tubes are avoided during turning by careful patient positioning (Fig. 3.11). Turning and positioning the patient may increase pleural drainage from dependent lung regions.

Tracheal Tubes

Tracheal tubes may obstruct with prone patient positioning for postural drainage. In order to prevent this prob-

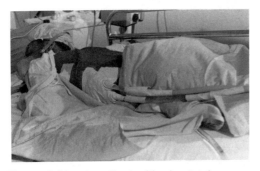

Figure 3.11. A patient with chest tubes may be positioned prone. The tubes are carefully positioned without tension or kinking.

lem, a large roll is placed under the upper thorax. This allows adequate space for the tracheostomy tube and ventilator tubing (Fig. 3.7). In order to minimize tracheal trauma, the patient may be disconnected from the ventilator while being turned. Patients with large intrapulmonary shunts that require high fractional inspired oxygen concentration (FIO_2) and positive end-expiratory pressure to maintain adequate arterial oxygenation are an exception to this general rule. In these patients, instead of disconnection, an additional person assists with turning by manipulating the ventilator tubing. This regimen of turning the intubated and mechanically ventilated patient has been found most satisfactory. Patients with tracheal tubes may be positioned prone routinely when this position is clinically indicated for chest physiotherapy. To prevent agitated patients from removing their tracheal tube, hand restraints or sedation are used before treatment and the tracheal tube is well secured.

Feeding Tubes

Patients in the ICU may receive nutritional support intravenously or through orogastric, nasogastric, or gastrostomy feeding tubes. It is important for the clinician altering a patient's position to be aware of the type of feeding an individual patient is receiving. Bolus feedings usually require coordination of physiotherapy treatment with the feeding schedule. Chest physiotherapy is given before or 30 min after a feeding. Continuous feedings can be stopped for physiotherapy treatment and resumed when the patient is no longer positioned head-down.

Gastroesophageal reflux, a malfunction of the distal esophagus causing regurgitation of stomach contents into the esophagus, may be associated with aspiration of gastric contents into the lungs. This condition is seen in infants and children and presents a dilemma to the therapist performing chest physiotherapy. Nutritional support must be coordinated with prevention and treatment of aspiration. The recommended medical treatment is the semierect position (head elevated 30–60°) (Herbst and Myers, 1981;

Ocha, 1981), especially 30–45 min after feedings. Chest physiotherapy is indicated to areas of suspected or confirmed aspiration. Treatment should be coordinated with feedings and administered either before meals or no sooner than 1 hr after meals, to minimize chances of regurgitation (De Ceasare, 1985). Positioning should be done judiciously and the patient's response to position changes should be closely monitored. If increased vomiting is noted after treatment, therapeutic positioning to minimize reflux, or a modified postural drainage position may be required. Therapeutic positioning for children with recurrent reflux is described in the literature. The prone upright position with partial neck flexion (Hewitt, 1976; Zimmerman and Oder, 1981) is thought to promote drainage of regurgitated secretions from the mouth and eliminate aspiration into the lungs. The right side-lying position may be beneficial to increase gastric emptying (Wood, 1979). A prone lyer may be used successfully in infants with severe central nervous system dysfunction associated with gastroesophageal reflux and aspiration. The infant is placed in the prone lyer head up 30–45 min prior to feedings. Tracheal aspiration and the need for routine chest physiotherapy treatment may be eliminated (Imle, 1983). The goal of treatment for patients with gastroesophageal reflux is to provide adequate nutritional support and pulmonary hygiene. Each patient should be individually assessed to determine if therapeutic positioning is adequate. If adventitial breath sounds and clinical signs of chest infection persist chest physiotherapy is indicated.

Sump Drains

Intraabdominal sump drains do not interfere with patient positioning. Care should be taken not to pull or disconnect intraabdominal tubes when moving the patient. Dislodging the sump may lead to hemorrhage or peritonitis.

Turning the Patient with a Urinary Catheter

Urinary catheters do not interfere with patient positioning. It is important to clamp the tubing between the collection bag and patient before turning patients. This prevents drainage of stagnant urine into the bladder, which may lead to urinary tract infection. The collection bag is moved to the side of the bed that the patient faces after turning. To promote urine drainage the collection bag should be kept in the dependent position, moved to the head or foot of the bed, depending on the patient's head-up or head-down position.

PATIENTS WITH HEAD INJURY

The two major problems of performing chest physiotherapy in patients with head injury are turning and obtaining the head-down position.

Turning the Patient with Head Injury

Use of Intracranial Pressure (ICP) Monitoring

ICP measurement by a subarachnoid screw or intraventricular catheter is extremely helpful to enable administration of chest physiotherapy to the patient with head injury. Intracranial pressure and cerebral perfusion pressure (CPP) limits are set, and when these are not exceeded, treatment is administered to appropriate lung lobes or segments. Monitoring of ICP and CPP, therefore, may allow chest physiotherapy to be performed; without it there could be no certainty that it was not detrimental to cerebral perfusion. Postural drainage and routine nursing procedures, such as turning and suctioning, may cause marked increases in ICP (See pp. 363–366). Once noxious stimulation has ceased, ICP returns to baseline, provided the patient has a high cerebral compliance. Therefore, after turning a patient, the therapist should wait a few minutes for the ICP to decrease spontaneously, rather than immediately returning the patient to the baseline position if increased pressures occur. Once the patient is turned and positioned, the head may need to be propped on a roll or intravenous bag to avoid pressure on the ICP monitoring device and to decrease ICP. Percussion and vibration do not increase ICP (see Chapter 8 and Appendix for details of patients with head injury treated with chest physiotherapy).

Turning the Patient with Abnormal Muscle Tone

Decerebration or decortication may make turning the patient with head injury difficult. Change of body position to minimize abnormal muscle tone allows both increased joint range of motion and improved positioning for chest physiotherapy (Bobath, 1974). Spasticity is often affected by the position of the neck. Although full cervical flexion may be limited for example, by a tracheostomy tube, even a small amount of flexion may minimize extensor spasticity. The uppermost shoulder, hip, and knee may then be flexed and restrained. Flexing the hip and knee may allow patients with increased lower extremity extensor muscle tone to assume the lateral position. Restraints are often required to keep the patient optimally positioned (Figs. 3.6 and 3.12). Once the patient with a head injury is breathing spontaneously, more

extensive physiotherapy is initiated, and this may reduce spasticity.

Turning Patients with a Craniotomy

After a craniotomy, patients require proper head positioning to minimize pressure on the operative side, especially if a bone flap was removed. Placement of 500-ml intravenous infusion bags above and below this area support the head and prevent undue pressure (Fig. 3.13).

Obtaining the Head-Down Position

After turning the patient, the therapist should wait a few minutes for the ICP to return to resting level. If this is below the set limit (usually 25 torr), the patient is lowered into the head-down position while the ICP and CPP are observed on the bedside monitor. Often the ICP is greater during positioning than when the patient is relaxed in the head-down position. CPP is usually > 50 mm Hg with these transient increases in ICP.

If the ICP or CPP exceeds the acceptable limits elevation of the head on a roll may result in a decreased ICP and increased CPP. The thorax may then be lowered. Once the secretions reach the upper airway, they may be suctioned even with the head elevated. If increased ICP is a major problem, patients can be sedated before treatment in an attempt to keep the pressure as low as possible. Barbiturates and lidocaine may be used (see Chapter 8).

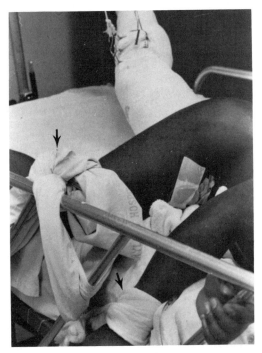

Figure 3.12. A sheet tied around the thigh and a wrist restraint *(arrows)* allow this patient to be maintained lying sideways. Neufeld traction is used to permit turning.

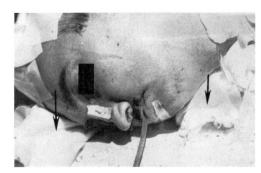

Figure 3.13. Following craniotomy the patient's head may be supported on two intravenous infusion bags *(arrows)* to prevent pressure on the operative site when the patient is turned or placed in a head-down position.

Case History 3.1. An 18-year-old male was admitted following a motor vehicle accident. He was unconscious and had a parietotemporal and basilar skull fracture, fractured mandible, multiple facial lacerations, a ruptured spleen and a lacerated liver.

An ICP monitor was inserted on admission. His chest X-ray remained clear throughout the first week of hospitalization. Because the intracranial pressures were greater than 15 torr when sitting up, and greater than 25 torr with turning and positioning, chest physiotherapy was not administered for 48 hr. Arterial blood gases at 8 A.M. on 60% FIO_2 by mechanical ventilation with 10 cm H_2O of PEEP were as follows: PaO_2, 73; pH, 7.45; and $PaCO_2$, 24. Total lung/thorax compliance (C_T) before therapy was 32 ml/cm H_2O. It was decided that aggressive chest physiotherapy should be given because of deteriorating clinical signs, including rhonchi and decreased air entry over the right middle and lower lobes. The chest x-ray remained clear, although arterial oxygenation had worsened. One hour of chest physiotherapy was given to the right middle and lower lobes, during which ICP varied between 25 and 35 torr. Treatment produced copious amounts of viscid secretions. Air entry improved over the right base and right middle lobe; rhonchi diminished. Repeat arterial blood gases with the same ventilator settings were as follows: PaO_2, 304; pH, 7.65; $PaCO_2$, 24. Inspired oxygen was decreased to 43%, and shorter daily routine treatments were given, provided the patient was productive of secretions. C_T at 2 P.M. following chest physiotherapy was 46 ml/cm H_2O. This case history demonstrates that marked decreases in arterial oxygenation may occur and C_T may worsen due to retained lung secretions despite repeatedly clear chest x-rays. Oxygenation and C_T may be increased with chest physiotherapy.

ORTHOPEDIC INJURIES

Positioning the Patient with Long-Bone Injury

Some patients may be difficult to position because of traction and splinting devices or specific injuries. The therapist must be familiar with the several different types of fixation before turning a patient with these devices. Devices that allow full patient turning and mobilization are preferred.

Closed femoral fractures that cannot be fixed by internal fixation within the first several hours of injury may be placed in Neufeld traction. This is a flexible traction system that allows patients to be turned equally to the right and left. Appropriate traction is still maintained at the fracture site (Fig. 3.14). Neufeld traction therefore enables nearly all the correct postural drainage positions to be obtained. The patient may be moved out of bed and seated in a chair. Ambulation training, usually non-weight-bearing, can also begin. Since turning is restricted with bilateral Neufeld traction (Browner et al., 1981), on admission, patients with bilateral closed femur fractures require internal or external fixation of at least one of the fractures.

Tibial fractures, some humeral and pelvic fractures, and an occasional open femur fracture may be managed with exoskeletal fixation. With the exception of the pelvic fixater these devices allow turning in all positions (Fig. 3.15). Pelvic fixation permits turning 90° to either side (Fig. 3.16). Alternately, a turning frame may be used for severe pelvic fractures with or without external fixation and allows chest physiotherapy (see Case History 8.1) (Fig. 3.17). External fixation of fractures allows frequent dressing changes, whirlpool cleansing, and debridement in patients with massive soft-tissue injuries. It also allows patients with pelvic, femoral, tibial, and fibular fractures to begin early sitting and ambulation training (Hoffmann, 1954; Fellander, 1963; Karlstrom and Olerud, 1975; Edwards et al., 1979; Brumback et al., 1986; Burgess and Mandelbaum, 1987). Patients with a fractured acetabulum or hip dislocation are commonly placed in Bucks traction (Shands and

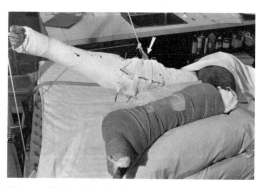

Figure 3.14. Neufeld traction *(arrow)* allows the patient with a fractured femur to be turned 90° to either side.

Figure 3.15. Exoskeletal fixation for a fractured left femur and right tibia allows prone positioning.

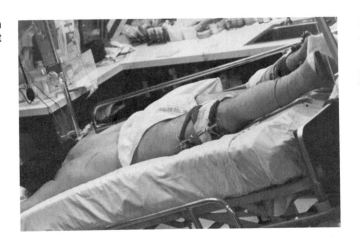

Raney, 1967). This form of skin traction need not interfere with patient positioning for postural drainage when there is close communication between the orthopedic and therapy staff. For acetabular fractures, a small roll may be placed under the iliac crest, and a second roll below the greater trochanter, to avoid pressure on the acetabulum. With severe fractures the patient may be turned prone by turning over the opposite hip to avoid pressure on the involved hip. The Bucks traction is adjusted during turning to pull parallel to the patient's hip.

Splints applied for preserving range of motion or immobilization of minor fractures do not interfere with patient positioning. Extremities with fractures treated with plaster casts are easily maneuvered once the plaster has dried.

Soft-tissue injury alone does not interfere with positioning the multiple-trauma patient. Dislocations, for example, are commonly seen following trauma. With posterior hip dislocation,

hip flexion and adduction are avoided. Anterior shoulder dislocations require minimizing shoulder external rotation and abduction. Patients with subluxation, dislocation, and ligamentous injury are therefore moved with caution to avoid motion similar to that causing the original injury.

The following case study demonstrates the need for flexible orthopedic traction devices that allow the patient to be mobilized.

Case History 3.2. A 24-year-old male was admitted following an auto accident in which he sustained a fractured first left rib, liver lacerations, a retroperitoneal hematoma, an oblique fracture of the left acetabulum, and a comminuted subtrochanteric fracture. Initially, for management of the pelvic and proximal femoral fractures, the patient was placed in 90–90 traction (hip flexion, 90°; knee flexion, 90°). Maximum turning was 70° to the right, and it was impossible to turn the patient onto the left side. The admission chest x-ray was clear. Four days later, repeat chest x-ray showed

Figure 3.16. External fixation allows patients with severe pelvic fractures to be turned 90° to either side.

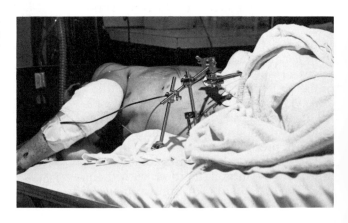

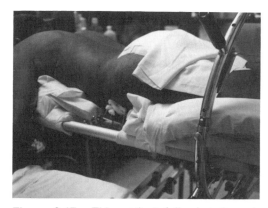

Figure 3.17. This patient following thoracic spine and pelvic injuries was managed on a turning frame to facilitate skin care and chest physiotherapy treatment.

right upper lobe atelectasis that persisted throughout the following day (Fig. 3.18A). On the sixth morning the patient also developed a left lung infiltrate (Fig. 3.18B). At this time it was decided that a more flexible traction system was necessary to assist management of the patient's pulmonary pathology. The patient was started on antibiotics, and the traction was lowered to allow turning (Fig. 3.18C). Chest physiotherapy was given to the right upper and lower lobes as well as the left lower lobe. Copious amounts of viscid brownish secretions were suctioned from the patient's tracheostomy tube. There was clearing of the radiological lung infiltrates (Fig. 3.18D).

This case history demonstrates that, in the trauma patient, priorities need to be established in patient management. The traction that allowed turning was not ideal, but the patient's

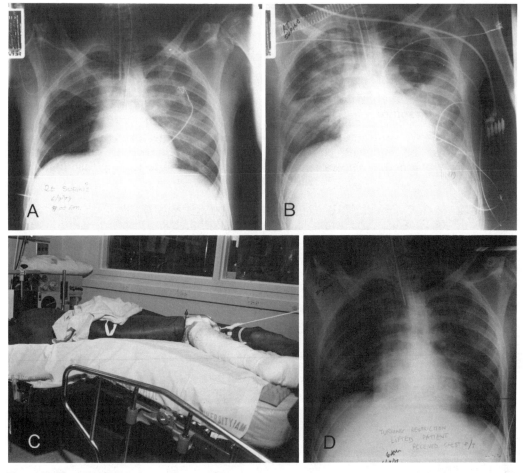

Figure 3.18. **(A)** Chest x-ray 4 days after admission shows a right upper lobe atelectasis. **(B)** On the sixth day after admission a left lung infiltrate had developed in addition to the persistent right lung infiltrate. **(C)** The traction was lowered to permit turning and chest physiotherapy. **(D)** Following chest physiotherapy treatment, the lung infiltrates have cleared.

pulmonary status improved and the patient survived.

One inflexible traction system is the Thomas splint and Steinmann pin. This was traditionally used to manage femoral shaft fractures prior to the routine use of internal and external fixation devices. The pin provided a point for skeletal traction. This skeletal traction makes turning a patient greater than 45° to either side almost impossible (Fig. 3.19). If turning is restricted to 45°, this prevents bronchial and segmental drainage of the posterior segment of the right upper lobe, the apical posterior segment of the left upper lobe, and the superior and posterior segments of both lower lobes. This is a serious restriction as, in our experience, the posterior segments of the lower lobes are the most commonly atelectatic lung segments (Appendix). More flexible traction systems are preferred for patients with femoral fractures and multiple trauma.

Positioning the Patient with Spinal Fracture

Patients with cervical fractures requiring traction can be managed routinely with a special board that allows side to side turning and upright positioning (Fig. 3.20). A turning frame may be used prior to surgical spinal stabilization for patients with major neurological deficit (see p. 268). Patients who cannot be turned fully on an orthodox bed can assume the prone and supine head-up and head-down positions on a turning frame (Table 3.2). Halo vests and body casts are used for stable fractures or after surgical fixation. Halo vests are preferred to body casts because they do not restrict costal or diaphragmatic excursion, radiological interpretation, sitting to 90°, or skin inspection. Chest physiotherapy can be adequately performed on patients with a Halo vest by opening the jacket. Percussion and vibration may be given to the nondependent lung in the lateral position or to both lungs posteriorly when the patient is in the prone position. The vest should be opened only after the patient is appropriately positioned. Taping the opened vest to the bedrails improves thoracic expansion and permits percussion and vibration to most lung segments (Fig. 3.21). Patients with polytrauma and complete neurological deficit may develop pulmonary problems if placed in a vest too early. Respiratory complications may occur due to inadequate chest expansion as noted in the following case history.

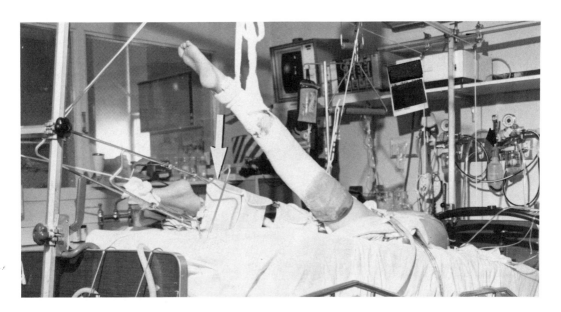

Figure 3.19. This patient with multiple injuries, including a pneumothorax, extensive liver and bowel injuries, and a fractured right femur and left tibial plateau, can only be turned 45° to either side due to the Thomas splint *(arrow)*, with traction applied to the femur by a Steinmann pin.

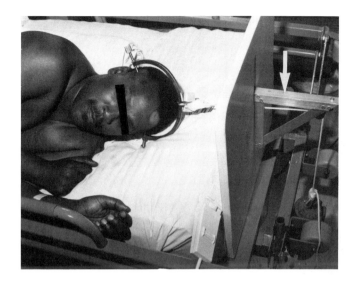

Figure 3.20. This quadriplegic patient following subluxation and an open-book pelvic fracture was managed in a regular bed and turned 90° to either side prior to receiving a halo vest. (Note special board and traction (arrow), which allow side-to-side turning and upright positioning.)

Case History 3.3. After being hit by a truck, a 45-year-old male was admitted with the following diagnoses: C3–C7 spinous process fractures with neurological deficit at C4, LeForte I fracture, and chest injury with seventh to ninth right rib fractures. The patient was placed on a turning frame for 8 days, and he received chest physiotherapy; his chest x-ray remained clear (Fig. 3.22A). On the eighth day after admission, it was decided to place the patient in a halo vest. His pulmonary status had stabilized, although he continued to need mechanical ventilation due to phrenic nerve paralysis. Chest x-ray the following morning showed infiltrates in both lower lobes, which became progressively worse (Fig. 3.22B). Three days after the patient was placed in a halo vest, he was returned to the turning frame and continued on aggressive chest physiotherapy (which may not have been adequate while in the halo vest). Repeat chest x-ray the following morning showed some improvement, which continued throughout the following day (Fig. 3.22C). This patient remained on the turning frame for several months due to his respiratory dependency secondary to lack of diaphragmatic function. The patient was later transferred to a rehabilitation center.

BEDS

Modifications for Postural Drainage

The high incidence of respiratory complications in the ICU makes pulmonary care a major patient management priority. The type of bed has a significant impact on the ability to perform adequate chest physiotherapy. Beds that achieve a 30° or greater head-down postural drainage position are preferred (Fig. 3.23). Gaskell and Webber (1973) advocate an 18-inch elevation of the foot of the bed for drainage of the anterior, lateral, poste-

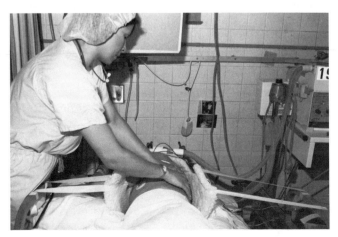

Figure 3.21. The halo jacket can be easily opened to permit percussion and vibration over appropriate lung segments. Skin integrity can also be evaluated.

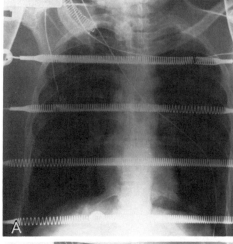
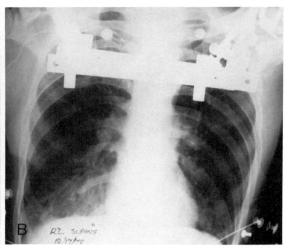
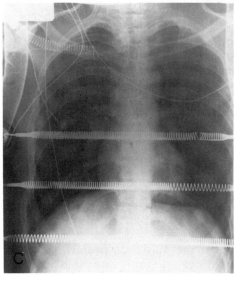

Figure 3.22. (**A**) Clear chest x-ray following 8 days of chest physiotherapy given to the patient on a turning frame. (**B**) Bilateral lower lobe infiltrates developed within 24 hr of placement in the halo jacket. (**C**) The lower lobe infiltrates have cleared since the patient was placed back on the turning frame and received vigorous chest physiotherapy.

rior, and medial segments of the lower lobes, and an elevation of 14 inches for the right middle lobe and lingula. The length of the bed and patient's position should be taken into consideration because they alter the tilt of the bronchial tree. Most standard beds can be placed in a 15° head-down position as a unit. Beds in which the head can be lowered to obtain an additional tilt of the bronchial tree are preferred. Shock blocks may be used with beds that do not provide an adequate head-down tilt (Fig. 3.24). During the past 10 years there has been a marked increase in the usage of specialty beds with minimal evidence to substantiate their usage. Frequently used specialty beds include turning frames, low air loss beds, air fluidized beds, kinetic turn-

ing beds, and beds specifically designed for the obese patient. The need for specialty beds is primarily dependent on the nurse to patient ratio, training of the nursing staff regarding turning and positioning difficult patients, patient skin integrity, and size of the patient. Turning frames and kinetic beds are often recommended for the spinal injury patient requiring traction, although a standard bed can be adapted to provide cervical traction that allows the patient to be turned 90° to either side and sit up in bed for pulmonary care (see Fig. 3.20). With this system spinal stabilization is adequate for management of cervical flexion injuries (Frederick Geisler MD, personal communication). It is the author's opinion that the turning frame allows better

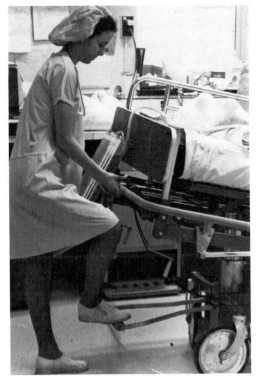

Figure 3.23. Hydraulic beds are easily placed in the head-down position.

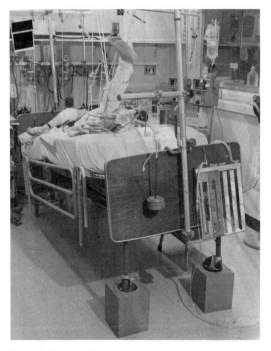

Figure 3.24. This electric bed is placed on shock blocks to promote more adequate postural drainage.

skin inspection, chest physiotherapy treatment, and early rehabilitation than a kinetic bed. Proponents of all specialty beds claim improved skin condition compared to a standard bed, although studies evaluating turning frequency and body position on standard versus specialty beds are minimal. It has been the author's personal observation that low air loss beds and flotation beds are often utilized to replace side to side turning. Turning affects all body systems, not just skin pressure. Air fluidized beds offer contact pressures lower than capillary closing pressures. Decreased capillary pressure is thought to lower the incidence of tissue breakdown and aid healing. Hargest (1977) states that pneumonia has not developed in patients on air fluidized beds whose primary problem is lack of movement. It is our experience and that of others (Smoot, 1986) that retained secretions and pneumonia do develop in trauma patients while on an air fluidized bed. Sitting upright and performing postural drainage are extremely difficult on this bed (Fig. 3.25).

The continuous movement of kinetic beds is thought to minimize tissue breakdown and secretion retention. Schimmel et al. (1977) demonstrated use of the kinetic bed to change ventilation–perfusion relationships. In a patient with a gunshot wound to the chest, a right lung contusion cleared, but a left lower lobe atelectasis was apparent on the chest x-ray taken within 8 hr of admission. Attempts to perform chest physiotherapy on patients in this bed demonstrate that adequate treatment can be given only for four lung segments: the anterior segments of both upper lobes, the right middle lobe, lingula, and anterior segments of both lower lobes. Seven postural drainage positions for the other lung segments therefore cannot be obtained, as the bed limits turning. In practice, the patient cannot be positioned with the affected lung uppermost for the most commonly atelectatic lung segments. The manufacturer advocates removal of the posterior chest portion of the bed to allow chest physiotherapy treatment. However, percussion and vibration without the use of segmental postural drainage is likely to be ineffective (see Chapter 4). Patients

Figure 3.25. The height and depth of the low air loss bed make mobilizing patients in and out of bed very difficult. Five staff members are required to lift this mechanically ventilated multiple trauma patient from the low air loss bed to a chair.

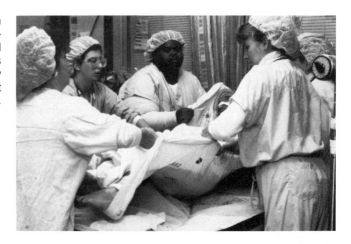

who do not tolerate positioning and turning on a turning frame because of increased ICP or agitation also do not tolerate treatment on the kinetic bed. For patients with increased ICP, a 45° head-elevated position is difficult to achieve. Table 3.2 compares standard and specialty beds. The following case history demonstrates the disadvantages of the kinetic bed for a patient with severe chest trauma.

Case History 3.4. A 19-year-old female was admitted to the trauma center following a motorcycle accident. She had a right pneumothorax, lung contusion, rib and clavicular fractures, and a torn right main stem bronchus. She was taken to the operating room for reanastomosis of the torn bronchus and a laparotomy. Liver lacerations were found and repaired.

After surgery the patient was placed on a kinetic bed. Repeat chest x-ray 8 hrs after admission showed the bilateral alveolar-interstitial infiltrates of respiratory distress syndrome (Fig. 3.26). This pattern persisted during the patient's hospital stay. The kinetic bed was used according to manufacturer's instructions when the patient was stable hemodynamically. No chest physiotherapy was given because of inability to achieve proper bronchial drainage positions. Chest x-ray 4 days after admission showed complete right lung atelectasis (Fig. 3.27). The patient's PaO_2 was 45 on an FIO_2 of 1.00. Bronchoscopy was performed; copious amounts of retained secretions were noted. The anastomosis in the right main stem bronchus remained intact. Cardiopulmonary arrest developed following bronchoscopy secondary to hypoxemia. The patient expired after numerous attempts at resuscitation, including open cardiac massage.

The kinetic bed was unable to prevent the development of complete right lung atelectasis in this patient with chest trauma. Chest physiotherapy performed with the patient turned into the postural drainage positions described in this chapter may have prevented some of the aspiration of blood and secretion retention. Once complete atelectasis and hypoxemia developed, they were irreversible.

This bed did not result in a favorable outcome with this patient. It may be advantageous for quadriplegic patients in a chronic facility, who have recurrent chest infections and decubitus ulcers. Often at home or in these facilities there is insufficient help for adequate patient turning. Bedridden quadriplegic patients who experience severe shoulder pain with side-to-side turning may prefer the kinetic bed. Results similar to the manufacturer's claims of treating acute atelectasis are obtained with chest physiotherapy (see Case History 6.1).

When working in a critical care unit it must be realized that any time a therapeutic intervention interferes with the operation of a specialty bed the cited benefits are eliminated. Many patients require bedside medical therapy, special studies, and transportation from the ICU for special procedures. Proponents of the rotating bed claim that the hazards of immobility are minimized and eliminated, although the bed is often immobile (Trammel et al., 1985), particularly when used for critically injured trauma patients (see Appendix, pp. 361-362). Initial claims by the manufacturer that kinetic therapy eliminates the hazards of immo-

Table 3.2
Comparison of Standard and Specialty Beds

Criteria	Standard Bed	Large Person	Turning Frame	Low Air Loss	Air Fluidized	Kinetic
Recommended patient population	All	When body weight exceeds standard bed weight requirements, 700 lb limit	Spinal injury or patients requiring inspection and treatment posteriorly, 250 lb limit	Immobilized patients, except spinal injury, tissue breakdown, burns	Burns, severe skin lesions, immobilized patient up to 260 lb. Not recommended with cardiac disease, reduced lung function, or disoriented patients (Kalaja, 1984)	Spinal injury requiring traction, immobilized patients, skin pressure sores, questionable for patients with elevated ICP. Patient must be able to tolerate rotation 18 hr/day
Patient evaluation and inspection	All body surfaces are exposed with side to side turning	Same	Same	Same	Same	Only anterior body surface is exposed. Pad placement restricts inspection
Bedside diagnostic tests	Allows 90° upright and lateral positioning for bedside x-rays and special procedures	Same, 90° upright easier to obtain	Cannot obtain true upright position	Same	Cannot obtain true upright position, difficult for placing cassettes to take bedside x-rays, more difficult to interpret x-rays	Cannot obtain true upright; abdominal and chest films are more difficult to obtain and interpret. Cassette rack placement is not ideal due to varying patient size
Turning ease and frequency	Dictated by the patient's medical status, usually every 2–3 hrs, 1–2 persons for routine turning, 3 for obese patients or prone positioning	Same, 3–4 persons may be required	Manufacturers suggest 1 person, in ICU 2 persons every 2 hrs, prone and supine positions	Same	Manufacturers claim these beds eliminate the need for patient turning although turning is necessary for most body systems (see Chapter 6); nursing staff often neglects necessary turning (Smoot, 1986)	124° every 3.5 min while rotating. One person required to operate bed
Patient comfort	Subjective, normal environmental stimulation	Subjective	Subjective, some patients do not like prone position	Subjective	Subjective, disorientation has been reported (Smoot, 1986; Lucke and Jarlsberg, 1985; Rath and Berger 1982). Patients have requested to be removed from bed (Bolyard et al., 1987) and complained of weightlessness, inability to move freely, and elevate head of bed (Nirmille and Storm 1984)	Subjective, manufacturers and Keane (1977) claim better than the Stryker frame; 4 stroke patients found confinement intolerable (Kelley et al., 1987); increased agitation has been noted in head injured patients; 30% patients on bed requested it be stopped (Trammell et al., 1985)

Table 3.2 (Continued)
Comparison of Standard and Specialty Beds

Criteria	Standard Bed	Large Person	Turning Frame	Low Air Loss	Air Fluidized	Kinetic
Pulmonary care	Suctioning: no interference	Suctioning: same	Suctioning: same, prone position assists oropharyngeal drainage	Suctioning: same	Suctioning: same	Suctioning: manufacturers claim the body position changes improve cannulation of the left mainstem bronchus. This is not substantiated in the literature (Kirimli et al., 1970; Kubota et al., 1980) Postural drainage: allows 12° head-down position; 4/11 positions can be obtained. Results same as documented by Mackenzie et al. (1985). Pulmonary complications may be reduced in spinal injury patients not easily turned (Reines and Harris, 1987) Decreased atelectasis, pneumonia, in trauma patients although frequency of turning on a conventional bed is not documented (Gentilello et al., 1988)
	Postural drainage: all postural drainage positions	Postural drainage: 5/11 drainage positions obtained. Does not go into head-down position	Postural drainage: 7 of 11 postural drainage positions, prone position assists drainage of posterior and most frequently involved lung segments	Postural drainage: same	Postural drainage: More difficult to obtain the 11 positions; head-down and sitting positions are not optimal. Atelectasis and decreased lung function documented (Smoot, 1987; Kalaja, 1984)	
Spinal alignment	Maintained through standard traction or special board, (see Fig. 3.20)	Same	Adequate for most spinal injuries	Not recommended for spinal stabilization	Not recommended for spinal stabilization	Proponents claim better than turning frame, not documented by controlled studies
Intracranial pressure	Head may be raised as necessary to lower ICP	Same	Head can be elevated to reduce ICP	Same	Difficult to maintain upright position; when patient is upright, posterior thorax does not receive benefit of bed	Kelley et al. (1987) found increased transtentorial herniation compared to standard bed, ICP not significantly altered by stationary bed positions (Gonzalez-Arias et al., 1983). Affect while rotating unkown

Pressure sores	Minimal with good nursing care	Unknown although bed has a very firm mattress which may lead to increased pressure sores	Decreased compared to kinetic bed (Trammell et al., 1985)	Decreased, reported to increase healing, contact pressure less than 27 mm Hg at any point, lower than standard bed (Beaver, 1986; Redfern et al., 1973)	Fluidized pressure 15–30 mm Hg (Lucke and Jarlsberg, 1985). Manufacturers and Micheels and Sorensen (1987) claim pressure relief and bactericidal effects prevent ulcers and promote healing, particularly with skin grafts and burns; heel and occipital ulcers reported (Parish and Witowski, 1980; Smoot, 1986)	Manufacturers and some authors claim decreased sores compared to standard bed (Green, 1980). Authors have noted heel and decubitus ulcers. Firm bed surface may lead to pressure sores when bed is not rotating
Mobility and functional activities	Normal	Upright position is easily obtained for self-care, bed can be adapted for easier transfer to the standing position	Allows self-feeding while prone; not appropriate for patients who can be mobilized out of bed	ADL easier than kinetic and air fluidized beds. Manufacturers claim shearing forces minimized when moving patient in bed	Upright positioning, bed to chair transfers, and ambulation require additional personnel, 3 or more personnel to lift patient out of bed (Fig. 3.25)	Spinal injury patients with upper extremity function are limited in ADL. Positioning to prevent shoulder and elbow contractures is difficult. Normal progression of mobilizing the ICU patient out of bed is cumbersome unless a special kinetic bed is used
Range of motion (ROM) exercises	Access to all joints for necessary exercises and bed positioning	Same	Same; allows positioning of SCI patients to prevent shoulder, elbow, ankle contractures	Same	More difficult to maintain and perform therapy for shoulders, elbows, and hips. Appear to develop more shoulder contractures (Smoot, 1986). Positioning is more problematic, when splinting is required to maintain joint ROM the effect of the bed is eliminated under splints. Shoulders cannot be appropriately positioned for burn victims (Lucke and Jarlsberg, 1985)	Many pads must be removed for range of motion exercises, full hip and shoulder extension cannot be obtained. Active exercise of all dorsal muscles is difficult

Table 3.2 (*Continued*)
Comparison of Standard and Specialty Beds

Criteria	Standard Bed	Large Person	Turning Frame	Low Air Loss	Air Fluidized	Kinetic
Deep vein thrombosis thrombophlebitis	Variable in the literature	Unknown in the obese population in this bed; improved ability to ambulate and mobilize the obese patient is thought to have a beneficial effect	Unknown	Unknown	Unknown	Proponents of the bed claim decreased venous stasis, decreased with heparin and support stockings (Kelley et al., 1987). Emhoff et al. (1987) documented deep vein thrombosis in a patient on a kinetic bed
Infection	Not specifically influenced by bed	Unknown	Unknown	Unknown	Controversial; Scheidt and Drusin (1983) report contamination of sheets in heavily infected burn patients; Bolyard et al. (1987) noted negligible difference to standard bed of air contamination in ulcer and pain patients	Decreased in stroke victims using bed (Kelley et al., 1987). Bed has many parts to be cleaned between patients
Safety/resuscitation	Board required	Same	Patients positioned prone must be turned supine for resuscitation	Rapid deflation of the sacs provide a flat, firm base for resuscitation	Can be rapidly defluidized for a firm surface	One person can stop bed for resuscitation, firm surface permits resuscitation
Mortality	Effect of bed unknown	Unknown	Inconclusive: reported by Brackett and Condon (1984) in a retrospective study to be increased for SCI patients	Unknown effect	Decreased mortality reported in burn victims (Scheuler and Munster, 1983)	Inconclusive: increased when compared to standard bed in controlled study of stroke victims. (Kelley et al., 1987). Brackett and Condon (1984) reported decreased mortality over the turning frame in a retrospective

Ease of transportation	Easier to move for special studies or transfer to the operating room than speciality beds other than the turning frame	Patient must be transferred to a stretcher for transport	Easier to move for special studies than other speciality beds	Some air loss beds have several bulky control units. Transportation more difficult than standard bed	Patient must be transferred to a stretcher for transportation	Very bulky, difficult to transport for special procedures
Expense (approximate)	No additional patient charge	$8000, $90/day		$50–60/day	$65–$80/day. Purchase not recommended by manufacturer because of comprehensive infection control guidelines; $39.20 per day over standard bed and decreased nursing care reported	$135/day
Hazards					Dehydration, increased insensible water loss, hypernatremia (McNabb and Hyatt, 1987; Micheels and Sorensen 1987; Rath and Berger 1982). Malfunction of thermal control, leaky nylon sheets, corneal abrasions. Ceramic beads may need to be changed more frequently than recommended by company. (Nirmille and Storm, 1984).	Lines and nasogastric tubes may be pulled out by rotating bed. Documented mechanical failure (Trammell et al., 1985)
Other					Thought to conserve body nitrogen through reducing body protein breakdown (Jones et al., 1985; Ryan, 1983)	

Figure 3.26. Chest x-ray taken within 8 hrs of admission, showing bilateral alveolar-interstitial infiltrates and a right lung contusion.

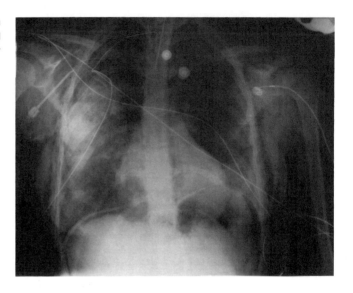

most patient populations have not been documented. Proponents of the bed now claim it does not replace routine nursing care (Green et al., 1983). Current literature, except for the studies by Kelley et al. (1987) and Gentilello et al. (1988) do not, in a controlled and detailed fashion, compare patient turning, mobilization, and pulmonary care to standard beds or a turning frame. Table 3.2 demonstrates documented advantages and disadvantages of specific beds. Specific criteria based on the results of well-designed studies need to be developed to justify the cost of specialty beds compared to traditional ones. The bed chosen for an

Figure 3.27. Complete right lung atelectasis developed after 4 days of treatment on a kinetic bed.

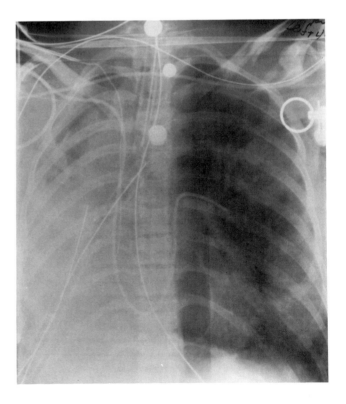

individual patient should include the ability to provide adequate pulmonary hygiene, splinting and range of motion exercises, normal environmental stimulation, and allow easy access for diagnostic tests and transfers to a bedside chair.

In our opinion the low air loss beds are the most practical of the specialty beds for the patient at high risk for tissue breakdown. Adequate patient mobility, comfort, orientation, and positioning can all be obtained. The exception is spinal injury patients who are managed quite well on a turning frame. The large person bed is very practical for the obese patient, although the major limitation is the inability to achieve the head-down position. Future clinical studies may determine the efficacy of the low air loss versus air fluidized beds.

BREATHING EXERCISES

Breathing exercises have been used since the 1890s to improve respiratory function (Nicholson, 1980). They are commonly taught to patients with chronic lung disease and neuromuscular disease, as well as to patients after surgery. The patient with chronic lung disease is often taught "breathing control" or "breathing retraining" exercises. Exercises used clinically include diaphragmatic and costal excursion exercises, the forced expiration technique, pursed lip breathing, and, more recently, the introduction of inspiratory muscle training (Leith and Bradley, 1976). In addition, segmental breathing exercises are frequently described in standard texts (Irwin and Tecklin, 1985; Frownfelter, 1987). Research has not documented these exercises to provide additional benefit over costal excursion exercises. As it is unlikely that a specific "segmental" breathing exercise can direct regional ventilation to a specific lung lobe or segment, these exercises are, therefore, not advocated.

The main goals of breathing exercises are to

1. Assist removal of secretions
2. Improve respiratory muscle strength and endurance
3. Increase thoracic cage mobility and tidal volume
4. Promote relaxation.

Studies evaluating lung ventilation with diaphragmatic and lateral costal excursion exercises show little or no change in the distribution of ventilation. It was found that ventilation is determined by body position and is greatest in dependent lung zones (Shearer et al., 1972; Bake et al., 1972; Sackner et al., 1974; Grimby et al., 1975; Martin et al., 1976; and Brach et al., 1977). This was true in normal subjects with unilateral lung disease (see pp. 93–94), and patients with chronic lung pathology. However, at high flow rates at functional residual capacity Roussos et al. (1977) and Fixley et al. (1978) found that in normal subjects abdominal inspiration increased gas distribution to the dependent lung, while intercostal inspiration gave a more even distribution of ventilation, preferentially to the nondependent lung zones. Hughes (1979) suggested that changes in thoracoabdominal shape could influence regional blood flow after measuring changes in segmental oxygen and carbon dioxide concentrations through a bronchoscope.

Recent studies continue to question the benefit of diaphragmatic breathing exercises for the patient with chronic lung disease. Williams et al. (1982) and Willeput et al. (1983) were unable to document a beneficial effect from thoracoabdominal breathing that was used to decrease paradoxical chest movements and improve exercise performance.

When studying the surgical patient, decreased postoperative pulmonary complications and hospital stay have been documented with chest physiotherapy treatment that included breathing exercises (Warren and Grimwood, 1980; Thoren, 1954; Morran et al., 1983; Wilklander and Norlin, 1957). Data are still inconclusive regarding the use of breathing exercises compared to other chest physiotherapy treatment components. It is difficult to separate the effects of coughing, position change, manual techniques, and breathing exercises because of the lack of standardization of chest physiotherapy treatment among acute care centers. Breathing exercise techniques used in patients who are hypoventilating due to intercostal muscle weakness or incisional pain after surgery require further investigation.

Breathing Exercises for the Patient with Obstructive Airway Disease

Diaphragmatic

For the patient with obstructive airway disease, diaphragmatic "breathing control" is advocated as a means of achieving relaxation and coordinated breathing patterns. It is often used with pursed lip breathing. Greater tidal volumes achieved with diaphragmatic breathing may improve overall ventilation (Brach et al., 1977). Use of an electronic respiration stimulator (Motley, 1963), a mechanical vibrator (Barach and Dulfano, 1968), and mechanical chest and abdominal compression (Petty and Guthrie, 1971) also demonstrated increased tidal volume and decreased respiratory rate in patients with chronic airway obstruction. Although an immediate decrease in respiratory rate and increased tidal volume are demonstrated, long-term beneficial effects are not substantiated (see pp. 119) (Miller, 1954; Becklake et al., 1954; McNeill and McKenzie, 1955; Campbell, 1955; Emirgil et al., 1969; Petty and Guthrie, 1971, Willeput et al., 1983; Williams et al., 1982).

Pursed Lip Breathing

Pursed lip breathing, used in conjunction with breathing retraining and diaphragmatic breathing, is often taught to the patient with chronic obstructive pulmonary disease. Temporary benefits include increased tidal volume, decreased respiratory rate, reduction in $PaCO_2$ levels, and improved PaO_2. Subjective benefit is reported by many patients (Thoman et al., 1966; Mueller et al., 1970; Barach, 1973; Motley, 1963; Tiep et al., 1986). Ingram (1967) demonstrated that symptomatic relief may occur before alveolar ventilation is altered. Although

the underlying physiological mechanism is not known, pursed lip breathing appears to be a beneficial noninvasive maneuver for some patients with chronic pulmonary disease. It can be taught in the hospital and the response of the patient monitored with ear oximetry. Temporary improvement in oxygen saturation is noted when pursed lip breathing is compared to relaxation. Tiep et al. (1986) believe pursed lip breathing may improve patient confidence and decrease anxiety by providing some temporary control over oxygenation.

Breathing Control

Breathing control is taught to asthmatics and patients with chronic lung disease for use when in mild to moderate distress. These patients may require the side-lying, head-elevated, or forward-leaning posture to achieve relaxation instruction.

Changes in posture alter respiratory function more dramatically than breathing retraining. Leaning forward posture, and, less frequently, the supine or head-down positions alter minute ventilation, expiratory reserve volume, minimize accessory muscle activity, relieve dyspnea, and correct paradoxical abdominal motion (Delgado et al., 1982; Sharp et al., 1980; Barach, 1974). The leaning forward posture is also adopted by long distance runners (Haas et al., 1982). In these healthy individuals who are stressing the respiratory system and in patients with chronic pulmonary disease, diaphragmatic function is thought to be improved by altering the muscle length–tension relationship when leaning forward. When teaching breathing retraining it may be necessary to utilize the optimum position for an individual patient (leaning forward, supine, or head down) and provide a manual stretch to the diaphragm. This would place the diaphragm in a position to facilitate optimum length–tension relationship. Kigen (1984) reports dramatic relief of dyspnea, improved walking ability, and minimal use of accessory muscles with a manual stretch applied to the diaphragm. In one recent study exercise reconditioning and breathing retraining led to significantly greater exercise tolerance, decreased respiratory rate, increased tidal volume, and improved PaO_2 when compared to exercise alone (Casciari et al., 1981). Electromyogram and biofeedback were used to monitor relaxation of the accessory muscles. Magnetometry and biofeedback were utilized to synchronize movement of the abdomen and thorax. One difference in this study and previous studies not substantiating a benefit of breathing retraining (Williams et al., 1982; Booker, 1984) is that objective measurements were taken and utilized in conjunction with the breathing exercises. For some patients biofeedback and magnetometry may be necessary to achieve the desired effects of breathing retraining in conjunction with a change in posture. Improved throacoabdominal motion noted clinically may actually induce paradoxical chest motion and induce hypoventilation during breathing exercise training (Willeput et al., 1983). Paradoxical chest motion may therefore appear abnormal but actually be beneficial for some patients. Asynchronous chest motion detected through magnetometers may be an indicator of exercise tolerance (Delgado et al., 1982). This may have clinical significance in the ICU when breathing exercises are used in conjunction with weaning the chronic lung disease patient from mechanical ventilation.

While teaching breathing control Innocenti (1966) advocated avoiding full expiration and beginning inspiration sooner than usual. In theory, prolonged expiration does not achieve significant emptying of emphysematous bullae but does compress and hamper ventilation of normal lung, Gandevia (1960), Miller (1967), Gaskell and Webber (1975), and Cash (1975) state that expiration should be controlled, but not forceful, to avoid increased airway resistance caused by premature airway closure and progressive air trapping. Webber (personal communication) believes avoiding full expiration and controlled expiration are essentially the same. Becklake et al. (1954). Dorinson (1955), and Campbell et al. (1986) emphasize prolonged expiration. It is our opinion that a controlled expiration, at times through pursed lips, followed by maximal inspiration is most beneficial.

Forced Expiration Technique

The forced expiration technique is described in the European and Australian literature as a breathing exercise that may minimize or eliminate the need for manual or mechanical techniques when used in conjunction with postural drainage. This breathing exercise is used most often with stable cystic fibrosis, although it may be employed with chronic lung disease, and possibly after surgery. The forced expiration technique consists of controlled diaphragmatic breathing exercises interspersed with "huffing" (forced expirations from mid-lung to low-lung volume) (see pp. 162). Currie et al. (1986) believe the forced expiration technique (four deep breaths with relaxed expiration followed by diaphragmatic breathing and forced expirations, diaphragmatic breathing, and one to two coughs) performed in appropriate postural drainage positions replaces the manual techniques of percussion and vibration. Sutton and colleagues (1983, 1984) found the forced expiration technique was more effective than directed coughing with the most sputum obtained when it was used in conjunction with postural drainage. In a later study Sutton et al. (1985) documented this exercise was more effective than manual techniques that were used with postural drainage to the affected lung. Faulk and colleagues (1984) found greater sputum production in cystic fibrosis patients using a face mask to deliver positive expiratory pressure in conjunction with postural drainage when compared to chest physiotherapy that included the forced expiration technique.

Documented benefits of the forced expiration technique include decreased time required for postural drainage and increased patient independence (Pryor et al., 1979a,b; Murphy et al., 1983; Webber et al., 1985). This may be a very cost-effective maneuver for patients with lung disease requiring life-long assistance to remove excessive tracheobronchial secretions.

Ventilatory Muscle Training

Since the initial work of Leith and Bradley in 1976 that demonstrated an increase of inspiratory muscle strength and endurance in normal subjects with training, breathing with inspiratory resistance is used in COPD, muscular dystrophy, severe kyphoscoliosis, acid maltase deficiency, following spinal cord injury, and with cystic fibrosis (Fig. 3.28). The majority of research includes subjects with chronic lung disease and cystic fibrosis and results are variable (Table 3.3). Training is prescribed for improving ventilatory muscle strength, endurance, or both. Strength training is accomplished by subjects breathing through a narrow tube that offers inspiratory resistance. The size of the tube orifice is determined by the patients tolerance, usually for 5–15 min (Kim 1984; Jederlinic et al., 1984; Dimarco et al., 1985; Belman et al., 1986; Hornstein and Ledsome, 1986). Endurance training is usually thought to be accomplished through isocapnic exercise that affects both the inspiratory and expiratory muscles. In this type of training subjects train for up to 15 min while the maximum sustained ventilatory capacity is measured under isocapnic conditions. Pardy et al. (1981b) and Sonne and Davis (1982) documented endurance with inspiratory muscle training as the amount of resistance that could be tolerated for

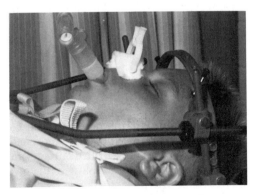

Figure 3.28. This quadriplegic patient uses inspiratory muscle training during acute hospitalization.

10 min, or the time a patient could sustain a critical level of resistance. Currently the inspiratory muscle training devices are more practical than isocapnic exercise for clinical and home use. Training benefits occur after 15–30 min of exercise daily for four to eight weeks. As noted in Table 3.3, research is inconclusive as to whether these breathing exercises consistently improve respiratory muscle strength and endurance (Pardy et al., 1988). Controlled studies where a training stimulus is chosen to achieve a desired response with larger patient populations are needed to determine the worth of inspiratory muscle training. Specific patient populations to be studied include cystic fibrosis, chronic lung disease, muscular dystrophy, and quadriplegia comparing the response of training to diaphragmatic breathing and general conditioning exercises. The advantage of this type of training compared to other approaches is the ability to exercise regularly at home with minimal equipment that is inexpensive.

Breathing Exercises for the Patient after Surgery

The incidence of postoperative pulmonary complications remains at 12–22% despite advances in postoperative pulmonary care (Ford and Guenter, 1984). The majority of complications occur following thoracic or upper abdominal surgery. Chest physiotherapy is routinely prescribed following surgery and at times preoperatively. Tarhan and colleagues (1973) documented that preoperative pulmonary preparation decreased postoperative pulmonary complications without altering mortality in 190 men and 37 women requiring thoracic and abdominal surgery. Recently Castillo and Haas (1985) studied preoperative chest physiotherapy that included breathing exercises and documented a decrease in overall complications and atelectasis. This patient population included 200 upper abdominal and thoracic surgical patients over age 65. Respiratory therapy that includes breathing exercises has significantly decreased the incidence of pneumonia and atelectasis following surgery (Campbell et al., 1986; Morran et al.,

Table 3.3
Studies Evaluating Ventilatory Muscle Training[a]

Reference	Population Studied	Training	Results
Smith et al. (1988)	8 Duchenne muscular dystrophy	2×/day—tolerable load for 10–15 min; 5 weeks—blinded; crossover method	No ↑ VC or MI max
Abelson and Brewer (1987)	1 COPD, 3 quadriplegic who failed weaning from mechanical ventilation	bid, 15 min at initial tidal volume; 21–71 days	↑ VC; ↑ PImax; ↑ endurance
Clanton (1987)	16 swimmers	8 controls, 8 IMT; 50–60% PI max ≅10 min, 3× week, 10 weeks	No additional benefit of IMT over a conditioning program
Hornstein (1987)	2 severe kyphoscoliosis	bid, 15 min when tolerated	↑ functional ability ↑ PI max, 1 subject ↑ endurance
McKeon et al. (1986)	18 severe COPD after optimum conventional therapy	10 subjects; orifice sizes 5–2.5mm; three 15 min sessions/day, 6 weeks; 8 trained with placebo	No ↑ in inspiratory muscle strength (PI max); ↑ tolerance of resistance; no ↑ mean exercise capacity
Belman et al. (1986)	10 COPD	One orifice smaller than orifice patient could sustain for 15 min, 15 min bid, 6 weeks	No change spirometric, pulmonary volumes, PI max, MEP, maximum sustained ventilatory capacity
Hornstein and Ledsome (1986)	20 acute quadriplegics	Resistance tolerated for 15 min, 15 min bid	↑ PImax 10 subjects, safe for acute stage quadriplegia
Larson et al. (1986)	22 COPD	Threshold breathing device 30 min/day, 2 mos; 12–15% PImax; 10–30% PImax	↑ endurance; ↑ inspiratory muscle strength; ↑ 12 min walk test; group exercising at 30% PImax
Aldrich and Karpel (1985)	4 chronic respiratory failure patients who failed weaning	Max tidal airway pressure 15–20% PNIP, 5–30 min, 10–24 days	↑ PNIP in 3 patients, successful weaning
Clanton et al. (1985)	8 normal females	Resistance adjusted to maintain adequate tidal volume, 10 weeks, 25 min/week	↑ PImax, ↑ endurance time
Dimarco et al. (1985)	11 muscular dystrophy	As tolerated for 5–15 min, 15 min bid, 6 weeks	↑ VC, ↑ PI max, ↑ FEV₁, ↑ duration of hyperpnea
Ambrosino et al. (1984)	16 stable COPD	Breathing exercises, 3–10 min sessions daily of inspiratory training; compared to medical treatment alone; fatigue measured clinically and by EMG	No added benefit measured in pulmonary function tests, blood gases, or exercise tolerance

Table 3.3 (*Continued*)
Studies Evaluating Ventilatory Muscle Training[a]

Reference	Population Studied	Training	Results
Jederlinic (1984)	6 normals, 19 COPD	4 weeks, resistor at 1 setting below max, 30 min daily	↓ SaO$_2$, no training effect
Larson and Kim. (1984)	9 stable COPD	15 min bid, 1 month	↑ PImax, ↑ sputum expectoration, no change 12 min walk test
Martin (1983)	1 acid maltase deficiency patient	bid, 15 min; 6, 21, 46, cm H$_2$O/liter/sec	↑ SaO$_2$; ↓ O$_2$ during sleep; ↑ endurance
Asher et al. (1982)	11 cystic fibrosis, moderately severe airflow limitation	Max resistance tolerated for 10 min, 4 weeks bid	↑ PImax and endurance, little effect on exercise performance
Sonne and Davis (1982)	6 severe COPD	Resistance tolerated 10 min, 30 min daily, 6 weeks	↑ endurance (amount inspiratory resistance tolerated for 10 min), ↑ max respiratory exercise capability
Pardy et al. (1981a)	17 patients with chronic airflow limitation	Compared IMT 30 min daily to exercises 3×/week, 2 months	IMT showed ↑ endurance time in distance walked in 12 min
Pardy et al. (1981b)	12 moderate to severe COPD	Resistance adjusted to minimal resistance with a sustained decrease H/L ratio noted in 2 of 3 respiratory muscles, 15 min bid, 2 months	↑ inspiratory muscle endurance documented by EMG and 12 min walk test, no change strength

Study	Subjects	Protocol	Results
Belman (1981)	2 COPD with acute respiratory failure	15 min hyperpnea 3–6× daily during weaning	↑ MSVC; ↑ ventilatory muscle endurance
Belman and Mittman (1980)	10 stable COPD	15 min MSVC, 6 weeks	Significant ↑ in MSVC, ↑ arm and leg exercise tolerance
Gross et al. (1980)	6 chronic quadriplegics	Resistance determined by EMG signs of fatigue, 30 min daily, 8–16 weeks	↑ PI Max and PmCrit, strength and endurance
Bradley and Leith (1978)	12 normals (4 strength, 4 endurance, 4 control)	Measured O_2 consumption during sustained voluntary normocapneic hyperpnea	↑ aerobic endurance of respiratory muscles with endurance training
Keens et al. (1977)	4 normals, 4 cystic fibrosis patients	Maximal sustainable ventilatory capacity 25 min/day, 5 days/week; normocapnic hyperpnea 4 weeks; 1.5 hr/day physical training	Upper body endurance exercise is as effective at increasing ventilatory muscle endurance as specific training
Leith and Bradley (1976)	12 normals	4 trained 30 min daily, 5 days week, 5 weeks, strength training at 20% intervals of VC, 4 trained for endurance through "ventilatory sprints"	↑ VC, ↑ TLC in strength training, ↑ maximal voluntary ventilation in endurance training

[a] H/L ratio, electromyogram ratio, amplitudes of high and low frequency; PNIP, peak negative inspiratory pressure; EMG, electromyogram; PmCrit, critical mouth pressure; MSVC, maximum sustained ventilatory capacity; MIN, minutes; MEP, maximum expiratory pressure; MAX, maximum; IMT, inspiratory muscle training; VC, vital capacity; TLC, total lung capacity; FEV_1, forced expiratory volume in 1 sec and; SaO_2, arterial oxygen saturation; PI max, maximum inspiratory pressure.

1983; Celli et al., 1984; Castillo and Haas, 1985). Diaphragmatic and lateral costal breathing exercises with vibration were shown to decrease chest infection when studying 102 patients following cholecystectomy (Morran et al., 1983). Campbell et al. (1986) demonstrated that hand-delivered positive expiratory pressure (PEP) and breathing exercises delivered to 71 abdominal surgery patients decreased respiratory complications. Smoking appeared to increase the incidence of respiratory complications; due to a larger number of smokers in the control group it is not known if PEP is of additional benefit compared to breathing exercises alone. Celli and colleagues (1984) found deep breathing exercises to be as effective as incentive spirometry and intermittent positive pressure breathing (IPPB) in 172 patients who had abdominal surgery.

Following pediatric surgery the institution of breathing exercises and postural drainage demonstrated a significant decrease in the incidence of atelectasis (Strandberg, 1956). Postural drainage was not differentiated from the use of breathing exercises in this study. Breathing exercises for patients following cardiothoracic procedures were studied by Vraciu and Vraciu (1977). In high-risk patients, breathing exercises resulted in a significant decrease in pulmonary complications, suggesting that they were more effective than postural drainage with percussion. However, patients intubated for greater than 48 hrs and those in whom additional chest physiotherapy was ordered were excluded. The group of patients in whom postural drainage and percussion may be of greatest benefit was therefore eliminated.

After coronary artery by-pass procedures Dull and Dull (1983) measured pulmonary function in 49 adults randomly assigned to a breathing exercise, incentive spirometry, or early mobilization group. Neither form of breathing exercise showed benefit over early patient mobilization. Hallbook and colleagues (1984) also documented patient mobilization to be as effective as chest physiotherapy in 154 patients after gallbladder surgery. Based on our clinical experience patient mobilization may replace routine breath-

ing exercises and chest physiotherapy after upper abdominal or thoracic surgical procedures except when there is a specific clinical indication for chest physiotherapy (see Chapter 6). Breathing exercises and postural drainage with manual techniques are necessary for the more acutely ill patient who cannot be optimally mobilized or who does not deep breathe and cough spontaneously.

The effects of deep breathing on arterial oxygenation were studied by Ward et al. (1966) and Hedstrand et al. (1978). Ward et al. studied ten normal subjects breathing 100% oxygen. Maximal inspiration, with and without a 5 sec hold, and 12 successive deep breaths were evaluated by arterial blood gas analysis. The greatest increase in arterial oxygenation was found with maximal inspiration and a 5-sec hold. There is controversy surrounding whether breathing 100% oxygen increases intrapulmonary shunt (McAslan et al., 1973), but it is a frequently stated opinion that it causes microatelectasis due to denitrogenation. These conclusions, therefore, may not be justified. Breath holding, which causes positive pressure in the lungs, is presumably the most effective of the three methods studied in reversing this process. Hedstrand et al. (1978) investigated 45 patients with several types of deep-breathing devices, which included incentive spirometry, the Bird asthmatic insufflator, and a paper coil. All produced essentially the same improvement in arterial oxygenation. Deep breathing with instruction by a physical therapist gave the same improvement in PaO_2 without the use of any mechanical devices.

Maneuvers designed to decrease pulmonary complications after surgery are unable to completely eliminate atelectasis and pneumonia. This may be due to a reduction of diaphragmatic function after thoracic or upper abdominal surgery (Ford et al., 1983; Simonneau; et al., 1983). It remains unclear whether breathing exercises can alter diaphragmatic dysfunction that is thought to cause the adjacent lung to retain secretions (Ford and Guenter, 1984). Current studies suggest that diaphragmatic contractility is not altered after surgery but diaphragmatic dysfunction is secondary to decreased afferent input of the phenic nerve. Diaphragm activity spontaneously returns 24 to 48 hr after operation (Dureuil et al., 1986), Ford and Guenter, 1984). Block of this afferent stimulation may be used in conjunction with diaphragmatic breathing exercises. Pain and anaesthesia may not contribute as greatly to postoperative pulmonary complications as previously thought (Craig, 1981).

Benefits gained from breathing exercises such as diaphragmatic, and lateral costal exercises, which are traditionally taught by physiotherapists, may be the same as the benefits gained from deep breathing alone. Improvement in pain-limited chest wall mobility is thought to be seen following breathing exercises when they are given to the patient after surgery (Grimby, 1974). Whether improved chest wall movement necessarily has any long-term benefit to ventilation of the underlying lung is not determined.

It is our opinion that breathing exercises are beneficial when used for spontaneously breathing patients to assist in removal of secretions. They are used independently or in conjunction with other chest physiotherapy techniques. The addition of chest percussion and postural drainage depends on evaluation of the results of the breathing exercises for spontaneously breathing patients. If decreased or adventitial breath sounds do not improve with deep breathing and coughing, chest physiotherapy is carried out to the clinical and radiological area of involvement.

Methods of Teaching Breathing Exercises

Diaphragmatic Breathing

The techniques of teaching breathing exercises are well described by Gaskell and Webber (1973), Cash (1975), Irwin and Tecklin (1985), and Frownfelter (1987). Diaphragmatic breathing exercises are used primarily to increase tidal volume, to assist in the removal of secretions, and for relaxation.

The following technique is used to teach diaphragmatic breathing:

1. The postoperative patient is positioned relaxed in the sitting position with the back of the head supported. The COPD patient may lean forward or assume a position to enhance respiratory function.
2. The therapist should oberve the patient's breathing pattern and note whether it is primarily abdominal, upper chest, or lateral costal.
3. The therapist's hand should be placed either just below the xiphoid process or over the costal cartilages of the lower ribs (Fig. 3.29).
4. The patient is encouraged to exhale and then "fill out your waist," or to "push the therapist's hand up" during inspiration. Simple commands and demonstration are usually most effective. Relaxation of the upper chest and shoulders is encouraged.
5. This maneuver is carried out with the patient's hand placed over the upper abdomen (Fig. 3.30).
6. It is repeated until adequate expansion is achieved.

Costal Excursion Exercises

Costal excursion exercises are used to mobilize the thoracic cage, especially in patients with intercostal weakness. They may also relieve splinting from incisional or abdominal pain and may promote deep breathing in all postural drainage postions. The hands are placed over the area

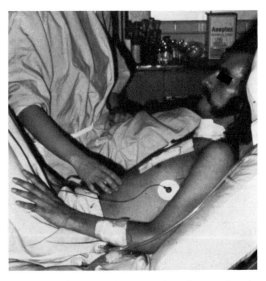

Figure 3.29.   A patient receives instruction in diaphragmatic breathing exercises.

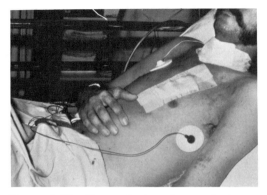

Figure 3.30. The patient performs diaphragmatic breathing independently after instruction.

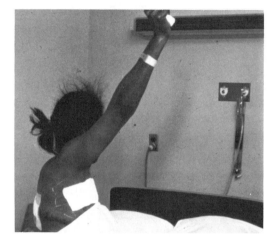

Figure 3.32. After thoracotomy this patient is performing active shoulder range of motion exercises.

of the lung being treated. Lateral costal excursion and diaphragmatic breathing exercises are the most frequently used breathing exercises.

The following technique is used to teach lateral costal excursion exericses:

1. The palm of the therapist's hand is placed over the seventh to tenth ribs laterally.
2. The patient is encouraged to take an active deep inspiration, pushing the lower ribs outward against the therapist's hands.
3. The therapist gradually increases resistance to this movement, as much as can be tolerated by the patient (Fig. 3.31).
4. The patient exhales, and the maneuver is repeated.

Once the patient has mastered chest wall movement, inspiration may be coordinated with shoulder flexion and abduction exercises and expiration may be coordinated with shoulder adduction and extension exercises. Incisional or referred pleuritic pain from chest tubes often limits shoulder motion. In these patients, active range of motion exercises may be administered within the limits of pain (Fig. 3.32). This maintains scapular mobility and reduces the chances of adhesions forming in the joint capsule. No problems with dislodgment of the chest tube have been noted during range of motion exercises. However, all chest tubes are sutured into place. Trunk flexion, extension and rotation exercises may also be added depending upon the individual patient's limitation of motion (Fig. 3.33).

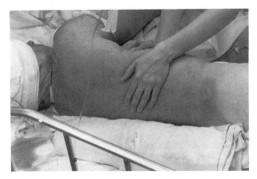

Figure 3.31. A patient receiving lateral costal excursion exercises in conjunction with postural drainage of the right lower lobe.

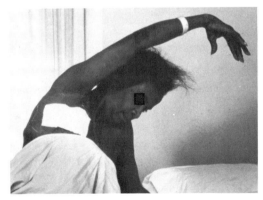

Figure 3.33. Lateral trunk flexion exercises are incorporated with breathing exercises to improve thoracic cage mobility.

SUMMARY

Chest physiotherapy is best performed in optimum bronchial drainage positions, even when positioning is difficult. The type of bed will influence the ability to properly position patients for postural drainage. Standard beds that achieve a 15° or greater head-down position are preferred. A turning frame and low air loss bed allow better positioning than kinetic and air fluidized beds. In spontaneously breathing patients, breathing exercises are used to increase tidal volume and aid removal of secretions. Chest wall movement is encouraged by use of costal excursion exercises in patients who have incisional pain, intercostal muscle weakness, or poor inspiratory force. Diaphragmatic breathing, lateral costal excursion exercises, or encouragement to breathe deeply and cough precede chest physiotherapy in spontaneously breathing patients. The forced expiration technique may replace manual techniques in cystic fibrosis and COPD. For spontaneously breathing patients without clinical or radiological evidence of retention of secretion, diaphragmatic breathing exercises the forced expiration technique, or inspiratory muscle training may be all that is required for prophylaxis. The COPD patient may benefit from breathing exercises in the leaning forward or head-down position. Early patient mobilization after minor surgical procedures may replace the need for chest physiotherapy.

References

Abelson H, Brewer K: Inspiratory muscle training in the mechanically ventilated patient. *Physiother Can* 39(5):305–307, 1987

Aldrich TK, Karpel JP: Inspiratory muscle resistive training in respiratory failure. *Am Rev Respir Dis* 131:461–462, 1985

Ambrosino N, Paggiaro PL, Roselli MG, Contini V: Failure of resistive breathing training to improve pulmonary function tests in patients with chronic obstructive pulmonary disease. *Respiration* 45:455–459, 1984

Asher MI, Pardy RL, Coates AL, Thomas E, Macklem P: The effects of inspiratory muscle training in patients with cystic fibrosis. *Am Rev Respir Dis* 126:855–859, 1982

Arborelius M, Granqvist U, Lija B, Zanner CW: Regional lung function and central haemodynamics in the right lateral body position during hypoxia and hyperoxia. *Respiration* 31:193–200, 1974

Bake B, Fugl-Meyer AR, Grimby G: Breathing patterns and regional ventilation distribution in tetraplegic patients and in normal subjects. *Clin Sci* 42:117–128, 1972

Barach AL, Dulfano MJ: Effect of chest vibration in pulmonary emphysema: A Preliminary report. *Ann Allergy* 26:10–17, 1968

Barach AL: Physiologic advantages of grunting, groaning, and pursed-lip breathing: Adaptive symptoms related to the development of continuous positive pressure breathing. *Bull NY Acad Med* 49(8):666–673, 1973

Barach AL: Chronic obstructive lung disease: Postural relief of dyspnea. *Arch Phys Med Rehabil* 55:494–504, 1974

Barrell SE, Abbas HM: Monitoring during physiotherapy after open heart surgery. *Physiotherapy* 64:272–273, 1978

Bateman J, Newman S, Daunt K, Sheahan N, Pavia P, Clarke S: Is cough as effective as chest physiotherapy in the removal of excessive tracheobronchial secretions? *Thorax* 36:683–687, 1981

Beaver M: Mediscus low air loss beds and the prevention of decubutus ulcers. *Crit Care Nurse* 6:32–39, 1986

Becklake M, McGregor M, Goldman HI, Braudo JL: A study of the effects of physiotherapy in chronic hypertrophic emphysema using lung function tests. *Dis Chest* 26:180–191, 1954

Belman MJ: Respiratory failure treated by ventilatory muscle training. *Eur J Respir Dis* 62:391–395, 1981

Belman MJ, Mittman C: Ventilatory muscle training improves exercise capacity in chronic obstructive pulmonary disease patients. *Am Rev Respir Dis* 121:273–280, 1980

Belman MJ, Thomas SG, Lewis M: Resistive breathing training in patients with chronic obstructive pulmonary disease. *Chest* 90:662–669, 1986

Bobath B: *Adult Hemiplegia, Evaluation and Treatment*, p 79. William Heinemann Medical Books, London, 1974

Bolyard EA, Townsend TR, Horan T: Airborne contamination associated with in-use air-fluidized beds: A descriptive study. *Am J Infect Control* 15(2):75–78, 1987

Booker HA: Exercise training and breathing control in patients with chronic airflow limitation. *Physiotherapy* 70(7):258–260, 1984

Brach BB, Chao RP, Sgroi VL, Minh VD, Ashburn WL, Moser KM: Xenon washout patterns during diaphragmatic breathing. *Chest* 71:735–739, 1977

Brackett TO, Condon N: Comparison of the wedge turning frame and kinetic treatment table in the acute care of spinal cord injury patients. *Surg Neurol.* 22:53–56, 1984

Bradley ME, Leith DE: Ventilatory muscle training and the oxygen cost of sustained hyperpnea. *J Appl Physiol: Respir Environ Exercise Physiol* 45(6):885–892, 1978

Browner BD, Kaneja S, Edwards CC: The use of modified Neufeld traction in the management of femoral fractures in polytrauma. *J Trauma* 21:778–786, 1981

Brumback KJ, Bosse MJ, Poka A, Burgess AK: Intramedullary stabilization of humeral shaft fractures in patients with multiple trauma: *J Bone Joint Surg* 68(1):960–969, 1986

Bryan AC: Comments of a devil's advocate. *Am Rev Respir Dis* 110(2):143–144, 1974

Burgess AR, Mandelbaum BR: Acute orthopedic injuries. In *Trauma Emergency Surgery and Critical Care*, edited by J Siegel, p 1062. Churchill Livingston, 1987

Buscaglia AJ, St Marie MS: Oxygen saturation during chest physiotherapy for acute exacerbation of severe chronic obstructive pulmonary disease. *Respir Care* 28:1009–1013, 1983

Campbell EJM, Friend J: Action of breathing exercises in pulmonary emphysema. 1:325–329, 1955

Campbell T, Ferguson N, McKinlay RGC: The use of a simple self-administered method of positive expiratory pressure (PEP) in chest physiotherapy after abdominal surgery. *Physiotherapy* 72(10):498–500, 1986

Casciari RJ, Fairshter RD, Harrison A, Morrison JT, Blackburn C, Wilson AF: Effects of breathing retraining in patients with chronic obstructive pulmonary disease. *Chest* 79:393–398, 1981

Cash JE: *Chest, Heart and Vascular Disorders for Physiotherapists*, pp 121–127. JB Lippincott, New York, 1975

Castillo R, Haas A: Chest physical therapy: Comparative efficacy of preoperative and postoperative in the elderly. *Arch Phys Med Rehabil* 66:376–379, 1985

Celli BR, Rodriquez KS, Snider G: A controlled trail of intermittent positive pressure breathing, incentive spirometry, and deep breathing exercises in preventing pulmonary complications after abdominal surgery. *Am Rev Respir Dis* 130:12–15, 1984

Chang S, Kwang JC, Chun J, Williams MH, Blaufos D: Positional effects on distribution of ventilation in chronic obstructive pulmonary disease. *Ann Intern Med* 105(3):346–350, 1986

Chulay M, Brown J, Summer W: Effect of postoperative immobilization after coronary artery bypass. *Crit Care Med* 10:176–179, 1982

Clanton TL, Dixon GF, Drake J, Gadek JE: Effects of swim training on lung volumes and inspiratory muscle conditioning. *J Appl Physiol* 62(1):39–46, 1987

Clanton TL, Dixon G, Drake J, Gadek J: Inspiratory muscle conditioning using a threshold device. *Chest* 87:62–66, 1985

Clauss RH, Scalabrini BY, Ray JF, Reed GE: Effects of changing body position upon improved ventilation-perfusion relationships. *Circulation*(Suppl 2)37:214–217, 1968

Craig DB: Postoperative recovery of pulmonary function. *Anesth Analg* 60:46–52, 1981

Currie DC, Munro C, Gaskell D, Cole PJ: Practice, problems and compliance with postural drainage. A survey of chronic sputum producers. *Br J Dis Chest* 80:249–253, 1986

DeCesare J: Physical therapy for the child with respiratory dysfunction. In *Cardiopulmonary Physical Therapy*, edited by S Irwin and J Tecklin, p 336. Mosby, St. Louis, 1985

Delgado HR, Braun SR, Skatrud JB, Reddan WG, Peglow DF: Chest wall and abdominal motion during exercise in patients with chronic obstructive pulmonary disease. *Am Rev Respir Dis* 126:200–205, 1982

Dhainaut JF, Bons J, Bricard C, Monsallier JF: Improved oxygenation in patients with extensive unilateral pneumonia using the lateral decubitus position. *Thorax* 35:792–793, 1980

Dimarco A, Dimarco M, Jacobs I, Shields R, Altose M: The effects of inspiratory resistive training on respiratory muscle function in patients with muscular dystrophy. *Muscle Nerve* 8:284–290, 1985

Dorinson SM: Breathing exercises for bronchial asthma and pulmonary emphysema. *JAMA* 156:931–933, 1955

Douglas WW, Rehder K, Beynen FM, Sessler AD, Marsh HM: Improved oxygenation in patients with acute respiratory failure: The prone position. *Am Rev Respir Dis* 115:559–566, 1977

Dull JL, Dull WL: Are maximal inspiratory breathing exercises or incentive spirometry better than early mobilization after cardiopulmonary bypass? *Phys Ther* 63(5):655–659, 1983

Dureuil B, Viires N, Cantineau JP, Aubier M, Desmonts JM: Diaphragmatic contractility after upper abdominal surgery. *J Appl Physiol* 61(5):1775–1780, 1986

Edwards CC, Jaworski MF, Solana J, Aronson B: Management of compound tibial fractures by external fixation. *Am Surg* 45:190–203, 1979

Emhoff T, Wedel S, Geisler FH, Gens D. The occurrence and detection of deep venous thrombosis and pulmonary embolism in the spinal cord injured patient. (abstract) *Crit Care Med* 15(4):428, 1987

Emirgil C, Sobol BJ, Norman H, Moskowitze: A study of the long term effect of therapy in chronic obstructive pulmonary disease. *Am J Med* 47:367–376, 1969

Faulk M, Kelstrup JB, Anderson JB, Kinoshita T, Falk P, Stovring S, Gothgen I: Improving the ketchup bottle method with positive expiratory pressure, PEP, in cystic fibrosis. *Eur J Respir Dis* 65:423–432, 1984

Fellander M: Treatment of fractures and pseudoarthrosis of the long bones by Hoffmann's transfixation method. *Acta Orthop Scand* 33:132–143, 1963

Fixley MS, Roussos CS, Murphy B, Martin RR, Engel LA: Flow dependence of gas distribution and the pattern of inspiratory muscle contraction. *J Appl Physiol* 45:733–741, 1978

Ford GT, Whitelaw WA, Rosenal TW, Cruse PJ, Guenter CA: Diaphragm function after upper abdominal surgery in humans. *Am Rev Respir Dis* 127:431–436, 1983

Ford GT, Guenter CA: Toward prevention of postoperative pulmonary complications. *Am Rev Respir Dis* 130:4–5, 1984

Froese A, Bryan AC: Effects of anesthesia and paralysis on diaphragmatic mechanics in man. *Anesthesiology* 41:242–255, 1974

Frownfelter D: *Chest Physical Therapy and Pulmonary Rehabilitation, an Interdisciplinary Approach*, pp 239–259. Year Book, Chicago, 1987.

Gandevia B: The treatment of chronic bronchitis and bronchiectasis. *Med J Aust* 47:700–703, 1960

Gaskell DV, Webber BA: *The Brompton Hospital Guide to Chest Physiotherapy*, 2nd ed., pp 5–9, 13–15, 22–23. Blackwell Scientific Publications, London, 1973

Gentilello L, Thompson P, Tonnesen A, Hernandez D, Kapadia A, Allen S, Houteher SB, Miner M: Effect of a rotating bed on the incidence of pulmonary complications in critically ill patients. *Crit Care Med* 16:783–786, 1988

Glaister DH: The effect of posture on the distribution of ventilation and blood flow in the normal lung. *Clin Sci* 33:391–398, 1967

Gonzalez-Arias SM, Goldberg ML, Baumgartner R, Hoopes D, Ruben B: Analysis of the effect of kinetic therapy on intracranial pressure in comatose neurosurgical patients. *Neurosurgery* 13:654–656, 1983

Green BA, Green KL, Klose KJ: Kinetic nursing for acute spinal cord injury patients. *Paraplegia* 18:181–186, 1980

Green BA, Green KL, Klose K; Kinetic therapy for spinal cord injury. *Spine* 8(7):722–728, 1983

Grimby G: Aspects of lung expansion in relation to pulmonary physiotherapy. *Am Rev Respir Dis* 110:145–153, 1974

Grimby G, Oxhoj H, Bake B: Effects of abdominal breathing on distribution of ventilation in obstructive lung disease. *Clin Sci Mol Med* 48:193–199, 1975

Gross D, Ladd HW, Riley EJ, Macklem PT, Grassino A: The effect of training on strength and endurance of the diaphragm in quadriplegia. *Am J Med* 68:27–35, 1980

Haas F, Simnowita M, Axen K, Gaudino D, Haas A: Effect of upper body posture on forced inspiration and expiration. *J Appl Physiol* 52(4):879–886, 1982

Hallbook T, Lindbald B, Lindroth B, Wolff T: Prophylaxis against pulmonary complications in patients undergoing gallbladder surgery: A comparison between early mobilization, physiotherapy with and without bronchodilation. *Ann Chir Gynaecol* 73:55–58, 1984

Hargest TS: Buoyant support systems: Their effect on cardiovascular and pulmonary function. *CVP* May/June, 1977

Heaf DP, Helms P, Gordon I, Turner HM: Postural effects of gas exchange in infants. *N Engl J Med* 308:1505–1508, 1983

Hedstrand U, Liw M, Rooth G, Ogren CH: Effect of respiratory physiotherapy on arterial oxygen tension. *Acta Anaesthesiol Scand* 22:349–352, 1978

Herbst JJ, Myers WF: Gastroesophageal reflux in a child. *Pediatr Case Rep Gastrointestinal Dis* 1(3):1–4, 1981

Hewitt VM: Effect of posture on the presence of fat in tracheal aspirate in neonates. *Aus Paediatr J* 12:267–271, 1976

Hoffmann R: Osteotaxis, osteosynthese externe par fiches et rotules. *Acta Chir Scand* 107:72–81, 1954

Hornstein S, Inman S, Ledsome JC: Ventilatory muscle training in kyphoscoliosis. *Spine* 12(9)809–863, 1987

Hornstein S, Ledsome J: Ventilatory muscle training in acute quadriplegia. *Physiother Can* 38(3):145–149, 1986

Hughes RL: Does abdominal breathing affect regional gas exchange? *Chest* 76(3):288–293, 1979

Ibanez J, Raurich M, Abizanda R, et al.: The effect of lateral positions on gas exchange in patients with unilateral lung disease during mechanical ventilation. *Intensive Care Med* 7:321–324, 1981

Imle PC: The physical therapy management of gastroesophageal reflux and its pulmonary sequelae in a child with central nervous system dysfunction. Masters Thesis, Johns Hopkins University, April 1983

Ingram RH, Schilder DP: Effect of pursed lips expiration on the pulmonary pressure-flow relationship in obstructive lung disease. *Am Rev Respir Dis* 95:381–388, 1967

Innocenti PM: Breathing exercises in the treatment of emphysema. *Physiotherapy* 52:437–441, 1966

Irwin S, Tecklin J: *Cardiopulmonary Physical Therapy*, pp 205, 376–377, 263, 231–235, 295–298. Mosby, St. Louis, 1985

Jederlinic P, Muspratt JA, Miller M: Inspiratory muscle training in clinical practice. Physiologic conditioning of habituation to suffocation? *Chest* 86(6):870–873, 1984

Jones GA, Clague MB, Ryan DW, Johnston ID: Demonstration of a reduction in postoperative body protein breakdown using the Clinitron fluidized bed with an ambient temperature of 32 degrees C. *Br J Surg* 72(7):574–578, 1985

Kalaja E: Clinical results of treatment of patients in the air-fluidized bed during a one-year period. *Scand J Plast Reconstr Surg* 18(1):153–154, 1984

Kane IJ: Segmental postural drainage in pulmonary disease. *Dis Chest* 23:418–427, 1953

Kaneko K, Milic-Emili J, Dolovitch MB, Dawson A, Bates DV: Regional distribution of ventilation and perfusion as a function of body position. *J Appl Physiol* 21:767–777, 1966

Karlstrom G, Olerud S: Percutaneous pin fixation of open tibial fractures. *J Bone Joint Surg* 57:915–924, 1975

Keane FX: Pain and cervical traction variation during manual turning. *Paraplegia* 15:343–348, 1977–78

Keens TG, Krastins IRB, Wannamaker EM, Livison H, Crozier DN, Bryan AC: Ventilatory muscle endurance training in normal subjects and patients with cystic fibrosis. *Am Rev Respir Dis* 116:853–860, 1977

Kelley RE, Vibulsresth S, Bell L, Duncan RC: Evaluation of kinetic therapy in the prevention of complications of prolonged bed rest secondary to stroke. *Stroke* 18(3):638–642, 1987

Kigin CM: Advances in chest physical therapy. In *Current Advances in Respiratory Care*, edited by W O'Donohue, pp 37–71. American College of Chest Physicians, Park Ridge Ill, 1984

Kim, MJ: Respiratory muscle training: Implications for patient care. *Heart Lung* 13(4):333–339, 1984

Kirimli B, King JE, Pfaeffle HH: Evaluation of tracheo bronchial suction techniques. *J Thorac Cardiovasc Surg* 59:340–344, 1970

Kubota Y, Margaribuchi T, Ohara M, Fujita M, Toyoda Y, Asada A, Harioka T: Evaluation of selective bronchial suctioning in the adult. *Crit Care Med* 8:748–749, 1980

Larson JL, Kim MJ: Respiratory muscle training with the incentive spirometer resistive breathing device. *Heart Lung* 13:341–345, 1984

Larson JL, Kim MJ: Sharp JT: Inspiratory muscle training with a threshold resistive breathing device in patients with chronic obstructive pulmonary disease. *Am Rev Respir Dis* 133:100–103, 1986

Leith DE, Bradley M: Ventilatory muscle strength and endurance training. *J Appl Physiol* 41(4):508–516, 1976

Lucke D, Jarlsberg C: How is the air fluidized bed best used? *Am J Nurs* 85(12):1338–1340, 1985

Mackenzie CF, Shin B: Cardiorespiratory function

before and after chest physiotherapy in mechanically ventilated patients with post-traumatic respiratory failure. Crit Care Med 13(6):483–486, 1985

Maloney FP, Fernandez E, Hudgel DW: Postural drainage effect after bronchial obstruction. Arch Phys Med Rehab 62:452–455, 1981

Marini JJ, Tyler ML, Hudson LD, Davis BS, Huseby JS: Influence of head dependent positions on lung volume and oxygen saturation in chronic air-flow obstruction. Am Rev Respir Dis 129:101–105, 1984

Martin RJ, Sufit RL, Ringel SP, Hudgel DW, Hill PL: Respiratory improvement by muscle training in adult-onset acid maltase deficiency. Muscle Nerve 6:201–203, 1983

Martin CJ, Ripley H, Reynolds J, Best F: Chest physiotherapy and the distribution of ventilation. Chest 69:174–178, 1976

McAslan TC, Matjasko-Chiu J, Turney SZ, Cowley RA: Influence of inhalation of 100% oxygen on intrapulmonary shunt in severely traumatized patients. J Trauma 13:811–821, 1973

McKeon JL, Turner J, Kelly C, Dent A, Zimmerman PV: The effect of inspiratory resistive training on exercise capacity in optimally treated patients with severe chronic airflow limiation. Aust NZ J Med 16:648–652, 1986

McNabb LJ, Hyatt J: Effect of an air-fluidized bed on insensible water loss. Crit Care Med 15(2):161–162, 1987

McNeill RS, McKenzie JM: An assessment of the value of breathing exercises in chronic bronchitis and asthma. Thorax 10:250–252, 1955

Menkes H, Britt J: Physical therapy, rationale for physical therapy. Am Rev Respir Dis 122(2):127–131, 1980

Micheels J, Sorensen B: The physiology of a healthy normal person in the air-fluidized bed. Burns 9:158–168, 1987

Miller W: Rehabilitation of patients with chronic obstructive lung disease. Med Clin North Am 5:349–361, 1967

Miller WF: A physiologic evaluation of the effects of diaphragmatic breathing training in patients with chronic pulmonary emphysema. Am J Med 17:471–473, 1954

Morran CG, Finlay IG, Mathieson M, McKay AJ, Wilson N, McArdle CS: Randomized controlled trial of physiotherapy for postoperative pulmonary complications. Br J Anaesth 55:1113–1116, 1983

Motley HL: The effects of slow deep breathing on the blood gas exchange in emphysema. Am Rev Respir Dis 88:484–491, 1963

Mueller RE, Petty TL, Filley GF: Ventilation and arterial blood gas changes induced by pursed lips breathing. J Appl Physiol 28:784–789, 1970

Murphy MB, Concannon D, Fitzgerald MX: Chest percussion: Help or hindrance to postural drainage? Irish Med J 76(4):189–190, 1983

Newhouse MT, Rossman CM: Effect of chest physiotherapy on the removal of mucus in patients with cystic fibrosis. (letter) Am Rev Respir Dis 127:391, 1984

Nicholson J: A course of lessons on the art of deep breathing giving physiological exercises to strengthen the chest, lungs, stomach, back, etc. Health Culture Co., London, 1890

Nirmille E, Storm H: Five years experience with the air-fluidized bed in the care of burned patients. Scand J Plast Reconstr Surg 18(1):149–151, 1984

Nye RE: The control and distribution of ventilation. Phys Ther 48:431–438, 1968

Ochoa JB: Diagnosis and management of gastroesophageal reflux in children. Surg Annu 31:123–137, 1981

Oldenburg FA, Dolovich MB, Montgomery JM, Newhouse MT: Effects of postural drainage, exercise and cough on mucus clearance in chronic bronchitis. Am Rev Respir Dis 120:739–745, 1979

Pardy RL, Rivington RN, Despas PJ, Macklem PT: Inspiratory muscle training compared with physiotherapy in patients with chronic airflow limitation. Am Rev Respir Dis 123:421–425, 1981a

Pardy RL, Rivington RN, Despas PJ, Macklem PT: The effects of inspiratory muscle training on exercise performance in chronic airflow limitation. Am Rev Respir Dis 123:426–433, 1981b

Pardy RL, Reid WD, Belman MJ: Respiratory muscle training. Clin Chest Med 9(2):287–296, 1988

Parish LC, Witowski JA: Clinitron therapy and the decubitus ulcer: Preliminary dermatologic studies. Int J Dermatol 19(9):517–518, 1980

Petty TL, Guthrie A: The effects of augmented breathing maneuvers on ventilation in severe chronic airway obstruction. Respir Care 16:104–113, 1971

Pierce AK, Robertson J: Pulmonary complications of general surgery. Annu Rev Med 28:211, 1977

Piehl MA, Brown MS: Use of extreme position changes in acute respiratory failure. Crit Care Med 4:13–15, 1976

Prokocimer P, Garbino J, Wolff M, Regnier B: Influence of posture on gas exchange in artifically ventilated patients with focal lung disease. Intensive Care Med 9:69–72, 1983

Pryor JA, Webber BA: An evaluation of the forced expiration technique as an adjunct to postural drainage. Physiotherapy 65:304–307, 1979a

Pryor JA, Webber BA, Hodson ME, Batten JC: Evaluation of the forced expiration technique as an adjunct to postural drainage in treatment of cystic fibrosis. Br Med J 2:417–418, 1979b

Rath T, Berger A: Treatment of severe burn cases in the air fluidized bed. Burns 9:115–117, 1982

Redfern SJ, Jeneid PA, Gillingham ME: Local pressures with ten types of patient-support system. Lancet 11:277–280, 1973

Reines DH, Harris RC: Pulmonary complications of acute spinal cord injuries. Neurosurgery 21(2):193–196, 1987

Remolina C, Khan AU, Santiago TV, Edelman NH: Postional hypoxemia in unilateral lung disease. N Engl J Med 304(9):523–525, 1981

Rivara D, Artucio H, Arcos J, Hiriart C: Positional hypoxemia during artificial ventilation. Crit Care Med 12(5):436–438, 1984

Roussos CS, Fixley M, Genest J, Cosio M, Kelly S, Martin RR, Engel LA: Voluntary factors influencing the distribution of inspired gas. Am Rev Respir Dis 116:457–466, 1977

Ryan DW: The influence of environmental temperature (32°C) on catabolism using the clinitron fluidized bed. Intensive Care Med 9:279–281, 1983

Sackner MA, Silva G, Banks JM, Watson DD, Smoak WM: Distribution of ventilation during diaphragmatic breathing in obstructive lung disease. Am Rev Respir Dis 109:331–337, 1974

Scheidt A, Drusin LM: Bacteriologic contamination in an air-fluidized bed. *J Trauma* 23(3):241–242, 1983

Scheuler JA, Munster A: Clinitron air fluidized support: An adjunct to burn care. *J Burn Care Rehab* 4(4):10–12, 1983

Schimmel L, Civetta JM, Kirby RR: A new mechanical method to influence pulmonary perfusion in critically ill patients. *Crit Care Med* 5:277–279, 1977

Seaton D: Effect of body position on gas exchange after thoracotomy. *Thorax* 34:518–522, 1979

Shands AR, Raney RB: *Handbook of Orthopaedic Surgery*, p 464. Mosby, St. Louis, 1967

Sharp JT, Drutz WS, Moisan T, Foster J, Machnach W: Postural relief of dyspnea in severe chronic obstructive pulmonary disease. *Am Rev Respir Dis* 122:201–211, 1980

Shearer MO, Banks JM, Silva G, Sackner MA: Lung ventilation during diaphragmatic breathing. *Phys Ther* 52:139–147, 1972

Siegel J: *Trauma: Emergency Surgery and Critical Care*, p 629. Churchill, Livingston, New York, 1988

Simonneau G, Vivien A, Sartene R, Kunstlinger F, Samii K, Noviant U, Duroux P: Diaphragm dysfunction induced by upper abdominal surgery. *Am Rev Respir Dis* 128:899–903, 1983

Smith P, Coakley J, Edwards R: Respiratory muscle training in duchenne muscular dystrophy. *Muscle Nerve* 784–785, 1988

Smoot EC: Clinitron bed therapy hazards (letter). *Plast Reconstr Surg* 77(1):165, 1986

Sonne LJ, Davis JA: Increased exercise performance in patients with severe COPD following inspiratory resistive training. *Chest* 81(4):436–439, 1982

Sonnenblick M, Melzer E, Rosin AJ: Body positional effect on gas exchange in unilateral pleural effusion. *Chest* 83(5):784–786, 1983

Strandberg B: The incidence of atelectasis after heart operations with and without breathing exercises. *Ann Phys Med* 3:18–20, 1956

Sutton PP, Parker RA, Webber BA: Assessment of the forced expiration technique, postural drainage and directed coughing in chest physiotherapy. *Eur J Respir Dis* 64:62–68, 1983

Sutton PP, Lopez-Vidriero MT, Newman SP, Clarke SW: Effect of chest physiotherapy on the removal of mucus in patients with cystic fibrosis (letter). *Am Rev Respir Dis* 127:390–391, 1984

Sutton PP, Lopez-Vidriero MT, Pavia D, Newman SP, Clay MM, Webber B, Parker A, Clarke SW: Assessment of percussion vibratory shaking and breathing exercises in chest physiotherapy. *Eur J Respir Dis* 66:147–152, 1985

Tarhan S, Moffitt EA, Sessler AD, Douglas WW, Taylor WF: Risk of anesthesia and surgery in patients with chronic bronchitis and chronic obstructive pulmonary disease. *Surgery* 74(5):720–726, 1973

Tiep BL, Burns M, Kae D, Madison R, Herrera J: Pursed lips breathing training using ear oximetry. *Chest* 90(2):218–221, 1986

Thoman RL, Stoker GL, Ross JC: The efficacy of pursed lips breathing in patients with chronic obstructive pulmonary disease. *Am Rev Respir Dis* 93:100–106, 1966

Thoren L: Postoperative pulmonary complications. Observations of their prevention by means of physiotherapy. *Acta Chir Scand* 107:193–204, 1954

Trammel TR, Reed DB, Goodwin CB: Controlled mobilization of patients undergoing reconstruction spinal surgery: Preliminary comparison of the kinetic therapy vs the Foster frame. *Orthopedics* 8(12):1489–1491, 1985

Vraciu J, Vraciu R: Effectiveness of breathing exercises in preventing pulmonary complications following open heart surgery. *Phys Ther* 57:1367–1370, 1977

Wagamen MJ, Shutack JG, Moomjian AS et al.: Improved oxygenation and lung compliance with prone positioning of neonates. *J Pediatr* 94:787–791, 1979

Ward RJ, Danziger F, Bonica JJ: An evaluation of postoperative respiratory maneuvers. *Surg Gynecol Obstet* 123:51–54, 1966

Warren CPW, Grimwood M: Pulmonary disorders and physiotherapy in patients who undergo cholecystectomy. *Can J Surg* 23:384–386, 1980

Webber B, Parker R, Hofmeyr J, Hodson M: Evaluation of self-percussion during postural drainage using the forced expiration technique. *Physiother Practice* 42–45, 1985

West JB: Regional differences in gas exchange in the lung of erect man. *J Appl Physiol* 17:893–898, 1962

Wilklander O, Norlin U: Effect of physiotherapy on postoperative pulmonary complications: A clinical and roentgenographic study of 200 cases. *Acta Chir Scand* 112:246–250, 1957

Willeput R, Vachaudez JP, Lenders D, Nys A, Knoops T, Sergysels R: Thoracoabdominal motion during chest physiotherapy in patients affected by chronic obstructive lung disease. *Respiration* 44:204–214, 1983

Williams IP, Smith CM, McGavin CR: Diaphragmatic breathing training and walking performance in chronic airways obstruction. *Br J Dis Chest* 76:164–166, 1982

Wong JW, Keens TG, Wannamaker EM, Douglas PT, Levinson H, Aspin N: Effects of gravity in tracheal transport rates in normal subjects and in patients with cystic fibrosis. *Pediatrics* 60:146–152, 1977

Wood LA: *Nursing Skills for Allied Health Services*, Vol 3, p 315, 319. Saunders, Philadelphia, 1979

Zack MB, Pontoppidan H, Kazemi H: The effect of lateral positions on gas exchange in pulmonary disease. *Am Rev Respir Dis* 110:49–55, 1974

Zausmer E: Bronchial drainage, evidence supporting the procedures. *Phys Ther* 48:586–591, 1968

Zimmerman JE, Oder LA: Swallowing dysfunction in acutely ill patients. *Phys Ther* 61(12):1755–1763, 1981

Zinman R: Cough versus chest physiotherapy, A comparison of the acute effects on pulmonary function in patients with cystic fibrosis. *Am Rev Respir Dis* 129:182–184, 1984

CHAPTER 4

Percussion and Vibration

P. Cristina Imle, M.S., P.T.

Literature Review
Percussion
Vibration
Mechanical Vibrators and Percussors

Percussion and vibration are specific maneuvers developed for use in conjunction with postural drainage. They are thought to facilitate both large and small airway clearance by advancing secretions centrally so they can be expectorated or suctioned. It is theorized that manual percussion and vibration decrease overall treatment time by enhancing the gravitational effects of bronchial drainage (Petty, 1974). Little research has been done on the mechanism of action or optimal methods of performing these manual techniques. The literature on percussion and vibration, though scarce and conflicting, is addressed in this chapter. An explanation of the various methods of performing these manual techniques is reviewed, along with the associated indications and precautions. Information is presented on the use of mechanical vibrators and percussors as aids to chest physiotherapy treatment.

LITERATURE REVIEW

It is widely accepted that percussion and vibration, when used with postural drainage, assist secretion removal from the large airways. The effect of these techniques on the smaller airways is more controversial. Radiological clearing of segmental, lobar, and multilobar atelectasis following postural drainage, percussion, vibration, and coughing or suctioning is well documented in both pediatric and adult patients (Roper

et al., 1976; Ayella, 1078; Mackenzie et al., 1978; Finer et al., 1979; Marini et al., 1979; Ciesla et al., 1981; Hammon and Martin, 1981). These chest x-ray changes provide some evidence of improved clearance of both peripheral and central secretions when manual techniques are used on patients with acute lung pathology.

The successful removal of radioactively labeled secretions from central, intermediate, and peripheral airways following chest physiotherapy maneuvers on patients with chronic lung disease has been reported by Bateman et al. (1979, 1981). In 1981, they found peripheral secretion removal to be better enhanced by physiotherapy techniques of postural drainage, percussion, vibration, and cough compared with cough alone. This contrasts with Rossman et al. (1982), who also measured radioaerosol clearance. These investigators found both directed cough and chest physiotherapy (consisting of drainage, percussion, vibration, and cough) to be more effective than a control period, postural drainage alone, or in combination with mechanical percussion. Chest physiotherapy also resulted in the largest volume of sputum. Postural drainage with coughing was evaluated with and without the use of deep breathing, vibration, and percussion by Sutton et al. (1985). No difference was found in radioaerosol clearance from the central, intermediate, or peripheral lung zones with any treatment. However, the wet and dry weights of sputum were increased significantly by the addition of deep breathing with percussion or vibration. Percussion with tidal breathing significantly increased the dry sputum weight.

There are some important similarities between the studies by Rossman et al. (1982) and Sutton and co-worker (1985). Both used subjects with chronic lung disease and in both investigations only 10% of the inhaled particles were deposited in the peripheral lung zones (Sutton et al., 1984). It is difficult to show clearance of radioaerosols from the lung periphery if only a small fraction is deposited there. It seems logical that the aerosols that were deposited in the peripheral zones would be deposited preferentially in the patent airways. Removal of secretions from the obstructed airways, perhaps with percussion and vibration, could explain the significant increase in sputum production but not aerosol clearance found in both studies. This theory is supported by the findings of Wollmer et al. (1985), which are discussed on p. 136. Van der Schans et al. (1986) neither confirmed nor negated this possibility in their study of radioaerosol clearance in nine patients with stable chronic airflow obstruction. No significant difference in central or peripheral aerosol clearance was found when percussion was added to a regimen of postural drainage, coughing, and breathing exercises. There was no information on sputum production or the proportion of tracer deposition in the peripheral or central lung zones. Only the supine, head-down position was used in this study compared to the others (Rossman et al., 1982; Sutton et al., 1985; Wollmer et al., 1985).

As in the preceding group of studies, most investigations on the efficacy of percussion and vibration have been carried out on patients with chronic lung disease. De Boeck and Zinman (1984) studied nine subjects with stable cystic fibrosis. They compared vigorous cough to 25 min of chest physiotherapy, which included 2 min of percussion and vibration in 11 postural drainage positions. They found chest physiotherapy to be of limited significant benefit over cough in terms of altering pulmonary function

tests (PFT). They noted that some patients responded better to cough and others to physiotherapy. No correlation was found between the volume of sputum expectorated and improved flow rates. These findings are similar to those of DeCesare and co-workers (1982), who used krypton scintigraphy on nine cystic fibrosis patients to measure the efficacy of drainage with cough, percussion, and vibration on peripheral ventilation. Percussion was again limited to 2 min and vibration to five exhalations in each postural drainage position. No significant changes were noted in PFT or peripheral ventilation. This is not surprising as the subjects varied widely in the amount of sputum produced, severity of disease (mild to severe), and phase of disease (acute exacerbation to routine outpatient visit). Also treatment time to each lung segment was short and not directed toward areas of specific pathology, which may have been evident from pretreatment scintigraphy.

In 16 cystic fibrosis patients during acute exacerbation of pulmonary infection, Webber and co-workers (1985) looked at the effect of self-percussion when added to a regimen of breathing exercises, forced expiratory technique (FET), and postural drainage. Self chest compression (vibration) was combined with FET in both groups if found helpful. They found no significant difference in forced expiratory volume in 1 sec (FEV_1) or forced vital capacity (FVC) between the two groups concluding that self-percussion may not provide added benefit to a treatment including drainage and FET. Zapletal and associates (1983) also studied the effects of chest physiotherapy (drainage, percussion, vibration, and cough stimulation) on 24 cystic fibrosis patients with a mean age of 12. There was no improvement in PFT following 30 min of treatment where only 2–10 ml of sputum was produced. Similar findings were reported by Kerrebijn et al. (1982) when chest physiotherapy (drainage with percussion, virbration, and coughing) was compared with no treatment or was preceded by N-acetylcysteine aerosol. Sputum volume was not measured in this study.

In 1984, Falk et al. reported a decrease

in FVC and skin oxygen tension (PsO₂) when postural drainage (for 4–5 min in seven different positions) with percussion and vibration was performed on 14 patients with cystic fibrosis. When face mask positive expiratory pressure (PEP) was applied either with or without drainage, these findings were reversed and sputum production was also better using PEP than with FET or drainage, percussion, and vibration. No patients had acute pathological findings on chest x-ray and no radiographical changes were noted with any therapy. This article is interesting, in part, because of its apparent bias. The investigators stated that "percussion should be stopped in patients who beforehand are close to the knee of the oxygen dissociation curve." This comment is opinion at best, since Falk et al. did not specifically look at percussion efficacy. It is also in conflict with others reporting on percussion in patients with chronic lung disease (Buscaglia and St. Marie 1983; Mazzocco et al., 1985; Wollmer et al.) FET is also described in this study as unacceptable and exhausting to cystic fibrosis patients, which is in direct opposition to the findings of others (Pryor et al., 1979; Sutton et al., 1983; Hofmeyer et al., 1986). However, these reports by Kerrebijn, Zapletal, and Falk et al. cast some doubt on the benefits of chest phsiotherapy, including manual percussion and vibration, to improve PFT in patients with stable cystic fibrosis.

Mazzocco and associates (1985) studied 13 subjects with stable chronic bronchitis. They failed to find either improvement or deterioration in FVC, FEV₁, or peak expiratory flow (PEF) following 10 min of postural drainage alone and then 10 min of drainage with percussion. No significant decrease in arterial oxygenation or heart rate was reported for patients whose sputum production ranged from 0 to 110 ml during this treatment. The authors concluded that drainage and percussion were both safe and helpful in mobilizing secretions in persons with bronchiectasis. These findings conflict with those of Wollmer and associates who studied patients with chronic bronchitis during acute exacerbation. The 10 subjects served as their own control; receiving postural drainage for 5 min in

three different positions both with and without percussion. A small but statistically significant decrease in FEV₁ was noted when percussion was added, although there was no difference in VC or oxygen saturation. Scintigraphic measurements showed a better penetration of inhaled aerosol after percussion and drainage than with drainage alone. Similarly, peripheral clearance of the tracer was higher when percussion was used. These findings did not reach statistical significance, perhaps because of the large particle size and the relatively poor peripheral deposition. Interestingly, the two patients with high sputum production (100–130 ml) had substantially higher isotope clearance when percussion was included. As noted by others, sputum volume did not correlate with particle clearance.

Another study of 10 patients during an acute exacerbation of severe chronic lung disease (bronchitis/emphysema) was done by Bascaglia and St. Marie. They found no significant changes in oxygen saturation during 12° head-down positioning, while supine and prone, or before and after 12 min of percussion and vibration in these two position. All subjects were spontaneously breathing and six required nasal oxygen prior to the study to maintain baseline oxygen tensions ≥60 mm Hg. Sputum production was not addressed, and none of the subjects had radiographic evidence of atelectasis or pneumonia, so it is unclear what the indications for treatment were. The authors conclude that Trendelenburg, prone, and supine positioning with percussion and vibration does not produce hypoxemia in acutely ill patients with COPD.

Few studies are available on the effect of percussion or vibration on the postoperative or posttraumatic patient. Case reports on such patients with a variety of diagnoses showed marked improvement in chest radiograph appearance, breath sounds, and arterial blood gases after chest physiotherapy that included lobar and segmental drainage, percussion, vibration, and cough or suctioning (Ciesla et al.; Hammond and Martin, 1981). The specific contributions of percussion or vibration were not addressed. Retained setions, atelectasis, and pneumonia were indications for treatment in the seven patients presented.

Three recent studies evaluated the routine use of chest physiotherapy to prevent postoperative pulmonary complications. Morran and associates (1983) studied 102 patients for up to 4 days after elective cholecystectomy. In addition to encouragement to cough and breathe deeply by the nursing and medical staff, 51 of the patients were given 15 min of breathing exercises, assisted cough, and chest wall vibration (CPT). The frequency of postoperative pulmonary complications (atelectasis) was similar in both groups and was attributed to the effects of anesthesia and pain. However, the incidence of chest infection was significantly less in the group receiving CPT, suggesting that breathing exercises, cough, and vibration prevent or reverse the progression of atelectasis to infection. Hallbook et al. (1984) also studied patients undergoing elective cholecystectomy. One hundred thirty-seven patients randomly received mobilization (walking and arm exercises, two times daily) or chest physiotherapy (mobilization plus breathing exercises, drainage, and coughing) both with and without bronchodilator medication. All patients were given effective pain relief by means of an intercostal nerve block. Postoperative pulmonary complications occurred in 36% of the patients and were similar in all three study groups. No added benefit was found with chest physiotherapy, perhaps because of the low incidence of pulmonary infection (three patients). Chest physiotherapy did not include either percussion or vibration in this study.

These studies contrast with those of Torrington et al. (1984), who studied 49 morbidity obese patients for 48 hr after gastric stapling. All patients received (1) intermittent positive pressure breathing (IPPB) every 4 hr, (2) incentive spirometry (IS) every 4 hr spaced between IPPB, (3) nebulized mist by face mask for 30 min following each IPPB or IS session, and (4) deep breathing and coughing after each session. Additionally, at 4-hr intervals, 24 of the patients were given 5–10 min of percussion while positioned head down and supine or side-lying (CPT). It is not clear if any attempt was made to direct the CPT toward the area of lung pathology. The investigators reported no differences in PaO_2, FVC, sputum production, chest x-ray findings, or hospital stay between the two groups; only a small but statistically significant difference in mean postoperative temperature (0.4–0.6°F) was found. The researchers report that CPT caused patient discomfort. However, if CPT was more painful than the vigorous control treatment, this suggests that it was improperly performed and/or not coordinated with appropriate postoperative analgesia. Pain with chest physiotherapy was not reported by Morran et al., (1983), who had a large number of obese patients (37) in their study but did not include postural drainage. Although Torrington and co-workers reported an average hospital stay of nearly 7 days, they did not monitor signs of pulmonary pathology beyond 48 hr after surgery. Therefore, no information was available on the differences in lung infection rates compared with pulmonary complications between the two regimens.

In 47 posttrauma patients requiring mechanical ventilation and positive end expiratory pressure (PEEP), Mackenzie and co-workers (1978) showed a marked improvement in auscultation and chest x-ray appearance after chest physiotherapy that included percussion and vibration. On 42 similar patients, significant increases in total lung/thorax compliance lasting for up to 2 hr after chest physiotherapy were reported (Mackenzie et al., 1980) (see p. 218). In both studies, indicators for treatment included atelectasis, lung contusion, pneumonia, and respiratory distress syndrome. In 1985, Mackenzie and Shin reported on the effects of postural drainage, percussion, vibration, and suctioning (CPT) on 19 patients requiring mechanical ventilation and PEEP for management of posttraumatic respiratory failure. They found an immediate improvement in intrapulmonary shunt and an increase in total lung/thorax compliance 2 hr after CPT. Chest physiotherapy treatment time was determined by the clearance of adventitial breath sounds and ranged from 30 to 105 min. No cardiac dysrhythmias or changes in dead space, cardiac output, or arterial blood gases were recorded. The findings of these three studies—improved air entry by auscultation, increased compliance, and decreased intrapulmonary shunt with no change in dead space— suggest an increase in the number of ventilated alveoli. This, along with the results of others (Bateman et al., 1979, 1981; Sutton et al., 1985), provides evidence that in adults, percussion and vibration, performed with postural drainage and cough or suctioning, are effective in removing secretions from the more peripheral as well as larger airways.

Klein et al. (1988) reported hemodynamic and metabolic changes in 23 postoperative patients during chest physiotherapy. These changes were not sustained after the chest therapy was completed and most were attenuated by administering short acting narcotics. In this study chest physiotherapy consisted of side-to-side turning, percussion, vibration, and suctioning. The therapy was not directed to a specific lung pathology and was not performed by a physical therapist. Mackenzie and associates (1978, 1980, 1985) did not measure PaO_2, lung compliance, cardiac output, or other indices during chest physiotherapy, as positional changes alone are known to alter cardiorespiratory function (see p. 26). Differences due to postural changes may help to explain the findings of Barrell and Abbas (1978) who studied spontaneously breathing patients within 24 hr of mitral valve replacement. Decreased cardiac output and $P\overline{V}O_2$ were noted during chest physiotherapy (side lying, percussion, vibration, breathing exercises, and supported cough). These parameters returned to baseline values within 15 min after therapy. In this study, supplemental oxygen was recommended as a means to minimize $P\overline{V}O_2$ changes in spontaneously breathing patients receiving chest physiotherapy. Significant decreases in PaO_2 are reported in critically ill patients receiving chest physiotherapy (postural drainage and percussion). Interestingly, a regression analysis of the PaO_2 changes showed that patients with lower baseline values had a less dramatic fall in PaO_2 during therapy. Based on this finding, the investigators recommended that chest physiotherapy need not be withheld in patients with a $PaO_2 < 60$ mm Hg but that careful monitoring was indicated during treatment (Tyler et al., 1980). Percussion and vibration alone are not proven to contribute to hypoxemia. However, in most studies these techniques are used along with bronchial drainage. Postural changes do cause alterations in cardiorespiratory function (see p. 94). These may become significant in patients with pulmonary or cardiac pathology and are perhaps the cause of the hypoxemia or other types of deterioration reported by some investigators in association with chest physiotherapy.

Chest physiotherapy techniques, including percussion and vibration, are also used on pediatric and neonatal patients. Conditions such as idiopathic respiratory distress syndrome, meconium aspiration, bronchopulmonary dysplasia, neonatal pneumonia, and postoperative pulmonary complications have led to more aggressive respiratory care, including intubation and mechanical ventilation in this age group (Crane, 1981). In infants, acute lung collapse unresponsive to other methods of treatment, including IPPB, has been reported to respond to chest percussion and vibration by reinflation (Mellins, 1974). Etches and Scott (1978) corroborated Mellins' clinical findings of increased secretion clearance after postural drainage with percussion and vibration compared with suctioning alone in a study of six neonates. Unless these maneuvers in themselves cause an increase in the production of lung secretions (which has not been documented), it may be assumed that the increase in sputum is a result of percussion and vibration loosening and advancing small airway secretions more centrally. This is supported by Finer and Boyd (1978), who compared the effect of postural drainage alone and in conjunction with "contact heel" percussion on arterial blood gases in 20 neonates with respiratory distress. They found a significant increase in PaO_2 when percussion was added to drainage. In 1979, Finer and associates investigated the role of postural drainage, vibration, and suctioning (chest physiotherapy) in preventing and reversing postextubation atelectasis in 85 neonates. The right upper lobe was the most commonly reported site of lung collapse. A significant decrease in atelectasis was found in the infants receiving chest physiotherapy. This occurred despite the fact that the control subjects were frequently put in postural drainage positions for the right upper lobe. These findings do not support the clinical opinions of some (Meier, 1979) that drainage alone may prevent or treat atelectasis in the sick neonate.

Curran and Kachoyeanos (1979) looked at the effect of percussion/vibration on six neonates suffering respiratory distress. Two subjects received 1 min of mechanical chest vibration with an electric toothbrush; another two were given 1 min of manual percussion with a padded nipple; and two served as controls. Treatments were given every other hour and were followed by suctioning. No indications for treatment were given. The authors concluded that the neonates receiving chest vibration with the toothbrush had increased PaO_2 and $PaCO_2$ along with improved breath sounds and skin color compared with the others. However, arterial blood gases were drawn at random times in reference to therapy, and changes in the blood gases were not compared with baseline values (which may well have varied greatly with only two subjects in each group). Breath sounds were poorly evaluated (clear, some or heavy congestion). Clinicians know that although rhonchi sound "worse" than rales, they are more easily treated. Possibly the only finding worth noting in this study is that suctioning rather than either form of therapy was responsible for most of the deleterious effects noted during the study.

Crane and associates (1978) tried to assess the isolated effects of manual techniques in 24 infants with hyaline membrane disease. They studied percussion and then vibration with the head down and bed flat. The subjects were also suctioned using supplemental O_2 in all four study situations. No bradycardia or apnea was noted, but there were significant increases in heart rate, respiratory rate, and systolic pressure following all four treatments with suctioning. Neither percussion nor head-down positioning was found to increase systolic blood pressure in adults (White and Mawdsley, 1983). It is unclear if the increases reported by Crane et al. were the result of the treatments, of suctioning or a combination of both.

In 1980, Tudehope and Bagley studied the effects of three types of chest physiotherapy on 15 premature infants requiring mechanical ventilation for respiratory distress. All babies randomly received each of the following treatments 2 hr apart: contact heel percussion, manual percussion using a face mask, or chest vibration with an electric toothbrush. Each treatment was performed for 3 min in four different postural drainage positions followed by suctioning. Indications for treatment were not given. Manual percussion and, to a lesser degree, contact heel percussion, resulted in significant rises in PaO_2, which were maintained for up to 1 hr after therapy. Both manual techniques were better tolerated than vibration with the mechanical toothbrush. The authors theorize that the loosened terminal airway secretions were responsible for the improved PaO_2 found with both types of manual percussion.

O'Rorke and co-workers (1984) studied the effects of chest physiotherapy on tidal volume (V_t) changes in six infants requiring intermittent mandatory ventilation (IMV). No indications for treatment were noted. Baseline V_t measurements were compared with those during percussion and vibration while sidelying. Percussion and, to less extent, vibration resulted in significant decreases in V_t, which rapidly returned to baseline values after treatment. No detrimental effects were associated with the drop in V_t. Unfortunately, the authors did not report V_t changes associated only with position change. It appears that some of the decrease in V_t may have been due to sidelying, in which case prone positioning increased inspired volume or a change in the mode of ventilation may be appropriate if chest physiotherapy is indicated.

In most of the chest physiotherapy research, postural drainage, cough, suctioning, and breathing exercises were included along with the manual techniques of percussion and vibration, making it difficult to assess the efficacy of each treatment component. As noted in the previously cited work, attempts to evaluate the specific contribution of either percussion or vibration are both rare and conflicting. To add further confusion, various forms of mechanical, manual, and self-percussion and vibration have been studied. A few researchers have tried to look at percussion or vibration as isolated treatments. Their findings are discussed in the subsequent sections of this chapter. Manual techniques have not been used historically as a treatment in and of themselves; rather, they have been considered adjuncts to postural drainage, breathing exercises, coughing, and suctioning. Therefore, it appears important to assess the added effects of percussion or vibration rather than examine their isolated role, if any. If the major benefit of manual techniques is merely to expedite the gravitational effects of bronchial drainage, this is an important finding. It would suggest that the addition of percussion or vibration is of limited value to the more stable patient; yet, in the critically ill or unstable patient, these techniques could shorten treatment time considerably while providing improved efficacy.

To the clinician, it is generally accepted that the appropriate postural drainage positions should be achieved prior to initiating percussion or vibration (see Chapter 3). It is possible that manual techniques may assist secretions to move more peripherally if combined with improper patient positioning (Howell and Hill, 1972). Whether this occurs is not known; however, transbronchial aspiration of mucus from one area to another does happen, particularly when copious secretions are present (Imle, 1983) (see Case History 7.1). Therefore, a knowledge of the segmental pulmonary anatomy and the overlying anatomical landmarks is essential for effective percussion and vibration (see Fig. 2.1). Note that the medial segment of the right lower lobe has minimal to no surface accessible for percussion; therefore, postural drainage accompanied by coughing or suctioning may be used when treating this segment. For other segments, percussion should be given directly over the area of lung involvement. Normally, during maximal inspiration the lungs do not extend below the tenth thoracic vertebra posteriorly or below the level of the xiphoid process anteriorly. Diaphragmatic descent is often less in patients with postoperative pain, weakness, or abdominal distension. Manual techniques should be limited to those areas with underlying lung.

PERCUSSION

The percussion technique consists of rhythmic "clapping" with cupped hands over the involved lung segment (Fig. 4.1). It was first described by Linton in 1934 (Zadai, 1981). Percussion should produce a hollow sound, not a slapping sound. It

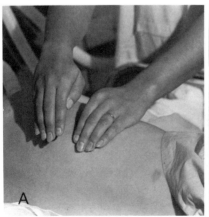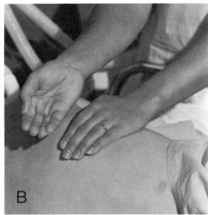

Figure 4.1. Percussion should be performed with cupped hands and fingers adducted as shown in **A.** The correct position of the palmar survace of the hand is demonstrated in **B.**

should impart an energy wave transmitted through the chest wall to cause a loosening of bronchial wall secretions (Sutton et al., 1982). The hand should create an "air cushion" on impact, which, it is proposed, aids in dislodging pulmonary secretions (Petty, 1974). This is confirmed by bronchoscopy (Kigin, 1984). Percussion is performed during both inspiration and expiration and should not result in undue pressure on the soft tissues of the chest. Manual percussion is normally performed at a rate of 100–480 times per minute and is reported to produce between 2 and 4 foot pounds and 58 and 65 Newtons of force on the chest wall (Flower et al., 1979a; Gray, 1980; Hammon and Martin, 1981; Murphy et al., 1983; White and Mawdsley; et al., 1985; Van der Schans et al.).

Percussion may be performed over rib fractures without any known complications (see p. 331). This is based on the author's experience of providing chest physiotherapy for 60 patients with clavicular or scapular fractures and 226 patients with rib fractures during a 34-month period. Over 80% of the rib fractures were multiple or bilateral (Appendix I, Table A1.8). Clinically, most patients with multiple rib fractures or flail chest require ventilatory support during the acute stage. It is theorized that controlled mechanical ventilation actually helps stabilize the fracture site by preventing negative intrathoracic pressures. Mechancial ventilation may act as a form of internal fixation of the fracture sites by encouraging synchronized rib cage and soft-tissue motion. Assisted ventilation (AV) or IMV often leads to more movement at the rib fracture site since negative intrathoracic pressures are generated by the patient. PEEP is frequently used in the management of patients with rib fracture and lung contusion. Percussion is shown to effect intrathoracic pressure changes of 5–15 cm H_2O (Flower et al., 1979a), which approximates the levels of PEEP used in this patient population. When properly performed, percussion should cause less pressure over the thorax and ribs than coughing or lying on the side of involvement. In addition, it probably causes less rib motion than occurs during spontaneous breathing, AV,

or IMV. Percussion appears to be a safe procedure for patients with rib fractures, however, it should not be performed by the novice therapist.

Chest percussion should not cause undue pain to the patient and need not be forceful (Gaskell and Webber, 1980). Some of the conflicting data surrounding the use of percussion may result from the misguided belief that this technique is routinely carried out in a painful manner, often referred to as pummelling (Reines et al, 1982; Holoday and Goldberg, 1982; Demers, 1986). Postoperative pain is a well-recognized side effect of surgery and it is frequently exacerbated by deep breathing, moving, turning, and coughing. However, no clinician would recommend withholding these maneuvers as a means of decreasing pain. Instead, they would recommend appropriate analgesia. The many methods of pain relief are discussed on p. 341. In general, analgesia should be used as indicated, according to the severity of injury or disease. Medication to reduce pain is given prior to treatment to aid patient comfort, particularly for patients with long-bone fractures or multiple rib fractures and for those who have undergone thoracic and abdominal surgery.

In addition to analgesia, patients with severe head injuries often require sedation to minimize abnormal responses that lead to raised intracrainal pressure (ICP). Sedation is usually given prior to treatment, so effective chest physiotherapy can be performed without compromising the patient's overall condition. Paralyzing agents or barbiturates may also be needed during the acute phase to minimize brain injury (Matjasko, 1986). It is generally thought that head-down positioning and manual techniques increase ICP. For this reason, chest physiotherapy is often withheld from a patient population at great risk for pulmonary infection. However, percussion is not normally associated with elevated ICP (see Fig. 8.2) and may actually lead to a decrease in this parameter (Gerradd and Bullock, 1986). The short period of increased ICP that may occur with chest physiotherapy may not be detrimental unless it precipitates a decrease in cerebral perfusion pressure (Hammon et al., 1981; Imle et al., 1988 see p. 259). In infants with head injuries that require ICP monitoring, spontaneous movements are found to result in the greatest increases in ICP (Tomney and Finer, 1980). It is the author's experience that, in most patients, complaints of pain, changes in vital signs, or increases in ICP are a result of the position changes, coughing, or suctioning, which are necessary aspects of routine care after surgery. The pain and changes in vital signs are not just specific to chest physiotherapy intervention and should not be viewed in isolation from the patient's total needs.

Percussion is thought to cause bronchospasm, which is evidenced by a fall in FEV_1 in some studies of patients with chronic lung disease (Campbell et al., 1975; Wollmer et al.). In most cases this decrease is both small and short lived. Others have reported no change or an increase in FEV_1 after chest physiotherapy techniques (Clark et al., 1973; Cochrane et al., 1977; Newton and Stephenson, 1978; May and Munt, 1979; Feldman et al., 1979; DeCesare et al.; Kerrebijn et al.; Zapletal et al.; deBoeck and Zinman; Falk et al.; Mazzocco et al.; Webber et al). It remains unclear if percussion is responsible for the decrease in FEV_1 noted by some following chest physiotherapy. A drop in FEV_1 by less than 10% may not be clincially significant (but may reach statistical significance) (Rivington-Law et al., 1979). Because this pulmonary measurement is effort dependent and forced expiration can affect bronchoconstriction, it is difficult to determine the cause of a fall in FEV_1. If wheezing or other signs of bronchospasm are present prior to or occur during chest physiotherapy, vibration and the FET may be more appropriate techniques to use than percussion.

Egan (1977) states that percussion must be performed over the bare skin. It is our belief that chest percussion should be preferentially performed directly over the thorax. Experience has shown that many less experienced therapists often attempt to percuss over bulky towels or pads. Aside from covering anatomical landmarks, towels often require that a greater force be applied to achieve the same cupping effect, since much of the "air cushion" is lost in the toweling. In addition, any covering over the thorax prevents the therapist from noting skin erythema or petechiae. Towels may also interfere with detection of previously undiagnosed rib fractures or subcutaneous emphysema.

If skin redness or petechiae occur with percussion, it is usually a result of improper technique, most commonly slapping or of not enough air being trapped between the hand and the chest wall (Tecklin, 1979). The trapped air creates the hollow cupping sound, cushions the blows, and is believed to be responsible for loosening the secretions. Patients with coagulopathies after massive blood tranfusions may also develop petechiae. When chest physiotherapy is indicated in these patients, percussion should be performed with care to minimize this effect and still clear the retained secretions. Patients with burns or large areas of skin loss or abrasion may benefit from the use of a sterile drape over the area being treated. Sterile precautions should be used when indicated, and gloves may be worn during percussion. For modesty or in the presence of sensitive skin, a thin hospital gown or drape may be beneficial. Thicker coverings, such as towels or blankets, should not be used. Obesity is believed to decrease the effect of chest percussion in much the same way as bulky dressings or towels. Chest tube or surgical dressings that cover the thorax should be kept to a minimum so they do not hinder percussion or chest wall expansion (see p. 74).

The use of chest tubes for either hemothorax or pneumothorax is not a contraindication to chest percussion or vibration. In fact, chest tubes are often necessary as a result of thoracic surgery or chest trauma and consequently indicate that chest physiotherapy may be necessary. Extrapleural hematomas are not a precaution to percussion, nor are they an apparent sequelae of this technique, as shown in a study of 250 patients, most having multiple rib fractures (Ciesla et al., 1987). Patients having subcutaneous emphysema also respond favorably to chest physiotherapy. They do not complain of increased discomfort with percussion or vibration, nor has increased emphysema been noted following such treatments (Ciesla et al., 1981). If a mechanically ventilated patient has subcutaneous emphysema and no chest tubes, the physical therapist should have confirmation that no pneumothorax is present before proceeding with therapy. Any increase in subcutaneous emphysema either during or between treatments should be noted and brought to the physician's attention promptly. Subcutaneous emphysema may be associated with pneumothorax, chest tube leakage and other complications discussed on p. 327.

A lung abscess or bronchopleural fistual is not a contraindiction to postural drainage, percussion, or vibration. For healing to occur, the connecting bronchi should be cleared of secretions by chest physiotherapy. In the case of brochopleural fistula, the pleural space is drained by open or closed thoracotomy. These patients may complain of pain associated with the chest tube site, empyema, or a cellulitis accompanying the fistula. These infectious processes should not interfere with postural drainage, but slight modification of percussion and vibration around the area of cellulitis helps alleviate discomfort. For the spontaneously breathing patient, breathing exercises are used in conjunction with manual techniques. Patients with gross unilateral infection resulting from a lung absecess or bronchopleural fistula require prophylactic treatment of the uninvolved lung following treatment of the involved side. This minimizes possible contamination or infection of the uninvolved lung. If subsequent resection is expected, treatment may be concentrated on the uninvolved areas of the lungs to prevent or lessen the spread of infection.

A single case of fatal pulmonary hemorrhage was reported by Hammon and Martin (1979) in a patient with squamous cell carcinoma and lung abscess. The patient received bronchial drainage and "light" percussion for 15 days. Hemoptysis was noted both during and independent of chest physiotherapy treatment. On the sixteenth day during drainage with percussion, the patient suffered massive hemoptysis and died. From this the authors concluded that percussion is contraindicated in patients with significant hemoptysis. However, hemoptysis occurs from other causes such as lung contusion or aspiration, for which percussion with postural drainange is not contraindicated. Also, bloody expectorate is not uncommon in lung abscess because of tissue and vessel destruction. Fatal pulmonary hemorrhage does occur as a consequence of lung cancer. Caution is needed in establishing cause and effect based on a single case study, especially since the role of cough is unclear and both disease processes place the patient at risk for spontaneous fatal hemorrhage (Kigin, 1984). A more appropriate conclusion may be that, in a patient with decreased platelet count and significant hemoptysis from carcinoma or lung abscess, the expected benefit should be weighed against the potential risk.

Due to the increasing number of pediatric and neonatal intensive care units, interest in chest physiotherapy for this population has grown. Because lung segments are small in an infant, various adaptations to manual percussion have been suggested in the literature (Tecklin; Curran and Kachoyeanos; Tudehope and Bagley; Parker, 1985; Irwin and Tecklin, 1985). Three objects commonly modified for chest percussion are shown in Figure 4.2. They include an infant-sized anesthesia mask with the smaller opening of the mask occluded by the therapist's hand or by tape. This device requires minimal adaptation of readily available equipment in a pediatric intensive care unit. Normally the bell end of a stethoscope has rubber padding and need not be altered for percussion. When using a 30-ml medicine cup, the rim should be covered and padded. Rubber nipples are also used, both with and without padding. Another percussion technique for neonates and infants is called "tenting"; this consists of overlapping the second finger over the first and third, as seen in Figure 4.3. Only the fingers are used for percussion. Contact-heel percussion, described for use in neonates with respiratory distress by Finer and Boyd (1978), uses the thenar and hypothenar eminences to apply percussion at a rate of 40 times a minute. The force varied to achieve a thoracic displacement of 1–2

Figure 4.2. Objects used in performing percussion on pediatric patients include (from *left* to *right*) the bell end of a stethoscope, a neonatal anesthesia mask, and a padded medicine cup.

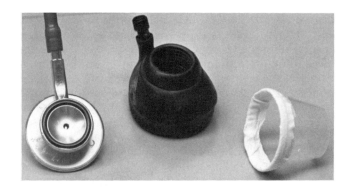

cm. It is not known if any one of these techniques is more advantageous than another. One study (Tudehope and Bagley, 1980) found the face mask to be superior to contact-heel percussion, but both techniques resulted in significant increases in PaO_2 and were superior to mechanical vibration.

In the neonatal population, one case of rib fractures following chest physiotherapy is reported (Purohit et al., 1975). This premature infant received at least one

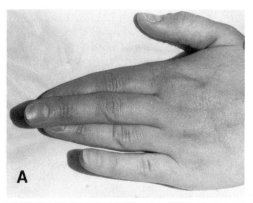

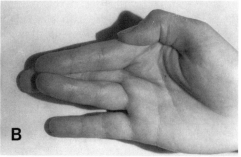

Figure 4.3. Tenting, a type of percussion used on pediatric patients, is demonstrated in **A** and **B**. Only the area from the metacarpalphalangeal joints, distally, is used for percussion.

month of either manual percussion or mechanical vibration (CPT) every 2 hr. No fractures or apparent detrimental effects were noted. A few weeks later, when atelectasis recurred, CPT (using the same techniques) was reinstituted. Subsequent to this second treatment period, rib fractures were noted and CPT was suggested as the cause. The authors correctly point out that stress fractures or neonatal rickets are reported in infants with prolonged respiratory distress. From a single infant it is difficult to determine if percussion was to blame, and whether manual or mechanical techniques were the culprit. As in all ICU settings, the experience and skill of the personnel directly treating patients are important factors.

A decreased platelet count is a very important finding in the patient with acute leukemia and coagulopathy. In the pediatric population, it is suggested that percussion can be expeditously performed if the platelet count is greater than 50,000 ml^3 of blood. Postural drainage with vibration is recommended with counts between 20,000 and 50,000; drainage with breathing exercises and coughing are continued with lower platelet levels (Irwin and Tecklin, 1985). These guidelines from one institution imply that for the patient with coagulopathy, percussion is potentially more hazardous than vibration and that both of these techniques pose more of a risk than postural drainage, breathing exercises, and coughing. It is the author's opinion that the amount of force used with either percussion or vibration is a greater determinant of potential complication than which type of manual technique is applied. Cough is very forceful and produces large fluctuations in thoracic, abdominal, and intracrainal pressure (see Chapter 5). It is likely that breathing exercises, percussion, vibration, FET, and alternative methods of expectoration present less risk than coughing to a patient with decreased platelet count. Research is needed to evaluate the effects of manual techniques and cough on patients with thrombocytopenia.

VIBRATION

Chest vibration, like percussion, is used in conjunction with postural drainage. Although it is stated that chest wall vibration often dislodges the most stubborn secretions in both large and small airways (Wade, 1973), no data have been found to support the claim that vibration alone mobilizes secretions from the small airways. At our institution, when postural drainage and vibration were performed during bronchoscopy, it was noted that secretions became visible in the larger segmental bronchi during vibration. This was also observed by others (Opie and Spalding, 1958; Thacker, 1959; Kigin 1981, 1984). Denton (1962) reported that during bronchoscopy under general anesthesia, vibration given during expiration squeezed the secretions from the bronchioles into the larger bronchi. However, fiberoptic bronchoscopy in trained hands was only reported to reach the fourth generation bronchi with 74% success (Kovnat et al., 1974). Therefore, information on the effects of vibration, as confirmed by bronchoscopy, pertains to the larger airways.

Vibration is an intermittent chest wall compression performed primarily during expiration. It may be initiated just before the expiratory phase and extended to the beginning of the inspiratory phase. This technique can be used during voluntary or ventilator-controlled expiration and should be performed over the involved area of the lung. If vibration is performed on a spontaneously breathing patient, encouragement toward a maximal inspiratory effort should precede chest wall vibration. Maximal inspiration is followed by shaking of the chest wall in the direction that the ribs and soft tissues of the chest normally move during expiration

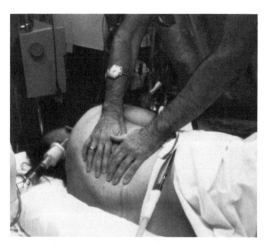

Figure 4.4. Vibration involves shaking the chest wall. It can be performed with one hand placed posteriorly and the other anteriorly, or the hands may be placed more laterally as shown.

(Fig. 4.4). Various sources describe differing types of vibration as "rib springing" or "chest shaking." All are more or less vigorous forms of the same general technique, with "vibration" usually refering to a gentler, more oscillatory treatment than the other terms. Frequencies of 12–20 Hz are reported for manual vibration, and 2 Hz is noted for chest shaking (Gormezano and Brainthwaite, 1972; Bateman et al., 1981; Sutton et al., 1985).

The forcefullness or method of vibration used on a particular patient is dictated by the physical therapist's bias and knowledge of the patient's injuries, diagnosis, and general condition. For the elderly or anxious patient, gentler or more rhythmical vibration may be applied. Initially, asthmatics tend to relax more with vibration techniques and breathing exercises than with percussion. Percussion may be added to the treatment regimen later. Because percussion has been noted by some to cause bronchoconstriction, wheezing, or a decrease in FEV_1 in patients with chronic lung disease (Campbell et al., 1975; Feldman et al.; Wollmer et al.), vibration may be of greater benefit in this patient population. However, these side effects have not been reported in patients with acute lung disease or normal subjects (Rivinton-Law et al.).

Subacute head-injured patients or

heavily sedated patients who are difficult to arouse and have shallow respiration may benefit from more vigorous vibration, with a hold or pause applied until the patient starts to initiate inspiration. It is thought that the increased tactile stimulation associated with vibration may improve the inspiratory effort in these patients. In the quadriplegic patient, thoracic vibration, as well as splinting of the abdominal musculature, may be beneficial (see Fig. 8.8). "Bag squeezing" to hyperventilate the lungs in association with vibration has been described in the literature. As with "sighing," the efficacy of this technique is unproven for patients receiving adequate mechanical ventilation. Hyperinflation with vibration usually requires the use of two persons and is associated with significant and deleterious increases in ICP (Garradd and Bullock) and fluctuations in cardiac output (Laws and McIntyre, 1969). In spontaneously breathing patients who cannot take a deep breath but who have artificial airways, an 800–1000 cm^3 manual resuscitator bag may be used as an adjunct to vibration and before and after suctioning (Fig. 4.5).

Although the ribs and normal anatomy of the thoracic spine provide inherent

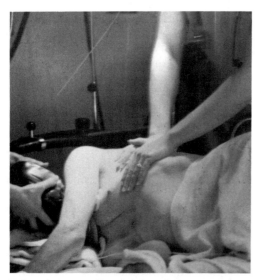

Figure 4.5. When patients are tracheally intubated, yet spontaneously breathing, a manual resuscitator bag may be used to augment the patient's inspiratory effort, thus making vibration more effective.

stability to the thorax, vigorous vibration over unstable thoracic spine injuries is not advised. Because of the shaking aspect of vibration, the author does not recommend its use on patients with known rib or sternal fractures. This is in contrast with others who believe vibration is more comfortable than percussion and does not effect rib motion (Kigin, 1981), 1984). Provided that the patient has an indication for chest physiotherapy, either technique (or both) appears to be safe in the hands of those therapists skilled in modifying treatment to individual patient needs. Elderly patients or persons who have used steroids over a long period of time may have varying degrees of osteoporosis. Chest vibration on these patients should be performed with this in mind.

MECHANICAL VIBRATORS AND PERCUSSORS

Mechanical percussors and vibrators were develop primarily to assist in the home care physiotherapy of patients with chronic pulmonary pathology. More recently, they were introduced into the intensive care unit. Because these mechanical devices may produce vertical or rotary movements, or a combination of both, some studies refer to them as vibrators and some as percussors. Research on the effectiveness of mechanical vibrators compared with manual vibration is limited, and only one study pertains to patients in the intensive care setting. Most of the information on mechanical percussors is available through companies producing or marketing such devices and thus is of questionable objectivity. The data behind claims such as the G5 massage apparatus provide "directional stroke action to help mobilize muscus in a selected direction rather than relying solely on gravity for flow" (General Physiotherapy, 1986) and many similar statements remain unsubstantiated.

In studying patients undergoing bronchopulmonary lavage for alveolar proteinosis, Hammond and co-workers (1980, 1983, 1984) compared the effects of manual percussion, manual vibration, mechanical percussion, and mechanical vibration. The number of patients in each study was small, but in all cases manual techniques were signifcantly more effective than mechanical means at removing proteinaceous-lipid material from the alveoli. Neither mechanical percussion nor vibration was superior to no treatment. It is noteworthy that, during bronchopulmonary lavage, the patient is positioned so that the dependent lung receives percussion or vibration while it is filled with saline, which is in contrast to normal chest physiotherapy techniques.

However, similar conclusions are reported by Rossman et al. in patients with cystic fibrosis. They found that postural drainage was not enhanced by mechanical percussion and that manual techniques were superior in terms of aerosol clearance and sputum production. In patients with chonic bronchitis, the effect of mechanical vibration at 41.0 $\pm$ 5.4 Hz on lung clearance in the semierect position was evaluated (Pavia et al., 1976). Comparison of sputum production and clearance rates between patients given no vibration and those receiving mechanical vibration showed no significant differences. These findings are in contrast to those of Holody and Goldberg (1981), who studied the effect of 30 min of mechanical chest vibration followed by tracheal suctioning in 10 hospitalized patients with lung pathology on chest x-ray. They reported significant increases in PaO_2 at 30 and 60 min after treatment. The vibration frequency was not reported. Appropriate postural drainage was not used in either study.

Although the results of animal studies should not be assumed to be valid for humans, Rowe et al. (1973) investigated the effect of mechanical vibration on 38 piglets following thoracotomy. The use of postural drainage was not specified, but radiographically the piglets given vibration showed an 89% improvement compared with a 71% improvement in the nonvibrated group. While investigating the mechanism for high-frequency oscillation, Bitterman et al. (1983) looked at the role of high-frequency vibration (10–50 Hz) applied to the chest wall of paralyzed cats and found that lateral and prone positions were optimal for vibration. Frequencies from 20–35 Hz were equally effective in maintaining adequate gas exchange during tracheal insufflation. They theorized that vibration may assist air flow to lung regions that are poorly ventilated during high-frequency, low-pressure oscillations. Bitterman et al. (1983) did not investigate the role of vibration during spontaneous breathing or as an adjunct to conventional ventilation. Their aim was to evaluate gas exchange with vibration rather than mucus clearance.

King and co-workers (1983) studied the effect of vibration, called high-frequency chest wall compression (HFCWC), on tracheal mucus clearance (TMC) in nine anesthetized dogs. Chest vibration was performed by oscillating the pressure in a circumferentially applied thoracic cuff. TMC was enchanced by 2 min of HFCWC at rates between 5 and 17 Hz, reaching a peak increase of 340% at 13 Hz. The authors discussed two mechanisms for the dramatically improved TMC: HFCWC may stimulate vagal release of acetylcholine, thus augmenting the frequency of ciliary beating; alternatively, HFCWC may enhance the amplitude of cilia motion since the peak of 13 Hz closely corresponds to known mammalian ciliary beat frequencies. This article does not shed light on bronchial or more peripheral mucus clearance. However, it does establish a peak beneficial range of vibration at 11–15 Hz for TMC in dogs. These findings are in conflict with Radford et al. (1982) who studied in vitro mucociliary transport using excised rabbit tracheas. They reported that optimal mucociliary transport occurred between 25–35 Hz.

In humans, George and associates (1985) studied the effect of orally applied oscillations (8–12 Hz) on mucociliary clearance. They found significantly improved tracheobronchial clearing using vibration (oscillation) compared with a control period. No postural drainage was used in this study and none of the subjects had pulmonary pathology. Because of the size of the radioaerosol and the low penetraction index, it was assumed that the majority of the tracer particles were deposited in the larger airways. The authors theorize that the improved mucociliary clearance was due to an alteration in viscoelasticity caused by vibration. These two studies in dogs and humans provide three possible mechanisms of action for vibration. They also provide evidence of improved tracheobronchial clearing using frequencies consistent with the manual vibration reported to be of benefit in humans with lung pathology (Bateman et al., 1981; Sutton et al., 1985).

The physical response of the human lung and thorax to vibration at various frequencies has not been evaluated; therefore, it is not known which frequencies are best able to dislodge mucus from the airways. This uncertainty may explain the varying results found in the literature. Mucus is thought to be best mobilized at resonant frequencies of 5–6 Hz (Mellins) and 8–12 Hz (George et al.). Flower et al. (1979a) recommended using a mechanical percussor at frequencies of about 15 Hz with a force of 58–65 Newtons. They reported that a higher and more constant intrathoracic pressure (25–30 cm H_2O) is achieved when the percussor is placed firmly on the chest to the degree that voice quiver is produced (Dalek effect). Flower and co-workers also stated that the force needed to produce voice quiver varied greatly depending on the size of the patient, the surface on which they lie, and the area of the thorax receiving treatment. Intrathoracic pressures rose as high as 112 cm H_2O (Flower et al., 1979b). External chest force is not reported in this study but is assumed to be excessive to produce such high intrathoracic pressures. In view of these conflicting opinions, it appears that further study is needed to determine which levels of vibration are most effective on the varying airways of infants and adults, diseased or normal lungs and mechanically ventilated or spontaneously breathing patients (Mellins; Kirilloff et al., 1985).

Manual percussion can be performed at varying frequencies, depending on the experience of the therapist and whether it is carried out using one or two hands. The frequency selected for mechanical percussion or vibration often is not specified in the literature. Ranges of 3–65 Hz are documented (Denton; Pavia et al.; Maxwell and Redmond, 1979; General Physiotherapy; Flower et al., 1979a; Murphy et al., 1983).

al. recommended their use in the absence of a well-trained chest physical therapist. Thibeault (1979) described specifically how to adapt an electrical toothbrush for use as a neonatal mechanical vibrator. Curran and Kachoyeanos reported some benefit from using an electric toothbrush compared with a padded nipple in two neonates. These findings are in direct contrast with others who consider mechanical devices ineffective and inferior to manual techniques (Parker; Tudehope and Bagley). The authors also report better patient tolerance of manual techniques in terms of agitation with extensor posturing, skin color, and bradycardia. They conclude that, in infants, skin-to-skin contact often has a comforting effect. In neonates, W.W. Fox (personal communication) recommended using mechanical percussors in place of manual techniques because of the possibility of causing rib fractures. However, in the only published case history associating rib fractures with chest physiotherapy an electric toothbrush was used as part of the treatment (Purohit et al., 1975). It is hard to accept that mechanical devices applied manually to the thorax produce less chest wall pressure than properly performed manual percussion. It appears that the key to minimizing complications and performing effective chest percussion is not through the use of mechanical devices on neonates but, rather, through utilizing specially trained individuals.

Mechanical devices are also used in the home care of the pediatric patient to decrease the parental burden and encourage patient independence (*Lancet*, 1979). However, Maxwell and Redmond found that the youngest child capable of using such a percussor independently was 13 years old. Flower and associates (1978) studied the domiciliary use of prototype mechanical percussor (Salford) on 28 children with cystic fibrosis. They found self-administration to be appropriate to the front and, to a less degree, the sides of the chest. Interestingly, increased paternal involvement was noted with the addition of the mechanical aid.

Mechanical devices are also used in the pediatric intensive care unit. Rowe et

In comparing manual to mechanical techniques, most studies have been on adolescents or adults with cystic fibrosis. Pryor and co-workers (1981) found a significant increase in FEV_1 and FVC with manual therapy but no difference in sputum weight. In small samples of patients, others have found no difference in the two techniques in terms of pulmonary function or sputum volume (Hartsell, 1978; Maxwell and Redmond; Murphy et al., 1983).

Drawbacks specific to mechanical devices include the weight, sensation, noise level, and cost of the device (Maxwell and Redmond; Tecklin; Pryor et al., 1981; Murphy et al.). In the literature, both the type of equipment available and the cost tend to vary considerably. Prices from $375 to $995 are common, with additional costs for accessory parts and applicators (General Physiotherapy).

In treating patients after surgery or trauma who require intensive pulmonary care, it is the author's experience that "manual techniques" have the following advantages over mechanical devices. (1) Rib and sternal fractures that are not detected on routine chest x-rays may result from trauma or thoracic surgery. These fractures may be noted during chest physiotherapy evaluation and treatment, requiring the modification in manual techniques described earlier. (2) Manual palpation and visual inspection during treatment of the thorax allows the therapist to monitor important changes in the patient's response to treatment, such as a change in skin color, chest excursion, subcutaneous emphysema, or tactile fremitus. (3) The manual techniques of percussion and vibration may be adapted to fit the patient's need or tolerance; mechanical devices are adjustable only within the preset range of their manufacturers. (4) Some benefit may result from the direct skin contact that occurs with manual techniques. (5) No existing data demonstrate any advantages of mechanical devices over manual percussion and vibration, and some research suggests that manual techniques are more effective (Tudehope and Bagley; Hammon et al., 1980; Pryor et al., 1981; Rossman et al; Hammon, 1983; Hammon and Freeman,

1984). Therefore, mechanical devices involve both purchase and maintenance costs, provide no documented benefit, and still require the presence of a therapist to administer the care in the hospital setting.

SUMMARY

Based on limited research, it appears that percussion and vibration in conjunction with postural drainage are effective in mobilizing retained secretions. The literature also suggests that these techniques aid mucus clearance in both peripheral and more central airways and may be more effective in patients with acute lung pathology. Although the mechanisms of action are not clear, it is assumed that percussion and vibration augment gravity. Therefore, it is questionable if these techniques are of benefit in the absence of postural drainage. Complications of percussion or vibration are very rarely reported and may be due to poor technique. The frequencies of percussion and vibration that are most beneficial to mucus clearance have not been established. There is limited evidence in animals and humans to suggest that optimal frequencies range between 8 and 15 Hz. This area requires further investigation. As a result of the positive effects attributed to manual percussion and vibration, mechanical devices have been introduced. These devices collectively demonstrate wide ranges in both operational frequencies and cost; yet mechanical percussors have not been found to be more effective than manual percussion. Unless mechanical devices can be proven more effective than the manual techniques, the added cost, with no corresponding decrease in personnel or treatment time, is unwarranted.

References

Ayella RJ: *Radiologic Management of the Massively Traumatized Patient*, pp. 114–123. Williams & Wilkins, Baltimore, 1978
Barrell SE, Abbas HM: Monitoring during physiotherapy after open heart surgery. *Physiotherapy* 64:272–273, 1978
Bateman JRM, Newman SP, Daunt KM, Pavia D, Clarke SW: Regional lung clearance of excessive bronchial secretions during chest physiotherapy in patients with stable chronic airways obstruction. *Lancet* 1:294–297, 1979

Bateman JRM, Newman SP, Daunt KM, Sheahan NF, Pavia D, Clarke SW: Is cough as effective as chest physiotherapy in the removal of excessive tracheobronchial secretions? *Thorax* 36:683–687, 1981

Bitterman, H. Kerem DH, Shabtai Y, Gavriely N, Palti Y: Respiration maintained by externally applied vibration and tracheal insufflation in the cat. *Anesth Analg* 62:33–38, 1983

Buscaglia AJ, St Marie MS: Oxygen saturation during chest physiotherapy for acute exacerbation of severe chronic obstructive pulmonary disease. *Resp Care* 28:1009–1013, 1983

Campbell AH, O'Connell JM, Wilson F: The effect of chest physiotherapy upon FEV_1, in chronic bronchitis. *Med J Aust* 1:33–35, 1975

Ciesla ND, Klemic N, Imle PC: Chest physical therapy to the patient with multiple trauma: Two case studies. *Phys Ther* 61:202–205, 1981

Ciesla N, Rodrieguez A, Anderson P, Norton B: The incidence of extrapleural hematomas in patients with rib fractures receiving chest physical therapy (abstract). *Phys Ther* 67:766, 1987

Clarke SW, Cochrane GM, Webber BA: Effects of sputum on pulmonary function (abstract). *Thorax* 28:262, 1973

Cochrane GM, Webber BA, Clarke SW: Effects of sputum on pulmonary function, *Br Med J* 2:1181–1183, 1977

Crane L: Physical therapy for neonates with respiratory dysfunction. *Phys Ther* 61:1764–1773, 1981

Crane LD, Zombek M, Krauss AN, Auld PAM: Comparison of chest physiotherapy techniques in infants with HMD (abstract). *Pediatr Res* 12:559, 1978

Curran CL, Kachoyeanos MK: The effects on neonates of two methods of chest physical therapy. *MCN* 4:309–313, 1979

deBoeck C, Zinman R: Cough versus chest physiotherapy a comparison of the acute effects on pulmonary function in patients with cystic fibrosis. *Am Rev Respir Dis* 129:182–184, 1984

DeCesare JA, Babchyck BM, Colten HR, Treves S: Radionuclide assessment of the effects of chest physical therapy on ventilation in cystic fibrosis. *Phys Ther* 62:820–825, 1982

Demers B: Contraindications for chest physiotherapy (letter). *Chest* 89:902–903, 1986

Denton R: Bronchial secretions in cystic fibrosis—the effects on treatment with mechanical percussion vibration. *Am Rev Respir Dis* 86:41–46, 1962

Egan D: *Fundamentals of Respiratory Therapy*, p. 473. CV Mosby, St. Louis, 1977

Etches PC, Scott B: Chest physiotherapy in the newborn: Effect on secretions removed. *Pediatrics* 62:713–715, 1978

Falk M, Kelstrup M, Andersen JB, Kinoshita T, Falk P, Stovring S, Gothger I: Improving the ketchup bottle method with positive expiratory pressure, PEP, in cystic fibrosis. *Eur J Respir Dis* 65:423–432, 1984

Feldman J, Traver GA, Taussig LM: Maximal expiratory flows after postural drainage. *Am Rev Respir Dis* 119:239–245, 1979

Finer NN, Boyd J: Chest physiotherapy in the neonate: A controlled study. *Pediatrics* 61:282–285, 1978

Finer NN, Moriartey RR, Boyd J, Phillips HJ, Stewart AR, Ulan O: Post extubation atelectasis: a retrospective review and a prospective controlled study. *J Pediatr* 94:110–113, 1979

Flower KA, Eden RI, Lomax L: A new mechanical aid to physiotherapy for patients with cystic fibrosis (oral presentation). Eighth European Working Group Cystic Fibrosis. Austria, 1978

Flower KA, Eden RI, Lomax L, Mann NM, Burgess J: New mechanical aid to physiotherapy in cystic fibrosis. *Br Med J* 2:630–631, 1979a

Flower KA, Mann MN, Lomax L: Intrathoracic pressure variations generated by mechanical percussion (oral presentation). Ninth European Working Group Cystic Fibrosis. The Netherlands, 1979b

Garradd J, Bullock M: The effect of respiratory therapy on intracranial pressure in ventilated neurosurgical patients. *Aust J Physiother* 32:107–111, 1986

Gaskell DV, Webber BA: *The Brompton Hospital Guide to Chest Physiotherapy*, p 25. Blackwell Scientific Publications, Boston, 1980

General Physiotherapy: *G5 Massage Apparatus*. General Physiotherapy, St Louis, 1986

George RJD, Johnson MA, Pavia D, Agnew JE, Clarke SW, Geddes DM: Increase in mucocilliary clearance in normal man induced by oral high frequency oscillation. *Thorax* 40:433–437, 1985

Gormezano J, Brainthwaite MA: Pulmonary physiotherapy with assisted ventilation. *Anaesthesia* 27:249–257, 1972

Gray L: Fatal pulmonary hemorrhage (letter). *Phys Ther* 60:343–344, 1980

Hallbook T, Lindblad B, Lindroth B, Wolff T: Prophylaxis against pulmonary complications in patients undergoing gall-bladder surgery. *Ann Chirurg Gynaecol* 73:55–58, 1984

Hammon WE: Manual versus mechanical percussion for clearance of alveolar contents (abstract). *Phys Ther* 63:756, 1983

Hammon WE, Freeman PC: Chest physical therapy research in the treatment of pulmonary alveolar proteinosis. *Cardiopulm Q (APTA)* 4:6–7, 1984

Hammon WE, Kirmeyer PC, Connors AF, McCaffree DR, Kaplan RJ: Effect of bronchial drainage on intracranial pressure in acute neurological injuries (abstract). *Phys Ther* 51:735, 1981

Hammon WE, Martin RJ: Fatal pulmonary hemorrhage associated with chest physical therapy. *Phys Ther* 59:1247–1248, 1979

Hammon WE, Martin RJ: Chest physical therapy for acute atelectasis. *Phys Ther* 61:217–220, 1981

Hammon WE, Martin RJ, Pennock B, Rogers RM: Percussion versus vibration for clearance of alveolar contents (abstract). *Phys Ther* 60:589, 1980

Hartsell M: The effects of postural drainage, manual percussion and vibration vs. postural drainage and mechanical vibration on maximal expiratory flows (abstract). *Am Rev Respir Dis* 177(suppl):204, 1978

Hofmeyer JL, Webber BA, Hodson ME: Evaluation of positive expiratory pressure as an adjunct to chest physiotherapy in the treatment of cystic fibrosis. *Thorax* 41:951–954, 1986

Holody B, Goldberg HS: The effect of mechanical vibration physiotherapy on arterial oxygenation in acutely ill patients with atelectasis or pneumonia. *Am Rev Respir Dis* 124:372–375, 1981

Holody B, Goldberg HS: More on the vibrating foot pad (letter). Am Rev Respir Dis 125:782–783, 1982

Howell S, Hill JD: Acute respiratory care in the open heart surgery patient. Phys Ther 52:253–260, 1972

Imle PC: Chest physical therapy guidelines for treating lung contusion. Cardiopulm Q (APTA) 4:5–6, 1983

Imle PC, Mars MP, Eppinghaus CE, Anderson P, Ciesla ND: Effect of chest physiotherapy (CPT) positioning on intracranial (ICP) and cerebral perfusion pressure (CPP) (abstract). Crit Care Med 16:382, 1988

Irwin S, Tecklin JS: Cardiopulmonary Physical Therapy pp 325–328, 358. CV Mosby Co, St. Louis, 1985

Kerrebijn KF, Veentjer R, Bonzet- VD Water E: The immediate effect of physiotherapy and aerosol treatment on pulmonary function in children with cystic fibrosis. Eur J Respir Dis 63:35–42, 1982

Kigin CM: Chest physical therapy for the acutely ill medical patient. Phys Ther 61:1724–1736, 1981

Kigin CM: Advances in chest physical therapy. In Current Advances in Respiratory Care, edited by WJ O'Donohue, pp 37–71. American College Chest Physicians, Park Ridge, 1984

King M, Phillips DM, Gross D, Vartian V, Chang HK, Zidulka A: Enhanced tracheal mucus clearance with high frequency chest wall compression. Am Rev Respir Dis 128:511–515, 1983

Kirilloff LH, Owens GR, Rogers RM, Mazzocco MC: Does chest physical therapy work. Chest 88:436–446, 1983

Klein P, Kemper M, Weissman C, Rosenbaum SH, Askanazi J, Hyman AI: Attenuation of the hemodynamic responses to chest physical therapy. Chest 93:38–42, 1988

Kovnat DM, Rath GS, Anderson WM, Snider GL: Maximal extent of visualization of the bronchial tree by fiberoptic bronchoscopy. Am Rev Respir Dis 110:88–90, 1974

Lancet Editorial: Mechanical chest physiotherapy. Lancet 2:729, 1979

Laws AK, McIntyre RW: Chest physiotherapy: A physiological assessment during intermittent positive pressure ventilation in respiratory failure. Can Anaesth Soc J 16:487–493, 1969

Mackenzie CF, Shin B: Cardiorespiratory function before and after chest physiotherapy in mechanically ventilated patients with post-traumatic respiratory failure. Crit Care Med 13:483–486, 1985

Mackenzie CF, Shin B, McAslan TC: Chest physiotherapy: The effect on arterial oxygenation. Anesth Analg (Cleve) 57:28–30, 1978

Mackenzie CF, Shin B, Hadi F, Imle PC: Total lung/thorax compliance changes following chest physiotherapy. Anesth Anal (Cleve) 59:207–210, 1980

Marini JJ, Pierson DJ, Hudson LD: Acute lobar atelectasis: A prospective comparison of fiberoptic bronchoscopy and respiratory therapy. Am Rev Respir Dis 119:971–978, 1979

Matjasko J, Pitts L; Controversies in severe head injury management. In Clinical Controversies in Neuroanesthesia and Neurosurgery, edited by J. Matjasko and J Katz, pp 200–212. Grune & Stratton, New York, 1986

Maxwell M, Redmond A: Comparative trial of manual and mechanical percussion technique with gravity assisted bronchial drainage in patients with cystic fibrosis. Arch Dis Child 54:542–544, 1979

May DB, Munt PW: Physiologic effects of chest percussion and postural drainage in patients with stable chronic bronchitis. Chest 75:29–32, 1979

Mazzocco MC, Owens GR, Kirilloff LH, Rogers RM: Chest percussion and postural drainage in patients with bronchiectasis. Chest 88:360–363, 1985

Meier P: CPT—Which method, if any? MCN 4:310–311, 1979

Mellins RB: Pulmonary physiotherapy in the pediatric age group. Am Rev Respir Dis 110(Suppl 2):137–142, 1974

Morran CG, Finlay IG, Mathieson M, McKay AJ, Wilson N, McArdle CS: Randomized controlled trial of physiotherapy for postoperative pulmonary complications. Br J Anaesth 55:1113–1116, 1983

Murphy M, Concannon D, Fitzgerald MX: Chest percussion: Help or hindrance to postural drainage? Ir Med J 76:189–190, 1983

Newton DAG, Stephenson A: Effect of physiotherapy on respiratory function. Lancet 2:228–230, 1978

Opie LH, Spalding JM: Chest physiotherapy during intermittent positive pressure respiration. Lancet 2:671–674, 1958

O'Rourke PP, Schena JA, Thompson JE: The effects of pulmonary physiotherapy on delivered tidal volume (abstract). Crit Care Med 88:286, 1984

Parker AE: Chest physiotherapy in the neonatal intensive care unit. Physiotherapy 71:63–65, 1985

Pavia D, Thomson ML, Phillipakos D: A preliminary study on the effect of a vibrating pad on bronchial clearance. Am Rev Respir Dis 113:92–96, 1976

Petty TL (ed): Intensive and Rehabilitative Respiratory Care, pp 106, 108. Lea & Febiger, Philadelphia, 1974

Pryor JA, Webber BA, Hodson ME, Batten JC: Evaluation of forced expiration technique as an adjunct to postural drainage in the treatment of cystic fibrosis. Br Med J 2:417–418, 1979

Pryor JA, Parker RA, Webber BA: A comparison of mechanical and manual percussion as adjuncts to postural drainage in treatment of cystic fibrosis in adolescents and adults. Physiotherapy 67:140–141, 1981

Purohit DM, Caldwell C, Levkoff AH: Multiple rib fractures due to physiotherapy in a neonate with hyaline membrane disease (letter). Am J Dis Child 129:1103–1104, 1975

Reines HD, Sade RM, Bradford BF, Marshall J: Chest physiotherapy fails to prevent post-operative atelectasis in children after cardiac surgery. Ann Surg 195:451–455, 1982

Rivington-Law B, Epstein SW, Thompson G: The effect of chest wall vibrations on pulmonary function in normal subjects. Physiother (Canada) 31:319–332, 1979

Roper PC, Vonwiller JB, Fisk GC, Gupta JM: Lobar atelectasis after nasotracheal intubation in newborn infants. Aust Paediatr J 12:272–275, 1976

Rossman CM, Waldes R, Sampson D, Newhouse MT: Effect of chest physiotherapy on the removal of mucus in patients with cystic fibrosis. Am Rev Respir Dis 126:131–135, 1982

Rowe MI, Weinberger M, Poole CA: An experimental study on the vibration in post operative tracheobronchial clearance. *J Pediatr Surg* 8:735–738, 1973

Sutton PP, Lopez-Vidriero MT, Pavia D, Newman SP, Clarke SW: Effect of chest physiotherapy on the removal of mucus in patients with cystic fibrosis (letter). *Am Rev Respir Dis* 127:390–391, 1984

Sutton PP, Lopez-Vidriero MT, Pavia D, Newman SP, Clay MM, Webber B, Parker RA, Clarke SW: Assessment of percussion, vibratory-shaking and breathing exercises in chest physiotherapy. *Eur J Respir Dis* 66:147–152, 1985

Sutton PP, Parker RA, Webber BA, Newman SP, Garland N, Lopez-Vidriero MT, Pavia D, Clarke SW: Assessment of the forced expiratory technique, postural drainage and directed coughing in chest physiotherapy. *Eur J Respir Dis* 64:62–68, 1983

Sutton PP, Pavia D, Bateman JRM, Clarke SW: Chest physiotherapy: A review. *Eur J Respir Dis* 63:188–201, 1982

Tecklin JS: Positioning, percussing, and vibrating patients for effective bronchial drainage. *Nursing '79* 9:64–71, 1979

Thacker EW: *Postural Drainage and Respiratory Control*, 2nd ed., p 19. Lloyd-Luke, Ltd., London, 1959

Thibeault DW, Gregory GA (eds): *Neonatal Pulmonary Care*, pp 248–250. Addison-Wesley Publishing, Menlo Park, 1979

Tomney PM, Finer NN: A controlled evaluation of muscle relaxation in ventilated neonates (abstract). *Crit Care Med* 8:228, 1980

Torrington KG, Sorenson DE, Sherwood LM: Postoperative chest percussion with postural drainage in obese patients following gastric stapling. *Chest* 86:891–895, 1984

Tudehope DI, Bagley C: Techniques of physiotherapy in intubated babies with respiratory distress syndrome. *Aust Paediatr J* 16:226–228, 1980

Tyler ML, Hudson LD, Grose BL, Huseby JS: Prediction of oxygenation during chest physiotherapy in critically ill patients (abstract). *Am Rev Respir Dis* 121(suppl):218, 1980

Van der Schans CP, Piers DA, Postma DS: Effect of manual percussion on tracheobronchial clearance in patients with chronic airflow obstruction and excessive tracheobronchial secretion. *Thorax* 41:448–452, 1986

Wade JF (ed): *Respiratory Nursing Care, Physiology and Technique*, p 105. CV Mosby, St. Louis, 1973

Webber B, Parker R, Hofmeyr J, Hodson M: Evaluation of self-percussion during postural drainage using the forced expiration technique. *Physiother Pract* 1:42–45, 1985

White DJ, Mawdley RH: Effects of selective bronchial drainage positions and percussion on blood pressure and healthy human subjects. *Phys Ther* 63:325–300, 1983

Wollmer P, Ursing K, Midgren B, Eriksson L: Inefficiency of chest percussion in the physical therapy of chronic bronchitis. *Eur J Respir Dis* 66:233–239, 1985

Zadai CC: Physical therapy for the acutely ill medical patient. *Phys Ther* 61:1746–1754, 1981

Zapletal A, Stefanova J, Horak J, Vavrova V, Samanek M: Chest physiotherapy and airway obstruction in patients with cystic fibrosis—a negative report. *Eur J Respir Dis* 64:426–433, 1983

CHAPTER 5

Methods of Airway Clearance: Coughing and Suctioning

P. Cristina Imle, M.S., P.T., and Nancy Klemic, B.S., P.T.

Ciliary activity may be impaired by a history of smoking, surgery, anesthesia, trauma, or preexisting lung disease. Pain and immobility accompany recovery and further impede secretion clearance and reduce lung volumes. Consequently, secondary techniques for airway clearance, such as coughing and suctioning, become increasingly important in the prevention of atelectasis and pulmonary infection. This chapter reviews the literature on coughing, addresses the etiology of cough suppression, and describes methods of cough stimulation. The techniques and hazards of suctioning are also considered. Pulmonary lavage and "bagging," or lung hyperinflation are reviewed as adjuncts to coughing and suctioning.

CILIARY ACTION

Coughing is considered an extremely important mechanism for the removal of lung secretions. Normally, coughing occurs infrequently, suggesting that this is not the only method active in secretion clearance. Phagocytosis and lymphatic drainage are the most peripheral mechanisms involved in secretion clearance, and these occur beyond the terminal bronchioles. The terminal airways are lined with surfactant that may also assist in airway clearance (Comroe, 1966; Leith, 1967). Cilia extend from the terminal bronchioles to the larynx. The rhythmical beating of these cilia is largely responsible for keeping the airways clear of excess mucus, and this provides adequate clearance in normal circumstances. Ciliary motion is continuous, initiating a wave-like action that carries the entire mucus blanket cephalad. Although the overall rate of clearance can vary, rates of up to 16 mm/min have been observed experimentally (Comroe). Under normal circumstances, phagocytosis, lymphatic drainage, and ciliary action keep the alveoli sterile.

Three major factors influence ciliary clearance: cilia length, density, and beat frequency, the quantity of mucus present, and the viscoelastic properties of mucus (King, 1980). Hypoxemia and dehydration can arrest ciliary action (Newhouse, 1973; Chopra et al., 1977). This adverse effect is usually reversible once the insult is removed. Dry gases such as supplementary oxygen or other vehicles used to deliver anesthetic agents have the same effect as dehydration unless adequate humidity is added (see Chapter 9). Anesthetic agents themselves can suppress ciliary activity. A history of smoking and most chronic lung diseases result in reduced ciliary function as shown in Figure 5.1 (Goodman et al., 1978; Mossberg et al., 1978; Puchell et al., 1980; Mossberg and Cramner, 1980). The rheological properties of sputum also affect mucociliary transport. Altering either the viscosity or elasticity diminishes normal sputum clearance. Interestingly, sputum that is either too thick or too runny decreases mucus transport. Mucociliary clearance is also significantly less in patients with purulent sputum (leukocyte count greater than 3500/mm) (Puchelle et al., 1980; King, 1980). Infection of the airways may increase secretion production, further impeding mucus flow. Chronic infection magnifies this by also

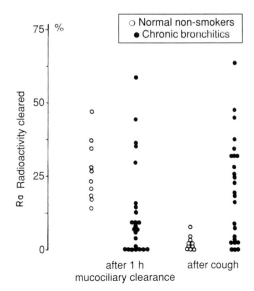

Figure 5.1. Comparison of the percentage of bronchial radioactivity eliminated after 1 hr by mucociliary clearance and coughing in healthy nonsmoking subjects and chronic bronchitics. (From Puchelle E: *Eur J Respir Dis* 61:254–264, 1980.)

causing cellular damage to the cilia and epithelium (Comroe).

A tracheal tube can impair ciliary flow while stimulating increased mucus production, due to its effect as a foreign object (Bucher, 1958; Leith, 1967). Secretions raised to the level of an artificial airway are reported to pool in this area due to the presence of the tracheal tube (Leith, 1967). The cuffs of artificial airways can additionally interfere with ciliary action and tracheal mucosal perfusion. This may lead to tissue necrosis or scarring and further decrease ciliary function. When mucociliary transport is impaired, cough can, in part, compensate for the loss (Mossberg and Cramner).

THE COUGH MECHANISM

Stages of a Cough

Coughing particularly affects the larger airways. It is most important in the removal of foreign bodies or excessive quantities of sputum and when normal ciliary activity is absent. The cough mechanism provides the most rapid means of secretion clearance. Coughing is usually considered a reflex controlled primarily by afferent stimulation of the vagus nerve, which leads to a complex series of muscular actions (see Fig. 5.2). It is normally triggered by mechanical or chemical stimulation of the larynx, carina, trachea, and large bronchi, in that order (Widdicombe, 1980). Cough can also be elicited experimentally by electrical and osmotic stimuli (Banner, 1986).

A normal cough consists of an inspiratory effort, glottic closure, and contraction of the expiratory muscles followed by opening of the glottis. Inhaling large volumes prior to a cough results in improved expiratory muscle function. At high lung volumes the length-tension relationships of the expiratory muscles are optimized and are therefore capable of generating greater the expiratory pressures and flows that increase cough effectiveness (Leith et al., 1986; McCool and Leith, 1987). However, the inspired volume at the beginning of a cough is variable. It is usually larger than a tidal breath and averages 2.5 liters (Leith,

1977; King et al., 1985). Cough is not always preceded by inspiration. If foreign material enters the larynx, it may immediately elicit a cough from the existing lung volume, thereby preventing impaction of the material deeper into the airway (Leith et al., 1986).

The glottic closure that ocurs along with expiratory muscle activity is often referred to as the compressive phase of cough and lasts for about 0.2 sec. The contraction of any or all of the expiratory muscles in the chest wall, abdomen, and pelvic floor interacts with inspiratory muscles to produce intrathoracic pressures as high as 200 cm H_2O. The expiratory phase of cough begins when the glottis opens and air is expelled. During this phase, compression of the central airways occurs and is associated with gas velocities of up to Mach 0.6. The high kinetic energy, shearing force, and acceleration of wave motion along the airway wall are thought to provide airway clearance, which is the major function of coughing (Leith, 1967, 1977, 1985; Guy-

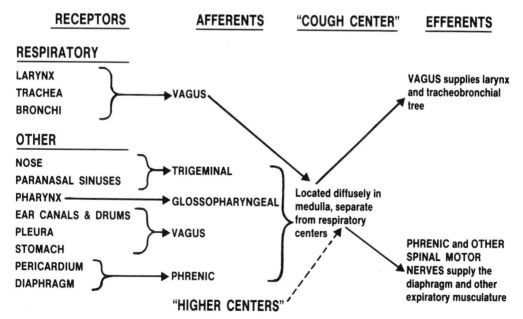

Figure 5.2. Anatomy of the cough reflex. Respiratory tract receptors are most numerous in the larger airways, least in the smaller airways, and none is present beyond the respiratory bronchioles. They respond to chemical and mechanical stimuli and adapt rapidly. Other receptors probably respond only to mechanical stimuli. "Higher centers" is included as afferent, since cough can be voluntarily initiated, postponed or suppressed. (From Irwin RS et al.: *Arch Intern Med* 137:1186–1191, 1977.)

ton, 1977; Irwin et al., 1977; Leith et al., 1986). Both airway compression and mechanisms of airway clearance are further described in this chapter.

Glottic Function

The role of the glottis during a cough is debated in the literature, but there appears to be agreement that its action is significant. Leith (1967) claims that glottic closure is important in achieving maximum positive airway pressure. It is the abrupt opening of the glottis following its closure that differentiates a cough from a forced expiration (Bucher; Leith et al., 1986). This distinction is used throughout the text. Ross et al. (1955) suggest that the reduction in lumen size differentiates a cough from a forceful expiration in which flow rates equivalent to those of a cough may be easily achieved. In normal subjects, no significant differences are found between the peak flow rates of forced expiration or coughing

(Leiner et al., 1966), nor is the ability to develop peak airway pressures found to depend upon glottic closure (Gal, 1980). Rather, it is the timing of both peak airway pressure and flow that differentiates a cough from a forced expiration (see Fig. 5.3). Glottic closure allows the expiratory phase of coughing to occur at higher lung volumes and at greater intrathoracic pressures than occur with forced expiration (Evans et al., 1975; Melissinos et al., 1976, 1978). The contractile force of the expiratory muscles, which control intrathoracic pressure during cough, are enhanced by glottic closure (Leith et al., 1986). With coughing, the closed glottis prevents air flow until considerable pressure develops and then the glottis opens. In forced expiration and in patients with artificial airways, flow begins and alters in relation to pressure changes. As a result, higher transpulmonary pressures and more marked tracheobronchial compression occur with coughing (Gal).

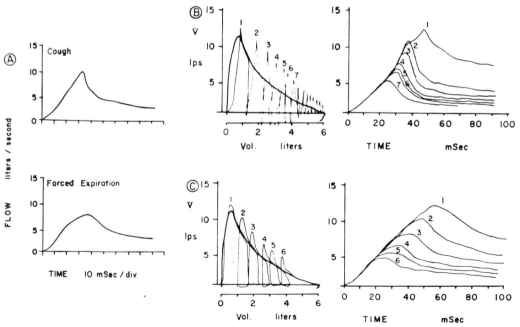

Figure 5.3. **(A)** Flow time representations of cough and forced expiration at the same lung volume in a normal subject. **(B)** On the left is a series of voluntary coughs beginning at total lung capacity and progressing sequentially down to vital capacity, superimposed on the subjects maximum expiratory flow–volume curve. On the right, the numbered coughs are represented as flow in time. **(C)** Series of brief rapid expiratory effects are depicted in the same manner as the coughs. All data shown are derived from the same normal subject. (From Knudson RJ et al.: *J Appl Physiol* 36:653–67, 1974.)

In a series of coughs, glottic closure allows pressure in the airways to equalize between coughs. It assists compressed airways in regaining normal size for that lung volume (Langlands, 1967; Gal). The glottis is also noted to oscillate violently during coughing, setting up pressure fluctuations that may play a part in loosening secretions from the airway walls. The rapid opening and closing of the glottis that may occur during the expiratory phase of coughing also cause changes in the airflow and pleural and abdominal pressure (Leith, 1967).

Airway Compression

The lungs are designed so that the cross-sectional area of the airways decreases as one moves from the alveolus to the mouth (McCool and Leith). When expiration begins, alveolar pressure is greater than ambient pressure, so air flows from the peripheral airways, along the pressure gradient and out of the lungs. Simultaneously, pleural pressure exceeds the pressure within the central airways, producing a rapid narrowing of the central air passages and a dramatic increase in air flow from the compressed areas mouthward (or downstream) (Leith, 1985). The high intrapleural pressure and smooth muscle activity are felt to be responsible for the changes in airway diameter noted during cough (Ross et al., Marshall and Holden, 1963; Leith, 1977; Gal). Tracheal narrowing occurs during both cough and forced expiration. Compression is limited to the posterior membranous portion of the trachea as the rest of the trachea is made up of rigid cartilage (see Fig. 2.6). The increased intrapleural pressure causes invagination of the posterior tracheal wall, thereby reducing the lumen caliber. A pressure gradient of 40 cm H_2O is reported as sufficient to reduce the cross-sectional area to roughly one-fifth its original size. This decrease generates a force of about 25 times that possible in the uncompressed trachea (Ross et al.). Tracheal narrowing of up to 80%, reported from bronchoscopic and bronchographic examination, could result in velocities of up to 25,000 cm/sec or three quarters the speed of sound (Leith, 1977). The degree of airway collapse is significant as decreasing the cross-sectional area by half produces a fourfold increase in the kinetic energy of the gas stream (Gal).

The location and extent of airway compression distal to the trachea and mainstem bronchi are debatable and poorly understood. Because glottic closure prevents air flow until peak pressure is reached, coughing is associated with more marked airway narrowing than forced expiration. The locations in the airways where peripheral flow is limited but where flow downstream is usually enhanced (by dynamic compression) are referred to in the literature as choke points, equal pressure points, or flow limiting segments (FLS) (Leith, 1977, 1985, 1986; Smaldone et al., 1979; Smaldone and Messina 1985a,b; Smaldone and Smith, 1985). There is general agreement that at high lung volumes (as normally precedes a cough), the FLS are confined to the trachea or mainstem bronchi. They are thought to move peripherally (an uncertain distance) as lung volume decreases (as with a series of coughs or forced expirations) (Leith, 1977, 1985). For this reason, coughing or forced expiratory efforts from progressively smaller lung volumes are suggested as methods to improve peripheral airway clearance due to upstream movement of the FLS (Meade et al., 1967; Pryor et al., 1979). However, in addition to lung volume, the location of the FLS depends on age, lung and airway geometry, elastic recoil, gas density and viscosity, and the presence of secretions or disease (Leith et al., 1986). Also, there is little evidence that FLS move outside of the central airways. Some researchers have suggested that they migrate as far as the fifth or sixth bronchial generations (trachea = 0) (Lambert et al., 1981, 1982). More recently, in studies of normal subjects, persons with chronic obstructive lung disease and mechanically ventilated patients with severe intracerebral injury, FLS failed to move beyond the fourth-generation bronchi with coughing or forced expiration at low lung volumes (Smaldone and Smith, 1985; Smaldone and Messina, 1985a,b).

Two-Phase Concurrent Flow

The clearance of secretions by coughing depends on the combined effect of secretions and air flow within the airways. This gas–liquid interaction is termed *two-phase concurrent flow*. Four proposed mechanisms are shown in Figure 5.4. Bubble flow is not relevant to cough. Slug flow is effective in removing large plugs of sputum from the central airways. The annular flow of mucus is thought to be slow despite the associated high air-flow velocities. Flow rates markedly decrease as energy is transferred into dragging the liquid layer of secretions mouthward. The waves that occur in the liquid layer with this annular flow probably enhance droplet formation, necessary for misty flow. Misty flow is thought to be the most important means of clearing secretions during cough. However, droplet formation, suspension, and clearance during cough are complex and poorly understood (Leith, 1967, 1977, 1985; Leith et al., 1986).

Cough, Forced Expiratory Technique, and Chest Physiotherapy

There is some debate on the efficacy of cough compared with chest physiotherapy in removing tracheobronchial secretions. Oldenburg and co-workers (1979)

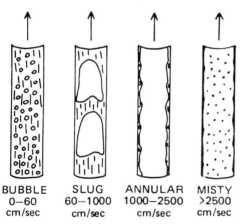

BUBBLE	SLUG	ANNULAR	MISTY
0–60	60–1000	1000–2500	>2500
cm/sec	cm/sec	cm/sec	cm/sec

Figure 5.4. Four main types of two-phase concurrent flow, with the corresponding superficial velocity of gas. (From Leith DL: Cough. In *Lung Biology in Health and Disease, Vol 5, Respiratory Defense Mechanisms,* edited by JD Brain, DF Proctor, and LM Reid, pp 545–592. Dekker, New York, 1977.)

evaluated the effect of cough, postural drainage, and exercise on the removal of radioaerosols in eight patients with chronic bronchitis. Coughing was prohibited during postural drainage. Aerosol clearance was better during cough than exercise and both were superior to postural drainage. The investigators claim that cough is effective in improving the peripheral clearance of secretions. However, the airways that they describe as peripheral (diameters approximately 2–4 mm) correspond to fifth- and six-order bronchi (Weibel, 1963). Their findings also contrast to more recent research showing that the effects of coughing (even at low lung volumes) are limited to the central airways and proximal to fifth-generation bronchi (Smaldone and Smith, 1985).

Three studies looked at the role of cough or forced expiratory technique (FET) in relation to chest physiotherapy techniques in patients with stable cystic fibrosis. Falk et al. (1984) found reduced sputum production, oxygen tension, and spontaneous cough in conjunction with postural drainage, percussion, and vibration than with positive expiratory pressure (PEP) or with FET (see p. 135). They conclude that both cough and FET affect only the more central airways whereas PEP also acts on the peripheral airways and collateral channels. No significant short-term benefit was found in pulmonary function tests or expectoration when cough was compared with postural drainage, percussion, and vibration with cough (deBoeck and Zinman, 1984). Similar findings were reported by Rossman and associates (1982), who measured mucus clearance using aerosol tracers. They reported no added benefit of combined chest physiotherapy maneuvers (postural drainage, percussion, and deep breathing with vibration) compared with cough. This is not surprising as the majority of the inhaled radioisotope was deposited in the large airways, where cough is particularly effective at removing excess secretions.

Bateman and colleagues (1981) compared the effect of cough alone and with chest physiotherapy (postural drainage, vibration, shaking, percussion, and cough) in patients with chronic bronchitis and bronchiectasis. Using inhaled radioaerosols, they found both regimens to be equally effective in clearing the central airways. Chest physiotherapy, but not cough, significantly enhanced peripheral lung clearance and increased sputum yield. These findings are supported by Sutton and associates (1983), who also measured inhaled radionuclide clearance in patients with copious sputum production (bronchiectasis, cystic fibrosis, and chronic asthma). They reported that FET alone and FET during postural drainage eliminated significantly more radioaerosol than either cough or a control period. In addition, more sputum was cleared with FET and postural drainage than any other treatment. The effect of postural drainage with cough was not compared with FET and cough in this study.

When evaluating the effects of chest physiotherapy on peripheral secretion clearance, it is neither logical nor relevant to separate the effects of cough (or FET) from other chest physiotherapy techniques. Distal secretions must be advanced centrally before they can be removed. If the most effective means of large airway clearance, cough, is prohibited, it is not surprising that chest physiotherapy appears relatively ineffective by comparison. Thus far, studies evaluating cough, FET, and chest physiotherapy involved patients with chronic lung diseases. The varying degrees of central, intermediate, and peripheral airway pathology in this population make both aerosol deposition and clearance of the distal airways difficult to assess. The results are not pertinent to patients with acute lung disease. From the existing research, it appears that both cough and FET enhance the removal of excess secretions from the larger, more central airways. Their effect in the intermediate (fourth- to sixth-order) bronchi is debatable. Neither cough nor FET alone is shown to improve mucus clearance in the peripheral airways (distal to sixth-generation bronchi). Therefore, mobilizing peripheral secretions to the central airways using postural drainage, percussion, vibration, ciliary action, or exercise enhances the effect of both cough and FET. Once in the upper airways, secretions should be promptly expectorated or suctioned before the effect of gravity causes peripheral migration or transbronchial aspiration as in the intubated or unconscious patient (see Case History 7.1).

Cough Suppression

Smaller airways are more sensitive to chemical stimuli, while the larger airways respond more readily to mechanical stimuli that elicit coughing. Both the large and small airways demonstrate adaptation to repeated stimulation. Apart from adaptation, the cough reflex can be both voluntarily and involuntarily suppressed, as is commonly observed in the intensive care unit. Any predisposing factor limiting the four stages of coughing (see p. 155) can interfere with its effectiveness.

Involuntary Cough Suppression

Involuntary cough suppression can result from decreased inspiratory effort, inability to close and then open the glottis, or diminished expiratory effort. Patients having recurrent laryngeal nerve palsy demonstrate difficulty in glottic or vocal cord closure (Innocenti, 1969). Diseases disrupting neuromuscular function commonly result in decreased cough effectiveness. In patients with quadriplegia, inspiration and particularly expiration are limited (as detailed in Chapter 8), yet glottic function is intact. The only forces of expiration present in the quadriplegic patient are provided by the elastic properties of the lung and thorax. Upper airway compression, normally seen during coughing, is minimal due to the low pressure gradients achieved (Siebens et al., 1964). Paraplegic patients primarily have the muscles of expiration affected, while inspiration is less involved.

Myasthenia gravis, Guillain-Barré syndrome, poliomyelitis, and demyelinating diseases may disrupt any or all aspects necessary for an effective cough, depending on the degree of involvement. Similarly, pharmacological neuromuscular blocking drugs interfere with all stages of coughing. Narcotics cause central nervous system depression, which can inhibit the cough mechanism. Patients with loss of consciousness or severe head injury may display diminished or absent cough reflexes for the same reason. Consequently, they are unable to protect their airway from possible aspiration. Tracheal intubation with a cuffed tube may be required. Apart from the pooling of secretions and diminished ciliary action discussed earlier, artificial airways mechanically prevent normal tracheal compression during coughing. As a result, higher flow rates are necessary to achieve the linear velocities required to clear secretions. Since tracheal tubes also cause increased resistance to air flow, higher lung volumes and excessive effort are required to clear the airways (Gal). Tracheal tubes additionally disrupt coughing by preventing glottic closure, making a cough resemble a forced expiration (Bucher; Gal).

It is our opinion, based on these findings, that to restore an effective cough, tracheal tubes should be removed as soon as ventilatory support is no longer necessary or when protective laryngeal reflexes return. The use of progressively smaller tracheostomy tubes to "wean" a patient from an artificial airway is not advisable as it leads to a compromised cough and increased ventilatory effort. The stoma left after tracheostomy tube removal diminishes cough effectiveness until wound closure occurs. Though glottic closure is not inhibited, the increased intrapleural pressures generated during a cough cause air to escape through the stoma. This can be prevented by sealing the stoma with an airtight dressing and instructing the patient to support the dressing manually during speaking and coughing (see Fig. 5.5). Fenestrated tracheostomy tubes are a compromise. In our opinion their use is very rarely justified, because, when they are present, secretion production is still stimulated, ciliary action and tracheal compression during coughing are still impeded, and airway resitance is still increased.

Posture also plays a role in coughing. In healthy individuals most lung volumes and functional residual capacity decrease as the person moves from sitting to supine to the head-down position. In a

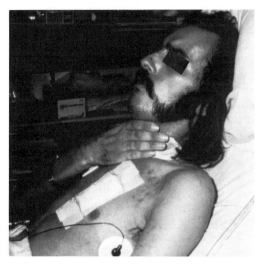

Figure 5.5. Following tracheostomy tube removal, an airtight dressing should be placed over the stoma. This must be supported during coughing, as illustrated.

study of 20 normal subjects, Curry and Van Eeden (1977) evaluated the effect of nine different positions on cough volume and flow rates. They found that cough efficacy increased as the posture was changed from side-lying to supine and from supine to progressively more upright sitting. Hip flexion also resulted in a larger volume and flow rate than coughing in the same position with the hips extended. These findings support the clinical impression that most patients have a stronger cough while sitting with the hips flexed. However, it is the authors' opinion and that of others that cough and FET should also be performed during postural drainage where gravity can assist these efforts in the clearance of mucus (Pryor et al., 1979; Hofmeyr et al., 1986). Further research is needed to evaluate the effects of coughing and FET in postural drainage positions in patients with pulmonary pathology.

Some controversy exists as to whether forced expiration or coughing is of greater benefit to the patient with obstructive pulmonary disease. Leiner et al. reported that peak expiratory flow rates were greater in patients with pulmonary obstruction, whereas most researchers found the reverse to be true. There is agreement that overall cough efficacy is reduced, as air flow obstruction allows less air to escape with each cough (Langlands, Leiner et al., Loudon and Shaw; Leith). Langlands also noted incomplete and inadequate glottic closure between successive coughs in patients with bronchitis. Lack of closure prevents compressed airways from reassuming their normal size between coughs. The rapid expiratory flow associated with coughing was found to reduce obstruction in some airways, while compromising clearance in others—notably in the patient with chronic obstructive pulmonary disease (Menkes and Britt, 1980). Because of the potential for increased airway obstruction, FET is often used in place of coughing for patients with chronic pulmonary disease.

Bouts of coughing may precipitate brief periods of dizziness and distress, particularly in patients with preexisting heart or lung disease. These responses are due to the increased transpulmonary pressure that accompanies coughing and causes decreased pulmonary, cardiac and cerebral blood flow (Langlands; Banner). The decreased cerebral blood flow or increased cerebral spinal fluid pressure that occurs during a cough is undesirable for patients with brain injury. In most cases, the deleterious response is transient and rapidly returns to baseline values. For some patients, the use of local or systemic medication may be necessary to control spasms of coughing. Other potential complications that may accompany cough are shown in Table 5.1. These associated findings may give rise to voluntary or involuntary cough suppression although they occur infrequently and usually in association with multiple coughing episodes. For these reasons, chest physiotherapy should not include repetitive coughing. In the intensive care unit both the effects and benefits gained from coughing should beassessed, and modifications made accordingly.

Voluntary Cough Suppression

Controlled suppression of the cough reflex is common, particularly in patients

Table 5.1
Complications of Cough[a]

Respiratory
  Bronchoconstriction
  Trauma to airways and larynx
  Barotrauma: pneumomediastinum, pneumothorax, interstitial emphysema
Hemodynamic
  Decreased venous return
  Transient systemic hypertension, hypotension
  Arrhythmias
Cerebral
  Syncope
  Apoplexy
Chest wall
  Rib fractures
  Ruptured rectus abdominus muscles
Miscellaneous
  Urinary incontinence
  Pulmonary emboli
  Kinking and knotting of venous catheters
  Fear attendant on loss of control

[a]From Banner AS: *Lung* 164:79–92, 1986.

following surgery. This is usually a result of fear or pain. Fear can often be minimized in the patient for elective surgery by instruction before the operation. This should include a general explanation of expected surgery and the importance of coughing despite discomfort after the operation (Thoren, 1954; Howell and Hill, 1972).

Pain after surgery cannot be eliminated but can be alleviated with analgesics, especially if administration is coordinated with the patient's efforts to cough. The pain following thoracotomy is particularly troublesome as these patients are at increased risk of postoperative pulmonary complications. Byrd and Burns (1975) used esophageal balloon pressures to assess cough efficacy in 24 adult males after thoracotomy. They found voluntary cough pressures to be reduced to 29% of preoperative values on the day of surgery and to still be only 50% of control values 1 week later. Cough induced by ultrasound mist resulted in higher cough pressures on the operative day (44%) and after 1 week (60%), indicating that pain, rather than neuromuscular function, was the limiting factor. However, administering narcotics did not consistently increase the patient's ability to cough. More selective types of analgesia may improve cough efforts by providing more appropriate pain relief (see Chapter 10). Yamazaki et al. (1980) also measured cough pressures in 20 patients following thoracotomy. They directly recorded intrapleural pressure by using a catheter inserted with the intraoperative chest tube. Although more accurate than using an esophageal balloon, this method did not allow for comparison of preoperative and postoperative values. However, intrapleural cough pressures were significantly improved in the supine position by epidural anaesthesia but not in the sitting position. As reported by others (Curry and Van Eeden), cough pressures were better in sitting than in supine positions. Interestingly, pressures in both positions were significantly improved by manual chest wall compression or supported coughing. This provides evidence for using assisted cough techniques after surgery. It is the authors' experience that pain may be decreased and voluntary cough improved by manual support of the surgical incision or area of rib fractures with a pillow or folded sheet (Fig. 5.6). Breathing exercises, as discussed in Chapter 3, may help to relieve anxiety and incisional pain. Again, an explanation of why coughing is important may improve the patient's ability and willingness to cough.

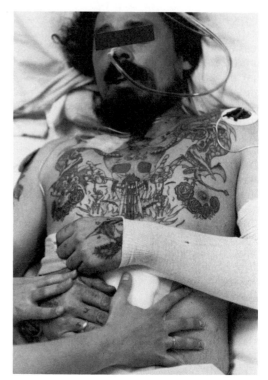

Figure 5.6. Incisional support may be manually applied by the patient or the therapist. Here both are supporting the incision (under the surgical dressing) while the patient coughs voluntarily.

METHODS OF COUGH STIMULATION

When voluntary control of coughing is absent, methods to stimulate this response become necessary. Suctioning is one of these and is discussed separately in this chapter. Another frequently used maneuver to improve cough effectiveness is "huffing." This consists of a single large inspiration followed by short expiratory blasts, interrupted by pauses. If secretions are mobilized centrally by previously mentioned maneuvers, this technique, which causes rapid changes in air flow, may oscillate the secretions and, hence, mechanically stimulate a normal cough. Huffing can be taught to the patient in the following manner. First, an inspiratory effort toward total

lung capacity should be encouraged. This is followed by active expiration during which the patient incorporates two or more pauses. Teaching the patient to say "huff, huff, huff," or "ha, ha, ha" during expiration (much as in laughing) may be helpful (Frownfelter, 1978; Hietpas et al., 1979). Huffing does not cause glottic closure and is reported to generate lower intrathoracic pressure than does coughing (Gaskell and Webber; Hietpas et al.). Therefore, this method may be specifically beneficial to patients with airway diseases, such as asthma, cystic fibrosis, and emphysema. The lower intrathoracic pressures may help decrease the small airway closure associated with coughing in patients with chronic obstructive pulmonary disease (Marshall and Holden; Hietpas et al.) Huffing is reportedly effective in mobilizing secretions more centrally as visualized by fiberoptic bronchoscopy (Hietpas et al.). It may be used with the previously described techniques, such as manual incisional support. Its use with controlled diaphragmatic breathing is termed "forced expiration technique" (Pryor and Webber, 1979) and is discussed on p. 121.

Vibration is reported to stimulate a spontaneous cough for much the same reason as huffing (Rowe et al., 1973). It is believed that either the movement of secretions into the larger airways, the increased tidal volume that follows a vibratory maneuver, or the rapid change in air flow during vibration may be sufficient to stimulate a cough mechanically (Belinkoff, 1976). Clinically, vibration seems particularly effective in producing a spontaneous cough in patients with decreased levels of consciousness. In the quadriplegic patient, manual pressure over the chest and abdomen during expiration causes increased expiratory force and may increase cough effectiveness (Siebens et al.). This is illustrated in Chapter 8.

Bucher states that the inspiratory effort preceding a normal cough is usually deeper than resting inspiration. Therefore, following surgery, instruction in deep breathing exercises may be beneficial to increase cough effectiveness. A series of three increasingly larger breaths, with the third followed by a voluntary cough, is found to render a previously ineffective cough productive. Similarly, patients with inspiratory muscle weakness, such as in quadriplegia, demonstrate an improved inspiratory effort using "summed breathing." This consists of three to five successive inspirations without an intervening expiration. It is based on the same principle as glossopharyngeal breathing (described in Chapter 8). The increased lung volume achieved by accumulated inspiratory effort may make a more effective cough possible. Repetitive coughing, however, should not be encouraged. In addition to the reasons stated earlier in this chapter, bouts of coughing are usually more fatiguing than controlled coughs or FET. Also Smaldone et al. (1979) reported that multiple coughs can retard and possibly arrest mucociliary transport in dogs. It is important to note that this finding was obtained after 50 to 100 coughs. In studying the effect of successive coughs in healthy

adults, Harris and Lawson (1968) found a progressive decline in efficiency.

External tracheal stimulation may be necessary in infants or patients who are unwilling to cough. This is achieved by applying manual pressure to the trachea above the manubrial notch (Ungvarski, 1971; Petty, 1974; Frownfelter). This creates partial tracheal compression, which often causes mechanical stimulation of the cough mechanism (Fig. 5.7). In children, mild compression over the superior sternum is found to be particularly effective in eliciting the same response.

When none of the above methods of cough stimulation is successful, stimulation of the oropharynx with a suction catheter or oral suction tube has been found to be effective. The catheter is inserted orally and advanced to the oropharynx until a gag or cough is elicited. Oropharyngeal suctioning may also be necessary in patients who have raised secretions to this level but are unable to expectorate them. Oropharyngeal stimulation should not be performed without short rest periods between attempts, especially if gagging is the most frequently obtained response. If vomiting occurs while in a postural drainage position, particularly in the head-down position (whether it be during the cough phase of treatment or not), the patient should be suctioned until the therapist is certain that the oropharynx is clear of vomitus. If the patient has an airway in place, this

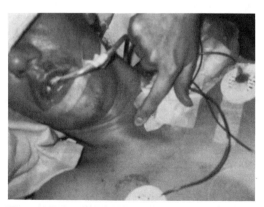

Figure 5.7. External tracheal compression may elicit a cough. It is achieved by applying gentle pressure to the anterior trachea between the cricoid cartilage and sternal notch, as shown.

should be suctioned prior to position change to prevent possible aspiration. The patient should NOT be turned supine or placed in the head-up position until proper suctioning is completed.

The use of transtracheal catheters to stimulate coughing following surgery was first reported in 1960. A short segment of polyvinyl tubing is introduced through a needle inserted into the cricothyroid membrane, and the needle is then withdrawn (Radigan and King, 1960; Pecora and Kohl, 1962; Kalinske et al., 1967; Hahn and Beaty, 1970; Pauker, 1970; Unger and Moser, 1973; Lourie et al., 1974; Ries et al., 1974; Schillaci et al., 1976). This is followed by the instillation of a respiratory tract detergent to encourage coughing. Alternately, administering short bursts of O_2 through a transtracheal catheter is described to stimulate coughing (Perel et al., 1988). Radigan and King advocated instilling fluid every 4 hr for 2–3 days after surgery or until the patient was able to cough effectively.

Despite its introduction as a simple and safe technique, literature reporting the complications associated with transtracheal aspiration has multiplied since 1970. Subcutaneous and mediastinal emphysema, transient hemoptysis, and bleeding at the puncture site are recorded by many authors (Spencer and Beaty, 1972; Ries et al.; Lourie et al.; Yoshikawa et al., 1974). Others reported vagal reflex stimulation following transtracheal puncture that caused cardiac dysrhythmia and death (Spencer and Beaty; Unger and Moser). Fatal and near-fatal hemoptysis are also recorded (Spencer and Beaty; Unger and Moser; Schillaci et al.), and fatal asphyxiation occurred due to hematoma formation (Pauker). Paroxysmal coughing attributed to transtracheal puncture is noted to result in bronchospasm, laryngospasm, and vomiting followed by aspiration of gastric contents and fatal rupture of esophageal varices (Radigan and King; Spencer and Beaty; Unger and Moser; Schmerber and Deltenre, 1978; Perel et al.). Parsons and associates (1976) reported mediastinal emphysema, pneumopericardium, and subsequent bilateral pneumothoraces after transtracheal aspiration. Cervical infections leading to

abscess formation up to 1 month following the procedure are also documented (Deresinski and Stevens, 1974; Yoshikawa et al.; Lourie, et al.). Therefore, transtracheal aspiration is a dangerous procedure that should be avoided.

Clinically, the necessity for transtracheal aspiration is shown to decrease or be eliminated by other less invasive procedures. Vraciu and Vraciu (1977) studied the effects of breathing exercises on patients in whom transtracheal catheters were frequently used following open heart surgery. These catheters were inserted based on the clinical findings of excessive secretions and an ineffective cough. Of the patients given assisted breathing exercises by a physical therapist, only 1 of 19 (5%) requires transtracheal puncture, as opposed to 7 or 14 (50%) of the controls, who were aided by the nursing staff in hourly turning, deep breathing, and coughing. Although in the early 1970s the use of transtracheal aspiration was employed by some of the surgical staff in our institute, it was replaced by appropriate chest physiotherapy and is no longer used.

Another technique developed for the treatment of sputum retention is the minitracheotomy. It was first described by Matthews and Hopkinson (1984) and consists of a 4-mm uncuffed pediatric endotracheal tube that is inserted into the trachea through a cricothyroid incision and then sutured to the skin. Suctioning with up to a 10 French catheter can be performed through the minitracheotomy, yet speech is preserved. Because of the small diameter of the suction catheter, there is a high resistance to flow; therefore, strong and long periods of suctioning are necessary to remove viscid secretions. As a result, supplemental oxygen is recommended (Charnley and Verma, 1986). The original minitracheotomy tubes did not have external airway adaptors and supplemental oxygen could only be given by face mask. More recent models have adaptors so resuscitator bags can be used in conjunction with suctioning. However, lung inflation is limited by the increased resistance to air flow through the small bore tube and the lack of a cuff. Tracheal contamination and the drying of tracheal secretions are not reported but are potential problems in the target population. Reported complications include fatal hemorrhage, spontaneous inhalation, and tracheal obstruction (Gwynn and Moustafa, 1984; Yeoh et al., 1985; Charnley and Verma). Experience with the minitracheotomy is limited. It appears to be a compromise treatment that needs further evaluation.

TRACHEAL SUCTIONING

Suctioning is performed routinely on intubated patients to aid in secretion removal and cough stimulation. The frequency of suctioning is determined by the quantity of secretions. With the exception of cardiogenic pulmonay edema, the more copious the lung secretions, the more frequently the patient requires suctioning. Secretions are commonly detected after turning or placing a patient in the head-down position. Patient mobilization usually causes secretions to gravitate from the peripheral to more central airways where they may be suctioned. This is also the objective of percussion and vibration in the postural drainage position. Suctioning is, therefore, a standard part of chest physiotherapy. Some authors consider suctioning and coughing the only important therapeutic maneuvers effective in removing retained lung secretions (Murray, 1979). However, when lung secretions are retained in the small airways, postural drainage with percussion and vibration appear necessary to mobilize them centrally, since the suction catheter can reach only the level of the main stem bronchi.

Aseptic technique is employed for tracheal suctioning, hands are washed before and after the procedure, and a sterile glove and sterile catheter are used. If the patient is monitored with an electrocardiograph, pulse oximetry and indwelling vascular catheters, these are observed during suctioning. The basic steps of the suctioning procedure shown in Figure 5.8A–E are as follows:

1. Provide the patient with supplemental oxygen before suctioning to increase arterial oxygenation (Fig. 5.8A). Patients receiving mechanical ventilation may not require this step (see p. 177). Patients with audible or copious secretions may not benefit from lung inflation or supplemental oxygen until after the secretions are removed.
2. Check the amount of negative pressure produced by the suction apparatus and, if necessary, adjust to 100–160 mm Hg.
3. Put a sterile glove on the dominant hand. Gloves should be worn on both hands to protect the clinician from contamination.
4. Expose the vent end of the catheter and connect it to the suction tubing. Any part of the catheter that may contact the patient's trachea must be kept sterile.
5. Slide the catheter out of its packaging, taking care not to cause contamination (Fig. 5.8B).
6. Disconnect the patient from the ventilator or oxygen source.
7. Gently insert the catheter into the tracheal tube. No suction is applied during insertion of the catheter (Fig. 5.8C).
8. If resistance to the catheter is present, pull the catheter back slightly and attempt to reinsert.
9. Apply suction by placing a finger over the vent. Turn the catheter slowly while withdrawing it, so that the side holes of the catheter are exposed to a greater surface area (Fig. 5.8D).
10. Reconnect the patient to the ventilator or oxygen source.
11. If the patient is not receiving mechanical ventilation, reinflate the patient's lungs with supplemental oxygen (Fig. 5-8E).

Steps 6 and 10 are omitted for patients suctioned through a port adaptor.

Difficulty in Passing a Suction Catheter

If there is difficulty passing a suction catheter through a tracheal tube, this should create concern, as it may be an early indication of occlusion of the airway. Some difficulty in passing the catheter may be due to kinking of a long tracheal tube. The remedy is to remove the excess length and use a more rigid cath-

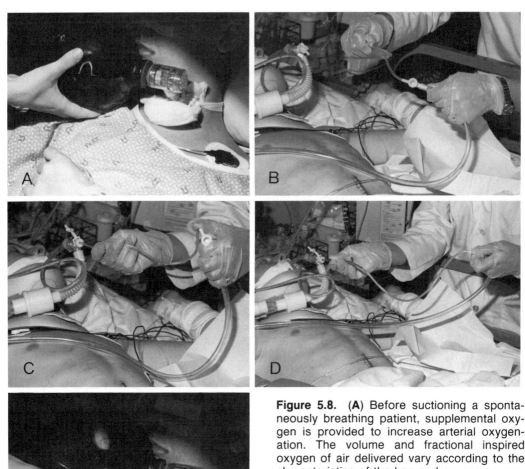

Figure 5.8. (**A**) Before suctioning a spontaneously breathing patient, supplemental oxygen is provided to increase arterial oxygenation. The volume and fractional inspired oxygen of air delivered vary according to the characteristics of the bag and oxygen source. (**B**) The suction catheter is removed from its packaging carefully so that the catheter is not contaminated. Catheters packaged in a straight position are found to be easier to handle without contamination. (**C**) Insertion of the suction catheter into the tracheal tube should be gentle but quick. Suctioning is preferentially performed through a port adaptor for patients receiving mechanical ventilation. Suction is not applied as the catheter is inserted. Loss of PEEP and tidal volume through the catheter may be prevented during insertion, if the catheter is kinked as shown with the left hand. (**D**) As the catheter is withdrawn, suction is applied by occluding the vent on the suction catheter, as shown. Removal of the suction catheter should be done without undue delay but slowly enough for secretion removal to be adequate. (**E**) After suctioning, lung reinflation is performed using the mechanical ventilator or a resuscitator bag in order to facilitate lung reexpansion and replenish the patient's oxygen supply.

eter. If resistance to the passage of the catheter is met soon after insertion, the patient may be biting on the tube. Proper placement of a bite block prevents this. When kinking and biting of the tracheal tube are excluded, obstruction to passage of a suction catheter may be due to improper positioning, viscous secretions, or debris, and a physician should be notified immediately. Airway obstruction in the patient receiving mechanical ventilation results in a significant elevation of airway pressures and a decrease in volume delivery. If difficulty is experienced when suctioning a patient with a tracheostomy, the tube may be occluded with secretions, malaligned in the trachea, or displaced into the subcutaneous tissues; this should be rectified immediately.

Difficulty Cannulating the Left Main Stem Bronchus

It is more difficult to pass a suction catheter into the left than the right main bronchus (Kirimli et al., 1970; Haberman et al., 1973; Fewell et al., 1979; Freedman and Goodman, 1982). In adults, the right main stem bronchus usually comes off at an angle of about 20° from a midline sagittal plane, whereas the left main stem bronchus has a more marked angle of about 35° and is longer (making the left more difficult to successfully cannulate). The usual anatomy is not always found (Fig. 2.5). Similar angles of bifurcation are noted in the neonate (24° for the right and 44° for the left) (Fewell et al.). Poor cannulation and suctioning of the left main stem bronchus inhibit secretion clearance in the upper airways of the left lung. This is clinically significant as secretion retention is more prevelant in the left lung of adults, particularly the left lower lobe (Sykes et al., 1976; Jaworski et al., 1989; Appendix I). A variety of techniques are described to facilitate left bronchial catheter placement. It is suggested that turning the head to the right (Haberman et al.) or tilting the body to the left (Salem et al., 1978) increases the chances of successful cannulation of the left bronchus. There is also evidence that turning the head to the right may facilitate entering the left main stem bronchus in neonates (Fewell et al., Placzak and Silverman, 1983). However, routine repositioning of the head or patient is not recommended as the research is inconclusive, the anatomy somewhat variable, and moving the head can increase laryngeal or tracheal irritation and alter tube placement, particularly in infants.

Curved-tip (coudé) catheters are thought to improve the chances of entering the left lung during suctioning (Opie and Smith, 1959). Kubota et al. (1980) found optimal selective cannulation with the head in midline when curved-tip catheters were used. Left bronchial cannulation is also more likely in adults

with tracheostomy rather than nasotracheal or orotracheal tubes when coudé catheters are used (Haberman et al.; Scott et al., 1977; Kabota et al., 1980; Freedman and Goodman). Selective entry of the left main stem bronchus with curved tip catheters ranges from 8 to 61% (Kirimli et al.; Scott et al.; Anthony and Sieniewicz, 1977; Kubota et al., 1980; Freedman and Goodman). Kubota and associates (1982, 1983) demonstrated success rates of up to 92% for left bronchial placement (compared with 98% for the right) when a longitudinal guide mark was added to the curved-tip catheter. Similar findings are reported by Placzek and Silverman using a marked coudé catheter in neonates. They also noted that stiff catheters were less likely to enter the left main bronchus than more flexible tubes. Using a controllable tip catheter originally designed for bronchography, Wang et al. (1976) achieved an 88% success rate in entering the left bronchus. Other methods of catheter modification are described but so far are of unproven benefit (Zaltzman, 1983; Kubota et al., 1983).

Differential auscultation is recommended as an adjunct to selective bronchial cannulation (Kubota et al., 1984; Krumpe and Denham, 1984). This method uses a stethoscope to determine the position of the catheter tip before suction is applied. It is thought to provide confirmation to the clinician that the appropriate bronchus will be cleared of mucus. The potential problems of longer suctioning time and cough stimulation are not addressed, nor is the fact that auscultation after suctioning should yield similar feedback. Based on the existing literature, curved-tip catheters appear indicated when suctioning a patient with left lung pathology. Other methods of catheter modification require further study as does the use of differential auscultation.

Suction Catheters

In addition to tip design, there are many other features of suction catheters to consider. Table 5.2 lists some desirable features of suction catheters. Catheters are typically made of polyvinyl chloride

Table 5.2
Desirable Characteristics of Suction Catheters

Material—polyvinyl chloride
Number of side holes—more than one
Size—half of the internal diameter of the tracheal or airway tube through which it is to be passed
Length—long enough to reach several inches beyond the end of the tracheal tube
Suction application vent—raised
Packaging—catheter straight; easy to open
Tip design—curved tip catheters for entering the left mainstem bronchus

or rubber. Polyvinyl chloride catheters are preferred, as they are less likely to cause irritation (O'Malley et al., 1979). Polyvinyl chloride allows visualization of the suctioned secretions because the catheter is clear; it is also easier to insert into a tracheal tube and may be directed more easily. Lubricating the polyvinyl chloride catheter before suctioning is usually unnecessary and only increases the possibility for contamination.

Suction catheters with more than one side hole or "eye" are preferable because secretion removal is more effective and results in less mucosal damage. During direct visualization of the suctioning process, Jung and Gottlieb (1976) observed that catheters with only one eye were not as effective in removing mucus as those with multiple eyes. This was confirmed by others who found that catheters with only one eye caused more mechanical damage to the trachea because they became adherent to the tracheal wall (Link et al., 1976).

The size of suction catheters ranges from 3.5 to 18 French gauge, and it is frequently proposed that the outer diameter of the catheter should not be greater than half of the inside diameter of the tube. This allows an adequate flow of air into the lungs around the catheter during suctioning (Rosen and Hillard, 1960, 1962). French size 10–14 catheters are most commonly used in adults. French size can be converted to millimeters on dividing by π. If a catheter is too small, secretion removal is less effective.

A suction catheter should be of sufficient length to be advanced several inches beyond the end of the tracheal tube. This allows entry into one of the main stem bronchi. If the length of the suction catheter is not monitored, the catheter may kink and effective suctioning may be hindered. This problem may be overcome by having increments of length marked on the catheter, indicating how much has been inserted (Scott et al.).

A catheter that has a raised vent for application of suction is preferred to one having a flush vent. The raised vent helps prevent clinician contact with secretions and is easier to locate during the suctioning procedure.

Catheters are packaged either coiled or straight; coiled catheters take up less storage space but are more difficult to handle, increasing the likelihood of contamination. Catheters packaged in a straight position may be more effective at entering the left main stem bronchus (Haberman et al.). Figure 5.9 illustrates three different suction catheters.

Figure 5.9. Three types of polyvinyl chloride suction catheters are shown. They are (from *top* to *bottom*) a standard, straight-tip catheter, a coudé tip catheter, which is designed to help enter the left main stem bronchus, and a catheter with a sleeve attached so that the operator is not required to wear gloves other than for self-protection.

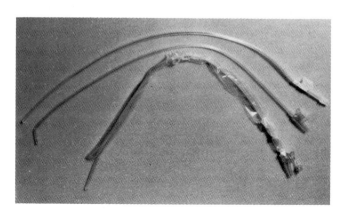

COMPLICATIONS OF TRACHEAL SUCTIONING

Hypoxemia

It is well documented that suctioning may lead to a significant decrease in arterial oxygenation. The hypoxemia associated with suctioning is usually more pronounced than that caused by apnea alone (Boutros, 1970; Adlkofer and Powaser, 1978; White et al., 1982). Presumably, this occurs when the catheter removes oxygen as well as secretions from the lungs. Many techniques are routinely performed in association with suctioning to ameliorate this problem. For clarity, the terms used in this text are defined in Table 5.3. The level of oxygenation prior to suctioning is an important factor in whether suctioning leads to significant hypoxemia (Taylor and Waters, 1971). Obviously, a patient with a PaO_2 of 150 mm Hg is better able to tolerate a 30 mm Hg drop in arterial oxygenation than a patient with resting PaO_2 of 80. Controversy exists over the optimal way to preoxygenate a patient prior to suction-

Table 5.3
Adjuncts Commonly Used with Suctioning

Term	Definition
Affects volume delivery	
Lung inflation	Inflating the lungs using a manual resuscitator bag or mechanical ventilator
	May be performed before or after suctioning
	Does not indicate a change in FIO_2, tidal volume, or respiratory rate above resting levels
Hyperinflation	Inflating the lungs with volume greater than a resting tidal volume
	May be performed before, during[a] and after suctioning using a manual resuscitator bag[b] or a mechanical ventilator[c]
	Does not indicate change in FIO_2
Affects oxygen delivery	
Preoxygenation	Administering an increased FIO_2[d] above resting levels before suctioning
	May be performed with a resuscitator bag or mechanical ventilator
	Does not indicate change in tidal volume or respiratory rate
Hyperoxygenation	Increasing the FIO_2[d] above resting levels before, during, or after suctioning
	May be performed with a manual resuscitator bag or a mechanical ventilator
	Does not indicate change in tidal volume or respiratory rate
Insufflation	Administering a continuous flow of oxygen, often simultaneously with suctioning, using a double lumen catheter, a modified catheter, or a side arm adaptor of an endotracheal tube
	Does not affect respiratory rate[e]
Affects respiratory rate	
Hyperventilation	Increasing the respiratory rate using a manual resuscitator bag or mechanical ventilator
	May be performed before or after suctioning
	Does not indicate change in FIO_2 or tidal volume

[a]It is not possible to hyperinflate during suctioning with a manual resuscitator bag. Theoretically, hyperinflation is possible with some mechanical ventilators. However, the actual volume delivered is unknown as air is continuously removed during suctioning.
[b]Hyperinflation with a bag is possible only if the bag delivers a larger tidal volume than the patient receives during resting ventilation.
[c]This is usually done by increasing the tidal volume or using the sigh feature.
[d]FIO_2 usually is increased to 1.0.
[e]The change in tidal volume that may occur with continuous insufflation is not known as gases are simultaneously removed during suctioning.

ing. Gold et al. (1981) found four large breaths of 100% oxygen (in 30 sec) as effective as administering 5 min of 100% oxygen to increase, both PaO_2 and arterial oxygen content in 22 adult surgical patients. Therefore, it appears that when preoxygenation is necessary, four breaths are adequate for most patients. Monitoring continuous arterial oxygen saturation is another way to assess the development of hypoxemia and the need for and effect of preoxygenation. Suctioning causes significant falls in mixed venous O_2 saturation that may be related to changes in cardiac output or oxygen consumption (Walsh et al., 1989). In patients demonstrating high intrapulmonary shunt or significant cardiovascular compromise, hypoxemia may lead to serious cardiac arrhythmias (Boba et al., 1959; Shim et al., 1969), and these patients should be closely monitored during suctioning.

The fall in PaO_2 that occurs with suctioning is directly related to the duration of suctioning; longer periods of suctioning lead to larger declines in PaO_2 (Boutros). Therefore, each suctioning procedure is limited to a total of 15 sec. However, there is no point in removing a patient from oxygen and having the patient undergo the mechanical trauma of suctioning if the procedure is performed so quickly that little, if any, secretions are removed. An effective but expedient suctioning technique should be used. The degree of subatmospheric pressure should also be controlled during suctioning. Vacuum pressures that are either insufficient or excessive can cause complications and should be avoided. If the suction is too low, longer periods of suctioning and repeated, but less effective, passes of the catheter may be necessary. Excessive suction may lead to an increase in mechanical trauma and hypoxemia, as air (as well as secretions) is more rapidly removed from the lungs. The American Society for Testing and Materials (1986) reports that static vacuum levels of up to 160 mm Hg for adults and 100 mm Hg for infants are regularly experienced in clinical practice during tracheal suctioning. They stress that suction levels should be based on clinical considerations. The amount of hypoxemia after

tracheal suctioning also depends on the patient's diagnosis, current medical status, and oxygen requirements. Patients with decreased cardiopulmonary reserve or PaO_2 may sustain a greater fall in arterial oxygenation during suctioning (Taylor and Waters, 1971). The patient's age is an additional consideration. Lung inflation after suctioning is particularly important in children and geriatric patients who have a high closing volume and are therefore more likely to develop small airway closure (Mansell et al., 1972). If retained secretions are a primary cause of hypoxemia, withholding suctioning because of the expected further decrease in PaO_2 only aggravates the situation.

Methods described to minimize or reverse the hypoxemia associated with suctioning are shown in Table 5.4. A review of the literature does not provide the reader with one obviously superior method. This is, in part, due to the divergent research designs, the variable methodology, and the different patient populations studied. Also, research and experience indicate that there are a variety of patient responses to suctioning. Yet, current practices in most hopsitals are rigid and follow guidelines that are based more on history and tradition than fact. A rigid suctioning protocol results in unnecessary (and possibly hazardous) treatment of some patients and suboptimal treatment of others who are usually at greater risk of hypoxemia. A flexible suctioning procedure is recommended to allow for optimal treatment of the patient, based on individual requirements and responses. However, flexibility can arise only from a sound theoretical and practical knowledge (Barnes and Kirchhoff, 1986). Table 5.5 reviews the current literature on hypoxemia and suctioning. A discussion of the methods used to prevent hypoxemia while suctioning spontaneously breathing and mechanically ventilated patients is provided.

Lung inflation is usually performed using a manual resuscitator bag for spontaneously breathing patients. The amount of inspired oxygen that is delivered varies according to the characteristics of the specific bag. Tidal volume is additionally affected by the operator's

Methods to Minimize Hypoxemia during Suctioning

Method	Researchers of Method	FIO₂ Delivered	Tidal Volume Delivered	Maintenance of PEEP	Ease of Use	Pressure Limit	Comments
Use of manual resuscitator bag	Cabal et al. (1979); Baker et al. (1980); Fitzmaurice and Barnes (1980); Brown et al. (1983), Pierce and Piazza (1987)	Varies according to bag design (often ↑ to 1.0); during disconnection times, patient is without O₂ source	Varies according to bag size and operator's ability	None maintained without a valve	May be difficult for one person to perform both suctioning and bagging functions adequately	May not be controlled	Requires ventilator disconnection and reconnection; may result in large fluctuations in PaO₂
Use of manual assist or sigh mode on ventilator	Bell et al. (1980); Brown et al. (1983); Benson and Pierson (1979); Brown et al. (1983); Pierce and Piazza (1987)	Same as presuctioning level unless ventilator settings are changed	Same as presuctioning level unless ventilator settings are changed	Same as presuctioning level unless ventilator settings are changed	Easy to use	Well controlled	May not be adequate for all patients; should consider ventilator "washout" time; operator may forget to reset ventilator settings when finished
Use of suction port adaptor on ventilator	Urban and Weitner (1969); Dryden et al. (1977); Belling et al. (1978); Cabal et al. (1979); Baker et al. (1980); Bell et al. (1980); Zmora and Merritt (1980); Jung and Newman (1982); Brown et al. (1983); Bodai et al. (1987); Durand et al (1989)	Presuctioning level maintained to some degree, exact level not known	Presuctioning level maintained to some degree, exact level not known	Presuctioning level maintained to some degree, exact level not known	Easy to use	Well controlled	Some port adaptor designs are not occlusive; complications may occur with low ventilator flow rates
Use of oxygen insufflation	Boba et al. (1959); Berman and Stahl (1968); Fell and Cheney (1971); Langrehr et al. (1981); Bodai et al. (1987); Graff et al. (1987)	Usually 1.0	Variable	None maintained	May restrict passage of suction catheter	Not known	May not be adequate for all patients
Use of additional ventilator	Skelley et al. (1980); Langrehr et al. (1981)	Can be set to optimal level	Can be set to optimal level	Can be set to optimal level	Easy to use	Well controlled	Impractical in most centers due to cost and space requirements

Table 5.5
Recent Studies on Preventing Hypoxemia during Suctioning [a,b]

Investigator	Subjects	Design	Adjuncts Used	Conclusions	Comments
Kelly et al. (1987)	38 adults anesthetized for open heart surgery, muscle relaxants were used	Compared 20 sec of conventional suctioning with 20 sec of suctioning with O_2 insufflation	Insufflation with 100% O_2 at 10 liters/min; No hyperoxygenation	O_2 insufflation significantly reversed hypoxemia and desaturation noted with conventional suctioning	Peak ↓ in PaO_2 and SaO_2 occurred 60 sec after suctioning and returned to baseline by 420 sec. Suction efficacy not addressed. Baseline FIO_2 not a good indicator of ↓ in PaO_2 or SaO_2, but baseline PaO_2 is
Bodai et al. (1987)	16 adults, moderate to severe respiratory failure, eliminated patients with baseline $PaO_2 > 100$ mm Hg	1. Compared preoxygenation/hyperinflation with and without O_2 insufflation 2. Compared preoxygenation/hyperinflation with suctioning to O_2 insufflation alone 3. Compared hyperinflation and suctioning through a port adaptor with and without O_2 insufflation	Preoxygenation Hyperinflation Insufflation at 100% O_2 at 10 liters/min	1. Both methods similarly prevented hypoxemia; hypoxemia noted in both groups 3. Hypoxemia was equally prevented by both methods; no added benefit from O_2 insufflation; preoxygenation/hyperinflation equally effective as using the port adaptor	Used intermittent suction. Suction included disconnecting from MV, instilling 3 ml of saline, 3 hyperinflations with O_2 or sighs, 3–15 sec passes of catheter within 1 min, reconnecting to MV. The different response to suctioning between 1 and 2 was thought to reflect individual differences. Recommend O_2 insufflation to replace bagging and recommend using an adaptor for patients on MV
Pierce and Piazza (1987)	30 adults, following open heart surgery	Compared postoxygenation using bag or sigh mechanism	? Hyperinflation Hyperoxygenation	No difference in PaO_2 using other method; pH ↓ with bagging but ↑ with sighing	Bagging performed with one hand. Sigh volume = 1000 ml. FIO_2 = 1.0 and 3 breaths given for both regimens. Recommend using adaptor
Graff et al. (1987)	20 newborns	Compared O_2 insufflation to	Preoxygenation ? Hyperinflation	O_2 insufflation resulted in less ↓	Suctioning included adaptor ↑ FIO_2 20% above

Source	Subjects	Method	Interventions	Results	Comments
Douglas and Larson (1985)	12 adults receiving MV > 24 hr and PEEP between 5 and 18 cm H_2O	conventional suctioning	O_2 insufflation at 4 liters/min	in $PtcO_2$, fastest recovery from hypoxemia, and less abnormal responses in $PtcO_2$; no difference in HR between groups	baseline, 0.5 ml saline instilled, bagging, suctioning for 5 sec and reconnected to MV or O_2 insufflation. Response considered abnormal if $40 < PtcO_2 < 90$ mm Hg or heart rate ↓ > 10%. Used intermittent suction
Gateley and Carson (1985)	11 adults after coronary artery bypass	Compared PaO_2 and SaO_2 levels using a port adaptor to a manual resuscitator bag; Compared hyperinflation with a bag to using a sigh; compared the use and lack of hyperoxygenation; compared using the port adaptor with not using it	Preoxygenation, Hyperoxygenation, Hyperinflation; Hyperinflation, Preoxygenation, Hyperoxygenation	No significant difference between groups; PaO_2 fluctuations and recovery time were greater with hyperoxygenation	Recommend not ↑ FIO_2. Noted ↑ contamination using the port adaptor
Schumann and Parsons (1985)	15 critically ill adults	Compared maintaining PEEP while bagging alone, before and after suctioning	Hyperinflation, Preoxygenation, Hyperoxygenation	Bagging with PEEP caused a significant ↑ in PaO_2	Used intermittent suctioning
Goodnough (1985)	28 patients, 4–6 hr after cardiac surgery; 26 were on MV	Four study procedures 1. ↑ FIO_2 before suctioning and hyperinflation after suctioning 2. ↑ FIO_2	Preoxygenation, Hyperoxygenation, Hyperinflation	Only procedure 3 had significant ↓ in PaO_2 during suctioning. Procedure 4 was associated with significantly less ↓ PaO_2 and 1 and 2 during suctioning. All procedures after	Hyperinflations = 150% of baseline V_t. FIO_2 was ↑ to 1.0 for 1 min pre- and/or postsuctioning. Hyperinflation should be aborted if hypotension or bradycardia occurs. Recommend 1 min of 100% O_2 before and

Table 5.5 (*Continued*)
Recent Studies on Preventing Hypoxemia during Suctioning [a,b]

Investigator	Subjects	Design	Adjuncts Used	Conclusions	Comments
		before and after suctioning 3. Hyperinflation before and after suctioning 4. ↑FIO$_2$ and hyperinflation before and after suctioning		suctioning were successful in restoring PaO$_2$ All procedures were equally effective at 5 and 10 min after suctioning	after suctioning
Brown et al (1983)	22 acutely ill patients, most with preexisting COPD	Phase I: compared no extra breaths to 4 prescutioning breaths, 4 postsuctioning breaths, and suctioning through an adaptor (all at baseline FIO$_2$) Phase II: compared suctioning using an adaptor to 6 presuctioning breaths and/ or 6 postsuctioning breaths at FIO$_2$ = 1.0 Phase III: compared 4 successive catheter passes using	Preoxygenation Hyperoxygenation Hyperventilation	Phase I: greatest desaturation occurred with no hyperventilation; desaturation significantly less with adaptors; recovery best using the adaptor or 4 postsuctioning breaths Phase II: significantly more desaturation occurred with only 6 postsuctioning breaths; adaptor equally effective to other two methods Phase III: adaptor equally effective at preventing desaturation	Used intermittent suctioning FIO$_2$ ↑ 1 min before extra breaths initiated Recommend using the adaptor without altering ventilator settings

Study	Subjects	Protocol	Interventions	Results	Comments
Jung and Newman (1982)	18 medical-surgical ICU patients with acute lung disease requiring MV and $FIO_2 \geq$ 0.4	an adaptor or 6 extra breaths before and after each catheter pass at $FIO_2 = 1.0$ Compared suctioning through a port adaptor with popping the patient off of MV	None	Desaturation significantly attenuated when using the port; in patients requiring PEEP, significantly less desaturation was noted with port use	All on IMV Instilled 10 ml of saline through the catheter prior to suctioning Used intermittent suctioning No patients developed arrhythmias Suctioning time is shorter using a port adaptor
Langrehr et al. (1981)	3 anesthetized mongrel dogs	O_2 insufflation flow rates less than, equal to, and greater than suction flow rates were compared; also, apnea, insufflation, and suctioning alone were compared	Hyperinflation Hyperoxygenation O_2 insufflation	Dog studies: When O_2 insufflation exceeded suction flow rates, PaO_2 was significantly maintained above baseline values	Used a bonded suction catheter-feeding tube for O_2 insufflation Suction applied for 15 sec at 18 liters/min with catheter fully inserted; no suction was applied while inserting or withdrawing the catheter When used, O_2 insufflation was continuous Used a second ventilator to deliver hyperoxygenation ($FIO_2 = 1.0$) and hyperinflation ($V_t = 150\%$)
	10 cardiac surgery patients within 10 hr of surgery	Hyperinflation/hyperoxygenation with 1 or 3 breaths was compared with O_2 insufflation at 10 and 15 liters/min	Hyperinflation Hyperoxygenation O_2 insufflation	Patient studies: Both O_2 insufflation rates prevented significant changes in PaO_2 Fall in PaO_2 greater following 1 breath than 3 breaths prior to suctioning	The greatest fall in PaO_2 with hyperinflation/hyperoxygenation occurred at 30 sec after suctioning O_2 insufflation may interfere with secretion removal

Table 5.5 (*Continued*)
Recent Studies on Preventing Hypoxemia during Suctioning [a,b]

Investigator	Subjects	Design	Adjuncts Used	Conclusions	Comments
Shelley et al. (1980)	3 anesthetized mongrel dog	Protocols for dog studies: 1. Suctioning without preoxygenation 2. 1 preoxygenation breath prior to suctioning 3. 3 preoxygenation breaths before suctioning 4. 1 preoxygenation breath without suctioning 5. 3 preoxygenation breaths without suctioning	Preoxygenation Hyperinflation Hyperoxygenation	Dog studies: Protocol 1 produced the greatest ↓ in PaO_2 20 sec after suctioning Both 2 and 3 protected the dogs from hypoxemia but were not different from each other Patient studies: Protocol 1 produced significant ↓ in PaO_2 30 sec after suctioning No significant difference between 1 and 2 PaO_2 was significantly better with protocol 3	112 Suction applied for 15 sec Total disconnect time = 23 sec Hyperoxygenation (FIO_2 = 1.0) and hyperinflation (V_t = 1.5) given via a second ventilator Patient response to suctioning is more variable than with dogs The effects of hyperinflation cannot be separated from hyperoxygenation in this study Recommend hyperoxygenation regardless of baseline PaO_2
	11 cardiac surgery patients within 12 hr of surgery	Patient studies: compared protocols 1, 2, and 3 above	Preoxygenation Hyperinflation Hyperoxygenation		

[a] In all studies, subjects served as their own control. Continuous suction was used unless noted.
[b] PEEP, positive end expiratory pressure; MV, mechanical ventilation; FIO_2, fraction of inspired oxygen; $PtcO_2$, transcutaneous oxygen; SaO_2, arterial oxygen saturation; V_t, tidal volume; IMV, intermittent mandatory ventilation; HR, heart rate.

ability to compress the bag. Airway pressure is not well controlled with a resuscitator bag. When a pressure valve is in place, the pressure limit may be too low for adequate patient ventilation (Hirschman and Kravath, 1982). However, if the relief valve is removed or not adequately functioning, pulmonary barotrauma may occur (Klick et al., 1978).

An alternative to bagging the spontaneously breathing patient is the use of a double-lumen catheter, whereby one lumen is used for oxygen insufflation and the other is used as a standard suction catheter. One inherent problem with using a double-lumen system is that the size of the port available for suctioning may be restricted and therefore less effective. Continuous oxygen delivery may also interfere with secretion aspiration (Langrehr et al., 1981). A variation of oxygen insufflation allows for oxygen delivery and suctioning through the same lumen. With this sytem, when suction is applied, oxygen is not simultaneously delivered (Bodai et al., 1987). Oxygen insufflation techniques depend on the patient's ability to breathe spontaneously, which may not be adequate in mechanically ventilated patients with compromised cardiorespiratory status or paralysis (Fell and Cheney, 1971). This problem may be overcome by another variation of insufflation advocated by Spoerel and Chan (1976), in which the second lumen is used to provide jet ventilation using a constant airway pressure. This variation is still under study.

In addition to using manual inflation or oxygen insufflation, suctioning can be performed in several ways for the mechanically ventilated patient. They include using the ventilator for lung inflation or suctioning through a port adaptor without disconnecting the patient from mechanical ventilation. Both methods may be used either with or without changing the ventilator settings. It is our opinion and that of others (Bell et al., 1980; Baker et al., 1980; Jung and Newman, 1982; Brown et al., 1983; Tyler, 1984; Bodai et al., 1987; Durand et al., 1989) that suctioning through a well-designed port adaptor without ventilator adjustment is the preferred method for most patients requiring mechanical ventilation. Since suctioning during chest physiotherapy is performed with the patient in a postural drainage position and requires multiple passes of the suction catheter, it is often difficult, if not impossible, for one clinician to quickly and effectively bag the patient without contaminating the suction catheter. The operator's ability to squeeze the resuscitator bag is also a factor, making both volume and pressure delivery variable. Many clinicians incorrectly assume that using a manual resuscitator bag produces lung hyperinflation. Frequently, this is not the case: bagging may produce a smaller volume than that delivered by the ventilator, particularly when the bag is compressed with one hand. Two other disadvantages of bagging are the interruption of positive end-expiratory pressure (PEEP) and the wide variations in oxygenation that can occur. Research indicates that suctioning through a port adaptor is equally effective or superior to bagging in minimizing arterial oxygen desaturation during suctioning (Bell et al.; Baker et al.; Jung and Newman; Brown et al.; Bodai et al.; Durand et al.).

There is a potential complication to using a port adaptor that is totally occlusive. Subatmospheric pressure develops if suction flow rates exceed ventilator delivery or if the patient is on controlled or assisted ventilation (Brown et al., 1983; Jung and Newman, 1982; Guthrie et al., 1983; Craig et al., 1984; Graff et al., 1987; Dickert, 1987; Taggart et al., 1988). The flow rates used for neonates may limit the widespread use of port adaptors for this population, although studies on the use of adaptors with infants are favorable (Cabal et al.; Zmora and Merrit, 1980; Gunderson et al., 1986; Graff et al.; Durand et al.).

In conjunction with suctioning through the port, a manual assist on some ventilators can be used to hyperventilate or the sigh feature can be used to increase volume delivery (hyperinflate). Hyperventilating a patient using the manual assist of the ventilator may be awkward for the therapist suctioning a patient turned away from the ventilator. Hyperinflation may have adverse hemodynamic effects, particularly in patients with serious lung disorders (Skelley et al., 1980; Langrehr et al.). For some patients whose cardiorespiratory status is very fragile, increasing oxygen delivery may be necessary. Elevating the FIO_2 (usually to 1.0) is indicated in patients prone to arrhythmias or exhibiting significant decreases in oxygen saturation. Whenever ventilator settings are adjusted, it is all too easy for the clinician to forget to return them to their proper level (Jung and Newman; Tyler). The effects of short duration but wide fluctuations in PaO_2 that occur with preoxygenation and hyperoxygenation are unknown. Leaving a patient on an FIO_2 of 1.0 is associated with complications that may be more detrimental than suctioning without hyperoxygenation.

Based on the research and our clinical experience, the use of an adaptor designed for simultaneous introduction of a suction catheter with continued mechanical ventilation is the most effective method of reducing hypoxic complications associated with suctioning. A port adaptor must be occlusive to allow for partial maintenance of FIO_2, tidal volume, and PEEP during suctioning. Ventilator flow rates must be adequate. Using an adaptor avoids the need for ventilator disconnection time. Also, ventilator settings normally do not need to be adjusted, preventing possible complications from accidental prolonged hyperoxygenation. The port adaptor is easy to use in all patient positions. Pressure regulation is optimal, allowing adequate ventilation in conjunction with a safeguard against barotrauma. The use of an occlusive port adaptor allows for improved maintenance of FIO_2, tidal volume, PEEP, and mean airway pressure.

An ideal method of minimizing hypoxemia, from a theoretical standpoint, would be connecting the patient to a second ventilator preset to provide appropriate hyperinflation, hyperventilation, or hyperoxygenation for the patient's needs (Skelley et al.,; Langrehr et al.). This is expensive and impractical in the clinical setting as well as unnecessary when other less dramatic methods are available.

Cardiac Dysrhythmias

Both the hypoxemia and tracheal stimulation that can occur during suctioning

are known to produce changes in cardiac function. Tracheal stimulation in normal subjects may produce increased sympathetic activity, resulting in tachycardia and hypertension. In neonates or when sympathetic control is lost (as in patients with spinal cord injury above T1), tracheal stimulation may induce bradycardia and even cardiac arrest (Cordero and Hon, 1971; Frankel et al., 1975). This may occur as a result of vasovagal reflex stimulation because the afferent fibers of the vagus nerve in the trachea and bronchi cause increased efferent vagal activity (Dollfus and Frankel, 1965; Frankel et al.). After the acute period of spinal shock is passed, there is a decrease in the vasovagal response associated with tracheal stimulation in spinal cord injury (Jennett, 1970).

Mechanical Trauma

Mechanical trauma to the tracheobronchial tree results from suctioning. Link et al. using catheters with more than one side hole observed that the mucosal damage occurred during insertion of the catheter rather than during mucosal "grabbing," even when vacuum pressures greater than 300 mm Hg were used. Similar findings are reported by Kleiber et al. (1988), who found tracheal damage after catheter insertion even when suction was not applied. The use of single-eyed catheters is reportedly more damaging because they cause a greater degree of mucosal invagination. Sackner (1978) and Sackner et al. (1973) advocate the use of a catheter with a beaded edge designed to prevent the side holes from coming in contact with, and irritating, the tracheobronchial mucosa. However, studies by Jung and Gottlieb and Link et al. did not find this catheter less irritating to the mucosa than traditional catheters. In neonates, there is some evidence that inserting a catheter a predetermined length may be less traumatic than inserting it until resistance is felt (Kleiber et al.). Suctioning efficacy was not evaluated using this technique. Atelectasis is cited by several sources as a mechanical complication of tracheal suctioning in infants. Lung reinflation after suctioning may remedy this problem (Brandstater and Muallem, 1969). However, others have suggested that in infants, increased right-to-left shunting is the cause of the hypoxemia, not atelectasis, since no change in total lung/thorax compliance or functional residual capacity is found after suctioning (Fox et al., 1978).

Bacterial Contamination

Tracheal suctioning causes bacterial contamination in three basic ways. First, incorrect suctioning technique may introduce bacteria into the tracheobronchial tree. This may be prevented through maintenance of strict asepsis during the procedure. It seems possible that increased tracheal contamination may occur with repeated passage of a suction catheter through a port adaptor. Dryden et al. described the use of a catheter with an attached sleeve so that aseptic technique may be maintained without using a sterile glove (see Fig. 5.9). Catheters with sleeves are commercially available and convenient to use. They are not as easily contaminated as traditional catheters, particularly when patients are turned for postural drainage. The user should wear gloves for additional self-protection. Second, suctioning equipment can produce a bacterial aerosol that may contaminate the patient and the patient care area. To help prevent bacterial transmission by suctioning equipment, Zelechowski (1980) suggests that a bacterial filter be used with the suction collection unit and that disposal of the unit occur in an area isolated from patient care. The third type of contamination directly involves the clinician. It is recommended that health care providers wear gloves on both hands during suctioning for self-protection. This prevents possible contact between the "nonsterile" hand and secretions. Hands should still be washed immediately after gloves are removed. Clinicians should also routinely use masks and protective eyewear to prevent mucous membrane exposure during procedures such as suctioning, which are likely to generate droplets of blood or body fluids (Centers for Disease Control, 1987). Intensive care unit staff require education in the dangers of bacterial contamination occurrring with the use of suctioning equipment.

Raised Intracranial Pressure

Suctioning is associated with elevations in intracranial pressure (ICP), which may be significant for patients with brain injury (see p. 259). Rises in ICP are more marked when coughing occurs with suctioning but are not routinely associated with decreased cerebral perfusion pressure. In almost all cases, ICP elevations due to suctioning are short lived, returning to baseline values within minutes (White et al.; Fisher et al., 1982; Perlman and Volpe, 1983; Parson and Shogan, 1984; Rudy et al., 1986; McQuillan, 1987; Imle et al., 1988; Durand et al.). Because preterm infants are predisposed to intraventricular hemorrhage, this population may be at increased risk of developing complications from suctioning-induced cerebral changes. However, many of the therapies used to treat brain injury and raised ICP (such as tracheal intubation, mechanical hyperventilation, barbiturates, and paralysis) put the infant and adult patient at increased risk of respiratory complication. Therefore, as with all medical procedures, the potential benefit of suctioning must be weighted against any potential complication.

Nasotracheal Suctioning

Nasotracheal suctioning of nonintubated infants and adults is traumatic and hazardous (Boba et al., Cordero and Hon; Sykes et al., Peterson et al., 1979; Gaskell and Webber, 1980). Several preferable alternative methods to stimulate coughing in the uncooperative patient are previously described in this chapter. The complications of nasotracheal suctioning are potentially more dangerous than suctioning through a tracheal tube. They include oxygen desaturation, hypoxemia, severe cardiac arrhythmias, apnea, and laryngeal spasm or bronchospasm. Should laryngeal spasm occur when the catheter is in the trachea during the nasotracheal maneuver, rapid deoxygenation and collapse of the lung can occur when suction is applied. The lung cannot be rapidly reexpanded in the nonintubated patient, so with laryngospasm, hypoxemia and death may result (Sykes et al.). Nasotracheal suctioning is specifically contraindicated in patients with stridor or suspected cerebrospinal fluid leak. Aside from precipitating possible central nervous system infection, nasotracheal suctioning can cause bacterial contamination of the trachea and more peripheral airways (LeFrock et al., 1976). Nasotracheal suctioning is frequently ordered for patients no longer in the ICU in whom events such as acute hypoxemia and cardic dysrhythmias may not be detected unless they are catastrophic (Peterson et al.).

The patient who cannot cough up secretions beyond the larynx has either a partial airway obstruction, an inadequate cough, or excessive secretions. Nasotracheal suctioning is not the appropriate therapy for these problems. Partial airway obstruction cannot be satisfactorily managed by a suction catheter. Trauma to an already edematous or narrowed larynx or stenosed trachea by repeated attempts to pass a catheter translaryngeally may precipitate complete airway obstruction. Vomiting is associated with nasotracheal suctioning, particularly in infants and persons with decreased levels of consciousness or a depressed cough reflex. The risks of aspirating vomitous into the lungs during this maneuver may be minimized by placing the patient in a sidelying position prior to suctioning (Gaskell and Webber). Such positioning is rarely observed in the ICU, where patients are invariably either supine or semierect when nasotracheal suctioning is attempted. Excessive secretions need ready, reliable, and repeated access for removal. Therefore, nasotracheal suctioning is not the appropriate treatment; rather the patient should be tracheally intubated with an artificial airway that allows passage of a suction catheter, lung reexpansion, and, if necessary, mechanical ventilation. All other methods to stimulate coughing and secretion removal should be attempted before nasotracheal suctioning is considered. This technqiue should never be performed without available oxygen and should al-

ways be viewed as a potentially life-threatening procedure.

OTHER ADJUNCTS TO COUGHING AND SUCTIONING

Lavage

The infusion of sterile saline into the lungs with the intent of washing out secretions or mucus plugs is used in some centers. Typically, small amounts (usually ≤10-ml increments) of sterile saline are instilled directly into the tracheal tube before suctioning. The effectiveness of the technique of using small-quantity tracheal lavage is not substantiated (Tyler; Ackerman, 1985) and should not be used as an adjunct to chest physiotherapy. The increased quantity of sputum often attributed to lavage may be due to aspiration of the lavage fluid itself or the effect of coughing. In fact, it is doubtful that lavage has therapeutic merit other than to stimulate a cough (see p. 162 for alternate methods of cough stimulation). Undesirable spasms of coughing may accompany lavage and are associated with increased ICP (White et al.). The limited research on the deposition of lavage reveals that most of it remains in the trachea and mainstem bronchi and that there is negligible distribution to the peripheral airways; deposition is not affected by lung hyperinflation (Hanley et al., 1978). Because lavage fluid is not instilled specifically into involved areas of the lung, if it remains in the airways and does move peripherally, it most likely goes to the dependent or unobstructed airways. Adequate patient hydration and humidification of inspired gases are the appropriate means of liquefying secretions. It is our opinion, and that of others, that the practice of instilling small quantities of lavage prior to suctioning should be abandoned (Hanley et al.; Tyler; Ackerman). It is not substantiated through research and does not remedy the underlying problem of dried secretions.

Many authors have described the use of larger amounts of saline (50–100 ml) lavage applied segmentally through a transtracheal polyethylene catheter (Ramirez et al., 1963) or a flexible bronchoscope (Weinstein et al., 1977; Reynolds, 1987). When used together, the therapeutic effects of bronchoalveolar lavage are difficult to differentiate from bronchoscopy alone. In a technique that is frequently cited, a double-lumen endobronchial tracheal tube allows lavage of the dependent lung with saline, while the untreated lung is ventilated with high inspired oxygen concentrations. Chest physiotherapy, including postural drainage and vigorous percussion and vibration, is then given following turning to enhance the mechanical effects of the lavage and hastened fluid removal (Kylstra et al., 1971). Lavage of an entire lung is beneficial for treatment of alveolar proteinosis (Ramirez, 1971; Reynolds) and chest physiotherapy technqiues are reported to improve the efficacy of lung lavage (see p. 146). This procedure may also be useful in the treatment of bronchial asthma (Kylstra et al.) and cystic fibrosis (Roger et al., 1972). The use of lung lavage in chronic obstructive lung disease and pneumonia is less conclusive (Rogers et al.). The role of bronchoalveolar lavage remains experimental in most diseases and may play a more important role in diagnosis than in the therapeutic management of lung pathology (Reynolds).

"Bagging"

Bagging is a means of providing artificial ventilation by use of a manual resuscitator bag, which is usually connected to an oxygen supply. If the patient is not intubated, a mask may be attached to the bag and placed over the patient's face, covering the nose and mouth. For the intubated pateint, the mask is removed and the bag is connected directly to the tracheal tube. Bagging is performed by squeezing the bag rhythmically, to deliver a volume of gas to the patient. Expiration is passive. Bagging is most frequently used for resuscitation, transportation of a patient requiring mechanical ventilation, and in conjunction with suctioning of spontaneously breathing patients.

Bag-Squeezing Method of Chest Physiotherapy

Many centers advocate the use of the bag-squeezing method of chest physiotherapy for intubated patients (Clement and Hubsch, 1968; Windsor et al., 1972). This consists of placing the patient in a modified postural drainage position and hyperinflating the lungs with a 2- to 5-liter bag. The chest is then vibrated during expiration, and the trachea suctioned.

This is not part of our practice because it considerably changes cardiac output, the method mimics the Valsalva maneuver and the respiratory effects are only short lived (Laws and McIntyre, 1969; Windsor et al.). Manual hyperinflation is also associated with rapid rises in ICP (Gerradd and Bullock, 1986). The technique also requires two people to perform. Our regimen of suctioning through a port adaptor or disconnecting and reconnecting the patient from the ventilator for suctioning requires only one therapist. It is doubtful whether lung hyperinflation in the already mechanically ventilated patient provides any additional benefit. Studies fail to show improvement in arterial oxygenation, gas exchange, and lung compliance with hyperinflation (Nunn et al., 1965; Housley et al., 1970; Novak et al., 1987). Secretion removal by chest physiotherapy techniques that do not include manual hyperinflation appears more effective at improving total lung/thorax compliance (Mackenzie, 1989). It is also noted that lung hyperinflation causes additional discomfort in awake patients and no lasting pulmonary benefits (Laws and McIntyre).

Manual Resuscitators or Bags

A manual resuscitation unit is typically composed of a self-inflating bag, a one-way valve or diaphragm to eliminate rebreathing and an adaptor to connect the unit to the tracheal tube or a face mask. Although apparently simple in design and use, there is a great deal of variability among different types of resuscitator bags. Familiarity with the bag's characteristics allows efficient and safe

Table 5.6
Important Design Characteristics of Manual Resuscitators

Bag capacity
Maximum and average stroke volume
Maximum oxygen concentration delivery
Performance of valves at high oxygen flow rates
Performance of bag when mucus is present
Presence of relief valve
Ease of use and cleaning
Durability

use. Important characteristics are noted in Table 5.6.

In 1975, Carden and Hughes examined the performance of eight commonly used bags and found several important deficiencies, including an inability to deliver adequate oxygen concentrations and malfunction of the valves when mucus was present (Carden and Hughes, 1975). After revision, these problems were eliminated in four of the bags (Carden and Friedman, 1977). However, some substandard bags may still be in use and should be replaced. Eaton (1984) reported oxygen delivery to range from 25 to 100% depending on the type of bag and if a reservoir was attached. A study by Priano and Ham (1978) suggested that the problem of low oxygen concentration delivery may be partly overcome by retarding reexpansion of the bag manually in order to obtain more oxygen entrainment. Oxygen delivery can be better controlled by adding a reservoir to the resuscitator bag, but this makes the bag more cumbersome to use (Barnes and Watson, 1982; Eaton). Manual resuscitators also provide a variable tidal volume. Bags are frequently compressed with one hand which provides volume delivery from 400 to 800 ml; a volume of at least 500 ml is recommended. Two-handed operation yields 500–1000 ml; maximal volume should not exceed 1500 ml (Hill and Eaton, 1983; Eaton). Since a spontaneous breath may exceed this volume, the inspiratory resistance of the bag should be low. Also, the spontaneous breath should come through the bag, rather than the atmosphere, if supplemental oxygen is required (Eaton). Rebreathing, leading to increased inspired CO_2, is another reported complication of some resuscitator bags (Hill and Eaton).

The most serious complication of bagging cited in the literature is barotrauma. In 1978, Klick and co-workers described a patient in whom incorrect assembly of a resuscitator bag led to pleural tears and multiple subpleural hematomas bilaterally. The situation occurred because the resuscitator bag was connected to a cuffed tracheal tube and high oxygen flow rates jammed the valve, causing transmission of high pressures to the patient's lungs. Klick warns against slowly releasing hand pressure on the bag, which may increase the likelihood of the valve remaining in the position of inspiration and prevent lung deflation. If this should occur, the bag must be disconnected immediately to allow emptying of the lungs. The pressure relief valve designed to limit barotrauma can also cause inadequate ventilation of the patient with intrinsic lung disease, pulmonary edema, or chest wall injury. Hirschman and Kravath (1982) describe this complication and suggest overriding this "safety" feature to ensure effective ventilation, particularly during resuscitation or when increased airway pressure is present. When the pressure relief system is deactivated, it is advisable that the operator be made aware of this fact by an audible or visual warning (Eaton).

SUMMARY

Phagocytosis and ciliary activity provide adequate airway clearance under normal conditions. Only in the presence of excessive secretions or foreign objects or when the primary mechanisms are altered is coughing of major importance. This is often the case following surgery, when ciliary activity may be impaired due to the effects of decreased humidity, diaphragm dysfunction, anesthetic agents, supplemental oxygen, or tracheal intubation. Incisional pain and fear also frequently accompany surgery or trauma, leading to voluntary cough suppression. Various conditions, such as neuromuscular disorders and chronic lung disease, may further impair cough efficacy. As a result, the methods outlined in this chapter may be necessary to stimulate the cough mechanism or improve its effectiveness. However, it is our opinion that nasotracheal suctioning is an avoidable and hazardous procedure and that transtracheal puncture should be abandoned as a method to clear secretions.

Safe and appropriate suctioning guidelines are summarized as follows: The clinician should use sterile technique. A coudé tip catheter is recommended for entering the left mainstem bronchus. Suction catheters should not be larger than one-half the internal diameter (ID) of the airway (e.g., 14 French gauge catheters are usually used with adults having 8- or 9-mm-ID airways). Lavage is not carried out during suctioning, and the "bag squeezing" method of chest physiotherapy is not routinely used. Supplemental oxygen is indicated if hypoxemia occurs with suctioning; suctioning time should be limited to 15 sec. Care should be taken to reexpand the lungs after suctioning by using a mechanical ventilator, a manual resuscitator bag, or a volitional deep breath. The clinician should be aware of the limitations and variations of resuscitator bags. Critically ill mechanically ventilated patients should be suctioned through a port adaptor whenever ventilator flow rates are adequate. This allows for shorter suctioning times and better maintenance of PEEP, FIO_2, and tidal volume delivery. Suctioning is an integral part of chest physiotherapy for the patient with a tracheal tube. The frequency of this procedure depends on secretion production and individual patient need.

References

Anthony JS, Sieniewicz DJ: Suctioning of the left bronchial tree in critically ill patients. Crit Care Med 5:161–162, 1977

Ackerman MH: The use of bolus normal saline instillations in artificial airways: Is it useful or necessary? Heart Lung 14:505–506, 1985

Adlkofer RM, Powaser MM: The effect of endotracheal suctioning on arterial blood gases in patients after cardiac surgery. Heart Lung 7:1011–1014, 1978

Baker PO, Baker JM, Koen PA: Effect of different suctioning technqiues on arterial oxygenation (abstract). Am Rev Respir Dis 121(Suppl):109, 1980

Banner AS: Cough: Physiology, evaluation and treatment. Lung 164:79–92, 1986

Barnes CA, Kirchhoff KT: Minimizing hypoxemia due to endotracheal suctioning: A review of the literature. Heart Lung 15:164–176, 1986

Barnes TA, Watson ME: Oxygen delivery performance of four adult resuscitation bags. Respir Care 27:139–146, 1982

Bateman JRM, Newman SP, Daunt KM, Sheahan NF, Pavia D, Clarke SW: Is cough as effective as chest physiotherapy in the removal of excessive tracheobronchial secretions? Thorax 36:683–687, 1981

Belinkoff S (ed): Introduction to Respiratory Care, p. 165, Little, Brown, Boston, 1976

Bell R, Fein A, Kimble P: Post suctioning hypoxemia: Is it preventable? (abstract). Am Rev Respir Dis 121(Suppl):111, 1980

Belling D, Kelley RR, Simon R: Use of a swivel adaptor aperture during suctioning to prevent hypoxemia in the mechanically ventilated patient. Heart Lung 7:320–322, 1978

Benson MS, Pierson DJ: Ventilator wash-out volume: A consideration in endotracheal suction preoxygenation. Respir Care 24:832–835, 1979

Berman IR, Stahl WM: Prevention of hypoxic complications during endotracheal suctioning. Surgery 63:586–587, 1968

Boba A, Cincotti JJ, Piazza TE, Landmesser CM: The effects of apnea, endotracheal suction and oxygen insufflation alone and in combination, upon arterial oxygen saturation in anesthetized patients. J Lab Clin Med 53:680–685, 1959

Bodai BI, Walton CB, Briggs S, Goldstein M: A clinical evaluation of an oxygen insufflation/suction catheter. Heart Lung 16:39–46, 1987

Boutros AR: Arterial blood oxygenation during and after endotracheal suctioning in the apneic patient. Anesthesiology 32:114–118, 1970

Brandstater B, Muallem M: Atelectasis following tracheal suctioning in infants. Anesthesiology 31:468–473, 1969

Brown SE, Stansbury DW, Merrill EJ, Linden GS, Light RW: Prevention of suctioning-related arterial oxygen desaturation. Chest 83:621–627, 1983

Bucher K: Pathophysiology and pharmacology of cough. Pharmacol Rev 10:43–57, 1958

Byrd RB, Burns JR: Cough dynamics in the post-thoracotomy state. Chest 67:654–657, 1975

Cabal L, Devaskar S, Siassi B, Plajstek C, Waffarn F, Blanco C, Hodgman J: New endotracheal tube adaptor reducing cardiopulmonary effects of suctioning. Crit Care Med 7:552–555, 1979

Carden E, Friedman D: Further studies of manually operated self-inflating resuscitation bags. Anesth Analg (Cleve) 56:202–206, 1977

Carden E, Hughes T: An evaluation of manually operated self-inflating resuscitation bags. Anesth Analg (Cleve) 54:133–138, 1975

Centers for Disease Control. Recommendations for prevention of HIV transmission in health care settings. MMWR 36(Suppl 2S):1–18, August 1987

Charnley RM, Verma R: Inhalation of a minitracheotomy tube. Intensive Care Med 12:108–109, 1986

Chopra SK, Taplin GV, Simmons DH, Robinson GD, Elam D, Coulson A: Effects of hydration and physical therapy on tracheal transport velocity. Am Rev Respir Dis 115:1009–1014, 1977

Clement AJ, Hubsch SK: Chest physiotherapy by the "bag squeezing" method. Physiotherapy 54:355–359, 1968

Comroe JH: The lung. Sci Am 214:56–58, 1966

Cordero L, Hon EH: Neonatal bradycardia following nasopharyngeal stimulation. J Pediatr 78:441–447, 1971

Craig KC, Benson MS, Pierson DJ: Prevention of arterial oxygen desaturation during closed-ariway endotracheal suction: Effect of ventilator mode. *Respir Care* 29:1013–1018, 1984

Curry LD, Van Eeden C: The influence of posture on the effectiveness of coughing. *S Afr J Physiother* 33:8–11, 1977

deBoeck C, Zinman R: Cough versus chest physiotherapy. *Am Rev Respir Dis* 129:181–184, 1984

Deresinski SC, Stevens DA: Anterior cervical infections: Complications of transtracheal aspirations. *Am Rev Respir Dis* 110:354–356, 1974

Dickert MS: Closed-system suctioning (letter). *Crit Care Nurse* 7:12–13, 1987

Dollfus P, Frankel HL: Cardiovascular reflexes in tracheostomised tetraplegics. *Paraplegia* 2:227–235, 1965

Douglas S, Larson EL: The effect of a positive end-expiratory pressure adaptor and oxygenation during endotracheal suctioning. *Heart Lung* 14:396–400, 1985

Dryden GE, Albrecht WH, Cummins DF, Link WJ: A nonhypoxemic system for sterile tracheal aspiration without gloves. *Anesth Analg (Cleve)* 56:449–450, 1977

Durand M, Sangha B, Cabal LA, Hoppenbrouwers T, Hodgman JE: —Cardiopulmonary and intracranial pressure changes related to endotracheal suctioning in preterm infants. *Crit Care Med* 17:506-510,1989.

Eaton JM: Adult manual resuscitators. *Br J Hosp Med* 31:67–70, 1984

Evans JN, Jaeger MJ: Mechanical aspects of coughing. *Pneumonologie* 152:253–257, 1975

Falk M, Kelstrup M, Anderson JB, Kinoshita T, Falk P, Stovring S, Gothgen I: Improving the ketchup bottle method with positive expiratory pressure, PEP, in cystic fibrosis. *Eur J Respir Dis* 65:423–432, 1984

Fell T, Cheney FW: Prevention of hypoxia during endotracheal suction. *Ann Surg* 174:24–28, 1971

Fewell J, Arrington R, Seibert J: The effect of head position and angle of tracheal bifurcation on bronchus catheterization in the intubated neonate. *Pediatrics* 64:318–320, 1979

Fisher DM, Frewen T, Swedlow DB: Increase in intracranial pressure during suctioning—stimulation vs rise in $PaCO_2$. *Anesthesiology* 57:416–417, 1982

Fox WW, Schwartz JG, Shaffer TM: Pulmonary physiotherapy in neonates: Physiologic changes and respiratory management. *J Pediatr* 92:977–981, 1978

Frankel HL, Mathias CJ, Spalding JM: Mechanisms of reflex cardiac arrest in tetraplegic patients. *Lancet* 2:1183–1885, 1975

Freedman AP, Goodman L: Suctioning the left bronchial tree in the intubated adult. *Crit Care Med* 10:43–45, 1982

Frownfelter DL (ed): *Chest Physical Therapy and Pulmonary Rehabilitation*, p. 184. Year Book Medical Publishers, Chicago, 1978

Gal TJ: Effects of endotracheal intubation on normal cough performance. *Anesthesiology* 52:324–329, 1980

Gaskell DV, Webber BA: *The Brompton Hospital Guide to Chest Physiotherapy*, 4th pp ed., 19-20, 94–95. Blackwell Scientific Publications, Boston, 1980

methods of supplementing oxygen in minimizing suction-induced hypoxemia (abstract). *Heart Lung* 14:293, 1985

Gerradd J, Bullock M: The effect of respiratory therapy on intracranial pressure in ventilated neurosurgical patients. *Aust J Physiother* 32:107–111, 1986

Gold MI, Duarte I, Muravchick S: Arterial oxygenation in conscious patients after 5 minutes and after 30 seconds of oxygen breathing. *Anesth Analg* 60:313–316, 1981

Goodman RM, Yergin BM, Landa JF, Golinvaux MH, Sackner MA: Relationship of smoking history and pulmonary function tests to tracheal mucous velocity in nonsmokers, young smokers, ex-smokers, and patients with chronic bronchitis. *Am Rev Respir Dis* 117:205–214, 1978

Goodnough SKC: The effects of oxygen and hyperinflation on arterial oxygen tension after endotracheal suctioning. *Heart Lung* 14:11–17, 1985

Graff M, France J, Hiatt M, Hegyi T: Prevention of hypoxia and hyperoxia during endotracheal suctioning. *Crit Care Med* 15:1133–1135, 1987

Gunderson LP, McPhee AJ, Donovan EF: Partially ventilated endotracheal suction. *Am J Dis Child* 140:462–465, 1986

Guthrie MM, Pardowsky BJ, Stephens JJ: Hazards of endotracheal suctioning through an adaptor while maintaining mechanical ventilation (abstract). *Am Rev Respir Dis* 127(Suppl):148, 1983

Guyton AC: Basic Human Physiology: *Normal Function and Mechanisms of Disease*, pp 400–401. WB Saunders, Philadelphia, 1977

Gwynn BR, Moustafa SM: Complications of a mini-tracheotomy. *J Royal College Surg Edinb* 29:381, 1984

Haberman PB, Green JP, Archibald C, Dunn DL, Hurwitz SR, Ashburn WL, Moser KM: Determinants of successful selective tracheobronchial suctioning. *N Engl J Med* 289:1060–1063, 1973

Hahn HH, Beaty HN: Transtracheal aspiration in the evaluation of patients with pneumonia. *Ann Intern Med* 72:183–187, 1970

Hanley MV, Rudd T, Butler J: What happens to intratracheal saline instillations? (abstract). *Am Rev Respir Dis* 101(Suppl):124, 1970

Harris, RS, Lawson TV: The relative mechanical effectiveness and efficiency of successive voluntary coughs in healthy young adults. *Clin Sci* 34:569–577, 1968

Hietpas BG, Roth RD, Jensen WM: Huff coughing and airway patency. *Respir Care* 24:710–713, 1979

Hill SL, Eaton JM: Rebreathing during use of the Air-Viva resuscitation bag: A hazard. *Br Med J* 287:583–584, 1983

Hirshman AM, Kravath RE: Venting vs ventilating. A danger of manual resuscitator bags. *Chest* 82(Suppl):69–70, 1982

Hofmeyr JL, Webber BA, Hodson ME: Evaluation of positive expiratory pressure as an adjunct to chest physiotherapy in the treatment of cystic fibrosis. *Thorax* 41:951–954, 1986

Housley E, Louzada N, Becklake MR: To sigh or not to sigh. *Am Rev Respir Dis* 101:611–614, 1970

Howell S, Hill JD: Acute respiratory care in the open heart surgery patient. *Phys Ther* 52:253–260, 1972

Imle PC, Mars MP, Eppinghaus CE, Anderson P, Ciesia ND: Effect of chest physiotherapy (CPT) positioning on intracranlal (ICP) and cerebral perfusion pressure (CPP) (abstract). *Crit Care Med* 16:382, 1988.

Innocenti DM: Chest conditions. *Physiotherapy* 55:181–189, 1969

Irwin RS, Rosen MJ, Braman SS: Cough: A comprehensive review. *Arch Intern Med* 137:1186–1191, 1977

Jaworski A, Goldberg SK, Walkenstein MD, Wilson B, Lippmann ML: Utility of immediate postlobectomy fiberoptic bronchoscopy in preventing atelectasis. *Chest* 94:38–43, 1988

Jennett S: The response of heart rate to hypoxia in man after cervical spinal cord transection. *Paraplegia* 8:1–13, 1970

Jung RC, Gottlieb LS: Comparison of tracheobronchial suction catheters in humans. Visualization by fiberoptic bronchoscopy. *Chest* 69:179–181, 1976

Jung RC, Newman J: Minimizing hypoxia during endotracheal airway care. *Heart Lung* 11:208–212, 1982

Kalinske RW, Parker RH, Brandt D, Hoeprich PD: Diagnostic usefulness and safety of transtracheal aspiration. *N Engl J Med* 276:604–608, 1967

Kelly RE, Yao FF, Artusio JF: Prevention of suction-induced hypoxemia by simultaneous oxygen insufflation. *Crit Care Med* 15:874–875, 1987

King M: Rheological requirements for optimal clearance of secretions: Ciliary transport versus cough. *Eur J Respir Dis* 61(Suppl):39–42, 1980

King M, Brock G, Lundell C: Clearance of mucus by simulated cough. *J Appl Physiol* 58:1776–1782, 1985

Kirimli B, King JE, Pfaeffle HH: Evaluation of tracheobronchial suction techniques. *J Thorac Cardiovasc Surg* 59:340–344, 1970

Kleiber C, Krutzfield N, Rose EF: Acute histologic changes in the tracheobronchial tree associated with different suction catheter insertion techniques. *Heart Lung* 17:10–14, 1988

Klick JM, Bushnell LS, Bancroft ML: Barotrauma, a potential hazard of manual resuscitators, *Anesthesiology* 49:363–365, 1978

Knudson RJ, Mead J, Knudson DE: Contribution of airway collapse to supramaximal expiratory flows. *J Appl Physiol* 36:653–667, 1974

Krumpe PE, Denham LC: Selective bronchial suctioning guided by differential auscultation (abstract). *Crit Care Med* 12:260, 1984

Kubota Y, Margaribuchi T, Ohara M, Fujita M, Toyoda Y, Asada A, Harioka T: Evaluation of selective bronchial suctioning in the adult. *Crit Care Med* 8:748–749, 1980

Kubota Y, Magaribuchi T, Toyoda Y, Marukawa M, Urabe N, Asada A, Fujimori M, Ueda Y, Matsurra H: Selective bronchial suctioning in the adult using a curve-tipped catheter with a guide mark. *Crit Care Med* 10:767–769, 1982

Kubota Y, Toyoda Y, Sawada S, Murakawa M: The utility of a handmade curve-tipped catheter on selective left bronchial catheterization (letter). *Crit Care Med* 11:765–766, 1983

Kubota Y, Toyoda Y, Ueda Y, Fugimori M, Mori K, Okamoto T, Yasuda T, Matsuura H: Device for determining location of an endotracheal catheter tip. *Crit Care Med* 12:125–126, 1984

Kylstra JA, Rausch DC, Hall KD, Spock A: Volume controlled lung lavage in the treatment of asthma, bronchiectasis, and mucoviscidosis. *Am Rev Respir Dis* 103:651–665, 1971

Lambert RK: The use of a computational model for expiratory flow to simulate the effects of two airway abnormalities. *Aust Phys Eng Sci Med* 4:100–108, 1981

Lambert RK, Wilsm TA, Hyatt RE, Rodarte JR: A computational model for expiratory flow. *J Appl Physiol: Respirat Environ Exercise Physiol* 52:44–56, 1982

Langlands J: The dynamics of cough in health and in chronic bronchitis. *Thorax* 22:88–96, 1967

Langrehr EA, Washburn SC, Guthrie MP: Oxygen insufflation during endotracheal suctioning. *Heart Lung* 10:1028–1036, 1981

Langrehr EA, Washburn SC, Guthrie MP: Oxygen insufflation during endotracheal suctioning. *Heart Lung* 10:1028–1036, 1981

Langlands J: The dynamics of cough in health and in chronic bronchitis. *Thorax* 22:88–96, 1967

Laws AK, McIntyre RW: Chest physiotherapy. A physiological assessment during positive pressure ventilation in respiratory failure. *Can Anaesth Soc J* 16:487–493, 1969

LeFrock JL, Kleiner AS, Wu WH, Turndorf H: Transient bacteremia associated with nasotracheal suctioning. *JAMA* 236:1610–1611, 1976

Leiner GC, Abramowitz S, Small MJ, Stenby VB: Cough peak flow rate. *Am J Med Sci* 251:211–214, 1966

Leith DE: Cough. *Phys Ther* 48:439–447, 1967

Leith DE: The development of cough. *Am Rev Respir Dis* 131(Suppl):S39–S42, 1985

Leith DE, Butler JP, Sneddon SL, Brain JD: Cough. In *Handbook of Physiology*, Vol III. *The Respiratory System*, edited by PT Macklem and J Mead, pp 315–336. American Physiological Society, Bethesda, MD, 1986

Leith DE: Cough. In *Lung Biology in Health and Disease*, Vol 5. *Respiratory Defense Mechanisms*, edited by JD Brain, DF Proctor, and LM Reid, pp 545–592. Dekker, New York, 1977

Link WJ, Spaeth EE, Wahle WM, Penny W, Glover JL: The influence of suction catheter tip design on tracheobronchial trauma and fluid aspiration efficiency. *Anesth Analg (Cleve)* 55:290–297, 1976

Loudon RG, Shaw GB: Mechanics of cough in normal subjects and in patients with obstructive respiratory disease. *Am Rev Respir Dis* 96:666–677, 1967

Lourie B, McKinnon B, Kibler L: Transtracheal aspiration and anaerobic abscess (letter). *Ann Intern Med* 80:417–418, 1974

Mackenzie CF: Do periodic hyperinflations improve gas exchange in patients with hypoxic respiratory failure? (letter). *Crit Care Med* 17:595-596,1988

Marshall A, Bryan C, Levison H: Airway closure in children. *J Appl Physiol* 33:711–714, 1972

Mansell A, Bryan C, Levison H: Airway closure in children. *J Appl Physiol* 33:711–714, 1972

Marshall R, Holden WS: Changes in calibre of the smaller airways in man. *Thorax* 18:54–58, 1963

Matthews HR, Hopkinson RB: Treatment of sputum retention by minitracheotomy. *Br J Surg* 71:147–150, 1984

McCool FD, Leith DE: Pathophysiology of cough *Clin Chest Med* 8:189–195, 1987

McQuillan KA: The effects of the trendelenburg position for postural drainage on cerebrovascular status in head injured patients (abstract). *Heart Lung* 16:327, 1987

Mead J, Turner JM, Macklem PT, Little JB: Significance of the relationship between lung recoil and maximum expiratory flow. *J Appl Physiol* 22:95–108, 1967

Melissinos CG, Bruce E, Leith D: Factors affecting pleural pressure during cough in normal man (abstract). *Clin Res* 25:421A, 1976

Melissinos CG, Leith DE, Brody JS, Bruce E, Mead J: Thoracoabdominal mechanics in spontaneous cough (abstract). *Am Rev Respir Dis* 117:372, 1978

Menkes H, Britt J: Rationale for physical therapy. *Am Rev Respir Dis* 122(Suppl 2):127–131, 1980

Mossberg B, Cramner P: Mucociliary transport and cough as tracheobronchial clearance mechanisms in pathological conditions. *Eur J Respir Dis* 61(Suppl 110):47–55, 1980

Mossberg B, Afzelius BA, Eliasson R, Camner P: On the pathogenesis of obstructive lung disease. *Scand J Respir Dis* 59:55–65, 1978

Murray JF: Editorial: The ketchup-bottle method. *N Engl J Med* 300:1155–1156, 1979

Newhouse MT: Factors affecting sputum clearance (abstract). *Thorax* 28:267, 1973

Novak RA, Shumaker L, Snyder JV, Pinsky MR: Do periodic hyperinflation improve gas exchange in patients with hypoxemic respiratory failure? *Crit Care Med* 15:1081–1085, 1987

Nunn JF, Bergman NA, Coleman AJ: Factors influencing the arterial oxygen tension during anesthesia with artificial ventilation. *Br J Anaesth* 37:898–914, 1965

Oldenburg FA, Dolovich MB, Montgomery JM, Newhouse MT: Effects of postural drainage, exercise and cough on mucus clearance in chronic bronchitis. *Am Rev Respir Dis* 120:739–745, 1979

O'Malley P, Zankofski MA, Beaumont E: Disposable suction catheters: A Nursing 79 product survey. *Nursing '79* 9:70–75, 1979

Opie LH, Smith AC: Tracheobronchial toilet through a tracheostome. *Lancet* 1:600–601, 1959

Parsons GH, Price JE, Auston PW: Bilateral pneumothorax complicating transtracheal aspiration. *West J Med* 125:73–75, 1976

Pauker SG: Transtracheal aspiration (letter). *Ann Intern Med* 73:142–143, 1970

Pecora DV, Kohl M: Transtracheal aspiration in the diagnosis of acute lower respiratory tract infection. *Am Rev Respir Dis* 86:755–758, 1962

Perel A, Pizor R, Fisher J, Goldberg M: Transtracheal oxygen to produce cough (letter). *Chest* 93:447–448, 1988

Perlman JM, Volpe JJ: Suctioning in the preterm infant: Effects on cerebral blood flow velocity, intracranial pressure, and arterial blood pressure. *Pediatrics* 72:329–334, 1983

Petersen GM, Pierson DJ, Hunter PM: Arterial oxygen saturation during nasotracheal suctioning. *Chest* 76:283–287, 1979

Petty TL (ed): *Intensive and Rehabilitative Respiratory Care*, p 108. Lea & Febiger, Philadelphia, 1974

Pierce JB, Piazza DE: Differences in postsuctioning arterial blood oxygen concentration values using two postoxygenation methods. *Heart Lung* 16:34–38, 1987

Placzek M, Silverman M: Selective placement of bronchial suction catheters in intubated neonates. *Arch Dis Child* 58:829–831, 1983

Priano LL, Ham J: A simple method to increase the FDO_2 of resuscitator bags. *Crit Care Med* 6:48–49, 1978

Pryor JA, Webber BA: An evaluation of the force expiration technique as an adjunct to postural drainage. *Physiotherapy* 65:304–307, 1979

Pryor JA, Webber BA, Hodson ME, Batten JC: Evaluation of the forced expiration technique as an adjunct to postural drainage in the treatment of cystic fibrosis. *Br Med J* 2:417–418, 1979

Puchelle E, Zahm JM, Girard F, Bertrand A, Polu JM, Aug F, Sadoul P: Mucociliary transport in vivo and in vitro. *Eur J Respir Dis* 61:254–264, 1980

Radigan LR, King RD: A technique for the prevention of postoperative atelectasis. *Surgery* 47:184–187, 1960

Ramirez J: Alveolar proteinosis: Importance of pulmonary lavage. *Am Rev Respir Dis* 103:666–678, 1971

Ramirez RJ, Schultz RB, Dutton RE: Pulmonary alveolar proteinosis. A new technique and rationale for treatment. *Arch Intern Med* 112:419–431, 1963

Reynolds HY: Bronchoalveolar lavage. *Am Rev Respir Dis* 135:250–263, 1987

Ries K, Levison ME, Kaye D: Transtracheal aspiration in pulmonary infection. *Arch Intern Med* 133:453–458, 1974

Rogers R, Braunstein MS, Shuman JF: Role of bronchopulmonary lavage in the treatment of respiratory failure: A review. *Chest* 62(Suppl):955–1106, 1972

Rosen M, Hillard EK: The use of suction in clinical medicine. *Br J Anaesth* 32:486–504, 1960

Rosen M, Hillard EK: The effects of negative pressure during tracheal suction. *Anesth Analg (Cleve)* 41:50–57, 1962

Ross BB, Gramiak R, Rahn H: Physical dynamics of the cough mechanism. *J Appl Physiol* 8:264–268, 1955

Rossman CM, Waldes R, Sampson D, Newhouse MT: Effect of chest physiotherapy on the removal of mucus in patients with cystic fibrosis. *Am Rev Respir Dis* 126:131–135, 1982

Rowe MI, Weinberger M, Poole CA: An experimental study of the vibrator in postoperative tracheobronchial clearance. *J Pediatr Surg* 8:735–738, 1973

Sackner MA: Tracheobronchial toilet. Weekly Update. *Pulm Med* 1–8, 1978

Sackner MA, Landa F, Greeneltch N, Robinson MJ: Pathogenesis and prevention of tracheobronchial damage with suction procedures. *Chest* 64:284–290, 1973

Salem MR, Wong AY, Mathrubhutham M, Ramilio J, Jacobs HK, Bennett EJ: Evaluation of selective bronchial suctioning techniques used for infants and children. *Anesthesiology* 48:379–380, 1978

Schillaci RF, Iacovoni VE, Conte RS: Transtracheal aspiration complicated by fatal endotracheal hemorrhage. *N Engl J Med* 295:488–490, 1976

Schmerber J, Deltenre M: A new fatal complication of transtracheal aspiration. *Scand J Respir Dis* 59:232–235, 1978

Schumann L, Parsons GH: Tracheal suctioning and ventilator tubing changes in adult respiratory distress syndrome: Use of a positive end-expiratory pressure valve. Heart Lung 14:362–367, 1985

Scott AA, Sandham G, Rebuck AS: Selective tracheobronchial aspiration. Thorax 32:346–348, 1977

Shim C, Fine N. Fernandez R, Williams MH: Cardiac arrhythmias resulting from tracheal suctioning. Ann Intern Med 71:1149–1153, 1969

Siebens AA, Kirby NA, Poulos DA: Cough following transection of spinal cord at C-6. Arch Phys Med Rehabil 45:1–8, 1964

Skelley BFH, Deeren SM, Powaser MM: The effectiveness of two preoxygenation methods to prevent endotracheal suction-induced hypoxemia. Heart Lung 9:316–323, 1980

Smaldone GC, Itoh H, Swift D, Wagner H: Effect of flow-limiting segments and cough on particle deposition and mucociliary clearance in the lung. Am Rev Respir Dis 120:747–758, 1979

Smaldone GC, Messina MS: Enhancement of particle deposition by flow-limiting segments in humans. J Appl Physiol 59:509–514, 1985a

Smaldone GC, Messina MS: Flow limitation, cough, and patterns of aerosol deposition in humans. J Appl Physiol 59:515–520, 1985b

Smaldone GC, Messina MS: Enhancement of particle deposition by flow-limiting segments in humans. J Appl Physiol 59:509–514, 1985a

Spencer CD, Beaty HN: Complications of transtracheal aspiration. N Engl J Med 286:304–306, 1972

Spoerel WE, Chan CK: Jet ventilation for tracheobronchial suction. Anesthesiology 45: 450–452, 1976.

Standard Specification for Medical and Surgical Suction and Drainage Systems American Society for Testing and Materials, Committee F-29, Subcommittee F-29.07.01, 1916 Race St., Philadelphia, PA 19103, 1986, p 8

Sutton PP, Parker RA, Webber BA, Newman SP, Garland N, Lopez-Vidriero MT, Pavia D, Clarke SW: Assessment of the forced expiration technique, postural drainage and directed coughing in chest physiotherapy. Eur J Respir Dis 64:62–68, 1983

Sykes MK, McNicol MW, Campbell EJM: Respiratory Failure, pp 153–157. Blackwell Scientific Publications, Boston, 1976

Taggart JA, Dorinsky NL, Sheahan JS: Airway pressures during closed system suctioning. Heart Lung 17:536–542, 1988

Taylor PA, Waters HR: Arterial oxygen tensions following endotracheal suction on IPPV. Anaesthesia 26:289–293, 1971

Thoren L: Post-operative pulmonary complications. Observations on their prevention by means of physiotherapy. Acta Chir Scand 107:193–204, 1954

Tyler ML: Nursing care of patients in acute respiratory failure. In Current Advances in Respiratory Care, edited by WJ O'Donohue, pp 137–148. American College of Chest Physicians, Park Ridge, IL, 1984

Unger KM, Moser KM: Fatal complication of transtracheal aspiration. Arch Intern Med 132:437–439, 1973

Ungvarski P: Mechanical stimulation of coughing. Am J Nurs 71:2358–2361, 1971

Urban BJ, Weitzner SW: Avoidance of hypoxemia during endotracheal suction. Anesthesiology 31:473–475, 1969

Vraciu JK, Vraciu RA: Effectiveness of breathing exercises in preventing pulmonary complications following open heart surgery. Phys Ther 57:1367–1371, 1977

Walsh JM, Vanderwarf C, Hoscheit D, Fahey PJ: Unsuspected hemodynamic alterations during endotracheal suctioning. Chest 95:162–165, 1989

Wang KP, Wise RA, Terry PB, Summer WR: A new controllable suction catheter for blind cannulation of the main stem bronchi. Crit Care Med 6:347–348, 1978

Weibel ER: Morphometry of the Human Lung, p. 139. Academic Press, New York, 1963

Weistein HG, Bone RC, Ruth WE: Pulmonary lavage in patients treated with mechanical ventilation. Chest 72:583–587, 1977

White PF, Schlobohm RM, Pitts LH, Lindauer JM: A randomized study of drugs for preventing increases in intracranial pressure during endotracheal suctioning. Anesthesiology 57:242–244, 1982

Widdicombe JG: Mechanism of cough and its regulation. Eur J Respir Dis 61(Suppl 110):11–15, 1980

Windsor HM, Harrison GA, Nicholson TJ: "Bag squeezing," A physiotherapeutic technique. Med J Aust 2:829–832, 1972

Yamazaki S, Owaga J, Shohzu A, Yamazaki Y: Intrapleural cough pressure in patients after thoracotomy. J Thorac Cardiovasc Surg 80:600–604, 1980

Yeoh NTL, Wells FC, Goldstraw P: A complication of minitracheostomy. Br J Surg 72:633, 1985

Yoshikawa TT, Chow AW, Montgomeriez JZ, Guze LB: Paratracheal abscess: An unusual complication of transtracheal aspiration. Chest 65:105–106, 1974

Zaltman JI; Selective left bronchial suctioning using a routine catheter with the programmed tip (letter). Crit Care Med 11:765, 1983

Zelechowski GP: Suction collection and its relation to nosocomial infection. Am J Infect Control 8:72–74, 1980

Zmora E, Merritt TA: Use of a side hole endotracheal tube adaptor for tracheal aspiration. Am J Dis Child 134:250–254, 1980

CHAPTER 6

Changes with Immobility and Methods of Mobilization

P. Cristina Imle, M.S., P.T., and Nancy Klemic, B.S., P.T.

THE EFFECTS OF IMMOBILIZATION

"The importance of immobilization has been part of medicine's body of knowledge for many, many years and can be accepted as fact. As with any fact, if not restated from time to time it tends to be forgotten.... Our advanced knowledge and technology by themselves cannot save the patient. Instead something so simple as turning the patient ... at least hourly, may make the difference between living and dying for the intensive care patient." (Bendixen, 1974)

The hazards of patient immbolization are often overlooked or not considered important enough to merit thorough discussion, particularly for patients in the intensive care unit (ICU). However, restriction to bed rest is known to alter the normal physiological function of all the organ systems described in this section. Most studies on the effects of immobility are performed on normal subjects. More delerterious findings can be assumed when bed rest is combined with trauma, malnutrition, decreased level of consciousness, or chronic disease. Immobilization of the acutely ill patient is often caused by a variety of factors such as those listed in Table 6.1. Restriction to bed rest includes maintaining the patient in the supine position rather than the normal erect position. The belief that the detrimental effects of bed rest and immobility can be better corrected once the patient is no longer acutely ill is not acceptable. Preventing secondary complications saves both time and money and may well affect the patient's recovery and quality of life. Methods of mobilizing patients are discussed after a systematic review of immobilization and its sequelae.

Cardiovascular System

The effects of immobilization on the cardiovascular system have been investigated since the 1940s. Table 6.2 summarizes the research in this area. The effects cited most frequently are decreased total blood volume, plasma volume, red blood cell mass, and hemoglobin concentration. There is also a decrease in maximal oxygen uptake and orthostatic tol-

**Table 6.1
Factors Leading to Immobilization of the
Intensive Care Patient**

Confinement to the intensive care unit
Confinement to bed rest
Administration of anesthesia, sedation and
neuromuscular blockers
Skeletal traction, casting and splinting
Neurological deficit including paralysis and
central nervous system depression
Pain
General debilitation, weakness and
malnutrition
Use of monitoring equipment

erance. Maximal and basal heart rates are increased during immobilization.

Physical Deconditioning

Following immobilization, the patient becomes deconditioned, as evidenced by a decreased ability to perform aerobic work and decreased endurance. Taylor et al. (1949) studied six normal men and found that after 3 weeks of bed rest, the heart rate was significantly higher with the same level of exercise. Oxygen intake during exercise decreased while oxygen debt and blood lactate concentration increased. Saltin et al. (1968) studied five normal young males before and after a 20-day period of bed rest. Their findings included an increased heat rate during a standardized level of exercise and decreased cardiac output with exercise and maximal work load. After studying 22 normal men who had undergone bed rest for 1 week, Friman (1979) determined that maximal oxygen uptake and work capacity decreased. These studies were done on previously normal patients. Therefore, it is not known what variations in deconditioning would occur in the intensive care patient with a history

**Table 6.2
The Effects of Immobilization on the Cardiovascular System**

Effect Found	Year/Researchers	Length of Immobilization	Population Studied
Decreased total blood volume	1945 Taylor et al.	3 wk	5 normal young men
	1967 Vogt et al.	14 days	4 normal young men
	1970 Triebwasser et al.	5 wk	8 normal adults
	1979 Friman	1 wk	22 normal men
Decreased plasma volume and red blood cell mass	1948 Deitrick et al.	6 or 7 wk	4 normal men
	1968 Georgiyevskiy et al.	20 days	4 normal men
	1967 Vogt et al.	14 days	4 normal men
	1968 Saltin et al.	20 days	5 normal men
	1979 Friman	1 wk	22 normal men
Decreased hemoglobin concentration	1964 Lamb et al.	2 wk	26 normal men
	1979 Friman	30 days	10 normal men
		1 wk	22 normal men
Increased maximal heart rate	1948 Deitrick et al.	6 or 7 wk	4 normal men
	1974 Bassey and Fentem	2 wk	9 postoperative knee surgery patients (male)
	1976 Stremel et al.	2 wk	7 normal young men
Increase in basal heart rate	1949 Taylor et al.	3 wk	6 normal young men
	1968 Georgiyevskiy et al.	20 days	3 normal young men
		62 days	3 normal young men
Decreased transverse diameter of heart	1949 Taylor et al.	3 wk	6 normal young men
	1969 Krasnykh	70 days	16 normal young women
Decreased maximum oxygen uptake	1949 Taylor et al.	3 wk	6 normal young men
	1968 Saltin et al.	20 days	5 normal men
	1979 Friman	1 wk	22 normal men
Decreased orthostatic tolerance	1949 Taylor et al.	3 wk	6 normal young men
	1963 Birkhead et al.	42 days	4 trained men
	1966 Chase et al.	15 days	18 normal young men
		30 days	18 normal young men

of preexisting disease or an acute multi-system insult. In addition, some degree of malnourishment is present in many patients confined to the ICU. Malnutrition results in increased muscle fatigability and an altered pattern of muscle contraction and relaxation (Lopes et al., 1982).

Decreased Orthostatic Tolerance

One effect of immobilization frequently seen in the clinical setting is a reduction in circulating volume, which may result in dizziness or fainting when the patient assumes the upright position. This happens because vasodilation occurs in the supine position. After prolonged bed rest, the blood vessels' ability to vasoconstrict is impaired; therefore, the upright position causes blood to pool in the lower extremities. This results in decreased cardiac filling pressures and decreased cardiac output and may produce mild cerebral hypoxemia (Browse, 1965). Orthostatic hypotension is particularly troublesome in the patient with quadriplegia.

Venous Thrombosis and Pulmonary Embolus

The incidence of venous thrombosis increases with the duration of bed rest (Sevitt and Gallagher, 1961). However, the etiology of venous thrombosis formation is not yet fully identified. Several factors are suggested, including changes in blood composition, loss of vessel wall integrity, and vascular stasis. The decreased circulating blood volume that occurs with immobility is due more to the loss of plasma than to the decrease in red blood cell mass. The net effect of increased blood viscosity may predispose the bedridden patient to thromboembolism (Wenger, 1982). While venous thrombosis is reportedly common in hospitalized (and immobilized) patients, over 80% of the detected thrombi are small, asymptomatic, confined to the calf, and probably clinically insignificant (Dalen et al., 1986). Dislodgment of a venous clot can lead to a pulmonary embolus, which may have severe, even fatal, consequences (Browse). The incidence of postoperative fatal pulmonary embolism in patients undergoing elective general surgery ranges from 0.1% to 0.8% (Dalen, et al.). Pulmonary embolus is difficult to diagnose clinically, since similar symptoms are often seen in patients sustaining multisystem injuries. In a 2-year period at our facility, only 1 trauma patient in 124 consecutive full autopsies demonstrated pulmonary emboli (Mackenzie et al., 1979). This low incidence of pulmonary embolus may be a result of early and aggressive patient mobilization since symptomatic pulmonary embolism is relatively uncommon in ambulant patients and fatal pulmonary embolism is very uncommon (Dalen et al.).

Respiratory System

Effects of Position Change

In normal subjects, changes in respiratory function occur only during the initial period of adjustment to the change in position from upright to supine (see Table 6.3). This position change may result in decreased total lung capacity with decreased vital capacity, functional residual capacity (FRC), residual volume, and forced expiratory volume. The shape of the rib cage and abdomen changes, with the anteroposterior diameter decreasing, while the lateral diameter increases. Pulmonary blood flow and ventilation distribution are altered. In the presence of lung pathology, the alteration in ventilation and perfusion due to position change may be dramatic (see p. 94). In normal subjects, alveolar size decreases and small airways close in dependent lung zones.

Of particular significance is the reduction in FRC that occurs in the supine position and the relationship of FRC to closing volume, which results in increased airway closure at resting tidal volumes. Craig et al. (1971) studied the relationship between airway closure and age and found that closing volume became greater than FRC at 49 years in the seated position and at 36 years of age in the supine position (see Fig. 6.1). A decrease in chest wall compliance also occurs with age (Estenne et al., 1985). Dynamic and static lung compliance also decrease and resistance to flow increases in normal

Table 6.3
The Respiratory Effects of Changing Position from Upright to Supine

Effect Found	Year/Researchers	Population Studied
Decreased total lung capacity	1957 Svanberg	25 normal people
	1971 Craig et al.	10 normal men
Decreased vital capacity	1951 Wade and Gilson	10 normal men
	1957 Svanberg	25 normal people
Decreased FRC[a]	1957 Svanberg	25 normal people
	1971 Craig et al.	10 normal men
Decreased residual volume	1957 Svanberg	25 normal people
	1971 Craig et al.	10 normal men
Decreased ERV	1983 Behrakis et al.	10 normal men
Decreased forced expiratory volume	1971 Craig et al.	10 normal men
Decreased static and dynamic lung compliance	1983 Behrakis et al.	10 normal men
Decreased rib cage compliance		
Increased diaphragm-abdomen compliance	1985 Estenne et al.	61 normal adults
Changes in pulmonary blood flow distribution	1970 Reed and Wood	Dogs
Closure of small airways in dependent regions	1970 LeBlanc et al.	80 normal subjects
	1971 Craig et al.	10 normal men
Decreased anteroposterior diameter and increased lateral diameter of rib cage and abdomen	1978 Vellody et al.	25 normal people
Decrease in size of dependent alveoli	1967 Glazier et al.	Greyhound dogs
	1983 Behrakis et al.	10 normal men
Decrease in PaO$_2$	1966 Ward et al.	50 elderly hospital patients

[a]FRC, functional residual capacity; ERV, expiratory reserve volume.

subjects When moving from siting to supine (Behrakis et al., 1983). Due to the changes in compliance, resistance, FRC, expiratory reserve volume, pulmonary blood flow, and closing volume while supine, pulmonary gas exchange is impaired; retention of secretions and atelectasis can develop. The trapping of secretions distal to areas of small airway closure, if not remedied, may lead to pulmonary infection.

Effects of Immobilization

While it appears that respiratory function in normal subjects may not be adversely affected by immobilization, critically ill patients may suffer severe respiratory complications from retention of secretions. This results from immobilization, coupled with inability to handle secretion clearance adequately. Effective clearance may be hindered in the criti-

cally ill by factors such as the presence of a tracheal tube, anesthesia or sedation, muscle weakness, neurological deficit including paralysis, chest trauma, and pain. As a result, secretions tend to accumulate peripherally in gravity-dependent positions, resulting in small airway closure. These secretions cannot be cleared with suctioning and frequently cause atelectasis. Therefore, specific positioning of the patient for postural drainage with percussion and vibration is required to mobilize secretions centrally where they can be suctioned. Research on the respiratory effects of immobilization is summarized in Table 6.4.

Mobilization of patients may aid in preventing the development of respiratory complications. Exercise has been shown to aid lung clearance of secretions in patients with chronic bronchitis (Oldenburg et al., 1979). The beneficial effects of mobilizing patients following sur-

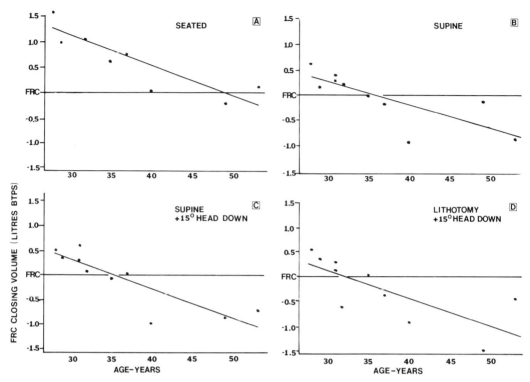

Figure 6.1. Closing volume in normal subjects becomes greater than functional residual capacity at 49 years in the seated position (**A**), at 36 years in the supine position (**B**), and progressively earlier in the head-down position (**C**, **D**). *BTPS,* body temperature and pressure saturation. (From D. B. Craig et al.: *Can Anaesth Soc J* 18:92–99, 1971.)

Table 6.4
The Effects of Immobilization on the Respiratory System

Effect Found	Year/Researchers	Length of Immobilization	Population Studied
Decreased A–aDO$_2$[a]	1967 Cardus	10 days	7 healthy young men
Increased pulmonary arteriovenous shunting	1974 Ray et al.	6–10 hr Varied	9 overhydrated dogs 2 overhydrated patients
Decreased PaO$_2$	1967 Cardus	10 days	7 healthy young men
	1968 Clauss et al.	Length of surgery time (hr)	13 open heart surgery patients
	1974 Ray et al.	6–10 hr Varied	9 overhydrated dogs[b] 2 overhydrated patients
Increase FRC	1986 Beckett et al.	11–12 days	18 healthy adults
Physical changes in dependent lung (by x-ray or exam on dissection)	1955 Lambert et al.	Length of time of thoracotomy (hr)	33 tuberculosis patients[b]
	1962 Craig et al.	Length of surgery time required (hr)	100 thoracic surgery patients (variety)[b]
	1974 Ray et al.	6–10 hr Varied	9 overhydrated dogs[b] 2 overhydrated patients

[a]A–aDO$_2$, alveolar–arterial oxygen gradient; FRC, functional residual capacity.
[b]Anesthetized.

gery is discussed in the second part of this chapter. Early operative fixation of long bone fractures in patients with multiple injuries allows early mobilization of these patients and has been cited as an important factor in reducing the incidence of fat embolus (Riska et al., 1977). In our experience over a 5-year period (1975–1980), only 2 patients of 3210 consecutive trauma admissions showed clinical signs of fat embolus, despite a multitude of orthopedic injuries. This low incidence is more impressive when it is realized that these patients with fractures were routinely and aggressively mobilized. Therefore, it is unlikely that early mobilization increases the incidence of a fat embolization.

Metabolic System

The metabolic consequences of immobilization during prolonged bed rest include increased excretion of nitrogen, calcium, potassium, magnesium and phosphorus (see Table 6.5). As a result, osteoporosis and kidney or ureteral stone formation may occur.

Osteoporosis

Osteoporosis, loss of bone integrity through demineralization and loss of bone matrix, is frequently seen during prolonged immobilization and is manifested by increased calcium excretion.

Possible etiological factors are decreased osteoblastic action, decreased blood flow to the bone, and increased osteoclastic activity (Browse). Osteoporosis may be painful for the patient and may lead to an increased incidence of bone fracture. Vertebral mineral bone loss of nearly 2% per week is reported following strict bed rest (Hansson et al., 1975). A mean decrease in lumbar mineral content of almost 1% per week is reported in 34 patients put on simple bed rest (mean, 27 days) during treatment for back pain. Reambulation reversed the demineralization but took nearly 4 months (Krolner and Toft, 1983).

Formation of Kidney or Ureteral Stones

As a result of increased calcium excretion through the kidneys and urinary tract, the incidence of stone formation may increase. The formation may be further enchanced when the patient lies in one position for too long, causing urine to stagnate in the kidney, pelvis, or bladder (Hirschberg et al., 1977).

Musculoskeletal System

The effects of immobilization on the musculoskeletal system include decreased muscle girth and strength, changes in periarticular and intraarticular connective tissue, and loss of bone density (see Table 6.6).

Table 6.5
The Effects of Immobilization on the Metabolic System

Effect Found	Year/Researchers	Length of Immobilization	Population Studied
Increased calcium excretion	1948 Deitrick et al.	6 or 7 wk	4 normal men
	1969 Donaldson et al.	30–36 wk	3 normal men
	1971 Hulley et al.	210 days	5 normal young men
Increased nitrogen excretion	1948 Deitrick et al.	6 or 7 wk	4 normal men
	1949 Taylor et al.	3 wk	6 normal young men
	1955 Heilskov et al.	16–18 days	3 normal young men
	1971 Hulley et al.	210 days	5 normal young men
	1973 Mack and Montgomery	14 days	5 normal young men
Increased phosphorus excretion	1948 Deitrick et al.	6 or 7 wk	4 normal men
	1969 Donaldson et al.	30–36 wk	3 normal men
	1971 Hulley et al.	210 days	5 normal young men
Increased magnesium excretion	1969 Donaldson et al.	30–36 wk	3 normal men
	1971 Hulley et al.	210 days	5 normal young men

Table 6.6
The Effects of Immobilization on the Musculoskeletal System

Effect Found	Year/Researchers	Length of Immobilization	Population Studied
Decreased muscle girth	1948 Deitrick et al.	6 or 7 wk	4 normal young men
	1963 Brannon et al.	60 days	30 normal young men
	1969 Patel et al.	4–38 wk	14 male patients (variety of disorders)
	1986 Grossman et al.	4 wk	23 rabbits
Decreased muscle strength	1948 Deitrick et al.	6 or 7 wk	4 normal young men
	1963 Brannon et al.	60 days	30 normal young men
	1969 Yeremin et al.	70 days	16 normal men
Increased creatinine clearance/ decreased muscle mass	1983 Krolner and Toft	11–61 days	34 adult patients
Changes in periarticular and intraarticular connective tissue	1963 Peacock	4 wk	8 dogs
	1972 Enneking and Horowitz	Varied more than 1 year	10 male patients (variety of disorders)
	1973 Akeson et al.	9 wk	10 male rabbits
	1974 Akeson et al.	1, 2, 4, 6, or 9 wk	40 male rabbits
Decreased tendon stiffness	1982 Amiel et al.	9 wk	10 male rabbits
Decreased bone density	1967 Burkhart and Jowsey	3–12 wk	30 adult dogs
	1969 Donaldson et al.	30–36 wk	3 normal men
	1983 Krolner and Toft	11–61 days	34 adult patients

Atrophied, Weak Muscles

After prolonged bed rest, muscles appear atrophied, and the patient may have substantial muscle weakness. Exercise causes muscle hypertrophy through increased amino acid transport, DNA and RNA protein synthesis, and decreased breakdown of protein (Goldberg, 1972). With prolonged bed rest, it is assumed that a reversal of these biochemical effects occurs. Immobility leads to diminished skeletal muscle mass, girth, and efficiency. Contractile strength may decrease by 10–15% within the first week of bed rest (Wenger). Less efficient muscle function results in an increased oxygen demand, which may be intolerable to the patient with cardiac or respiratory pathology. The malnutrition of many ICU patients can further impair skeletal muscle performance (Lopes et al., 1982).

Joint Contractures

Contractures are restrictions in joint range of motion following immobiliza-

tion caused by periarticular and intraarticular changes in connective tissue. An array of changes has been described. Akeson et al. (1961, 1973, 1974) found biochemical changes in the composition of canine connective tissue, which may alter the mechanism of cross-linking. Peacock (1963) determined that a significant increase in collagen production in connective tissue occurs in the popliteal space of dogs following 4 weeks of immobilization. Studying human knees that were immobilized for extended periods of time (at least 1 year), Enneking and Horowitz (1972) frequently detected obliteration of the joint space by fibrofatty connective tissue.

Decubitus Ulcers

Unrelieved pressure over an area where skin closely overlies bone can cause tissue necrosis. This can lead to decubitus ulcer formation, which not only results in damage to skin, muscle or even bones but also causes a great deal of expense, loss of rehabilitation time and infection (Kottke, 1966). However, decubitus ulcer formation is one of the most easily prevented secondary side effects of immobilization. Good patient care, including frequent turning with careful positioning, is necessary to eliminate this problem in the ICU. Specialty beds are not a substitute for good nursing care and optimal pressure relief (see Chapter 3).

Central Nervous System

Central nervous system function is altered by immobilization (see Table 6.7). Electroencephalogram activity slows. Emotional and behavioral changes develop, including emotional lability, regression in behavior to childlike patterns, increase in anxiety and depression, and decrease in attention span (Spencer et al., 1965). Psychomotor performance decreases in the areas of intellect, perception and coordination. Visual and auditory changes occur (Greenleaf and Kozlowski, 1982). Sleeping patterns change, with an increase in deep or delta sleep and an increased memory for dreams (Hammer and Kenan, 1980). Further impairment of central nervous system function is seen in the critically ill patient due to a variety of contributing factors, as outlined in Table 6.8.

METHODS OF PATIENT MOBILIZATION

To help prevent the detrimental sequelae of bed rest and immobilization, maximal patient mobility is initiated in the ICU. As the paitent progresses, following admission, activities may be modified accordingly. Passive positioning is almost always possible despite numerous intravascular lines and lifesustaining equipment. Active exercising while bedridden or sitting and early ambulation are encouraged. In this section, each stage of patient progression is addressed, as well as methods to facilitate patient mobility. Emphasis is placed on functional activities.

Bedridden Patients

Mobility of patients confined to bed is not as severely restricted as might be expected. Hospital beds allow patients to be passively positioned in many ways when the knee break, head elevation or head-down mechanisms are used. When bed position change is combined with posturing the patient over the range of supine to prone, a wide spectrum of possible movements become available. Even Stryker frames allow variations from either

Table 6.7
The Effects of Immobilization on the Central Nervous System

Effect Found	Year/Researchers	Length of Immobilization	Population Studied
Slowing of electroencephalogram activity	1963 Zubeck and Wilgosh	1 wk	22 male college students
		1 wk	32 male college students
	1966 Zubeck and MacNeill	62 days	6 healthy young men
	1968 Petukhov and Purakhin	5 wk	8 healthy young men
	1971 Ryback et al.		
Emotional and behavioral changes	1966 Zubeck and MacNeill	1 wk	32 male college students
			Not known
	1969 Boganchenko et al.	5 wk	8 healthy young men
	1971 Ryback et al.		
Decreased psychomotor performance	1953 Heron et al.[a]	Varied	Not known
	1963 Zubeck and Wilgosh	1 wk	22 male college students
		5 wk	8 healthy young men
	1971 Ryback et al.		
Changes in sleep patterns	1971 Ryback et al.	5 weeks	8 healthy young men

[a]This study combined immobilization with severe sensory deprivation.

Table 6.8
Factors Leading to Central Nervous System Impairment in the Critically Ill

Physical inactivity and restraint
Sensory deprivation
Loss of circadian light pattern
Anesthesia and sedation
Fever
Hypoxia
Electrolyte imbalance

supine to prone and head up to head down. Passive mobilization of patients may be coordinated with other necessary ICU procedures, such as linen or dressing changes and skin and wound examination. As illustrated in Chapter 3, a wide variety of both patient and bed positions can be assumed, despite the presence of monitoring equipment, intravascular lines and a mechanical ventilator.

Passive positioning is necessary to maintain normal joint and muscle ranges. It also helps to counteract some of the soft-tissue and vascular changes seen with prolonged bed rest. Based on this premise, the continuous passive motion (CPM) machine was developed to improve range of motion and tissue healing as well as decrease pain and edema following joint replacement or repair (Frank et al., 1984). It is our experience that the CPM machine can be applied to patients while in the ICU; it should not be considered a substitute for good bed positioning since CPM treatment to the lower extremity restricts the patient to lying supine. CPM therapy can be temporarily discontinued when postural drainage, bed positioning, or out-of-bed activities are necessary.

Exercise, ambulation, and altering a patient's bed position can have a profound effect on ventilation, particularly in the face of respiratory dysfunction as is often seen in the intensive care unit. It may even markedly reduce the need for chest physiotherapy. This is exemplified by the following case history:

Case History 6.1. A 17-year-old male was admitted with a cervical spine dislocation of C6. Initial respiratory dysfunction necessitated tracheal intubation and mechanical ventilation. Anatomical reduction of the spinal malalignment was established and maintained with a halo ring and cervical traction while on a Stryker frame. A manual muscle test following alignment revealed paralysis below C5 on the left and C6 on the right. For the first 2 weeks following admission, the patient's course was unremarkable. Chest roentgenograms remained free of pulmonary pathology, and chest physiotherapy was performed only prophylactically. Improved pulmonary capabilities allowed the patient to be extubated, following which a halo vest was applied to provide cervical stabilization. The patient was moved out of the ICU to a step-down unit. During this time the patient became progressively mentally depressed; watching television was his only interest.

Eighteen days following his injury the patient complained of shortness of breath and was tachypneic upon examination. A chest x-ray taken at that time demonstrated collapse of the left lung (see Fig. 6.2A), so chest physiotherapy was reinstituted. Prior to treatment, bronchial breath sounds were heard over the left upper lobe, while breath sounds were completely absent over the entire left lower lobe. The techniques used to treat this patient included segmental postural drainage, percussion, vibration, summed breathing and supportive coughing (as described in the preceding chapters). Due to the patient's dyspnea and fear, treatment was initially given to the anterior segment of the left upper lobe, the lingula and then the anterior segment of the left lower lobe. The patient tolerated the head-down position well but was unable to tolerate turning until the more anterior lung fields were clear to auscultation. During the 95 min of chest physiotherapy, all left lung segments were eventually treated as turning became better tolerated. However, the halo vest made percussion to the superior segment of the left lower lobe inadequate. Throughout the treatment, large amounts of sputum were expectorated, though no mucus plugs were noted. When breath sounds returned to normal, another chest x-ray was taken (see Fig. 6.2B).

During discussion after this treatment, it was discovered that the patient had been positioned either supine or lying on the left side, since this allowed him optimal viewing of his television. Subsequently, the television and the patient were both positioned from side to side (the patient was also placed prone and supine). These changes in the patient's daily care were enough to prevent further pulmonary complications throughout the rest of his hospital stay. There is little doubt that this incident and the need for vigorous chest physiotherapy could have been avoided altogether if adequate bed positioning and early patient mobilization had been performed.

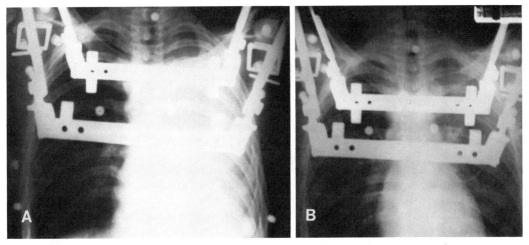

Figure 6.2. **(A)** A complete left lung atelectasis is shown in this radiograph taken just prior to treatment. **(B)** After 95 min of chest physiotherapy the left lung has cleared, and the diaphragmatic, hilar and superior mediastinal borders are visible. (The radiopaque device at the top of both x-rays is the metal portion of the halo vest. The rest of the vest is not apparent radiologically.)

Central nervous system injuries are often accompanied by abnormally increased muscular tone, which is seen particularly in the antigravity muscles of the neck, trunk, and limbs. When spasticity is present, the supine position is known to increase extensor tone (Bobath, 1974). Side-lying, as shown in Figure 6.3, has been found to diminish this abnormal tone (Peterkin, 1969). Although footboards and high-top tennis shoes are often recommended to prevent plantar flexion contractures, their use is discouraged in patients with upper motor neuron lesions. Footboards can often contribute to abnormal posturing by the patient, since they stimulate the plantar surface of the foot and can only be effectively used while the patient is supine. Tennis shoes do not maintain the ankle in neutral position and are associated with skin breakdown. Instead, passive positioning to maintain joint motion should be encouraged, particularly with the patient in the side-lying or prone position.

Serial casting is indicated to prevent

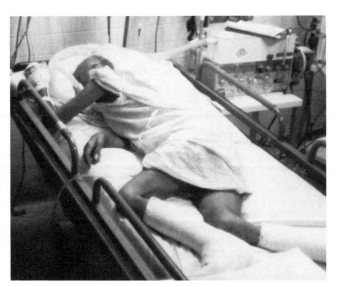

Figure 6.3. Side-lying is reported to decrease abnormal muscle tone in patients with central nervous system injuries. Despite requiring intracranial pressure monitoring and controlled mechanical ventilation, this patient demonstrates how range of motion can be altered passively.

contracture formation in brain-injured patients who demonstrate decreased ankle motion despite passive movement and positioning. Ankle casting can be used to maintain or regain functional joint position and may decrease abnormal muscle tone (see Fig. 6.3). For patients with severe head injury who were casted in the ICU, cylindrical casts are reported less likely to result in skin breakdown than bivalved casts (Imle et al., 1986). Dropout casts may also be used, particularly when casting is used along with muscle reeducation. Patients with peripheral nerve injuries or complete spinal cord lesions resulting in foot-drop may benefit from footboards. Splinting coordinated with range of motion exercises, is preferable to using a footboard with bedridden patients. Footboards are

usually fixed to the base of the bed. Therefore, when patients are moved toward the head of the bed or turned on the side, the footboard becomes nonfunctional. Ankle splints, on the other hand, are fixed to the patient and can provide joint support in all positions. Similarly, Stryker frames are fitted with adjustable footboards, which should be used to prevent foot-drop while the patient is supine (Fig. 6.4).

Quadriplegic and quadriparetic patients require specific bed positions to minimize or eliminate upper extremity contracture formation. Full shoulder external rotation and complete elbow extension are essential for wheelchair transfer activities in patients without triceps function. The Stryker frame can be easily adapted in the prone and supine

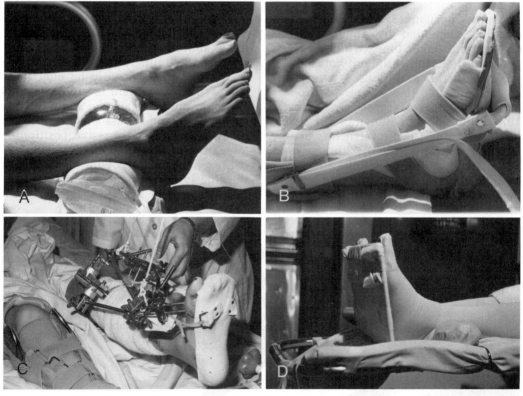

Figure 6.4. (**A**) Ankles passively assume plantar flexion in the bedridden patient. Though placing fluid bags under the ankles relieves calcaneal pressure, it can also accentuate plantar flexion. The footboard, just visible at the bottom of the bed, is of no benefit in maintaining dorsiflexion. (**B**) Splinting combined with passive ankle movement is effective in decreasing foot-drop in patients with peripheral nerve lesions. Prefabricated splints may be as effective and less expensive than custom-made splints. (**C**) A custom-made foot plate and metatarsal pins are used to maintain ankle and toe position in a patient with a peripheral nerve injury from an open compound tibial fracture. (**D**) The use of an adjustable footboard on a Stryker frame is helpful in maintaining ankle joint range.

positions for upper extremity placement. While the patient is in the prone position, the armboards can be moved as far cranially as necessary to maintain 90° shoulder abduction and full external rotation with elbow flexion. While the patient is in the supine position, placing the armboards caudally allows shoulder external rotation and full elbow extension (Fig. 6.5). Resting hand splints are also indicated initially, with complete neurological lesions above the C6–C7 level. Frequently, full elbow extension is difficult to maintain due to unopposed biceps activity. If this is the case, range of motion, exercises and positioning should stress maximal elbow extension as well as full movement of the other joints. Positioning of the shoulders and elbows to prevent contracture formation is a particular problem on the Roto rest bed (Imle and Boughton, 1987). Patients who are capable of independently performing upper limb range of motion exercises or functional activities do not require passive positioning to preserve adequate range of motion. For all complete neurological lesions, the ankles should be maintained as stated above; fluid bags under the ankle can reduce heel pressure effectively.

Wilson et al. (1974) found the range of motion capabilities, shown in Table 6.9, to be necessary for function in the quadriplegic patient. Guttman (1976) states that upper extremity contractures involving shoulder adduction and forearm pronation can be prevented in patients with spastic lesions of C5 and above. This is achieved by proper positioning of the arm in shoulder abduction and supination in the initial weeks following injury. While the quadriplegic patient is in the ICU, full, pain free range of motion should be preserved in both the upper and lower extremities. This can be done in conjunction with necessary chest physiotherapy maneuvers. Once the period of spinal shock is over, a more ac-

Table 6.9
Functional Ranges of Motion Necessary for Quadriplegic Patients [a]

Motion	C4,C5	C6
Shoulder		
Flexion	90°[b]	180°
Abduction	90°[b]	180°
Internal rotation	90°	70°
External rotation	30°	90°
Elbow		
Flexion	WNL,[c]150	WNL
Extension	0°	0°
Forearm		
Pronation	90°	
Supination	90°	
Wrist		
Flexion	40°	60°
Extension	40°	
Hip		
Flexion	95°	
Straight leg raises		100°[d]

[a]Adapted from Wilson et al. (1974).
[b]For C5 injured patients capable of using swivel bars for transfers, 160° of shoulder flexion and abduction are needed.
[c]WNL, within normal limits.
[d]Needed for dressing.

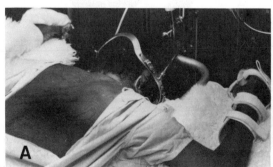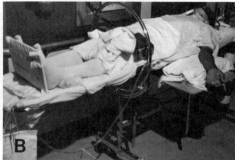

Figure 6.5. Quadriplegic patients require specific upper limb positioning to prevent contracture formation. The correct arm placement and use of resting splints while the patient is prone is illustrated in **A**. Proper extremity positioning of a supine patient is seen in **B**.

curate assessment of functional motor level and corresponding range of motion can be made. Our philosophy is in agreement with that of Etter (1968), who states that to save the life of a quadriplegic patient at the expense of further impairing already-limited function is to add an unnecessary burden to an already-devastating situation.

Passive range of motion should be maintained in bedridden patients. Once there is active participation in the desired motions, active exercising becomes possible. Because exercise increases both cardiovascular and respiratory demands, repetitive exercises to increase strength or endurance are not carried out in patients requiring high levels of FIO_2 and PEEP with mechanical ventilation and inotrophic support. However, these patients can perform active exercises; functional activities, such as rolling and positioning, should be encouraged (see Fig. 6.6). When the need for mechanical ventilation diminishes, more vigorous forms of exercise are possible even during bed restriction. Patients immobilized due to spinal fractures or skeletal traction are susceptible to respiratory problems and may benefit from active exercise programs. In addition to increasing range of motion, strength and endurance, these exercises may diminish the need for future chest physiotherapy.

Range of motion can be improved by the patient in two ways: stretching the area of limitation by actively contracting the opposing muscle groups or by passive stretch applied by another extremity.

The second method is particularly helpful in patients following thoracotomy who are hesitant to move their trunk and upper extremities. As a result, they are more likely to develop postural deformities and the frozen shoulder syndrome (Howell and Hill, 1972). To combat this, one arm may be used to assist the motion of the other, allowing increased shoulder mobility (shown in Fig. 6.7).

Strength may be improved by adding resistance to movement by using the effect of gravity (Fig. 6.8), manual resistance, or weights and pulleys. Weighted pulley systems allow resistance to be applied to motions that gravity normally assists (see Fig. 6.9), while weights alone increase the load applied by gravity (see Fig. 6.10). Manual resistance can be used to apply constant pressure throughout a wide range of movement or provide graded pressure at various points through an arch of motion. Pulleys may also be used to reduce the effect of gravity on a motion, thereby making it easier for the patient to actively achieve a greater range in a joint than would otherwise be possible (see Fig. 6.11). Endurance is improved by increasing the number of repetitions of any given exercise.

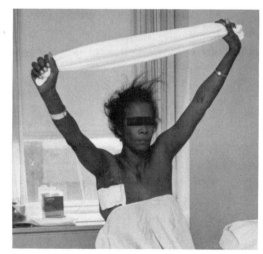

Figure 6.7. Following thoracic surgery, trunk and shoulder mobility must be encouraged to decrease deformity. By using a towel, this patient is able to assist her weaker arm (on the thoracotomy side) achieve increased range of motion.

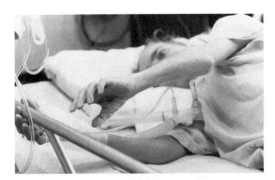

Figure 6.6. This mechanically ventilated patient is able to assist in her own bed positioning by using the side rails.

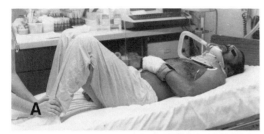
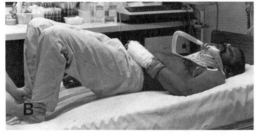

Figure 6.8. After sustaining an incomplete cervical spine injury, this patient exhibited upper extremity, trunk and pelvic weakness. Active hip extension with gravity acting to increase resistance is being performed in **A** and **B**.

Sitting

Patients can be passively positioned in a chair even during mechanical ventilation. Transferring a totally dependent patient to a chair usually involves a two-to-four-person lift (shown in Fig. 6.12). Chest tube connections, monitoring equipment, and intravascular lines should be checked to determine that there is sufficient slack before moving the patient. Patients should be temporarily disconnected from the mechanical ventilator while being transferred to prevent unnecessary trauma to the trachea. Some patients requiring lower extremity skeletal traction may transfer out of bed to a chair. Traction is maintained by a therapist as the patient performs a stand-pivot transfer or is lifted into the chair. The weights are then reconnected once the patient is seated, as in Figure 6.13.

Due to loss of sympathetic control, patients with spinal cord transection often

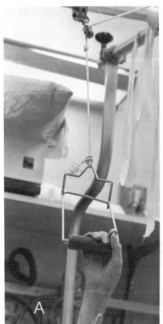
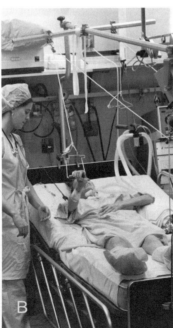
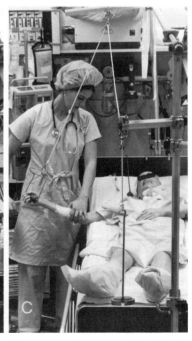

Figure 6.9. While supine, gravity normally assists shoulder and elbow extension, as well as shoulder horizontal abduction. Pulleys can be used to resist these motions. (**A**) A handle that allows movement through a wide range of motion is demonstrated. (**B**) Active shoulder and elbow extension is performed. (**C**) Instruction in horizontal abduction exercises is demonstrated.

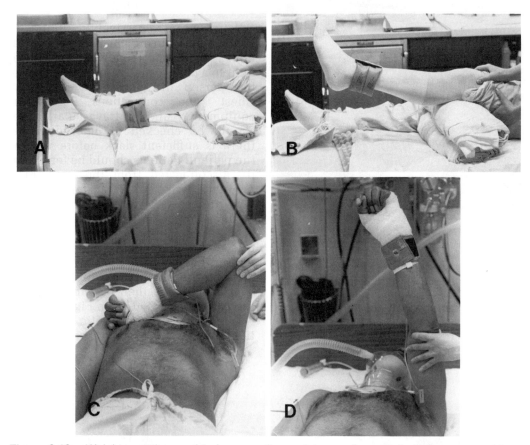

Figure 6.10.   Weights can be used to increase the resistance of gravity in both upper and lower limbs. Knee extensor muscles are being exercised in **A** and **B**. **C** and **D** demonstrate elbow extension exercises. Note that the presence of a left radial arterial line does not prohibit the use of cuff weights or exercise.

Figure 6.11.   The weight of orthopedic hardware or the strength required to move an extremity across bed linen may hinder active motion. Pulley systems can be used to decrease these effects, as illustrated in **A** and **B**, in which the patient performs active-assistive hip adduction and abduction.

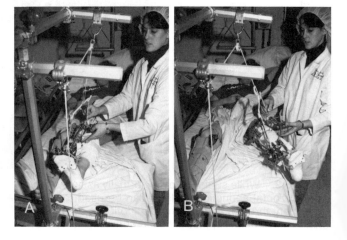

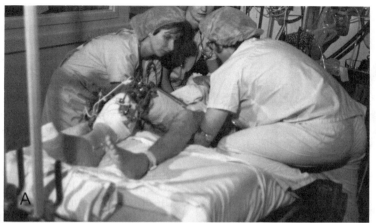

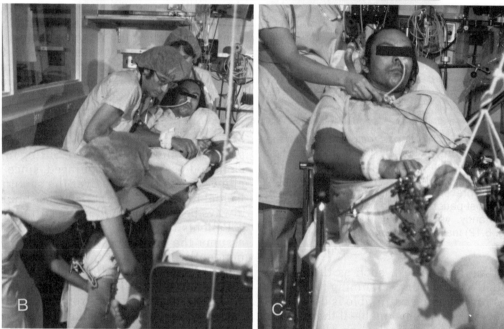

Figure 6.12. (A) Some patients are unable to assist with transfers because of their injuries. This patient sustained a severe brain injury and required abdominal surgery and orthopedic external fixation. To perform a dependent transfer, the patient is first moved to the side of the bed nearest the chair. Chairs may need to be placed on the same side of the bed as the mechanical ventilator to ensure adequate length of ventilator tubing. Elevation of the right leg is interrupted during the transfer. (B) With one person supporting the head and shoulders, another at the hips, and a third supporting the lower extremities, the patient can be lifted into a chair. Note that the patient is momentarily disconnected from the respirator during the transfer to minimize tracheal trauma. (C) As the patient is settled in the chair, mechanical ventilation is resumed and the right leg is again elevated to minimize edema.

exhibit hypotension when sitting is initiated. This response can be minimized by wrapping the lower extremities with elastic bandages from the toes to the groin before moving the patient. Abdominal binders or corsets may be used in patients with quadriplegia to provide trunk and abdominal support. When properly applied, binders may increase vital capacity, inspiratory capacity, and tidal volume, particularly when worn while sitting (Maloney, 1979; Goldman et al., 1986; McCool et al.,1986).

For patients who must spend a period

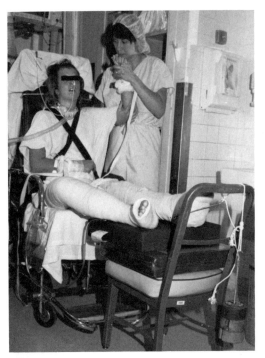

Figure 6.13. Traction is maintained while the patient is out of bed by placing the traction rope and weight over the back of a chair. The patient must be held securely in the seat at the hips to prevent slouching and loss of traction. For most patients, traction must be maintained constantly, yet extremity elevation (shown in Fig. 6.12) may be interrupted during a transfer.

of time on bed-rest, such as those with spinal cord injury, assuming the erect posture by using a tilt-table is described. However, it is questionable if there is any advantage, psychological or physical, to placing a patient who is not a candidate for ambulation in the standing position for short periods of time. Tilt-tables are not routinely found in the intensive care setting, are nearly as large as a bed, and can interfere with monitoring lines and equipment. Tilt-tables also maintain the lower limbs in a markedly dependent position, which may facilitate a hypotensive response. As a result, postponement of sitting, until a patient can be transported to a physiotherapy department having a tilt-table, may be detrimental and increase rehabilitation time. Instead, progressive sitting should begin in the ICU as soon as the patient with spinal cord injury is allowed to sit up. Following application of an abdominal binder and

elastic wraps (as described above), the head of the bed is elevated approximately 20°. In the absence of hypotension, the incline may be gradually increased until the limits of the bed are achieved. When this posture can be maintained for 30 min or longer, the patient is ready to be transferred to a reclining-back wheelchair. If at any stage the patient is unable to tolerate this progression to sitting, the head of the bed or back of the wheelchair may be reclined to an acceptable level. Initially, elevation of the lower extremities may be necessary. Once in a wheelchair, the time spent in this position may be increased by 30-minute intervals. Since skin sensation is decreased or absent, it is advisable to use a 4-inch high-density foam cushion to better distribute skin pressure and prevent decubitus ulcer formation. A cutout seat board may also be used to further reduce ischial weight bearing and improve trunk stability. Weight shifting from side to side or other methods of ischial pressure relief must be instituted. Sitting in a slouched position is discouraged, since it allows greater pressure over the sacrum. Ischial tuberosity and sacral areas should always be examined following sitting.

Patients in the ICU are encouraged to assume the sitting posture either independently or with assistance. Once a patient can maintain sitting balance over the side of the bed, as shown in Figure 6.14, transferring to and from a chair or bedside commode is possible. If a patient cannot coordinate moving from the bed to a chair, assistance may be necessary, as illustrated in Figure 6.15. Proper body mechanics should always be used by those persons transferring a patient. Assistive devices, such as a walker or overhead trapeze should be used as the patient's condition and the environment allow.

Once the patient is sitting, passive positioning or exercises may be performed to increase range of motion, strength or endurance. At rest, ankle joint motion should be passively maintained in a neutral position; footrests or stools may be helpful. Alternatively, if legs are elevated while the patient is sitting, tight hamstring or low back extensor muscles may be stretched passively. However, pa-

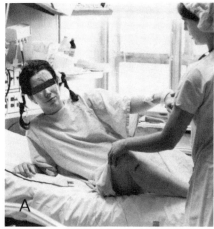
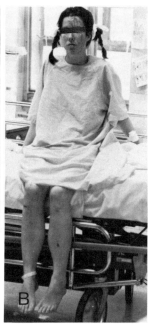
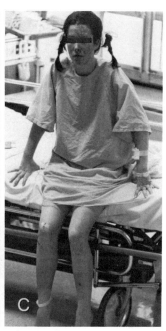

Figure 6.14. (**A**) Sitting up from a supine position may require assistance. Unassisted sitting balance (**B** and **C**) is necessary prior to performing independent transfers to a chair or bedside commode.

tients with increased extensor tone should be seated with the hips and knees in at least 90° of flexion to minimize this effect. Serial casting of the ankles may still be necessary. These patients also tend to demonstrate hip adductor tightness, which may be reduced by placing a rolled sheet or blanket between the patient's thighs. Again, slouched sitting should not be allowed. In addition to causing sacral pressure, it may result in increased trunk and lower extremity extensor tone and the likelihood of the patient sliding out of the chair. To encourage upright sitting and for patient safety, a securing strap can be placed across the hips and around the chair (it should not be positioned around the waist). Chair inserts are indicated for many patients with brain injury and abnormal muscle tone. The inserts should be fitted with adjustable trunk and head supports to improve sitting posture and stability. For patients with poor balance reactions, proper placement of a bedside table may provide additional trunk support, encourage normal equilibrium responses, and increase proprioceptive input by allowing some weight bearing through the elbows and shoulders (see Fig. 6.16).

Exercises to increase strength and endurance while the patient is sitting are similar to those described for use while the patient is bedridden. Weights or manual resistance may be used to increase the work being performed. Again, the effect of gravity can be used to increase resistance. Patients should be instructed to perform chair push-ups to relieve ischial tuberosity pressure and strengthen the upper extremities. Armrests are necessary to perform chair push-ups in which the patient bears minimal to total body weight on the armrests, then extends the elbows and depresses the shoulders, lifting the gluteal area from the seat of the chair. This exercise is especially beneficial for patients with spinal cord injury or those in whom future use of crutches or a walker is indicated.

Standing and Ambulating

When allowed, standing and ambulation should be encouraged. In general, patients who are unable to maintain sitting balance should not be expected to be able to walk without assistance. Standing balance is also a prerequisite for independent ambulation. For patients who cannot bear full weight on one lower extremity (for example, a patient with a lower limb fracture or soft-tissue injury), a walker or crutches may be used. Intra-

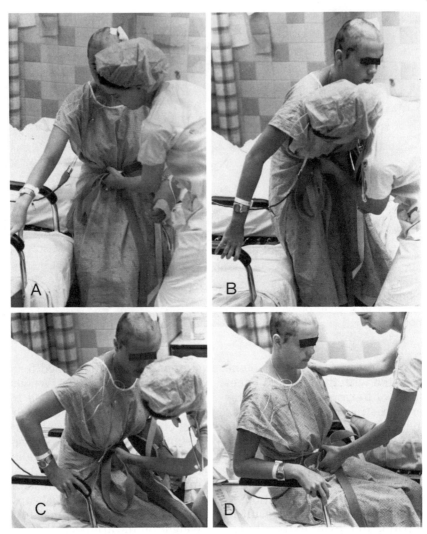

Figure 6.15. Following a craniotomy and upper extremity fracture, this patient requires assistance in transferring to a chair. (**A**) The therapist prepares to support the patient at the waist by means of a belt as the patient grasps the far armrest of the chair. (**B**) The patient stands with the support of the therapist and pivots until the chair is directly behind. (**C** and **D**) The therapist assists in lowering the patient onto the chair and then moving the hips back into the chair.

vascular lines do not prevent ambulation; they may be attached to a rolling intravenous (IV) pole. Electrocardiogram leads and arterial or central venous pressure lines may be temporarily disconnected from the recording module during ambulation. At the physician's discretion, chest tubes and abdominal sumps may be disconnected from wall suction to allow increased mobilization (see Fig. 6.17). As in other situations, collection bags from indwelling urinary catheters are always kept lower than the bladder.

They may be fixed to the base of the rolling pole or walker during ambulation (see Fig. 6.18). The need for supplemental oxygen or humidity does not hinder mobilization. Oxygen tanks with added humidification (as used in the transportation of patients) may be secured to a standard walker or IV pole (see Fig. 6.19). Walkers that provide attachments for oxygen tanks are available commercially; walkers fitted with IV poles, oxygen and respirators have been described in the literature (Burns and Jones, 1975).

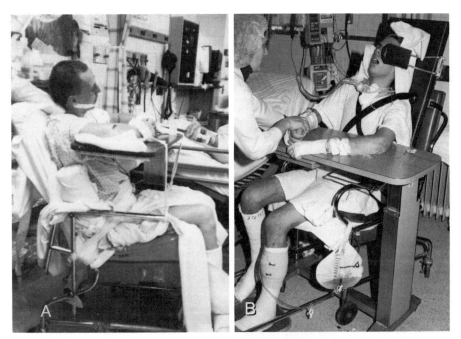

Figure 6.16. **(A)** The chair back is reclined to provide increased trunk support, yet 90° of hip and knee flexion are maintained by using a wedge in the seat and a roll under the feet. A bedside table is placed uner the arms and raised to provide greater trunk and shoulder stability, thereby improving the patient's head control. A sheet is tied across the hips for safety and to prevent slouching. **(B)** A seat insert is used for patients requiring additional support. Chest cross straps are applied in addition to a seat belt and lateral head supports are used. An effort is made to provide optimal support for the brain-injured patient during sitting. The goal is to decrease abnormal posture and muscle tone in order to allow more normal movement and respiratory patterns.

It has been our experience that early mobilization of patients often diminishes the need for long or vigorous chest physiotherapy. Spontaneous coughing following exercise or exertion is common, and chest physiotherapy usually is not needed once routine walking is possible. In reviewing the study by Howell and Hill, it was noted that increased patient mobilization, following open heart surgery, coincided with a decreased need for chest physiotherapy. This same principle is alluded to by Sternweiler (1968) in the physiotherapy treatment of a patient following heart transplantation. A day after the patient was allowed to sit up, lung bases showed increased air entry and were free of crackles for the first time.

Chulay et al. (1982) reported a decrease in postoperative fever and ICU stay in patients who were turned every 2 hrs for the first day after coronary artery bypass surgery. In a similar patient population, neither deep breathing exercises nor incentive spirometry demonstrated benefit over the effects of early patient mobilization (Dull and Dull, 1983). Likewise, Frolund and Madsen (1986) found no added benefit from positive expiratory pressure over chest physiotherapy that primarily consisted of early mobilization and breathing exercises in 75 patients after thoracotomy. Both bed mobility and ambulation were included in the chest physiotherapy regimen used by Warren and Grimwood (1980). They reported fewer pulmonary complications in cholecystectomy patients who received chest physiotherapy. Patients undergoing hysterectomy who received breathing exercises toward maximal inspiration were found to have no additional benefit compared to those encouraged to breathe deeply and to ambulate (Giroux et al., 1987). Similarly, Schwieger et al. (1986) reported no added benefit from incentive

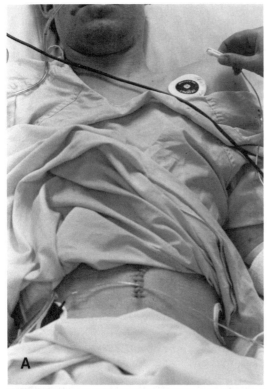

Figure 6.17. **(A)** In preparation for ambulation, electrocardiogram leads may be disconnected from the recording patches. **(B)** If arterial or central venous pressure catheters are used, the transducers can usually be unplugged from the manifold while the patient is walking. **(C)** Abdominal sumps or drains may also be disconnected from suction for short periods of time.

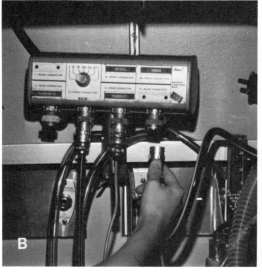

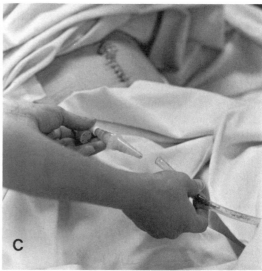

spirometry in 40 patients who were mobilized on the same day as their cholecystectomy. From these studies it appears that early patient mobilization, including ambulation, is a good form of prophylaxis against postoperative secretion retention.

For physical therapists, it is a routine finding that mobilizing a patient (from supine to sidelying or out of bed to a chair) often leads to spontaneous coughing and improved breath sounds. In some instances, retained secretions and their sequelae are unresponsive to both chest physiotherapy and other methods of clearance, yet pulmonary improvement

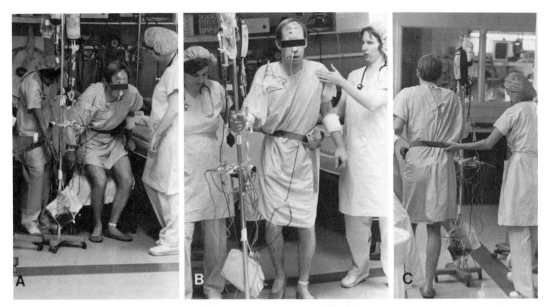

Figure 6.18. (A) Intravascular fluid bags are secured to a rolling IV pole prior to ambulation. Note that the urine collection bag is attached to the pole below the level of the bladder. (B) Proper posture is encouraged in this patient following surgery for liver lacerations and a ruptured diaphragm and spleen. (C) The patient's balance is controlled by using a waist belt while walking.

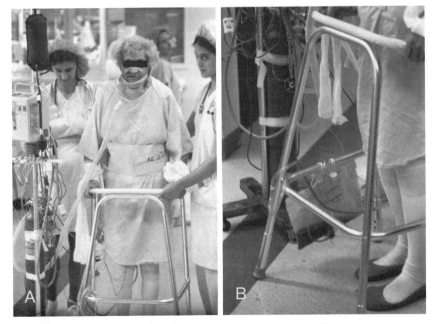

Figure 6.19. (A) Patients requiring supplemental oxygen and humidity can be ambulated. Walkers are helpful in improving patient stability, especially in the elderly and debilitated. (B) Oxygen tanks can be secured to rolling IV poles, as shown. The urine collection bag can also be attached to a walker below the level of the bladder.

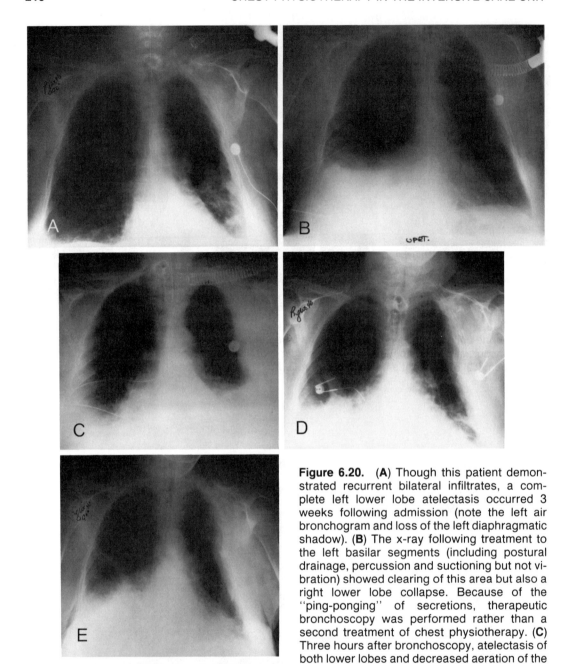

Figure 6.20. (A) Though this patient demonstrated recurrent bilateral infiltrates, a complete left lower lobe atelectasis occurred 3 weeks following admission (note the left air bronchogram and loss of the left diaphragmatic shadow). (B) The x-ray following treatment to the left basilar segments (including postural drainage, percussion and suctioning but not vibration) showed clearing of this area but also a right lower lobe collapse. Because of the "ping-ponging" of secretions, therapeutic bronchoscopy was performed rather than a second treatment of chest physiotherapy. (C) Three hours after bronchoscopy, atelectasis of both lower lobes and decreased aeration of the left lung were radiologically apparent. None of these events corresponded with temperature elevations. Throughout the following week the patient's chest roentgenogram remained as shown in **D**. Once the patient no longer required mechanical ventilation, the tracheostomy tube was removed, and walking was encouraged. (E) The following chest x-ray demonstrates improved aeration of both lung fields despite fluid persisting in the right major fissure.

has been noted to follow increased patient mobility. This is demonstrated by the following case history:

Case History 6.2. A 77-year-old-female was admitted following an automobile accident. Di-

agnoses of a closed head injury with intracerebral hemorrhage, bilateral multiple rib fractures with left flail chest, extrapleural hematoma, and fractured left clavicle were made. Respiratory management included tracheal intubation and use of intermittent mandatory ventilation with positive end-expiratory pressure throughout the patient's 1 month stay in the critical care unit. Neurological improvement was satisfactory, but generalized weakness resulted. During this same interval, intermittent infiltrates were present in both lung bases radiologically. These cleared periodically with chest physiotherapy and were unresponsive to fiberoptic bronchoscopy (see Fig. 6.20A–C). Although the patient was turned routinely and allowed to sit in a bedside chair, walking was not encouraged until ventilatory support was discontinued. On the same day that the patient began breathing independently, her tracheostomy tube was removed; the stoma was covered with an occlusive dressing. Cough effectiveness increased and ambulation with a walker also commenced. Subsequent roentgenograms showed increased aeration of both lower lobes (see Fig. 6.20D–E). Continued radiological evidence of improvement coincided with increased ambulation and mobilization of the patient.

Equipment Used for Mobilization

Minimal supplies, in addition to equipment normally found in an intensive care setting, are necessary to maximize patient mobilization. Plastic intravenous infusion bags, as well as cuff and dumbbell weights can be used to provide resistive exercises. Cuff weights are advantageous, when available, because they are easily applied and cannot be dropped by the patient. However, they are not a necessity. Pulley systems can be adapted from standard overhead traction units, along with the ropes, weights and pulleys normally utilized in applying orthopedic traction. Safety belts, used for transferring patients to a chair or when assisting ambulation, are available commercially and can be used repeatedly. Adjustable walkers and crutches can be measured and altered to fit different patients. Rolling IV poles and sources of supplemental oxygen and humidity are available to any ICU. Reclining-back wheelchairs with elevating leg rests are helpful for improving sitting tolerance in patients who demonstrate orthostatic hypotension. For facilities that normally treat patients with spinal cord and head injury, high-back chairs and adjustable inserts are recommended to increase trunk and head support.

SUMMARY

Physiological alterations and secondary disabilities occur with immobilization. In patients requiring intensive medical care, mobilization is found to be both possible and advantageous. With foresight, optimal patient mobility can be achieved without interruption of monitoring or life-sustaining equipment. Passive range of motion, postural changes and even active exercise can be incorporated into the care of the critically ill patient to minimize the detrimental effects of bed rest. Limited additional supplies are needed to provide these aspects of patient care. It should be emphasized that the methods of patient mobilization that are outlined not only counteract the complications addressed at the beginning of this chapter, but also decrease rehabilitation time and, therefore, the total hospital stay of a patient.

References

Akeson WH: An experimental study of joint stiffness. J Bone Joint Surg [Am] 43:1022–1034, 1961

Akeson WH, Woo SL, Amiel D, Coutts RD, Daniel D: The connective tissue response to immobility: Biochemical changes in periarticular connective tissue of the immobilized rabbit knee. Clin Orthop 93:356–362, 1973

Akeson WH, Woo SL, Amiel D, Matthews JV: Biomechanical and biochemical changes in the periarticular connective tissue during contracture development in the immobilized rabbit knee. Connect Tissue Res 2:315–323, 1974

Amiel D, Woo SL, Harwood FL, Akeson WH: The effect of immobilization on collagen turnover in connective tissue: A biochemical-biomechanical correlation. Acta Orthop Scand 53:325–332, 1982

Bassey EJ, Fentem PH: Extent of deterioration in physical condition during postoperative bedrest and its reversal by rehabilitation. Br Med J 4:194–196, 1974

Beckett WS, Vroman NB, Nigro D, Thompson-Gorman S, Wilkerson JE, Fortney SM: Effect of prolonged bed rest on lung volume in normal individuals. J Appl Physiol 61: 919–925, 1986

Behrakis PK, Baydur A, Jaeger MJ, Milic-Emili J: Lung mechanics in sitting and horizontal body positions. Chest 83:643–646, 1983

Bendixen HH: Editoral Comment. Arch Surg 109:541, 1974

Birkhead NC, Haupt GJ, Myers RN: Effect of prolonged bedrest on cardiodynamics. Am J Med Sci 245:118–119, 1963

Bobath B: Adult Hemiplegia: Evaluation and Treatment, p. 79. William Heinemann Medical Books, London, 1974

Boganchenko VP: State of psychic activity in subjects during prolonged confinement to bed. Probl

Kosm Biol 13:171–174, 1969 (as cited in Greenleaf et al., 1976)

Brannon EW, Rockwood CA, Potts P: The influence of specific exercise in the prevention of debilitating musculoskeletal disorders: Implication in physiological conditioning for prolonged weightlessness. *Aerospace Med* 34:900–906, 1963

Browse NL: *The Physiology and Pathology of Bedrest*, pp 29–31, 159–190. Charles C Thomas, Springfield, IL, 1965

Burkhart JM, Jowsey J: Parathyroid and thyroid hormones in development of immobilization osteoporosis. *Endocrinology* 81:1053–1062, 1967

Burns JR, Jones FL: Early ambulation of patients requiring ventilatory assistance (letter). *Chest* 68:608, 1975

Cardus D: O$_2$ alveolar-arterial tension difference after 10 days recumbency in man. *J Appl Physiol* 23:934–937, 1967

Chase GA, Grave C, Rowell LB: Independence of changes in functional and performance capacities attending prolonged bedrest. *Aerospace Med* 37:1232–1238, 1966

Chulay M, Brown J, Summer W: Effect of postoperative immobilization after coronary artery bypass surgery. *Crit Care Med* 10:176–179, 1982

Clauss RH, Scalabrini BY, Ray, JF, Reed GE: Effects of changing body positions upon improved ventilation-perfusion relationships. *Circ (Suppl 2)* 37:214–218, 1968

Craig DB, Wahba WM, Don H: Airway closure and lung volumes in surgical positions. *Can Anaesth Soc J* 18:92–99, 1971

Craig JO, Bromley LL, Williams R: Thoracotomy and the contralateral lung. A study of the changes occurring in the dependent and contralateral lung during and after thoracotomy in lateral decubitus. *Thorax* 17:9–15, 1962

Dalen JE, Paraskos JA, Ockene IS, Alpert JS, Hirsh J: Venous thromboembolism scope of the problem. *Chest* 89(Suppl):370S–373S, 1986

Deitrick JE, Whedon GD, Shorr E, Toscani V, Davis VB: Effects of immobilization upon various metabolic and physiologic functions of normal men. *Am J Med* 4:3–36, 1948

Donaldson CL, Hulley SB, McMillan DE, Hattner RW, Bayers JH: The effect of prolonged simulated non-gravitational environment on mineral balance in the adult male. *NASA Contract* CR-108314, 1969

Dull JL, Dull WL: Are maximal inspiratory breathing exercises or incentive spirometry better than early patient mobilization after cardiopulmonary bypass? *Phys Ther* 63:655–659, 1983

Enneking WF, Horowitz M: The intra-articular effects of immobilization on the human knee. *J Bone Joint Surg [Am]* 54:973–985, 1972

Estenne M, Yernault J, DeTroyer A: Rib cage and diaphragm-abdomen compliance in humans: Effects of age and posture. *J Appl Physiol* 59:1842–1848, 1985

Etter MF: *Exercise for the Prone Patient*, p 7. Wayne State University Press, Detroit, 1968

Frank C, Akeson WH, Woo SL, Amiel D, Dip.Ing MS, Coutts RD: Physiology and therapeutic value of passive joint motion. *Clin Orthop Rel Res* 185:113–125, 1984

Friman G: Effect of clinical bedrest for seven days on physical performance. *Acta Med Scand* 205:389–393, 1979

Frolund L, Madsen F: Self-administered prophylactic postoperative positive expiratory pressure in thoracic surgery. *Acta Anaesthesiol Scand* 30:381–385, 1986

Georgiyevskiy VS, Mikhaylov BM: Effect of hypokinesia on human circulation. *Kosm Biol Aviakosm Med* 2:48–51, 1968 (as cited in Greenleaf et al.)

Giroux JM, Lewis S, Holland LG, Black EE, Gow SA, Langlotz JM, Pomfret ME, Vanderkooy CL: Postoperative chest physiotherapy for abdominal hysterectomy patients. *Physioth Can* 39:89–93, 1987

Glazier JB, Hughes JM, Maloney JE, West JB: Vertical gradient of alveolar size in lungs of dogs frozen intact. *J Appl Physiol* 23:694–705, 1967

Goldberg AL: Mechanisms of growth and atrophy of skeletal muscle. In *Muscle Biology*, edited by RG Cassens, pp 89–118. Marcel Dekker, New York, 1972

Goldman JM, Rose LS, Williams SJ, Silver JR, Denison DM. Effect of abdominal binders on breathing in tetraplegic patients. *Thorax* 41:940–945, 1986

Greenleaf JE, Kozlowski S: Physiological consequences of reduced physical activity during bed rest. *Exerc Sport Sci Rev* 10:84–119, 1982

Greenleaf JE, Greenleaf CJ, Van Derveer D, Dorchak KJ: Adaptation to prolonged bedrest in men: A compendium of research. *NASA Tech Memo* TMX-3307, 1976

Grossman MR, Rose SJ, Sahrmann SA, Katholi CR: Length and circumference measurements in one-joint and multijoint muscles in rabbits after immobilization. *Phys Ther* 66:516–520, 1986

Guttman L: *Spinal Cord Injuries: Comprehensive Management and Research*, 2nd ed, p 565. Blackwell Scientific Publications, Oxford, 1976

Hammer RL, Kenan EH: The psychological aspects of immobilization. In *The Immobilized Patient*, edited by FV Steinberg, pp 123–149. Plenum Medical Book Company, New York, 1980

Hansson TH, Roos BO, Nachemson A: Development of osteopenia in the fourth lumbar vertebrae during prolonged bed rest after operation for scoliosis. *Acta Orthop Scand* 46:621–630, 1975

Heilskov NC, Schoriheyder F: Creatinuria due to immobilization in bed. *Acta Med Scand* 151:51–56, 1955 (as cited in Greenleaf et al.)

Heron W, Bexton WH, Hebb DO: Cognitive effects of a decreased variation to the sensory environment. *Am Psychol* 8:366, 1953

Hirschberg GG, Lewis L, Vaughan P: Promoting patient mobility and other ways to prevent secondary disabilities. *Nursing '77* 7:42–46, 1977

Howell S, Hill JD: Acute respiratory care in the open heart surgery patient. *Phys Ther* 52:253–260, 1972

Hulley SB, Vogel JM, Donaldson CL, Bayers JH, Friedman RJ, Rosen SN: The effect of supplemental oral phosphate on the bone mineral changes during prolonged bedrest. *J Clin Invest* 50:2506–2518, 1971

Imle PC, Eppinghaus CE, Boughton AB: Efficacy of non-bivalved and bivalved serial casting on head injured patients in intensive care (abstract). *Phys Ther* 66:748, 1986

Imle PC, Boughton AC: The physical therapist's role in the early management of acute spinal cord injury. *Top Acute Care Trauma Rehabil* 1:32–47, 1987

Kottke FJ: The effects of limitation of activity upon the human body. *JAMA* 196:825–830, 1966

Krasnykh IG: Influence of prolonged hypodynamia on heart size and the functional state of the myocardium. *Probl Kosm Biol* 13:65–71, 1969 (as cited in Greenleaf et al.)

Krolner B, Toft B: Vertebral boneloss: An unheeded side effect of therapeutic bed rest. *Clin Sci* 64:537–540, 1983

Lamb LE, Johnson RL, Stevens PM, Welsh BE: Cardiovascular deconditioning from space cabin simulator confinement. *Aerospace Med* 35:420–428, 1964

Lambert RL, Willauer G, Dasch FW: Postoperative status of dependent lung. *J Thorac Cardiovasc Surg* 30:713–718, 1955

LeBlanc P, Ruff F, Milic-Emili J: Effects of age and body position on "airway closure" in man. *J Appl Physiol* 28:448–451, 1970

Lopes J, Russell DM, Whitwell J, Jeejeebhoy KN: Skeletal muscle function in malnutrition. *Am J Clin Nutr* 36:602–610, 1982

Mack PB, Montgomery KB: Study of nitrogen balance and creatine and creatinine excretion during recumbency and ambulation of five young adult human males. *Aerospace Med* 44:739–746, 1973

Mackenzie CF, Shin B, Fisher R, Cowley RA: Two-year mortality in 760 patients transported by helicopter direct from the road accident scene. *Am Surg* 45:101–108, 1979

Maloney FP: Pulmonary function in quadriplegia: Effects of a corset. *Arch Phys Med Rehabil* 60:261–265, 1979

McCool FD, Pichurko BM, Slutsky AS, Sarkarati M, Rossier A, Brown R: Changes in lung volume and rib cage configuration with abdominal binding in quadriplegia. *J Appl Physiol* 60:1198–1202, 1986

Oldenburg FA, Dolovich MB, Montgomery JM, Newhouse MT: Effects of postural drainage, exercise and cough on mucus clearance in chronic bronchitis. *Am Rev Respir Dis* 120:739–745, 1979

Patel AN, Razzak ZA, Dastur DK: Disuse atrophy of human skeletal muscles. *Arch Neurol* 20:413–421, 1969

Peacock EE: Comparison of collagenous tissue surrounding normal and immobilized joints. *Surg Forum* 14:440–441, 1963

Peterkin HW: The neuromuscular system and the re-education of movement. *Physiotherapy* 55:145–153, 1969

Petukhov BN, Purakhin YN: Effect of prolonged bedrest on cerebral biopotentials of healthy subjects. *Kosm Biol Med* 2:56–61, 1968 (as cited in Greenleaf et al.)

Ray JF, Yost L, Moallemsanoudos GM, Villamena P, Paredes RM, Clauss RH: Immobility, hypoxemia, and pulmonary arteriovenous shunting. *Arch Surg* 109:537–541, 1974

Reed JH, Wood EH: Effect of body position on vertical distribution of pulmonary blood flow. *J Appl Physiol* 28:303–311, 1970

Riska EB, von Bonsdorff H, Hakkinen S, Jaroma H, Kiviluoto O, Paavilainen T: Primary operative

fixation of long bone fractures in patients with multiple injuries. *J Trauma* 17:111–121, 1977

Ryback RS, Lewis OF, Lessard CS: Psychobiologic effects of prolonged bed rest (weightless) in young, healthy volunteers (study II). *Aerospace Med* 42:529–535, 1971

Saltin B, Blomqvist G, Mitchell HH, Johnson RL Jr, Wildenthal K, Chapman CB: Response to exercise after bed rest and after training. A longitudinal study of adaptive changes in oxygen transport and body composition. *Circ (Suppl 7)* 38:1–78, 1968

Schwieger I, Gamulin Z, Forster A, Meyer P, Gemperle M, Suter PM: Absence of benefit of incentive spirometry in low-risk patients undergoing elective cholecystectomy. *Chest* 89:652–656, 1986

Sevitt S, Gallagher N: Venous thrombosis and pulmonary embolism. A clinicopathological study in injured and burned patients. *Br J Surg* 48:475–489, 1961

Spencer WA, Vallbona C, Carter RE: Physiologic concepts of immobilization. *Arch Phys Med Rehab* 46:89–100, 1965

Sternweiler MR: Physiotherapy and the South African heart transplant patient. *Phys Ther* 48:1399–1408, 1968

Stremel RW, Convertino VA, Bernauer EM, Greenleaf JE: Cardiorespiratory deconditioning with static and dynamic leg exercise during bedrest. *J Appl Physiol* 41:905–909, 1976

Svanberg L: Influence of posture on the lung volumes, ventilation and circulation in normals. *Scand J Clin Lab Invest* 25(Suppl):7–17, 1957

Taylor HL, Erickson L, Henschel A, Keys A: Effect of bedrest on the blood volume of normal young men. *Am J Physiol* 144:227–232, 1945

Taylor HL, Henschel A, Brozek J, Keys A: Effects of bedrest on cardiovascular function and work performance. *J Appl Physiol* 2:223–239, 1949

Triebwasser JH, Fasola AF, Stewart A, Lancaster MC: The effect of exercise on the preservation of orthostatic tolerance during prolonged immobilization. *Aerospace Med Assoc Preprints* 65–66, 1970

Vellody VP, Nassery M, Druz WS, Sharp JT: Effects of body position change on thoracoabdominal motion. *J Appl Physiol* 45:581–589, 1978

Vogt FB, Mack PB, Johnson PC, Wade L: Tilt table response and blood volume changes associated with fourteen days of recumbency. *Aerospace Med* 38:43–48, 1967

Wade OL, Gilson JC: The effect of posture on diaphragmatic movement and vital capacity in normal subjects with a note on spirometry as an aid in determining radiological chest volumes. *Thorax* 6:103–126, 1951

Ward RJ, Tolas AG, Benveniste RJ, Hansen JM, Bonica JJ: Effect of posture on normal arterial blood gas tensions in the aged. *Geriatrics* 21:139–143, 1966

Warren CPW, Grimwood M: Pulmonary disorders and physiotherapy in patients who undergo cholecystectomy. *Can J Surg* 23:384–386, 1980

Wenger NK: Early ambulation: The physiologic basis revisited. *Adv Cardiol* 31:138–141, 1982

Wilson DJ, McKenzie MW, Barber LM: *Spinal Cord*

Injury—A Treatment Guide for Occupational Therapists, p 24. CB Slack, Thorofare, NJ, 1974

Yeremin AV, Bazhanov VV, Marishchuk VL, Stepantsov VI, Dzhamgarov TT: Physical conditioning for man under conditions of prolonged hypodynamia. *Probl Kosm Biol* 13:192–199, 1969 (as cited in Greenleaf et al.)

Zubeck JP, MacNeill M: Effects of immobilization: Behavioural and EEG changes. *Can J Psychol* 20:316–336, 1966

Zubeck JP, Wilgosh L: Prolonged immobilization of the body: Changes in performance and in the electroencephalogram. *Science* 140:306–308, 1963

CHAPTER 7

Physiological Changes Following Chest Physiotherapy

Colin F. Mackenzie, M.B., Ch.B., F.F.A.R.C.S.

In this chapter the author's investigational approach to clinical measurement of the effects of chest physiotherapy is described, and the problems encountered are discussed. As a result of this experience and that of others, some generally accepted statements concerning chest physiotherapy are enumerated and possible mechanisms for chest physiotherapy action are postulated. The 1974 and 1979 American Thoracic Society-sponsored conferences on the scientific basis of respiratory therapy are summarized, and their conclusions concerning the requirements and methods of physiological measurement are discussed.

The need for objective assessment of maneuvers designed to remove secretions from the tracheobronchial tree is apparent from the variety of techniques and claims described in the literature. The ever-rising cost of these maneuvers and their increasing contribution to the overall cost of medical care make investigation of their benefits of great economic importance. However, before objective assessment can be made, the best indicators of beneficial change following these maneuvers must be decided. Once these indicators are identified, the factors that influence their measurement can be considered.

THE EFFECTS OF CHEST PHYSIOTHERAPY

Arterial Oxygenation in Mechanically Ventilated Patients

In 1975–76, 47 patients who were mechanically ventilated with positive end-expiratory pressure (PEEP) (5–10 cm H_2O) were prospectively studied before and after chest physiotherapy, to determine changes in arterial oxygenation (Mackenzie et al., 1978a). The 47 patients showed a variety of chest x-ray changes before therapy, including atelectasis, pneumonia, or lung contusion. Eight of the 47 patients were nontrauma cases and had multiple pathology, as can be seen in Table 7.1. The 39 patients who suffered trauma also showed other pathology, such as chronic lung or heart disease, but it was found less frequently than in the nontrauma group. No significant changes in partial pressure of arterial oxygen (PaO_2) could be found after analysis using the paired t-test (Fig. 7.1). There was also no difference in PaO_2 before and after physiotherapy, between patients with or without trauma or between those treated with or without head-down postural drainage.

For the last 14 patients studied, PaO_2 and total lung/thorax compliance (C_T) were simultaneously measured. The raw compliance data are shown in Table 7.2. As can be seen from the raw data, C_T rose immediately following chest physiotherapy in 8 of the 14 patients, in 1 patient there was no increase, and in 4 patients the increase did not take place until 1.5 hr after therapy ceased. The relationship of PaO_2 and C_T to an approximation of intrapulmonary shunt, partial pressure of arterial oxygen/fractional inspired oxygen (PaO_2/FIO_2), for the same 14 patients is shown in Figure 7.2. A PaO_2/FIO_2 of 250 is approximately equivalent to a 15% intrapulmonary shunt. A shunt of less than 15% (greater than 250 PaO_2/FIO_2) is one of the prerequisites often used for weaning from mechanical ventilation. It appears from the data that in some patients, PaO_2/FIO_2 is increased to above 250 with chest physiotherapy. If these indicators are used to determine the need for mechanical ventilation, chest physiotherapy should reduce the duration of mechanical support.

All of the 47 patients studied to determine PaO_2 changes also had portable chest x-rays taken before chest physiotherapy. Radiological follow-up occurred within 38 hr in all instances, although in the majority, chest x-ray was taken within 6 hr of the completion of chest physiotherapy. Unilobar lung pathology showed radiological improvement in 74% (20/27) and multilobar pathology improvement in 60% (12/20). These findings are similar to those obtained by fiberoptic bronchoscopy in patients resistant to routine respiratory therapy (Lindholm et al., 1974) and demonstrate that by using either technique, a localized lesion is more easily changed than a generalized one.

Although most of this information is not novel, it confirms our clinical impression that in patients who are mechanically ventilated with PEEP, chest physiotherapy produces radiological improvement without causing hypoxemia. There is, therefore, a very definite place for this therapy in the management of critically ill patients in whom the hypoxemia and hemodynamic changes associated with and occurring following bronchoscopy might be hazardous

Table 7.1
Other Pathological States Found in Trauma and Nontrauma Patients Treated with Chest Physiotherapy

Patient	Number	Mean Age (yr)	Male/ Female Ratio	Chronic Lung Disease	Renal Failure	Septic Shock	Chronic Heart Disease	Diabetes
Trauma	39	36	36/3	4	1	1	1	1
Nontrauma[a]	8	64	6/2	2	4	3	5	

[a]Multiple pathology present in nontrauma group.

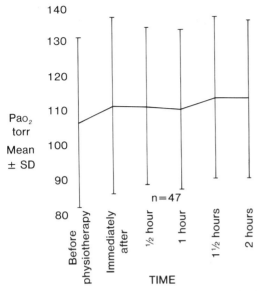

Figure 7.1. Arterial oxygen tension levels before and after chest physiotherapy. (From C. F. Mackenzie et al.: *Anesthesia and Analgesia (Cleveland)* 57:28–30, 1978a.)

(Lundgren et al., 1982). It appears that chest x-ray appearance improved equally successfully with chest physiotherapy as fiberoptic bronchoscopy in expert hands. This finding was confirmed by others (Marini et al., 1979). It was not known whether the falls in arterial oxygenation that were reported by others to occur following chest physiotherapy could be reversed by the use of PEEP.

Arterial Oxygenation in Spontaneously Breathing Patients

To determine if mechanical ventilation and PEEP were factors altering arterial oxygenation, 17 spontaneously breathing patients were studied before and after chest physiotherapy. All patients had indwelling arterial lines and were recovering from trauma. Six were breathing room air; the remainder received oxygen by face hood. No patient breathed with elevation of airway pressure above ambient pressure. Indications for chest physiotherapy included segmental atelectasis (7 patients), infiltrates (6 patients), lung contusion (3 patients), and pneumonia (1 patient). With the patient lying supine in bed, arterial blood gases (ABGs) were sampled before and immediately after chest physiotherapy and at half-hourly intervals for up to 2 hr after therapy. Figure 7.3 shows that there was no statistically significant change in arterial oxygenation. However, it is of interest to note that there is a larger standard deviation in PaO_2 values after therapy than before therapy. This suggests that the trend of unchanged arterial oxygenation in spontaneously breathing patients was not as obvious as in the patient who was mechanically ventilated with PEEP (Fig. 7.1). In the latter group, standard deviation progressively decreased, indicating conformity to the trend. This diversity in

Table 7.2
Raw C_T Data (ml/cm H_2O) in 14 Patients before, Immediately after, and for Half-Hourly Intervals for 2 hr after Chest Physiotherapy

Patient Number	Before Physiotherapy	Immediately after Physiotherapy	After Physiotherapy				Diagnosis
			0.5 hr	1 hr	1.5 hr	2 hr	
33	22	24	24	24	29	29	Pneumonia
34	33	43	35	43	43	43	Contusion
35	47	54	50	54	50	57	Pneumonia
36	47	47	48	75	75	54	Chronic lung disease
37	70	65	65	65	70	70	Atelectasis
38	52	65	56	56	56	56	Contusion
39	40	40	37	37	43	52	Atelectasis
40	40	37	37	37	52	52	Contusion
41	44	55	68	55	68	55	Contusion
43	47	62	51	51	51	51	Atelectasis
44	35	38	38	43	43	47	Atelectasis
45	38	38	38	38	41	41	Atelectasis
46	41	44	47	54	44	41	Contusion
47	58	43	58	58	72	72	Atelectasis

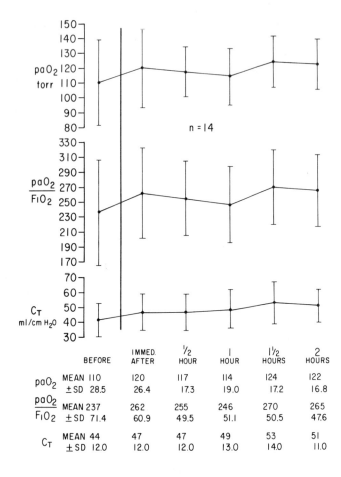

Figure 7.2. Simultaneous PaO_2, C_T, and PaO_2/FIO_2 for 14 mechanically ventilated patients before, immediately after, and at half-hourly intervals for 2 hr after chest physiotherapy.

		BEFORE	IMMED. AFTER	1/2 HOUR	1 HOUR	1 1/2 HOURS	2 HOURS
paO_2	MEAN	110	120	117	114	124	122
	±SD	28.5	26.4	17.3	19.0	17.2	16.8
$\dfrac{paO_2}{FIO_2}$	MEAN	237	262	255	246	270	265
	±SD	71.4	60.9	49.5	51.1	50.5	47.6
C_T	MEAN	44	47	47	49	53	51
	±SD	12.0	12.0	12.0	13.0	14.0	11.0

the spontaneously breathing patients is confirmed by consideration of individual patients. The greatest fall in PaO_2 recorded in a spontaneously breathing patient was from 95 to 56 torr, 2 hr after therapy. The greatest rise was from 59 to 181 torr. In an individual patient, arterial oxygenation may improve, remain unchanged, or get worse following chest physiotherapy. It was apparent from the study of 47 mechanically ventilated and 17 spontaneously breathing patients that no method was found that predicted which of these possibilities might occur.

Total Lung/Thorax Compliance (C_T)

The next step was to find a more objective indicator of the clinical and radiological improvement noted. Initial calculations suggested that C_T could quantitate any change in the small airways following chest physiotherapy. A similar calculation was previously described by Winning et al. (1975), in which the expiratory limb of a ventilator (Bennet MAI) was occluded and airway pressure was measured. However, this maneuver alters lung mechanics. Since no patient or ventilator adjustment is required to read end inspiratory pressure on the Engström

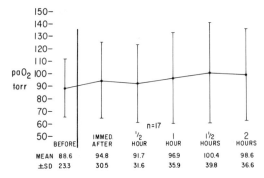

	BEFORE	IMMED. AFTER	1/2 HOUR	1 HOUR	1 1/2 HOURS	2 HOURS
MEAN	88.6	94.8	91.7	96.9	100.4	98.6
±SD	23.3	30.5	31.6	35.9	39.8	36.6

Figure 7.3. PaO_2 before, immediately after, and at half-hourly intervals for 2 hr after chest physiotherapy in 17 spontaneously breathing patients.

300, the physician or physical therapist can observe these changes at the bedside during therapy. The accuracy of the inspiratory pause read off the airway pressure gauge is great, and is not significantly exceeded by transducing the airway pressure wave form to a paper write-out (Mackenzie et al., 1979). Other more recently developed electronically driven ventilators, such as the MA2, Servo 900, Bear I, and Foregger 210, may be adjusted to give an inspiratory pause in the flow wave form. However, this does not appear as well defined in these ventilators as the mechanical, piston-driven Engström. Therefore, it may be advisable to use a paper trace of the airway pressure wave form to obtain the inspiratory pause pressure when using these other ventilators.

The initial results suggesting an increase in C_T following chest physiotherapy were confirmed (Fig. 7.4) by the results found following therapy in 42 mechanically ventilated patients who suffered trauma (Mackenzie et al., 1980). There appeared to be no difference in the C_T increase whether the patient had atelectasis, lung contusion, pneumonia, or respiratory distress syndrome. Nor did differences occur between patients ventilated with or without PEEP or between those treated for more or less than 1 hr. C_T changes when there are alterations in either the small airways or chest wall or in intraabdominal pressure. Since the latter two alterations generally change

slowly, C_T changes usually reflect an alteration of the small airways. The greatest C_T increase occurred 2 hr after therapy had ceased, which suggested that changes continue to occur even after the completion of therapy.

Airway Resistance (R)

R_{aw} is assessed by measurement of airway pressure during peak flow. The measurement is made in a mechanically ventilated patient by using a pneumotachygraph and a differential pressure transducer. Rubi et al. (1980) report that in volume-preset ventilators with a sine wave form and a fixed inspiratory/expiratory ratio of 1:2 (e.g., the Engstrom 300 series ventilators), the pneumotachygraph-derived airway resistance [R_{aw}) could be closely approximated ($r = 0.96$) by using the bedside measurement of peak (P_{max}) and end inspiratory (P_{IE}) airway pressures and applying the formula,

$$R_{aw} = [(P_{max} - P_{IE})$$
$$\times 10]/\text{minute ventilation.}$$

By using this approximation to R_{aw}, assessments were made on the same patient population at the same time that the compliance data (Fig. 7.4) were obtained. The results displayed in Figure 7.5 were analyzed by using the paired t-test and show that there was no significant change in R_{aw} for up to 2 hr after chest physiotherapy. In view of the significant increase in C_T in these same patients, the

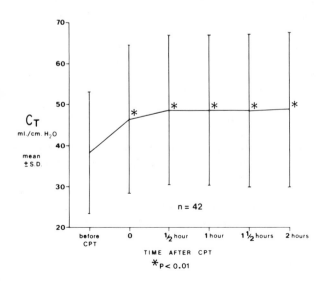

Figure 7.4. Changes in C_T in relation to a single treatment with chest physiotherapy *(CPT)* in 42 patients. [From C. F. Mackenzie et al.: *Anesthesia and Analgesia (Cleveland)* 59:207–210, 1980.]

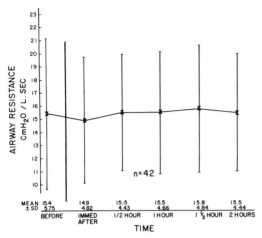

| MEAN ± SD | 15.4 5.75 | 14.9 4.82 | 15.5 4.43 | 15.5 4.66 | 15.8 4.84 | 15.5 4.44 |
| | BEFORE | IMMED AFTER | 1/2 HOUR | 1 HOUR | 1 1/2 HOUR | 2 HOURS |

TIME

Figure 7.5. Changes in R_{aw} in relation to a single treatment with chest physiotherapy from data obtained at the same time and in the same 42 patients as in Figure 7.4.

R_{aw} results might, at first, appear surprising. However, the unchanged R_{aw} confirmed that the larger airways were as clear before chest physiotherapy began as they were up to 2 hr afterward. In general, C_T monitors change in small airways, whereas R_{aw} reflects change in large airways. If C_T is increased and R_{aw} is unchanged following chest physiotherapy, the secretions were removed from the small rather than the large airways.

From a practical point of view, measurement of P_{max}, as described by Rubi and colleagues (1980), has more sources of error than measurement of P_{IE}. Reading P_{max} is more difficult; it is affected by secretions in the tracheal tube, the internal diameter of the tube, and changes in patient sedation or intra-abdominal pressure. These variables do not normally affect P_{IE}, which occurs during a no-flow state that holds the pressure constant long enough for equilibration to take place. Even though both maneuvers are only approximations, they are useful bedside monitors. C_T may be used to confirm clinical improvement or to determine an end point for treatment.

Sputum Volume Production in Tracheally Intubated Patients

The volume of expectorated sputum is often used to assess the efficacy of chest physiotherapy in patients with chronic lung disease. Whether the quantity of sputum obtained following chest physiotherapy correlates well with improvement in respiratory function remains controversial. It is generally agreed that sputum should be produced for the therapy to be of benefit, but there are doubts about the volume required, the accuracy of sputum measurement (Bateman et al., 1979), and the importance of its viscoelastic properties and distribution in the tracheobronchial tree (Clarke et al., 1973). To our knowledge, there is only one report in the literature in which sputum is measured in some intubated patients with acute lung pathology (Connors et al., 1980). Tracheal intubation with a cuffed tube removes two sources of error in sputum volume measurement: addition of saliva, and swallowed sputum.

To determine the relationship between the quantity of sputum removed and changes in arterial oxygenation, PaO_2/FIO_2, C_T and R_{aw} were calculated after a single treatment with chest physiotherapy; 15 sets of measurements were made in 10 patients (no measurements were less than 2 days apart) who had a mean age of 36.6 years. All patients were intubated and mechanically ventilated for at least 12 hr before study. PEEP with a mean of 9 cm H_2O (range, 2–20 cm H_2O) was applied in 5 patients. Nine treatments were performed for left lower lobe, 4 for right lower lobe and 2 for right upper lobe segmental or lobar atelectasis. Three patients had multilobar pathology. Treatment time was 49 ± 24.2 min (mean ± SD). Average sputum volume produced by chest physiotherapy was 9 ± 10.2 ml. Nine treatments produced 5 ml or less of sputum (Group A). The changes following chest physiotherapy in Group A were compared to the remaining six treatments (Group B), which produced 19 ± 11.8 ml of sputum (Table 7.3). The C_T and R_{aw} changes following chest physiotherapy in Group A and Group B are compared in Figure 7.6.

The Group B treatments resulted in no change in R_{aw} or C_T. Following Group A treatments, R_{aw} was unchanged, but PaO_2 increased ($p < 0.05$), and C_T rose significantly ($p < 0.05$) immediately, 0.5 hr, and 1 hr after chest physiotherapy. PEEP was

Table 7.3
Comparison of Variables between Group A (Treatments Producing Less Than 5 ml of Sputum) and Group B (Treatments Producing More Than 5 ml Sputum) and Their Significance

	Group A	Group B	Significance
PEEP (cm H_2O)	7 ± 3.5[a]	11 ± 5.3	$p < 0.05$
Duration of therapy (min)	41 ± 13.8	62 ± 31.9	NS[b]
Age (yr)	45 ± 21.0	29 ± 12.5	NS
PaO_2			
Before	126 ± 35.8	127 ± 29.9	NS
After	140 ± 34.3*	143 ± 65.5	NS
PaO_2/FIO_2			
Before	338 ± 131.7	242 ± 56.1	NS
After	379 ± 137.5	286 ± 112.0	NS
Volume of sputum (ml)	3.8 ± 1.3	18.8 ± 11.8	—

[a]Mean ± SD.
[b]NS, not significant.
*$p < 0.05$. Before and after values in Group A.

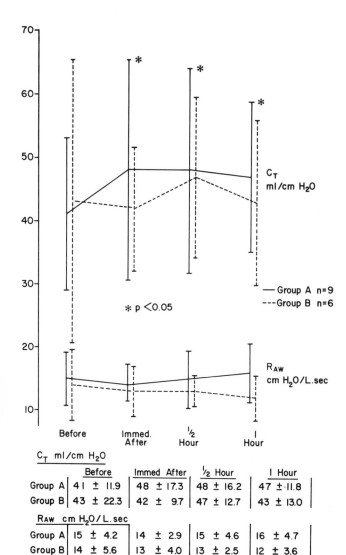

Figure 7.6. C_T and R_{aw} changes after treatments producing less than 5 ml of sputum (Group A) and more than 5 ml of sputum (Group B).

C_T ml/cm H_2O

	Before	Immed After	½ Hour	I Hour
Group A	41 ± 11.9	48 ± 17.3	48 ± 16.2	47 ± 11.8
Group B	43 ± 22.3	42 ± 9.7	47 ± 12.7	43 ± 13.0

R_{AW} cm H_2O/L.sec

	Before	Immed After	½ Hour	I Hour
Group A	15 ± 4.2	14 ± 2.9	15 ± 4.6	16 ± 4.7
Group B	14 ± 5.6	13 ± 4.0	13 ± 2.5	12 ± 3.6

221

higher ($p < 0.05$), and mean duration of therapy was longer, in the group producing the greater quantity of sputum. The increase in compliance and PaO_2 in Group A suggests that beneficial effect following sputum removal depends not on the volume of sputum removed, but rather on the area of the tracheobronchial tree from which it is obtained. If the larger airways are already clear, any sputum removed comes from the smaller airways.

Benefit, after removal of a given quantity of sputum, is additionally determined by the relation of the sputum volume removed to that still in the tracheobronchial tree. If the majority of the sputum is removed, a favorable outcome can be expected. If a large quantity of sputum is obtained, yet a large quantity remains, the benefit is likely to be limited. The relationship between the volume of sputum removed and the volume remaining and radiological evidence of benefit is clearly shown in Case History 7.1.

Case History 7.1. A 47-year-old male was admitted following an automobile accident in which he sustained a right lung contusion, fractured ribs 1–7 on the right, and a fractured right clavicle. He also had a base of the skull fracture and a wedge fracture of the body of T6 and required a laparotomy for repair of a liver laceration.

Nineteen days after admission an atelectasis of the left base and progressive atelectatic changes in the right base were noted on the 6 A.M. chest x-ray (Fig. 7.7). Chest physiotherapy, including postural drainage, percussion, vibration, and suctioning, was given to both lower lobes. Treatment time was 75 min. Six milliliters of sputum was suctioned while the patient was in the left lower lobe position, and 15 ml of blood tinged sputum was suctioned while in the right lower lobe bronchial drainage position (Fig. 7.8).

At 1:30 P.M. after therapy a chest x-ray was taken (Fig. 7.9). This showed a complete right upper lobe atelectasis with shift of the hilum and mediastinum to the right. The left lower lobe was completely reexpanded. Therefore, postural drainage, percussion, and suctioning were performed to the right upper and lower lobes for 45 min. Twenty-five milliliters of sputum was obtained from the right upper lobe (Fig. 7.8). Repeat chest x-ray at 5:05 P.M. showed clearance of the atelectasis with some residual loculated fluid in the right horizontal fissure (Fig. 7.10). Arterial oxygenation and minute ventilation changes during mechanical ventilation with a PEEP of 5 cm H_2O and an FIO_2 equal to 0.47 are shown in Table 7.4.

Case History 7.1 shows that transbronchial aspiration into the dependent lobe may occur with postural drainage. Therefore, the dependent lung should be examined and, if secretion retention is suspected, treated appropriately. This complication of postural drainage should always be considered if oxygenation fails to improve or lung/thorax compliance (not calculated in this case because expired minute ventilation was altered) is unchanged despite clinical evidence of clearance of secretions from the treated lung. Case History 7.1 also demonstrates that although 21 ml of sputum was removed from the left and right lower lobes (Fig. 7.8), little improvement resulted. After removal of 46 ml of sputum, arterial oxygenation was virtually unchanged, but there was radiological evidence of benefit.

It is possible that a given volume of sputum removed from a similar area of lung of the same patient may produce related changes in cardiac and respiratory function when it is obtained on two different occasions. It is, however, unlikely that there will be similar changes when the same volume of sputum is removed from different patients.

This point is illustrated by Case History 7.2 in which assessment of benefit following sputum removal was made by use of an indwelling, thermistor-tipped, pulmonary artery catheter.

Case History 7.2. A 48-year-old male was admitted following an accident in which a tree fell on his head and chest. The patient was unconscious. Multiple rib fractures and a lung contusion were seen on chest x-ray. Past medical history was uneventful. Three days after admission despite continuous mechanical ventilation, there was a steady deterioration in pulmonary and cardiovascular function. The patient was ventilated with a tidal volume of 16.5 ml/kg, a PEEP equal to 18 cm H_2O, and an FIO_2 of 0.61. Intrapulmonary shunt (Q_s/Q_t) was 29.4%, and $PaCO_2$ was 48 torr. Cardiac output (Q_t) was thought to be inadequate on the basis of a pulmonary capillary wedge pressure ($\bar{P}_{CWP}$) ranging from 20 to 25 torr and a mixed venous PO_2 ($P\bar{V}O_2$) of 15–30 torr. It was supported with

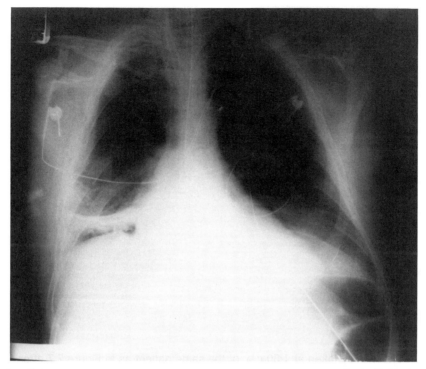

Figure 7.7. Six A.M. portable anteroposterior chest x-ray showing left and right lower lobe atelectasis and compensatory overdistension of both upper lobes. Multiple rib fractures and a clavicular fracture are shown on the right side.

dopamine (3 μg/kg/min) by continuous i.v. infusion.

Chest physiotherapy with postural drainage of both lower lobes was administered. Sixty milliliters of brownish-red watery secretions was obtained following percussion and suctioning while the patient was in the postural drainage position. The changes following 60 min of therapy are seen in Table 7.5.

In contrast, a 54-year-old male was admitted after he was trapped under a tractor trailer for 2 hr. The patient had multiple right-sided rib fractures, a pelvic fracture, a right radial, right patella, left fibula, and medial malleolar fractures and a fracture of L5. He required a laparotomy for multiple liver lacerations and for contusion and laceration of the small bowel. He had a lung contusion and an aortic arch he-

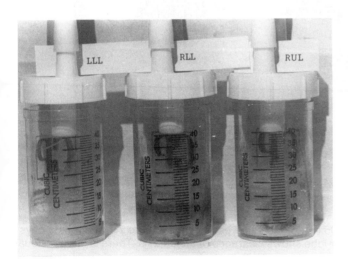

Figure 7.8. Sputum volumes (from *left* to *right*) obtained from the left lower lobe *(LLL)*, right lower lobe *(RLL)* and right upper lobe *(RUL)*. Note darker coloration (blood) in *RLL* specimen.

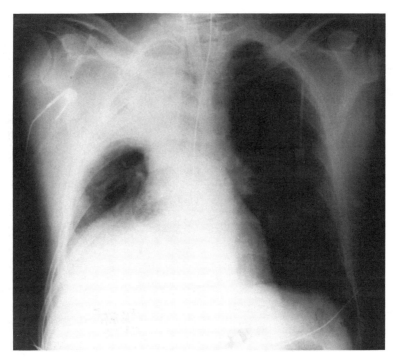

Figure 7.9.   Chest x-ray taken at 1:30 P.M. of the same patient as in Figure 7.7 after chest phys-iotherapy shows clearance of the left lower lobe atelectasis. There is now a complete right upper lobe and partial right lower lobe atelectasis.

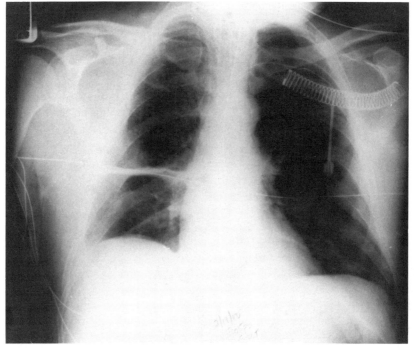

Figure 7.10.   Chest x-ray taken at 5:05 P.M. of the same patient as in Figure 7.7 after chest phys-iotherapy to right upper lobe and lower lobe shows clearance of atelectasis. There is still a residual quantity of fluid in the right horizontal fissure.

Table 7.4
Arterial Blood Gas Changes in a 47-Year-Old Male Patient after Sputum Removal

	PaO_2 (torr)	pH	$PaCO_2$ (torr)	V_E (liters/min)
Before first treatment	114	7.43	39	15
After removal of 21 ml of sputum	64	7.41	44	15
Before second treatment	75	7.53	31	18
After removal of 46 ml of sputum	123	7.58	27	18

matoma. Past medical history revealed that the patient had chronic obstructive pulmonary disease and previous pulmonary tuberculosis. He was also diabetic. Two days after admission he was given chest physiotherapy for 50 min. This produced copious (>30 ml) sputum and the cardiorespiratory changes that are shown in Table 7.6.

Despite the production of considerable quantities of sputum in both patients only the 48-year-old patient with previously normal lungs showed beneficial effects from sputum removal (Table 7.5). Q_s/Q_t, Q_t, pulse, and PaO_2 all fell in this patient but remained unchanged in the other (Table 7.6).

Cardiac and Respiratory Function

Both C_T and R_{aw} values shown in Figures 7.4 and 7.5 suggested that following chest physiotherapy, secretions were removed from the small airways. To investigate this possibility further and to quantitate the changes taking place with objective measurement, cardiac and respiratory function were measured before and after chest physiotherapy. Nineteen

trauma patients were studied (Mackenzie et al., 1985). Before investigation, all were mechanically ventilated for at least 6 hr with PEEP (Mean, 9 cm H_2O, range 5–18) and had indwelling arterial and thermistor-tipped, pulmonary arterial lines in position. Intrapulmonary shunt ($\dot{Q}_s/\dot{Q}_t$), dead space (V_d/V_t), cardiac output ($\dot{Q}_t$), and C_T were measured before, immediately after, and 2 hr after chest physiotherapy. The indications for therapy included secretion retention with segmental or platelike atelectasis (11 patients), lung contusion (6 patients), and respiratory distress syndrome (2 patients).

Respiratory failure following trauma may frequently result in high $\dot{Q}_s/\dot{Q}_t$ that requires increasing levels of inspired oxygen (FIO_2) and PEEP to maintain adequate oxygenation. If chest physiotherapy in the presence of retained secretions can reduce the requirements for high FIO_2 and PEEP, it is beneficial. It may also result in reduced morbidity and mortality from respiratory failure after trauma.

Table 7.5
Cardiorespiratory Changes in a 48-Year-Old Male Patient after 60 Min of Chest Physiotherapy

Variable[a]	Before Physiotherapy	Immediately after Physiotherapy	Two Hours after Physiotherapy
FIO_2	0.61	0.61	0.61
PaO_2 (torr)	47	71	138
$PaCO_2$ (torr)	48	32	33
a-$\bar{v}DO_2$(ml)	8.2	7.7	3.6
Pulse (beats/min)	125	110	100
$\bar{P}_{art}$ (torr)	68	80	95
$\bar{P}_{CWP}$ (torr)	25	20	24
$\dot{Q}_t$ (l/min)	8.7	6.0	5.4
R_{syst} (dynes/sec/cm^{-5})	405	800	1051
R_{pul} (dynes/sec/cm^{-5})	129	133	133
Q_s/Q_t (%)	29.4	17.3	20.7
C_T (ml/cm H_2O)	17	20	26
$\dot{V}O_2$ (ml/min)	656	460	194

[a]a-$\bar{v}DO_2$, arterial venous oxygen difference; $\bar{P}_{art}$, mean arterial pressure; R, resistance; $\dot{V}O_2$, oxygen consumption per minute.

Table 7.6
Cardiorespiratory Changes in a 54-Year-Old Male Patient after 50 min of Chest Physiotherapy

Variable	Before Physiotherapy	Immediately after Physiotherapy	Two Hours after Physiotherapy
FIO_2	0.54	0.54	0.54
PaO_2 (torr)	112	124	95
$PaCO_2$ (torr)	37	39	37
a-$\bar{v}DO_2$ (ml)	5.0	5.3	37
Pulse (beats/min)	125	122	125
$\bar{P}_{art}$ (torr)	95	90	100
$\bar{P}_{CWP}$ (torr)	21	21	18
$\dot{Q}_t$ (liters/min)	7.9	7.6	7.7
R_{syst} (dynes/sec/cm^{-5})	618	745	858
R_{pul} (dynes/sec/cm^{-5})	132	136	165
$\dot{Q}_s/\dot{Q}_t$ (%)	17.5	14.8	18.7
C_T (ml/cm H_2O)	48	36	41
$\dot{V}O_2$ (ml/min)	394	403	368

a-$\bar{v}DO_2$, arterial venous oxygen difference; $\bar{P}_{art}$, mean arterial pressure; R, resistance; $\dot{V}O_2$, oxygen consumption per minute.

Chest physiotherapy produced a significant fall in $\dot{Q}_s/\dot{Q}_t$. The greatest decrease in $\dot{Q}_s/\dot{Q}_t$ was from 36.3% to 16.5% and 13 patients showed a fall in $\dot{Q}_s/\dot{Q}_t$ immediately after therapy. In six patients there was a rise in $\dot{Q}_s/\dot{Q}_t$ (greatest from 14.8% to 23.5%) that persisted for at least 2 hr in three of the patients with lung contusion (Fig. 7.11). Dead space, $PaCO_2$, and PaO_2 were unchanged (Table 7.7). There was a significant overall increase in total C_T 2 hr after CPT. Eleven patients showed a rise in C_T immediately after and 2 hr after CPT. In three patients C_T was unchanged and in five C_T fell. The greatest C_T rise was from 34 to 51 ml/cm H_2O, while the greatest C_T decrease was from 48 to 36 ml/cm H_2O. In three patients, all treated

Figure 7.11. Individual plots of $\dot{Q}_s/\dot{Q}_t$ before, immediately after, and 2 hr after a single chest physiotherapy treatment. (From C.F. Mackenzie et al.: *Crit Care Med* 13:483-486.1985.)

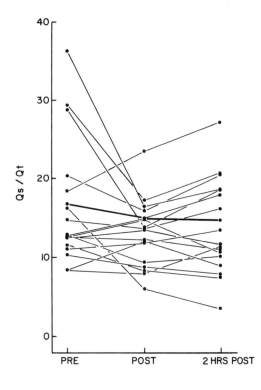

Table 7.7
Cardiorespiratory Function before, Immediately after, and 2 hr after CPT

	Before CPT	Immediately after CPT	Two Hours after CPT
CI (liters/min/m^2)	4.5 ± 1.35[a]	4.2 ± 1.23	4.0 ± 0.92
LVSWI (g/m/m^2)	65 ± 27.1	51 ± 27.7	63 ± 27.3
RVSWI (g/m/m^2)	19 ± 6.0	17 ± 6.6	18 ± 6.6
Ca-$\bar{V}O_2$ (ml/dl)	4.2 ± 1.36	4.2 ± 1.38	3.9 ± 0.91
Pulse (beats/min)	94 ± 23.2	95 ± 23.0	90 ± 23.5
Q_s/Q_t (%)	16.4 ± 7.55	13.2 ± 4.03*	14.5 ± 6.10
V_d/V_t	0.47 ± 0.16	0.46 ± 0.15	0.45 ± 0.13
C_T (ml/cm H_2O)	29 ± 11.3	32 ± 13.4	33 ± 11.7**
PaO_2 (torr)	128 ± 36.6	143 ± 31.5	137 ± 24.9
$PaCO_2$ (torr)	34 ± 7.4	35 ± 8.1	33 ± ·6.7

From C.F. Mackenzie et al.: *Crit Care Med* 13:483-486,1985.[a]
Mean ± SD.*
$p < 0.05$ before and immediately after.**
$p < 0.05$ before and 2 hr after.

for atelectasis, the fall in C_T persisted for 2 hr (Fig. 7.12). The mean values of cardiorespiratory function for the 11 patients with atelectasis were not clinically or statistically different from those of the six patients with lung contusion. There were no hemodynamically significant cardiac dysrhythmias during or 2 hr after CPT.

There was no significant change in cardiac function after CPT (Table 7.7). But no measurements were made during therapy because positional changes alter cardiac function (Rivara et al., 1984) and cause ventilation perfusion changes (Kaneko et al., 1966; Douglas et al., 1977; Zack et al., 1979; Remolina et al., 1981). Decreases in mixed venous oxygenation occur during suctioning (Bade et al., 1982) and together with change in position may explain the lack of significant change in PaO_2 despite a fall in Q_s/Q_t immediately after CPT. There are three other reports of cardiac function after CPT in the literature (Laws and McIntyre, 1969; Barrell and Abbas, 1978

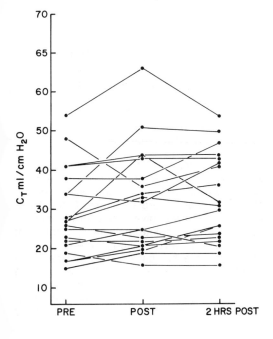

Figure 7.12. Individual plots of C_T before, immediately after, and 2 hr after a single chest physiotherapy treatment. (From C.F. Mackenzie et al.: *Crit Care Med* 13:483-486.1985.)

Klein et al, 1988). All reported detrimental effects. In the Laws and McIntyre study cardiac output (by dye dilution) increased by 50% with artificial coughs produced by lung hyperinflation. Barrell and Abbas found mixed venous oxygenation and cardiac output fell significantly during CPT but returned to baseline values within 10 min after the end of therapy. The differences may be accounted for by CPT techniques and patient population studied. Laws and McIntyre's patients had respiratory failure and received inflation pressures during the artificial cough of 60–100 cm H_2O, which many patients found distressing. Barrell and Abbas studied 14 patients who were extubated after mitral valve replacements. Despite the changes in cardiac output and mixed venous saturation, arterial oxygenation was unchanged. The same effects were not found in our study of 19 trauma patients. This difference may be because the trauma patients were young and did not have preexisting cardiac disease. In addition, falls in mixed venous saturation may only be transient and occur during CPT. All the trauma patients were ventilated with PEEP, which is known to restore functional residual capacity and improve oxygenation (McIntyre et al., 1969). The increase in C_T in 11 patients was probably secondary to the recruitment of more functioning alveolar units as a result of mobilization and clearance of secretions from small airways. The process of recruitment may have been assisted by PEEP and interdependence.

Klein et al. (1988) showed that cardiac output did rise by 50% over baseline values during chest physiotherapy in two unsedated patients. In patients who received continuous infusion of 3 μg/kg fentanyl there was still a 20–25% rise in cardiac output during chest physiotherapy that returned to baseline within 15 min after the end of therapy. With the analgesia there was no significant increase in heart rate or blood pressure but O_2 consumption and CO_2 production were still increased. The important questions about changes in cardiac function occurring during chest physiotherapy are: Are they clinically relevant? Are they associated with detrimental long

lasting effects? Can they be prevented with modifications of chest physiotherapy and use of analgesia and sedation?

While the decreased $\dot{Q}_s/\dot{Q}_t$ in three of the contusion patients may suggest an adverse effect of CPT, contusion is a recommended indication for CPT (Mackenzie and Shin, 1978b; Richardson et al., 1982). The greatest decrease in $\dot{Q}_s/\dot{Q}_t$ also occurred in a patient with lung contusion. The rise in $\dot{Q}_s/\dot{Q}_t$ may reflect transbronchial aspiration of bronchial secretions during positioning for CPT (see Case History 7.1). In patients with lung contusion, in whom coagulopathy complicates management, CPT should be given to the noncontused lung after therapy to the contused area. Alternatively, endobronchial intubation with a double lumen tube may prevent transtracheal aspiration of blood. This study confirmed our clinical impression that in critically ill patients, mechanically ventilated with PEEP, who have low lung compliance and increased $\dot{Q}_s/\dot{Q}_t$, CPT does not produce the deleterious cardiopulmonary changes that have been reported with bronchoscopy (Lundgren et al., 1982). CPT may be used to manage retained lung secretions due to acute posttraumatic respiratory failure, without producing hypoxemia.

Mass Spectrometry Analysis of Expired Gases

Mass spectrometry, as peviously described (McAslan, 1976), was used to analyze breath-by-breath end-tidal carbon dioxide ($P_{ET}CO_2$) and oxygen ($P_{ET}CO_2$) in mechanically ventilated patients. To determine the effects of chest physiotherapy on the uptake and excretion of O_2 and CO_2, analyses were obtained before, during, and after treatment.

Case History 7.3. An 18-year-old male was admitted following an automobile accident. He had a severe head injury, pulmonary edema, and had suffered cardiac arrests 8 and 10 hr previously. He was given chest physiotherapy because of a complete atelectasis of the right lower lobe and deterioration in arterial oxygenation while mechanically hyperventilated, with an FIO_2 of 0.6. The abnormal traces obtained by mass spectrometry before chest physiotherapy are shown in Fig. 7.13. Note the fluctuations seen in expired CO_2 during the latter

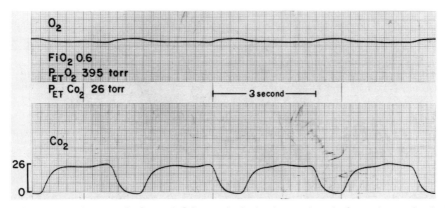

Figure 7.13. Breath-by-breath O_2 and CO_2 analysis in the patient before chest physiotherapy. Note the lack of alveolar plateau and the presence of a terminal peak in the CO_2 curve. $P_{ET}O_2$ and $P_{ET}CO_2$ values are shown.

part of expiration. ABG analysis showed a PaO_2 of 69, a pH of 7.51, and a $PaCO_2$ of 30.

After 45 min of chest physiotherapy to the right lower lobe and removal of copious secretions, there was clinical and radiological evidence of clearance of the atelectasis. The expired gas wave form now showed a plateau (Fig. 7.14). The trace in Figure 7.14 was made 1.5 hr after that in Figure 7.13. ABGs sampled at the same time as the mass spectrometry analysis in Figure 7.14 showed a PaO_2 of 148, a pH of 7.52, and a $PaCO_2$ of 34 despite unchanged ventilator settings and FIO_2.

The baseline traces obtained before therapy show a lack of constant "alveolar" CO_2, suggesting that the CO_2 tensions did not reach the same values as the pulmonary capillary CO_2 in all alveoli. Therefore, a considerable arterial alveolar CO_2 gradient (a–$ADCO_2$) would exist. $P_{ET}CO_2$ levels were inconsistent; well-ventilated alveoli emptied early; poorly ventilated units in which alveolar gas was trapped emptied later. There is a peak in the terminal plateau of the CO_2 curve (Fig. 7.13). Similar peaks in me-chanically ventilated patients may be abolished with PEEP (McAslan) or an expiratory retard (Ricker and Haberman, 1976). $P_{ET}CO_2$, in the presence of this terminal increase in expired CO_2, is unrepresentative of "average" mixed alveolar gas composition (McAslan, 1976). Therefore, the recorded a–$ADCO_2$ of 4 torr may be only an estimation of the gradient. This situation is thought to occur due to $\dot{V}/\dot{Q}$ imbalance and premature airway closure. If there is a large difference in the distribution of ventilation causing a spectrum of rates of emptying, the slope of the alveolar plateau increases. Time constants given as the product of regional lung compliance and airway resistance describe the rate of airway emptying during expiration. In obstruction, time constants increase so that no alveolar plateau may be visible on the expired CO_2 curve (Fig. 7.15). The abolition of the peak by chest physiotherapy (Fig. 7.14) and the change in shape of the expired CO_2 curve appeared to indicate that chest physiotherapy affected the small airways

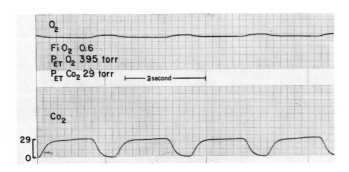

Figure 7.14. Following chest physiotherapy, an alveolar plateau is apparent, and the terminal peak in the CO_2 curve is abolished. Note the rise in the $P_{ET}CO_2$ value after chest physiotherapy.

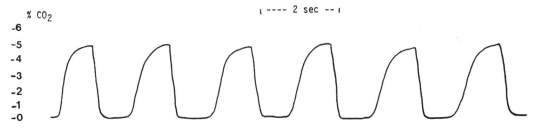

Figure 7.15. Expired CO_2 curve of patient with chronic bronchitis and emphysema. Note the lack of alveolar plateau suggesting inequality of emptying of alveoli and impaired distribution of ventilation.

and their ability to take part in gas exchange. The expired gas wave form after chest physiotherapy shows a plateau with a constant value for $P_{ET}CO_2$. The a–ADCO$_2$ of 5 torr is increased. This suggests that alveolar dead space is similarly increased after chest physiotherapy and removal of secretions.

The expired CO_2 curve of a patient out of phase with a mechanical ventilator shows a characteristic change (Fig. 7.16A). This occurs because the patient attempts to breathe in non-CO_2-containing gases while the ventilator is in the expiratory phase. This patient was thought to be out of phase because of lung secretion retention. Following chest physiotherapy and removal of these secretions, a normal CO_2 curve was produced (Fig. 7.16B).

Breath-by-breath analysis of CO_2 and O_2 curves during chest physiotherapy and chest wall vibration is shown in Figure 7.17. The CO_2 and O_2 analysis confirm that chest wall vibration causes changes in the expired gas wave form. These variations occur due to the ex-

pired air column oscillations found with chest vibration. Mass spectrometry demonstrates that chest physiotherapy produces changes in CO_2 and O_2 gas exchange. The more normal CO_2 curves found following chest physiotherapy suggest that the therapy has a favorable effect on the small airways.

ANALYSIS OF CHEST PHYSIOTHERAPY DATA

Factors Influencing Physiological Measurement in the ICU

Physiological measurement in the ICU is difficult. The patient, especially when unstable, undergoes continual and often dramatic changes in cardiorespiratory function. Because the patient may be critically ill, therapeutic intervention is frequently necessary, and this often alters cardiac or respiratory function. While it is usually quite easy to exclude such obvious cardiorespiratory changes as development of shock or tracheal in-

Figure 7.16. (**A**) Breath-by-breath CO_2 curve in a patient who was out of phase with mechanical ventilation. (**B**) CO_2 analysis on the same patient after chest physiotherapy shows a normal curve.

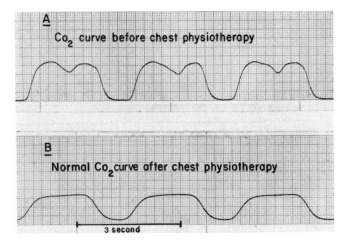

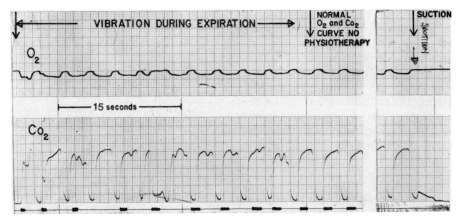

Figure 7.17. Breath-by-breath O_2 and CO_2 analysis during vibration chest physiotherapy, showing a normal curve when vibration ceased and loss of the curve with suctioning of the tracheobronchial tree.

tubation and mechanical ventilation, other more subtle variables may easily go undetected or be attributed to the therapy under study. This is one argument for using a control population. Investigation of chest physiotherapy in ICU patients is made especially difficult because there is no control or standardization of the therapy itself. Many reports of chest physiotherapy include the use of bronchodilating or mucolytic agents. Some centers do not use postural drainage, while others exclude chest vibration of percussion. The duration and frequency of therapy vary enormously (see p. 39).

What control should be used to compare with chest physiotherapy in critically ill patients? The commonly suggested control is side-to-side turning and tracheal suction (Murray, 1979b). However, when researching the effects of therapy in humans, both standards of care must be comparable and acceptable medical practice. In our experience, side-to-side turning and tracheal suctioning are not comparable therapy for treatment of conditions such as left lower lobe, posterior segment atelectasis. Long-term follow-up studies suggest that this regime did not prevent deterioration in chest x-ray appearance, PaO_2/FIO_2, and C_T (see pp. 233–237). Also, when side-to-side turning and suctioning are used, as occurred at our institution during a period of understaffing of physical therapists, atelectasis was not prevented. In October 1977, there was a physical therapy staff shortage and a large patient load. Twenty-one patients in the step-down (ICU) unit were not treated by physical therapists but, instead, received tracheal suctioning and side-to-side turning. In that month, there were 14 readmissions to the critical care recovery unit (CCRU) from the ICU because of deteriorating respiratory function that was documented by clinical examination, chest x-ray, and blood gas analysis (C. F. Mackenzie, personal communication to R. A. Cowley, M.D., Director MIEMSS, October 1977). In contrast, an average of three readmissions/month occurred during the remainder of the year. This strongly suggests that side-to-side turning and suctioning are not comparable or acceptable medical practice, compared to chest physiotherapy, when performed on ICU patients with acute lung pathology.

In addition to the ethics of using control groups in critically ill patients, and the difficulty of finding a comparable and clinically acceptable control, some standardization of chest physiotherapy should be achieved before physiological measurements can be truly claimed to reflect the effects of chest physiotherapy.

Factors Influencing Analysis of Data from Different ICUs

Therapist Variability

When comparisons are made of chest physiotherapy between different ICUs, is it possible to exclude such a subjective but very important factor as the clinical variability between one therapist's ability to clear an acute atelectasis and another's inability? It is our impression that physical therapists trained by staff experienced in ICU work are more successful in improving the patient's clinical and radiological signs than are nurses, respiratory therapists, or physicians. This impression is confirmed by the following case history.

Case History 7.4. A 23-year-old male was admitted with a head injury, cerebral contusion, and a ruptured spleen sustained in an automobile accident. He was tracheally intubated, mechanically hyperventilated ($PaCO_2 < 30$ torr) and given corticosteroids. Five nights after admission (that is, November 18) he developed a complete left lower lobe atelectasis. This was recognized following deterioration of arterial oxygenation and after a chest x-ray. The patient was suctioned, FIO_2 was increased, and the ABG analysis was repeated. Little improvement occurred as is shown in Table 7.8). After suctioning, a nurse gave chest therapy with the patient turned onto his right side. There was an increase in arterial oxygenation from 71 to 118 torr and of C_T from 44 to 60 ml/cm H_2O. The patient was treated 3 hr later by a chest physical therapist in the correct postural drainage position, after which arterial oxygenation further improved to 185 torr and C_T increased to 68 ml/cm H_2O.

The following morning (November 20), arterial oxygenation on the same ventilator settings had again deteriorated despite tracheal suctioning and "chest therapy" performed by the nurse. Chest physiotherapy by a physical therapist again produced improvement in arterial

oxygenation and increase in C_T. The patient, who regained consciousness, was placed on a T-piece and was successfully extubated.

Other investigators confirm that trained physical therapists produce a more favorable outcome than do nurses or physicians. Vraciu and Vraciu (1977) found that breathing exercises administered by a physical therapist reduced the incidence of pulmonary complications after open heart surgery, compared to turning, deep breathing, and coughing every hour assisted by nursing staff. Finer and Boyd (1978) noted that the improved oxygenation that occurred after chest physiotherapy in infants was related to a chest physiotherapist, rather than to the ICU nurses, performing chest physiotherapy. Lyager et al. (1979) thought that the reduction in pulmonary complications that they reported, compared to those noted by Bartlett et al. (1973), may have resulted from their use of specially trained physical therapists rather than residents or nursing staff. Application of a standard therapy, such as is advocated in this book, may help reduce therapist variability.

Patient Population

How can compensation be made for the variability between different patient populations? For example, can chest physiotherapy or any other therapy be compared between trauma and medical ICUs? Admission to a trauma unit is not

Table 7.8
ABG, C_T, and PaO_2/FIO_2 Changes Occurring over a 3-Day Period

Date	Time	PaO_2 (torr)	pH	$PaCO_2$	C_T (ml/ cm H_2O)	PaO_2/ FIO_2	Event
November 18	11:00	107	7.58	28	78	282	
	21:30	57	7.51	31	68	150	Left lower lobe atelectasis
	23:00	71	7.59	28	44	161	Suction, FIO_2 increased
November 19	05:00	118	7.58	27	60	268	Chest therapy by nurse
	10:00	185	7.60	28	68	420	Chest physiotherapy by physical therapist
	22:00	94	7.54	33	60	214	ABG fall at night
November 20							Chest physiotherapy by physical therapist
	09:40	146	7.57	31	78	348	ABG following chest physiotherapy
	10:45	122	7.56	35			Spontaneous respiration T-piece 40% O_2
	14:00	112	7.52	36			Extubated face tent O_2

determined by a history of preexisting pathology but usually by an acute insult to an otherwise-healthy individual. Application of physiotherapy is likely to have a different effect in the trauma patient than in the medical patient. It may be possible to overcome this variability by considering a large patient population studied over a long period.

Method of Mechanical Ventilation

Manufacturers of ventilators and advocates of different modes of mechanical ventilation and respiratory support claim that important differences result from use of one or other ventilator or methods of ventilation. If this is so, the outcome of chest physiotherapy in mechanically ventilated patients is likely to be different, even when the patient population and therapy are similar.

Variability in Anesthetic Techniques

Different anesthetic techniques produce different effects on the respiratory system. Regional anesthetic techniques are credited with causing fewer deaths after surgery than general anesthetic techniques (Beecher and Todd, 1954). However, there is a lack of controlled studies comparing regional anesthesia to modern general anesthetic techniques. Regional techniques are frequently not applicable, as, for example, in the management of a patient with multisystem trauma. Regional techniques such as epidural anesthesia are time consuming and require considerable expertise. Nonetheless, they are of enormous benefit for relief of pain after surgery, when an epidural catheter is left in place. Regional analgesia is more effective than narcotics for maintaining pulmonary function after surgery (Fairley, 1980). This may considerably alter the incidence of respiratory complications and the need for mechanical ventilation (see Chapter 10, p. 341 for details of pain relief in ICU).

General anesthesia with use of neuromuscular blockade (and an opiate, or low doses of inhalational agent) frequently produces a more awake patient, on reversal of the neuromuscular blockade, than occurs following the use of inhalational agents alone. The recovery period, to the point where the patient sits up, follows commands, and takes deep breaths and coughs, may be shortened when neuromuscular blockade is used. This may decrease the incidence of respiratory complications.

Water vapor loss may be reduced by use of a closed or semiclosed rebreathing circuit on the anesthesia machine. Alternatively, inclusion of a humidifier or nebulizer in the ventilator/anesthesia machine ensures humidification of dry anesthetic gases at all times. Lack of humidification during anesthesia or in the period after surgery may be an important determinant of subsequent respiratory complications in the ICU. (See Chapter 9 for more details on humidification.)

Therapeutic Intervention

In the long-term follow-up of patients in ICUs, can the numerous other clinically essential therapeutic interventions (such as intravenous fluids, vasoactive drugs, and analgesics) be excluded from influencing the effects and outcome of chest physiotherapy? Standardization of these therapies is unthinkable, yet pain relief is an important factor in the prevention of respiratory complications after surgery and patient acceptance of chest physiotherapy and mobilization. The duration, type, and frequency of interventions in four different types of patients over an 8-hr period are described in Appendix IV. In some institutions there are interventions that do not occur at others. For example, if there is variability between one surgical ICU and another in the morbidity and mortality associated with the same surgical procedure, how can this discrepancy in standard of care be accounted for when comparing chest physiotherapy at the two institutions? These are just a few of the difficulties of evaluating chest physiotherapy in the ICU. The solution, for the most part, remains unknown.

Long-Term Follow-up

A 2-hr follow-up of respiratory changes after chest physiotherapy may be too long, since, allowing 1 hr for chest physiotherapy and 2 hr for sampling and measurement, variables are assumed to be constant during a study period of about 3.5 hr. The number of interventions for four patients is shown in Appendix IV. The four patients studied demonstrate the care given to patients in a typical trauma ICU. They were observed from 8 A.M. to 4 P.M., and all interventions that caused alterations in cardiac or respiratory function or that made physiological study difficult were recorded.

The mean number of clinically required interventions was 59 (Table 7.9). These interventions took, on average, 298 min or 5 min for each intervention. The nonintervention time was, therefore, limited to a mean of 93 min in the whole 8 hr. The longest intervention-free period averaged 34.5 min, which represented only 9.1% of the total 8 hr. The duration of restricted access was 145 min on average. Restricted access was the term used to refer to situations that alter the ability to monitor (for example, patient 3 left the CCRU for hyperbaric O_2 therapy and whirlpool debridement), change the hemodynamic status (for example, patient 1 had dialysis that can cause considerable circulating volume shifts), or make comparative physiological measurement impossible (for example, patient 2 was, at times, rotated on the Roto-Rest bed). This alters hemodynamics, ventilation/perfusion relationships within the lung, and respiratory mechanics and function. The changes in heart rate, mean arterial blood pressure, mean P_A pressure, ICP and cerebral perfusion pressure (CPP) in patient 4 are shown graphically in Appendix IV. The clinically necessary adjustments to ventilation and cardiac function exclude

acutely ill patients from lengthy study of the effects of chest physiotherapy on these parameters.

An alternative to long follow-up of highly changeable parameters, such as pulse and cardiac output, is to record more nonspecific indicators. If these variables are recorded for a long period and in a large enough patient population, useful data may be generated concerning the effectiveness of chest physiotherapy. Information on daily 8 A.M. ABG, lung/thorax compliance, and chest x-ray appearance was, therefore, collected in 58 mechanically ventilated patients between August and October 1977. All received chest physiotherapy and had suffered multiple system injuries (see Appendix I, p. 352, Table A1.7 for definition of systems) and were admitted to the CCRU.

The patients were divided into groups based on whether they had chest injury, head injury and other injury, pelvic fracture, cervical spinal column injury, or extremity fracture (Table 7.10). Data were collected only in mechanically ventilated patients and the numbers in each category from which the data were obtained are shown at the top of Figures 7.18–7.20. Not all the data could be collected on every patient each day.

Chest X-Ray

The daily chest x-ray was assessed by using the following system: clear, 0; infiltrate or plate-like atelectasis, 1; atelectasis (segmental or lobar) or lung contusion, 2; and pneumonia, 3. The results are shown in Figure 7.18. On admission, the

Table 7.9
Duration and Frequency of Interventions Causing Changes in Cardiac or Respiratory Function in Three Critically Ill Patients[a]

	Direct Intervention (min)	Nonintervention (min)	Restricted or No Access Time (min)	Longest Period of Nonintervention (min)	Number of Interventions
Patient 1	448	32	359 (dialysis)	20	43
Patient 2	399	81	197 (rotation of Roto-Rest bed)	20	75
Patient 3	161	106	213 (hyperbaric chamber, whirlpool debridement)	28	29
Patient 4	183	154	35 (visitors)	70	89

[a]Full details of all interventions appear in Appendix IV; each patient was observed a total of 480 min.

Table 7.10
Injuries Sustained by 58 Long-Term Follow-Up Patients

Injury	Number of Patients	Average Number Body Systems Injured
Rib fractures; lung contusion	26	3.0
Pelvic fracture	31	2.9
Unconscious	16	2.7
Extremity fracture	29	2.7
Cervical spine fracture	13	2.1

patients with chest injury presented with the highest score, and those with head injury, with the lowest. Two of the 19 patients with chest injury developed a pneumonia-like process that lasted 9 and 3 days, respectively. On average, in patients with multisystem injury, chest physiotherapy was successful in prevention of major atelectasis or pneumonia (Fig. 7.18). Chest injury or pelvic fracture (or a combination) produced the highest score and the longest duration of chest x-ray changes despite chest physiotherapy. There is a lack of difference, after 4 days

of mechanical ventilation, between the chest-injured patients who received chest physiotherapy and the head-injured patients who received routine turning and tracheal suctioning, but no chest physiotherapy (unless the chest x-ray scored 2 or more). This suggests that chest physiotherapy prevented further deterioration in chest x-ray changes and that routine turning and suctioning did not.

PaO_2/FIO_2

The changes in PaO_2/FIO_2 are shown in Figure 7.19. The patients with head injury presented with the highest ratio (lowest intrapulmonary shunt), and the patients with chest and cervical spine injury, with the lowest. After 1 week, two distinct groups emerged; the patients with chest, pelvis and extremity injury had low PaO_2/FIO_2, and those with head and cervical spine injury had high PaO_2/FIO_2. The differences between these two groups receiving chest physiotherapy are likely to be the result of the injuries sustained by the different patient population rather than the chest physiotherapy. The

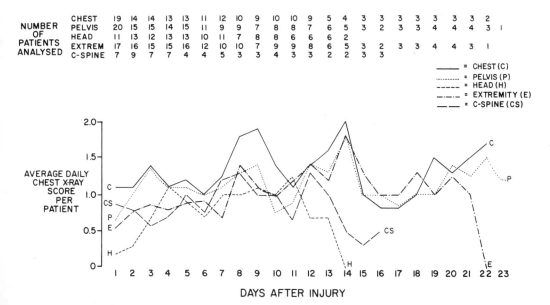

Figure 7.18. Long-term follow-up of daily morning chest x-ray changes following admission day (day 1). Assessment: clear, 0; infiltrate or plate-like atelectasis, 1; atelectasis (segmental or lobar) or lung contusion, 2; pneumonia, 3. Numbers of chest x-rays examined appears above graph; mean score is plotted. *C*, chest injury; *H*, head and other injury; *P*, pelvic fracture; *CS*, cervical spine injury; *E*, extremity fracture.

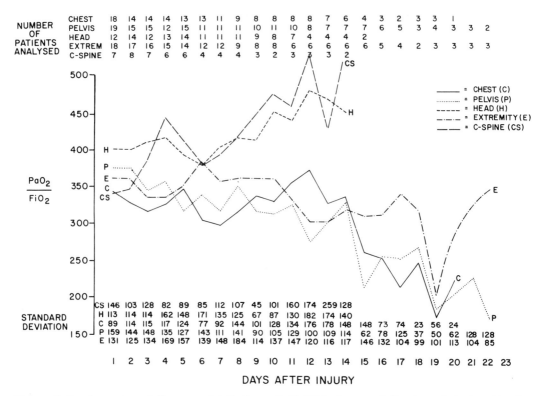

Figure 7.19. Long-term follow-up of daily 8 A.M. PaO₂/FIO₂ changes following admission. Number of values assessed appears above graph; mean value is plotted; standard deviation appears below graph. Symbols used are the same as in Figure 7.18.

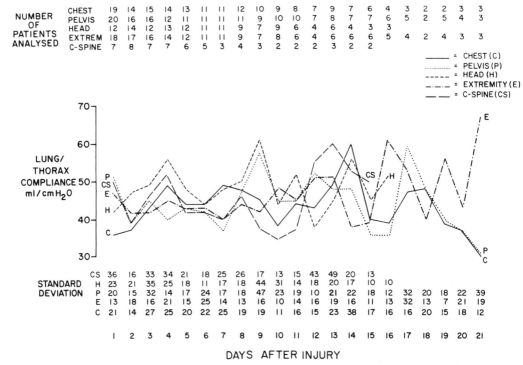

Figure 7.20. Long-term follow-up of daily 8 A.M. C$_T$ changes following admission. Number of values assessed appears above graph; mean value is plotted; standard deviation appears below graph. Symbols used are the same as in Figure 7.18.

former group were more susceptible to respiratory complications, although only those who were sick enough to require continued mechanical ventilation were sampled.

Total Lung/Thorax Compliance

The chest-injured patients presented with the lowest C_T although those with head injury also had decreased C_T (possibly because of spasticity). On average, despite chest physiotherapy, C_T was low in all the patients studied (Fig. 7.20). It was not until the third week of mechanical ventilation that deterioration below 30 ml/cm H_2O occurred in the group of patients studied. This is often considered the lowest C_T acceptable for weaning from mechanical ventilation. It is apparent from the study of Figures 7.18–7.20 that PaO_2/FIO_2 and C_T changes usually preceded chest x-ray changes.

Role of Collateral Ventilation in Gas Exchange with Obstructed Airways

Distal to a complete airway obstruction in the mainstem bronchus, alveolar gases rapidly achieve equilibration with mixed venous gas tension. The alveolar gas is absorbed, atelectasis develops, and no further gas exchange takes place. Consequently, any perfusion of this area increases intrapulmonary shunt. However, this does not occur if the obstruction is of a sublobar airway. Van Allen and Lindskog (1931) showed that collateral ventilation has the effect of preventing the formation of atelectasis after lobular but not lobar obstruction. The pores of Kohn, the interbronchiolar channels of Martin (Martin, 1966), and the alveolar bronchiolar channels of Lambert (Lambert, 1955) are suggested as pathways for collateral ventilation (Macklem, 1978) (Fig. 2.8, p. 61). Van Allen and Lindskog suggested that collateral ventilation assists bronchoelimination by maintaining a normal volume of air in the lung parenchyma beyond a mucus obstruction. Measurement of forces exerted by cough showed that they failed to eliminate mucus when absorption atelectasis occurred within 30 min of obstruction. Similarly, Van Allen and Lindskog suggested that the expelling forces of ciliary and peristaltic activity and of drainage by gravity also depended upon the presence of a normal content of air in the lung beyond an obstruction. Absorption of air resulted in atelectasis when no collateral ventilation was present. No matter how great a respiratory effort was made, without collateral ventilation, collapse rather than reexpansion occurred. Van Allen and Jung (1931) showed that binding of the chest did not decrease collateral flow but binding of the abdomen reduced tidal volume and collateral ventilation.

Baarsma et al. (1948) described two children, one of whom had a metal foreign body in the left lower main bronchus that resulted in atelectasis of the left lower lobe. The other aspirated a metal pellet that lodged tightly in a sublobar airway of the left lower lobe. There was no trace of atelectasis on chest x-ray of the second patient. They restate Van Allen and Lindskog's hypothesis that inspiration, without collateral ventilation, would increase subatmospheric transpulmonary pressures in the obstructed lung. Mucus would be moved more firmly into the bronchus. Baarsma et al. (1948) hypothesized that postoperative atelectasis was due to accumulation of mucus, shallow breathing, weak cough, and diminished collateral ventilation.

Chen et al. (1970) simultaneously recorded pressure in the trachea and collaterally ventilated airways of dogs with an obstructed airway. During inspiration, pressure was greater in the trachea than the obstructed pulmonary segment favoring inflation of the obstructed segment. During exhalation air flowed from the obstructed segment to the main airway through collateral channels, though the pressure difference was small. They suggest that this would favor the development of enough force to help dislodge an obstruction in a segmental bronchus and prevent atelectasis. Culiner and Reich (1961) suggested that segmental atelectasis was rare unless collateral ventilation was impeded by accumulation of bronchial and alveolar secretions.

Collateral Airway Resistance

The resistance to collateral flow was first measured in living subjects by Bartels (1972), and is influenced greatly by lung volume. Increases in lung volume above FRC were associated with dramatic decreases in collateral airway resistance in humans (Inners et al., 1979). The fall in resistance could be due to enlargement of the airways alone or enlargement together with recruitment of other collateral channels. It is possible that different channels provide collateral ventilation at differing lung volumes. Increasing lung volumes from 55% to 80% of total lung capacity were associated with a decrease in collateral resistance of 60% (Inners et al., 1979). Despite this the resistance in collateral airways is about 50–4000 times greater than normal airway resistance (Inners et al., 1979; Bartels, 1972) so that flow is preferentially through airways other than collateral channels. However, in disease states such as emphysema and when CO_2 retention occurs as in chronic lung disease, collateral airways resistance falls and may approach that of airways resistance. Kuriyama et al. (1984) examined the role of collateral ventilation in ventilation–perfusion balance and concluded that species with collateral ventilation have an auxiliary respiratory mechanism that could protect them from regional alveolar hypoxia. Collateral ventilation was found to be the first line of defense, before hypoxic pulmonary vasoconstriction, against regional hypoxia. Because air is less dense than blood, the ability to redistribute ventilation rather than perfusion would seem to be an efficient arrangement.

Traystman et al. (1978) found that CO_2 was a major determinant of collateral airways resistance. High CO_2 reduced resistance. If a portion of lung that has a low CO_2 is adjacent to a hypoventilating portion (with higher CO_2), the high CO_2 area facilitates collateral ventilation. A homeostatic mechanism was preserved for increasing ventilation to the poorly ventilated portion despite the adjacent hypocapnia. Traystman et al. (1978) also showed that the surrounding lung exerts significant control over the resistance to flow in collateral airways. Failure to consider the effects of this interdependence of bronchiolar channels and the surrounding lung erroneously suggests that alveolar pores of Kohn might be the major pathways for collateral ventilation (Mead, 1973). However, Traystman et al. (1978) conclude that bronchiolar channels of Lambert and Martin, because they have smooth muscle, are the sites of collateral ventilation.

Development and Role of Collateral Airways in Disease

Collateral ventilation appears to increase with age (Terry et al., 1987). Rosenberg and Lyon (1979) showed collateral ventilation in excised adult lungs but not in those of children. Martin (1963) also observed that pores of Kohn are absent in newborn animals but reach adult levels in 1 year (see Fig. 8.1). Macklin (1936) documented a reduced number of pores of Kohn in young humans. There is considerable variation in the amount of collateral ventilation in different regions of the lung. Specifically, there are less collateral ventilation channels in the middle lobe and lingula. The reason for this may be that the middle lobe and inferior segment of the lingula interface with only one segment while all other lung segments interface with at least two other segments (Terry et al., 1985).

Because the channels of Martin and Lambert contain smooth muscle their caliber and resistance to collateral flow vary. Collateral resistance mediated through parasympathetic stimulation changes with inhalation of common pollutants such as ozone, metacholine, histamine, cholinergic blockade, oxygen, CO_2, and atropine (Batra et al., 1981). Collateral airways were suggested by Kohn (1893) and others to be a means by which pneumonia infected adjacent lung segments. Loosli (1937) suggested that tumors may spread between alveoli by collateral airways. The frequent infections that occur in intralobar sequestrations may occur by entry through collateral airways.

In asthma, small airways are obstructed by inflammation and mucus plugging and up to half of an asymptomatic asthmatic's airways may be closed. The binodal distribution of ventilation–perfusion ratios seen in asthma is best explained by the presence of collateral ventilation. Asthmatics breathing 100%

oxygen do not develop increased shunt (Field, 1967). Prevention of shunting may be explained by effective collateral ventilation (Terry et al., 1985). Culiner and Reich (1961) suggest collateral ventilation may play an important role in development of emphysema because of a ball-valve-like arrangement that allows air to enter a segment through collateral airways but prevents its escape. Collateral airway resistance is low in emphysema and allows gas mixing in the lung periphery and maintenance of adequate blood gases (Filley et al., 1968). Terry et al. (1978) showed that in emphysematous patients airways closed at pressures of 3–8 cm H_2O above atmospheric pressure. However, flow through collateral airways occurred at 5 cm H_2O suggesting that air was rapidly distributed in the emphysematous lung at FRC.

Possible Therapeutic Effects of Collateral Ventilation

Andersen et al. (1979) showed in normal human lungs at autopsy that collapsed lung can be recruited through collateral airways using techniques that employ continuous positive airway pressure. Reexpansion was achieved by mechanical ventilation with and without PEEP by deep breathing simulation in a pletysmograph with CPAP (which caused an increasing FRC), but reexpansion did not occur with normal breathing at constant FRC. In six of the seven lungs studied, collateral reinflation required lower pressures than reinflation through normal airways. Andersen et al. (1979) explain this lower pressure by a difference in time constants between normal and collateral reinflation. During ordinary conditions of lung expansion the collateral time constant (product of airflow resistance and lung compliance) is longest because of the large collateral flow resistance. However, when the lung is collapsed the normal bronchial route is narrowed or closed by mucus, menisci formation, or contraction of elements in the wall (Macklem, 1971). All these factors increase the time constant for reinflation through normal air passages. If collateral time constants are longer during exhalation, which is thought to be so

(Andersen et al., 1971; Macklem, 1971), then more air would enter an obstructed but not collapsed lung segment during inspiration than could exit during exhalation. Pressure would build up in the obstructed segment forcing secretions more centrally.

Gravity changes collateral ventilation and body position affects the response of collateral channels to CO_2, O_2, and cholinergic blockade (Batra et al., 1981). Resistance in collateral airways increased 54% when the obstructed segment was rotated from a nondependent to dependent (segment down) position. Since pleural pressure is lower in nondependent lung, transpulmonary pressure (airway less pleural pressure) is increased, and regional volume is greater. Kaplan et al. (1979) showed that collateral airways resistance decreases 13% for each centimeter increase in transpulmonary pressure. Alternative suggestions for the mechanisms increasing resistance in the dependent lung include differences in $\dot{V}/\dot{Q}$ and intravascular volume. In normal, upright lung, $\dot{V}/\dot{Q}$ is greater in nondependent than dependent regions and O_2 tensions are higher but CO_2 tensions are lower. Because increased CO_2 has a more potent dilating effect on collateral airways than reduced O_2 has a constrictor effect, $\dot{V}/\dot{Q}$ changes are unlikely to be the cause. It is unlikely that vascular distension affected collateral airway resistance because even large changes in vascular pressure cause trivial effects (Batra et al., 1981). In addition, the dilating effects of CO_2 on collateral airways are more apparent in the nondependent (segment-up) position. This may be due to different local levels of CO_2 in the obstructed segment. The clinical importance of these changes is that postural drainage with the obstructed lung segment placed in a nondependent position optimized collateral airway flow by reducing its resistance and time constants for inflation of the obstructed segment as well as optimizing gravity-assisted drainage of mucus with coughing and exhalation. Since cholinergic blockade also dilates collateral airways (Batra et al., 1981) beneficial effects of bronchodilating drugs used in conjunction with chest physiotherapy should be greatest when the obstructed area is in the nondependent position.

Interdependence

Increasing pressure differences between adjacent lung regions promotes flow through collateral channels. In living subjects interdependence also increases collateral ventilation (Macklem, 1971; Menkes and Traystman, 1977). There is also interdependence between lung and chest wall (Zidulka et al., 1976) that may contribute to the effectiveness of deep breathing in reexpansion of atelectatic lung. Andersen et al. (1979) explain the effectiveness of application of subatmospheric pleural pressure during deep breathing, compared to using mechanical ventilation with PEEP by this mechanism of lung/chest interdependence. Transpulmonary pressure swings over an atelectatic area may be much greater than over a nonatelectatic area, and, if so, should increase collateral flow during inspiration. Chest/lung interdependence tends to promote homogeneous or synchronous ventilation throughout the lung. The chest wall increases the effects of interdependence between adjacent portions or the lung about 10-fold when the thorax is intact (Menkes and Traystman, 1977). With paralysis of respiratory muscles the magnitude of interdependence decreases (Sylvester and Menkes, 1975), The chest wall appears to affect interdependence by preserving the shape of the obstructed segment during inspiration. The chest wall prevents increases in elastic recoil of the segment that result when it is unrestrained by the thoracic cage.

When lung volume increases, regional interdependence decreases (Sylvester et al., 1975). When the volume of the obstructed segment is increased independently of the surrounding lung, interdependence appeared to increase. Sylvester et al. interpret the increased interdependence as indicating that elastic recoil of the obstructed segment and interdependence falls as it returns toward a homogeneous shape. Clearly, changes in shape of an obstructed segment alter collateral flow. Segmental-alveolar pressure differ-ence is determined by the amount of inhomogeneity. In respiratory distress syndrome interdependence is also likely to be reduced and to be a less effective mechanism of expanding atelectatic lung segments because of increased surface tension due to lack of surfactant. Interdependence between adjacent portions of lungs should maintain the caliber of collateral channels and maintenance of interdependence would be clinically very important if an obstructed segment tended to collapse.

Synthesis of Mechanisms of Action and Hypothesis for Benefit from Chest Physiotherapy

Around and within atelectatic lung segments there are areas of lung that are partially aerated. It is possible that these partially aerated areas are the focus of physiotherapy effect during percussion, vibration, and coughing in the postural drainage position. Collateral ventilation and interdependence increase the likelihood of reexpansion of such atelectatic lung using chest physiotherapy by the following mechanisms.

Increase in Transpulmonary Pressure

Deep breathing increases the alveolar–pleural pressure difference. This increases collateral flow by increasing the driving pressure between the atelectatic segment and open airways. There may be greater transpulmonary pressure swings over an atelectatic than nonatelectatic area. Increased rib cage expansion and diaphragmatic descent are encouraged during breathing exercises and increase transpulmonary pressure. Rib cage vibration is performed over the course of exhalation and is followed by release of the rib cage compression. The effect is of "springing the ribs" outward causing a sudden increase in transpulmonary pressure. Since collateral airways resistance falls 13% for each centimeter of water increase in transpulmonary pressure (Kaplan et al., 1979), flow is promoted into an obstructed segment through collateral airways.

Positioning of Atelectatic Segment Nondependently

Postural drainage places the previously identified atelectatic segment in the optimum position for gravity to assist the drainage of secretions from the segmental bronchi toward the trachea. Postural drainage, therefore, always places the affected segment nondependently. The major effects of nondependent positioning are (1) transpulmonary pressure is increased, (2) $\dot{V}/\dot{Q}$ is increased, (3) lung/thorax compliance of the nondependent hemithorax is increased, and (4) collateral airways resistance with cholinergic blockage is reduced, which is not apparent when the same segment is positioned dependently. The combination of postural drainage with maneuvers such as mechanical ventilation with PEEP probably increases the likelihood of reexpansion of a nondependent atelectasis because the uppermost hemithorax is preferentially ventilated and has a greater absolute volume. Bronchodilators are likely to be most efficacious in their action to reduce collateral airway resistance and promote flow into an atelectatic area when administered with the affected segment nondependent. CO_2 tension in an obstructed lung segment is equal to mixed venous CO_2 tension and is, therefore, usually about 4–6 mm Hg higher than arterial CO_2 tensions. Since CO_2 is a potent collateral airway dilator and it is present in higher tensions in obstructed than ventilated airways, the elevated CO_2 promotes flow into the obstructed segment.

Generation of Pressure Differences between Atelectatic Segment and Open Airways

During exhalation there is a pressure gradient from the alveoli to the mouth that promotes flow. During a cough, huffing maneuver, or the forced expiratory technique, described in the chest physiotherapy literature, the alveolar–mouth pressure difference is increased. With coughing from total lung capacity dynamic airways compression sometimes occurs limiting flow (see Chapter 5). With forced expiratory techniques or external chest vibration and percussion, pressure gradients between the peripheral airways and mouth are increased without dynamic compression of the airways. The increased pressure gradient between air that entered an atelectatic segment by collateral airways during inspiration and the more proximal airways tends to propel inspissated secretions in the obstructed segment more centrally during exhalation. Some flow occurs from the obstructed segment by collateral ventilation during exhalation. However, when high flows occur, resistance in the collateral airways increases and so does the time constant. It is thought that the time constant for inflation of an obstructed segment through collateral airways is shorter than that for deflation. For the time constant to be increased either compliance or resistance of the collateral airways must increase. Resistance could increase by compression, by contraction of smooth muscle in the collateral airways, or by a valve mechanism. Aerodynamic valving occurs independently of diameter changes in the airways. Valving may be a factor decreasing outward flow through collateral airways and promoting the expulsion of mucus or overcoming surface tension forces necessary to expand an atelectatic lung segment.

The effect of cough on clearance of secretions from the peripheral airways is still unresolved (Rochester and Goldberg, 1980; Bateman et al., 1981). Cough may play a role as a necessary adjunct to chest physiotherapy. It is quite possible that during the deep inspiration before coughing, resistance in the collateral channels falls sufficiently to allow retrograde aeration of obstructed airways. During a cough the accelerated flow propels mucus into more central airways. Percussion and chest vibration may assist the movement of mucus centrally by causing oscillations in the airflow and changes in transpulmonary pressure. Percussion vibrates alveoli, alveolar ducts, and bronchioles and may promote flow of air through collateral and small airways. Secretions loosened by these maneuvers may then be propelled into the larger airways. Chest wall vibration oscillates air in larger airways and causes changes in the expired gas wave form analyzed by mass spectrometry (Fig. 7.17). The effect is transmitted to speech causing different vocal pitches and variations in air flow.

Interdependence

The process of reexpansion of atelectasis is greatly assisted by interdependence, which promotes synchronous ventilation of all parts of the lungs. During a thoracotomy when the lung is collapsed, application of an expiratory resistance while the chest is open and the lung visualized shows that the peripheral airways appear to help each other open due to interdependence. Reexpansion occurs from the normally ventilated lung bordering atelectatic areas inward. Interdependence counteracts the inhomogeneity of ventilation found in an atelectatic segment and maintains the collateral airways open.

Generally Accepted Statements

Subjective

1. Removal of sputum from the tracheobronchial tree is thought to be beneficial.
2. Subjective benefits reported by patients cannot always be supported by any measurable objective data.
3. Clinical examination of the chest, chest x-ray changes, sputum volume, and breathlessness are subjective assessments.
4. In chronic lung diseases, copious sputum production is essential for the treatment to produce subjective improvement.

Arterial Oxygenation

1. Oxygenation improves, deteriorates, or remains unchanged after chest physiotherapy. There are no known predictors.
2. Marked changes in lung/thorax compliance are accompanied by little or no change in arterial oxygenation.
3. Treatment of lung contusion with chest physiotherapy reduces intrapulmonary shunt when there is no excessive bleeding into the bronchi.
4. Alteration in cardiac function and the body positions used during and after chest physiotherapy may change arterial oxygenation.

Sputum

1. Sputum removal from major airways is achieved by coughing or suctioning through a tracheal tube and by postural drainage.
2. Retrograde aeration of obstructed airways by collateral ventilation assists mobilization of mucus obstructions more centrally.
3. The more viscid and tenacious the sputum, the more difficult it is to remove.
4. Sputum volume collected is an unreliable indicator of the efficacy of a chest physiotherapy treatment for acute lung disease because of different pathophysiology of the pulmonary disorder, swallowing of sputum, and unexplained variations in sputum production independent of chest physiotherapy.

Cough

1. Ciliary action, not cough, is the usual mechanism for movement of secretions from the peripheral lung more centrally.
2. When mucociliary transport is impaired, cough assists secretion removal.
3. Repetitive coughing decreases mucus transport and narrows the airways.
4. There are many other less hazardous techniques of cough stimulation than nasotracheal suctioning and transtracheal catheters.

Chest X-Ray

1. Identification of segmental lung pathology by a recent chest x-ray increases the likelihood of correct positioning for postural drainage and treatment of the area of pathology.
2. Acute atelectasis appears to respond as favorably to chest physiotherapy as bronchoscopy, when it is evaluated by

chest x-ray and outcome in prevention of pneumonia.

3. When an air bronchogram is visible to the peripheral lung fields, bronchoscopy does not improve the radiological picture.

4. The silhouette sign is invaluable for identification of lung segments on a straight portable anteroposterior chest x-ray.

More Sophisticated Objective Measurements of Improvement

1. Lung compliance increases after chest physiotherapy and removal of retained secretions in mechanically ventilated patients.

2. Intrapulmonary shunt falls after removal of secretions from the peripheral airways.

3. Functional residual capacity measurement and closing capacity are objective measures of the effect of chest physiotherapy on ventilation to small airways.

4. $\dot{V}/\dot{Q}$ scans are expensive and radioactive, but measure localized changes in V/Q that can be quantitated. The multiple inert gas technique of Wagner et al. (1974) overcomes many of the disadvantages of radioisotopes and is more specific. Extensive investigation of chest physiotherapy remains to be carried out.

Chronic Versus Acute Lung Disease Treated with Chest Physiotherapy

1. No study has shown that the chronic lung disease processes can be reversed by chest physiotherapy. Several studies have shown reversal of acute atelectasis.

2. The results of chest physiotherapy in patients with chronic lung disease cannot be extrapolated to patients with acute lung pathology.

3. Because therapist training differs and treatment methods, duration, and use of adjuncts, such as bronchodilators, mucolytics, and intermittent positive pressure breathing (IPPB), vary, rarely can comparisons be made of results from different centers.

4. The results of secretion removal on

sputum production and mucociliary transport may be different in chronic and acute lung disease.

Acute Lung Pathology

Atelectasis

1. Chest physiotherapy produces clinical and radiological resolution in 70% of unilobar atelectasis with a single treatment in mechanically ventilated patients.

2. Resolution of acute atelectasis is not related to the volume of sputum produced by chest physiotherapy.

3. Mechanical aids to lung expansion, such as bronchoscopy, incentive spirometry, IPPB, PEEP, and pressure support, are frequently more expensive and less effective than chest physiotherapy in treating acute atelectasis.

Lung Contusion

1. On percussing, vibrating, and suctioning the tracheobronchial tree, a lung contusion produces blood, not sputum.

2. Radiological evidence underestimates the extent of lung contusion. Maximum radiological effect of lung contusion is commonly seen 12 hr or more after injury. Contusion can be present despite a lack of rib fractures. Rib fractures and external signs of injury correlate poorly with lung injury found at autopsy.

3. Bleeding from a lung contusion can cause a deterioration of intrapulmonary shunt after postural drainage. This can also cause transbronchial aspiration and confuse the radiological diagnosis by giving a segmental distribution.

4. Pulmonary edema seen with lung contusion is usually noncardiogenic.

Pneumonia

1. Well-established pneumonia does not resolve with chest physiotherapy or mechanical ventilation.

2. Systemic and local hydration and appropriate antibiotic therapy are the recognized treatments of pneumonia.

3. If retained secretions are allowed to remain with the lungs, pneumonia may develop.

4. If a pneumonia-like process is treated during its development, pneumonia may be prevented.

Despite the ability to make some generally accepted statements about chest physiotherapy there is still a great deal that is unknown or unproven. Because there is so much that is disputed, personal bias weighs heavily. The areas of dispute are summarized in Chapter 1, Table 1.3 together with our opinion and practice. In our environment, it is difficult to persuade a Human Volunteers Research Committee that it is ethically acceptable to withhold percussion, vibration, and postural drainage and substitute tracheal suction and side-to-side turning for the treatment of sick ICU patients, since the former therapy is so strongly advocated, and the latter was found to be ineffective in preventing respiratory complications. Equally, random allocation of two groups of patients to either chest physiotherapy or bronchoscopy would, in our opinion, subject the mechanically ventilated patient with low lung compliance, high minute ventilation, and PEEP to an unacceptable risk with bronchoscopy.

There is quite naturally a wish to use noninvasive techniques to assess respiratory function following chest physiotherapy maneuvers.

The techniques of choice include $\dot{V}/\dot{Q}$ scanning of the lungs with xenon and technetium tracers and the multiple inert gas indicator technique (Wagner et al., 1974). Radioactive safety procedures with xenon and technetium tracers prevent the routine use of the $\dot{V}/\dot{Q}$ scan in other than nuclear medicine departments, the laboratory, or a specifically designed side ward in the ICU. The Wagner–West technique requires expensive and sophisticated equipment but is quite suitable for use in the ICU provided the patient is stable for the period of study. The magnetometer derived Konno–Mead plot (1967) may be used to measure regional chest wall function. Together with pneumotadygraph-derived values of lung and chest wall compliance and resistance, this provides useful noninvasive information about the mechanics of the chest wall and abdomen. Other noninvasive techniques assessing cardiac and respiratory function are usually not as accurate or informative as the invasive techniques. For example, what use is a knowledge of cardiac output gained by impedance cardiography if intracardiac filling pressures and mixed venous blood gases are unknown? How accurate is trancutaneous oxygen analysis in the adult? Noninvasive assessments of respiratory function by means of nitrogen washout or lung/thorax compliance are more easily obtained, but they lack the regional specificity available with the $\dot{V}/\dot{Q}$ scan and Wagner–West multiple inert gas technique. If it is difficult to obtain objective evidence of benefit by using invasive techniques, one can expect a similar difficulty with less invasive procedures. The solution to some of these problems is, therefore, a laboratory approach using animals.

Suggested Questions That Need Answering

1. What measurements should be made to quantitate the efficacy of chest physiotherapy maneuvers?
2. What are the indications for chest physiotherapy?
3. Is chest physiotherapy better than simple postural drainage and suctioning in removal of retained lung secretions?
4. Which component of chest physiotherapy among postural drainage, breathing exercises, percussion, vibration, cough, and tracheal suction is most effective in clearing secretions from the small airways?
5. Are mechanical devices, such as incentive spirometers, electrical vibrators, and CPAP face masks as effective as therapist-assisted manual techniques in altering respiratory function?
6. How important is cough in clearance of secretions from the smaller airways?
7. How important is suction in clearance of secretions from the smaller airways?
8. What are the optimum frequencies for vibration and percussion of the chest wall?
9. Is sputum volume, viscosity, and rheology important?

10. Is postural drainage with specific segmental positioning better than turning from side to side?
11. Does duration of chest physiotherapy alter secretion clearance?

SUMMARY

Arterial oxygenation may increase, fall, or remain unchanged following chest physiotherapy in mechanically ventilated or spontaneously breathing patients. No method was found to predict which possibility might occur. C_T was found to be a useful assessment of benefit from chest physiotherapy and with clinical signs an end point for therapy. R_{aw} was not such a reliable indicator. Benefit after removal of sputum in the patient with acute lung pathology does not depend on the volume removed. Mechanically ventilated patients may show increased PaO_2 and C_T despite less than 5-ml sputum production during chest physiotherapy. Cardiac and respiratory function changes during and after chest physiotherapy suggested that secretions were moved from the larger and smaller airways, resulting in improved function apparent for up to 2 hr after therapy.

Many factors, such as postural and cardiorespiratory changes and therapeutic interventions, make long-term follow-up difficult in the critically ill patient. Differences in methods of ventilation, application of therapy, anesthetic techniques, and patient population make comparisons between ICUs questionable. Generally accepted statements about chest physiotherapy that appear on pp. 242–244 and areas of dispute considered in Table 1.3 summarize our opinion on some controversial points.

WHAT PHYSIOLOGICAL MEASUREMENTS ARE REQUIRED AND HOW SHOULD THEY BE MADE? NATIONAL HEART, LUNG AND BLOOD INSTITUTE CONFERENCES OF 1974 AND 1979

1974 National Heart and Lung Institute

In 1974, the National Heart and Lung Institute organized a conference on the scientific basis of respiratory therapy, which was sponsored by the American Thoracic Society. It is frequently referred to as the "Sugarloaf Conference" and was published as a supplement to the journal, *American Review of Respiratory Disease*. This conference was held because of the controversy about the effectiveness of various maneuvers designed to remove secretions from the tracheobronchial tree. It was necessary for some objective judgments to be made by experts in the field and for the state of the art to be defined. The conference had three objectives: (1) to assess the existing data concerning the efficiency of respiratory therapy in the treatment of patients with chronic obstructive pulmonary disease, (2) to determine the additional data required to assess various modes of respiratory therapy more adequately, and (3) to make these findings available to stimulate appropriate investigations. The modes of respiratory therapy examined were chest physiotherapy, and IPPB with mucolytic agents and aerosolized detergents.

Petty (1974b) introduced the section on physical therapy and asked some specific questions: How will benefit following respiratory therapy be measured? What will be measured? Will symptomatic improvement, reduction in dyspnea, or mobilization of increased volumes of sputum be considered beneficial? If these items are too subjective, can studies be designed with acceptable controls and identifiable and reproducible end points? Six years later, these questions have not been answered and are still being asked (Cherniack, 1980; Peters and Turnier, 1980).

Since the conference was specifically addressed to respiratory therapy in patients with chronic obstructive pulmonary disease, the state of the art presentation (Jones, 1974) and other papers in this conference made no mention of the patients with acute lung disease. Some of the questions posed were, nonetheless, relevant to chest physiotherapy in the ICU. A particular question that Jones asked was, "Does postural drainage, chest vibration and percussion increase peripheral airway sputum removal?" Sputum rheology and volume, and the relation of these to respiratory function, were discussed. It appeared that there might be some weak correlation between respiratory function and sputum viscosity. The effect of the volume of sputum removed on respiratory function was, and still is, controversial. The results of chest physiotherapy on the peripheral airways were discussed earlier (see p. 219). Grimby (1974) reviewed the knowledge on breathing exercises and stressed the importance of deep breathing in prevention of airway closure. Alteration in flow rates, achieved with breathing exercises, may alter distribution of ventilation, but this required further evaluation using different breathing patterns.

Mellins (1974) wrote on pulmonary physiotherapy in the pediatric age group and credits the beginning of physical means for removing secretions in this age group to the early obstetricians who percussed the buttocks, not the chest. He was one of the few discussants in this conference to comment on the apparent success of chest physiotherapy in reversing pulmonary complications in acute conditions. Success of therapy was based on subjective measures such as clinical appearance, chest x-ray, and auscultatory changes. In general, this 1974 conference was very thought provoking to those interested in respiratory therapy. It posed many questions, suggested many studies, and played the devil's advocate to many traditionally held views. The details should be read because there is still a lot that can be learned from it.

1979 National Heart, Lung and Blood Institute (NHLBI) Conference

The 1979 NHLBI conference on the scientific basis of in hospital respiratory therapy was published as a supplement to the November 1980 issue of the *American Review of Respiratory Disease*. It intended to establish what is known and accepted about respiratory therapy, what needs to be found out so that therapy can be more rationally given, and what studies should be done to fulfill the necessary research. The conference was aimed toward the use of respiratory therapy outside the ICU.

There was not much that was novel in this conference, compared to the 1974 version on the same topics. However, reviews such as this undoubtedly help by focusing attention on the problems and by providing a diversity of expert opinion. Many of the studies suggested in 1974 have still not been performed. The 1979 conference adds to this backlog. At least a further 23 groups of studies were suggested by the authors of the 1979 conference, who wrote on chest physiotherapy and mechanical aids to lung expansion. It appears, therefore, that it is the practitioner's obligation to complete this research before the next conference.

There are eight papers concerning chest physiotherapy and mechanical aids to lung expansion. The authors of these articles quote over 300 references, of which only about 40% were published since 1974. This lack of progress in research was not adequately addressed by any of the authors, and only two groups acknowledged restricting their comments to updating information gained since 1974 (Darrow and Anthonisen, 1980; Rochester and Goldberg, 1980). This is surely an important point. One reason why these studies were not performed may be that the suggested research required sophisticated techniques and equipment not available in the average hospital. Alternatively, the end points may not be well enough defined, or the nonstudy factors may be too variable, to determine any significant differences. The difficulties encountered in producing a steady state, allowing only study variables in a critically ill patient, were already addressed (see p. 234).

In the three sections dealing with mechanical aids to lung expansion in the 1979 NHLBI conference, incentive inspiratory spirometry was generally favored over expiratory spirometry, which was condemned (Pontoppidan, 1980). IPPB was also unfavorably compared to other techniques. However, Murray (1980) noted that it might be useful to alter lung compliance in patients with chronic lung disease. The assumption of all these techniques, and of the whole conference, was that the patient was fit and well enough to cooperate. This may be the case with a great many people who receive therapy outside the ICU, but the majority of critically ill patients who receive chest physiotherapy require tracheal intubation and ventilatory support. Frequently they are unconscious, making continuous positive airway pressure by face mask and incentive spirometry both impractical and hazardous. It is unfortunate that the conference did not include physiotherapy and other respiratory maneuvers for the sick, mechanically ventilated patient in the ICU. It is possible that this group of patients may benefit the most from these techniques.

Ingram (1980), in the summary on mechanical aids to lung expansion, suggests some very pertinent questions. The most notable are, Is supervised deep breathing as effective in producing acute pulmonary function changes as incentive spirometry, IPPB, or continuous positive airway pressure? Is the benefit gained by periodic hyperinflation sufficiently great to justify a major investigative effort? The incidence of these problems can be judged from the finding that 106 (1%) of 10,931 chest physiotherapy treatments given to critically ill patients in a 22-month period between September 1978 and June 1980 consisted of coughing and deep breathing exercises only. However, in this same period, 232 (30.2%) of the 769 patients treated were mobilized. Mobilization included ambulation and exercises (see Chapter 6). The low incidence (1%) of problems that were felt to be avoidable by use of breathing exercises alone reflects the aggressive approach to early mobilization and the fact that the majority of treatments were given to mechanically ventilated patients. In our experience, without the use of mechanical aids to lung expansion, breathing exercises supervised by the chest physical therapists are sufficient to reverse the problem in nonintubated patients who are conscious, cooperative, and breathing spontaneously.

The rationale for physical therapy discussed by Menkes and Britt (1980) is of great interest. It is one of the few papers presented at either conference that attempts to answer questions rather than pose them. These authors reviewed the importance of lung volume in affecting resistance to flow through the collateral channels, the factors that may affect regional distribution of ventilation, the responses to mucociliary clearance, and $\dot{V}/\dot{Q}$ changes that might take place follow-

ing chest physiotherapy. Some of the difficulties of using sputum volume, ABGs, and airways resistance as indicators of changes in peripheral airways were discussed.

The article by Peters and Turnier (1980) discussed indications for, and effects of, physiotheraphy in surgical patients. They reviewed the literature and listed some agents promoting collapse after surgery. Immobility and pain were stressed as important factors in the development of respiratory complications. They noted that a difference between mechanical aids, such as incentive spirometry and IPPB, and chest physiotherapy was the presence of a skillful, sympathetic therapist. This may be a vital determinant of whether secretions are cleared. Finally, these authors enumerated several problems in evaluation of chest physiotherapy effectiveness.

Techniques of respiratory therapy were divided into two functionally discrete entities by Rochester and Goldberg (1980): pulmonary physical therapy for patients with increased sputum production and breathing training for patients with dyspnea or poor exercise tolerance. The variation in techniques termed "chest physiotherapy" in the articles that they quoted was not discussed, nor were some of the different conclusions in the currently published literature resolved. However, their summary brings out important points concerning treatment of the patient with chronic bronchitis, bronchospasm, hypoxia or pneumonia. They suggest that failure to exclude the effect of cough may change some previously accepted conclusions of beneficial effects of pulmonary physiotherapy. Breathing exercises were thought to be best judged on the basis of respiratory muscle strength and endurance rather than on the basis of pulmonary function tests. They hypothesized that the patient's metabolic and nutritional status will affect the outcome of a breathing training program.

What did these experts consider the best indicators of benefit from chest physiotherapy? Cherniack (1980) recommended studies in three areas. First, the effectiveness of bronchial drainage should be compared to deep breathing and cough. The suggested indicators of benefit included volume of sputum produced, alterations in gas exchange, and mucociliary clearance. The techniques for assessing mucociliary clearance were not identified, but the gamma camera and radioactive tracers are the most advanced assessments presently available. Clearance of radioactive-labeled secretions of different viscosity, placed at various sites in the tracheobronchial tree, may be compared by using postural drainage, percussion, vibration, coughing, and huffing. The second area for study was to evaluate the balance between changes in energy cost and gas exchange following breathing exercises. Energy cost was not defined but would certainly include measurement of oxygen consumption and carbon dioxide excretion. Diaphragmatic and costal excursion exercise techniques may then be compared to determine if breathing retraining is of value. The importance of controlling other treatment variables that occur after surgery, including changes in nutritional and metabolic status, was stressed. Maximal inspiratory and expiratory and transdiaphragmatic pressures were suggested as relatively accurate assessments of respiratory muscle strength. However, specific respiratory muscle endurance tests were noted to be lacking. The third area recommended for study by Cherniack was pulmonary rehabilitation. The cost effectiveness, staffing, and impact of rehabilitation on the course of chronic respiratory disease should be determined and then evaluated. The methods of evaluation were not suggested, but patients with moderate respiratory dysfunction and employment were considered the best group to study.

References

Andersen JB, Qvist J, Kann T: Recruiting collapsed lung through collateral channels with positive end-expiratory pressure. Scand J Resp Dis 60:260–266, 1979

Aylward M: A between-patient, double-blind comparison of S-carboxymethylcysteine and bromhexine in chronic obstructive bronchitis. Curr Med Res Opin 1:219–227, 1973

Baarsma PR, Dirken MNJ, Huizinga E: Collateral ventilation in man. J Thorac Surg 17:252–263, 1948

Bade PL, McMichan JC, Marsh HM: Continuous monitoring of mixed venous oxygen saturation in critically ill patients. Anesth Analg 61:513–516, 1982

Barach A, Segal MS: The indiscriminate use of IPPB. JAMA 231:1141–1142, 1975

Barrell SE, Abbas HM: Monitoring during physiotherapy after open heart surgery. Physiotherapy 64:272–273, 1978

Barrett CR: Flexible fiberoptic bronchoscopy in the critically ill patient. Chest 73:746–749, 1978

Bartels M: Collateral ventilation beim menchen habihtation schnft ans der medizinischen. Thesis, Tübingen Universitätsklinik, 1972

Bartlett RH, Brennan ML, Gazzaniga AB, Hansen EL: Studies on the pathogenesis and prevention of postoperative pulmonary complications. Surg Gynecol Obstet 137:925–933, 1973.

Bateman JRM, Newman SP, Daunt KM, Pavia D, Clarke SW: Regional lung clearance of excessive bronchial secretions during chest physiotherapy in patients with stable chronic airways obstruction. Lancet 1:294–297, 1979

Batra G, Traystman R, Rudnick H, Menkes H: Effects of body position and cholinergic blockade on mechanics of collateral ventilation. J Appl Physiol 50:358–362, 1981

Beecher HK, Todd DP: A study of the deaths associated with anesthesia and surgery. Ann Surg 140:2–34, 1954

Chen C, Sealy WC, Seaber AV: The dynamic nature of collateral ventilation. J Thorac Cardiovasc Surg 59:518–529, 1970

Cherniack RM: Physical therapy. Am Rev Respir Dis 122(2):25–27, 1980

Clarke SW, Cochrane GM, Webber B: Effects of sputum on pulmonary function (abstract). Thorax 28:262, 1973

Cochrane GM, Webber BA, Clarke SW: Effects of sputum on pulmonary function. Br Med J 2:1181–1183, 1977

Connors AF, Hammon WE, Martin RI, Rogers RM: Chest physical therapy. The immediate effect on oxygenation in acutely ill patients. Chest 78:559–564, 1980

Culiner MM, Reich SB: Collateral ventilation and localized emphysema. Am J Roetgenol 85:246–252, 1961

Darrow G, Anthonisen NR: Physiotherapy in hospitalized medical patients. Am Rev Respir Dis 122(2):155–158, 1980

Dohi S, Gold MI: Comparison of two methods of postoperative respiratory care. Chest 73:592–595, 1978

Douglas WW, Rehder K, Beyneu FM, Sessler AD, Marsh HM: Improved oxygenation in patients with acute respiratory failure; the prone position. Am Rev Respir Dis 115:559–566, 1977

Fairley HB: Oxygen therapy for surgical patients. Am Rev Respir Dis 122(2):37–44, 1980

Feldman NT, Huber GL: Fiberoptic bronchoscopy in the intensive care unit. Int Anesthesiol Clin 14:31–42, 1976

Field GB: The effects of posture, oxygen, isoproterenol and atropine on ventilation. Clin Sci 32:279, 1967

Filley GF, Beckwitt HJ, Reeves JT, Mitchell RS: Chronic obstructive bronchopulmonary disease II: oxygen transport in two clinical types. Am J Med 44:26, 1968

Finer NN, Boyd J: Chest physiotherapy in the neonate: A controlled study. *Pediatrics* 61:282–285, 1978

General Physiotherapy: *G5 Massage Apparatus.* General Physiotherapy, St. Louis, 1979

Gold MI: Is intermittent positive-pressure breathing therapy (IPPB Rx) treatment necessary in the surgical patient? *Ann Surg* 184:122–123, 1976

Gormezano J, Branthwaite MA: Effects of physiotherapy during intermittent positive pressure ventilation. *Anaesthesia* 27:258–263, 1972

Graham WGB, Bradley DA: Efficacy of chest physiotherapy and intermittent positive-pressure breathing in the resolution of pneumonia. *N Engl J Med* 299:624–627, 1978

Grimby G: Aspects of lung expansion in relation to pulmonary physiotherapy. *Am Rev Respir Dis* 110(2):145–153, 1974

Hedstrand U, Liw M, Rooth G, Ogren CH: Effect of respiratory physiotherapy on arterial oxygen tension. *Acta Anaesthesiol Scand* 22:349–352, 1978

Ingram RH: Mechanical aids to lung expansion. *Am Rev Respir Dis* 122(2):23–24, 1980

Inners CR, Terry PB, Traystman RJ, Menkes HA: Effect of lung volumes on collateral and airway resistance in man. *J Appl Physiol* 46:67–73, 1979

Jones NJ: Physical therapy—present state of the art. *Am Rev Respir Dis* 110(2):132–136, 1974

Kaneko K, Millic-Emili J, Dolovich MD: Regional distribution of ventilation and perfusion as a function of body position. *J Appl Physiol* 21:767–782, 1966

Kaplan J, Koehler RC, Terry PB, Menkes HA, Traystman RJ: The effects of lung volume on collateral and small airways resistance in the dog. (Abstract) *Am Rev Respir Dis* 119:322, 1979

Klein P, Kemper M, Weissman C, Rosenbaum SH, Askanazi J, Hyman AI: Attenuation of the hemodynamic responses to chest physical therapy. *Chest* 93:38–42, 1988

Kohn HN: Zur histologie der indurirenden fibrenosa pneumonie. *Munch Med Wochensdir* 40:42–45, 1893

Konno K, Mead J: Measurement of the separate volume changes of the rib cage and abdomen during breathing. *J Appl Physiol* 22:407–422, 1967

Kuriyama T, Latham LP, Horwitz LD, Reeves JT, Wagner WW: Role of collateral ventilation in ventilation-perfusion balance. *J Appl Physiol* 56:1500–1506, 1984

Lambert MW: Accessory bronchiole-alveolar communications. *J Pathol Bacteriol* 70:311–314, 1955

Laws AK, McIntyre RW: Chest Physiotherapy: A physiological assessment during intermittent positive pressure ventilation in respiratory failure. *Can Anaesth Soc J* 16:487–493, 1969

Lindholm C-E, Ollman B, Snyder J, Millen E, Grenvik A: Flexible fiberoptic bronchoscopy in critical care medicine. *Crit Care Med* 2:250–261, 1974

Loosli CG: Interalveolar communications in normal and in pathologic mammalian lungs. *Arch Pathol* 24:743–767, 1937

Lundgren R, Haggmark S, Reiz S: Hemodynamic effects of flexible fiberoptic bronchoscopy performed under topical anesthesia. *Chest* 82:295–299, 1982

Lyager S, Wernberg M, Rajani N, Bøggild-Madsen B, Nielsen L, Nielsen HC, Andersen M, Møller J, Sil-

berschmid M: Can postoperative pulmonary conditions be improved by treatment with the Bartlett-Edwards Incentive Spirometer after upper abdominal surgery? *Acta Anaesthesiol Scand* 23:312–319, 1979

Mackenzie CF, Shin B, McAslan TC: Chest physiotherapy: The effect on arterial oxygenation. *Anesth Analg (Cleve)* 57:28–30, 1978a

Mackenzie CF, Shin B: Evaluation of physical therapy (letter). *N Engl J Med* 301:665–666, 1978b

Mackenzie CF, Shin B, Friedman S, Wai M: Evaluation of total lung/thorax vs static lung compliance. *Anesthesiology* 51:S381, 1979

Mackenzie CF, Shin B, Hadi F, Imle PC: Changes in total lung/thorax compliance following chest physiotherapy. *Anesth Analg (Cleve)* 59:207–210, 1980

Mackenzie CF, Shin B: Cardiorespiratory function before and after physiotherapy in mechanically ventilated patients with post-traumatic respiratory failure. *Crit Care Med* 13:483–486, 1985

Macklem PT: Airway obstruction and collateral ventilation. *Physiol Rev* 51:368–436, 1971

Macklem PT: Collateral ventilation. *N Engl J Med* 298:49–50, 1978

Macklin CC: Alveolar pores and their significance in the human lung. *Arch Pathol* 21:202–216, 1936

Marini JJ, Pierson DJ, Hudson LD: Acute lobar atelectasis. A prospective comparison of fiberoptic bronchoscopy and respiratory therapy. *Am Rev Respir Dis* 119:971–978, 1979

Martin HB: The effect of aging on the alveolar pores of Kohn in the dog. *Am Rev Respir Dis* 88:773–778, 1963

Martin HB: Respiratory bronchioles as the pathway for collateral ventilation. *J Appl Physiol* 21:1443–1447, 1966

May DB, Munt PW: Physiologic effects of chest percussion and postural drainage in patients with stable chronic bronchitis. *Chest* 75:29–32, 1979

McAslan TC: Automated respiratory gas monitoring of critically ill patients. *Crit Care Med* 4:255–260, 1976

McConnell DH, Maloney JV, Buckberg GD: Postoperative intermittent positive-pressure breathing treatments. *J Thorac Cardiovasc Surg* 68:944–952, 1974

McIntyre RW, Laws AK, Ramanchandran PR: Positive expiratory pressure plateau: Improved gas exchange during mechanical ventilation. *Can Anaesth Soc J* 16:477–486, 1969

Mead J: Respiration: pulmonary mechanics. *Ann Rev Physiol* 35:169–192, 1973

Mellins RB: Pulmonary physiotherapy in the pediatric age group. *Am Rev Respir Dis* 110(2):137–142, 1974

Menkes HA, Britt J: Rationale for physical therapy. *Am Rev Respir Dis* 122(2):127–131, 1980

Menkes H, Gardiner A, Gamsu G, Lempert J, Macklem PT: Influence of surface forces on collateral ventilation. *J Appl Physiol* 31:544, 1971

Menkes HA, Traystman RJ: State of the art. Collateral ventilation. *Am Rev Respir Dis* 116:287–309, 1977

Murray JF: Reply to correspondence on evaluation of respiratory physical therapy. *N Engl J Med* 301:666, 1979

Murray JF: Indication for mechanical aids to assist

lung inflation in medical patients. *Am Rev Respir Dis* 122(2):121–125, 1980

Newton DAG, Stephenson A: Effect of physiotherapy on pulmonary function. *Lancet* 2:228–230, 1978

O'Donohue WJ: Maximum volume IPPB for the management of pulmonary atelectasis. *Chest* 76:683–687, 1979

Opie LH, Spalding JMK: Chest physiotherapy during intermittent positive pressure respiration. *Lancet* 2:671–674, 1958

Pavia D, Thomson ML, Phillipakos D: A preliminary study of the effect of a vibrating pad on bronchial clearance. *Am Rev Respir Dis* 113:92–96, 1976

Peters RM, Turnier E: Physical therapy: Indications for and effects in surgical patients. *Am Rev Respir Dis* 122(2):147–154, 1980

Petty TL: A critical look at IPPB (editorial). *Chest* 66:1–3, 1974a

Petty TL: Physical therapy. *Am Rev Respir Dis* 110(2):129–130, 1974b

Pontoppidan H: Mechanical aids to lung expansion in non-intubated surgical patients. *Am Rev Respir Dis* 122(2):109–119, 1980

Remolina C, Khan AV, Santiago TV, Edelman NH: Positional hypoxemia in unilateral lung disease. *N Engl J Med* 304:523–525, 1981

Richardson JD, Adams L, Flint LM: Selective management of flail chest and pulmonary contusion. *Ann Surg* 196:481–485, 1982

Ricker JB, Haberman B: Expired gas monitoring by mass spectrometry in a respiratory intensive care unit. *Crit Care Med* 4:223–229, 1976

Rivara D, Artucio H, Arcos J, Hiriart C: Positional hypoxemia during artificial ventilation. *Crit Care Med* 12:436–438, 1984

Rochester DF, Goldberg SK: Techniques of respiratory physical therapy. *Am Rev Respir Dis* 122(2):133–146, 1977

Rosenberg DE, Lyons HA: Collateral ventilation in excised human lungs. *Respiration* 37:125–134, 1979

Rubi JAG, Sanartin A, Diaz GG, Apezteguia C, Martinez GT, Rubi JCM: Assessment of total pulmonary airway resistance under mechanical ventilation. *Crit Care Med* 8:633–636, 1980

Sackner MA, Wanner A, Landa J: Applications of bronchofiberscopy. *Chest (Suppl)* 62:70–78, 1972

Sackner MA: State of the art bronchofiberscopy. *Am Rev Respir Dis* 111:62–88, 1975

Sands JH, Cypert C, Armstrong R, Ching S, Trainer D, Quinn W, Stewart D: A controlled study using routine intermittent positive-pressure breathing in the post-surgical patient. *Dis Chest* 40:128–133, 1961

Schmerber J, Deltenre M: A new fatal complication of transtracheal aspiration. *Scand J Respir Dis* 59:232–235, 1978

Shim C, Fine N, Fernandez R, Williams MH: Cardiac arrhythmias resulting from tracheal suctioning. *Ann Intern Med* 71:1149–1153, 1969

Shim C, Bajwa S, Williams MH: The effect of inhalation therapy on ventilatory function and expectoration. *Chest* 73:798–801, 1978

Sinha R, Bergofsky EH: Prolonged alteration of lung mechanics in kyphoscoliosis by positive-pressure hyperinflation. *Am Rev Respir Dis* 106:47–57, 1972

Sylvester JT, Menkes HA: Pulmonary interdependence during spontaneous and artificial ventilation in the pig. (Abstract) *Am Rev Respir Dis* 111:942, 1975

Sylvester JT, Menkes HA, Stitik F: Lung volume and interdependence in the pig. *J Appl Physiol* 38:395, 1975

Terry PB, Menkes HA, Traystman RJ: Effects of maturation and aging on collateral ventilation in sheep. *J Appl Physiol* 62:1028–1032, 1987

Terry PB, Traystman RJ, Menkes HA: The clinical significance of collateral ventilation. Personal communication, 1985

Terry PB, Traystman RJ, Newball HH, Batra G, Menkes HA: Collateral ventilation in man. *N Engl J Med* 298:10–15, 1978

Thomson ML, Pavia D, Jones CJ, McQuiston TAC: No demonstrable effect of S-carboxymethylcysteine on clearance of secretions from the human lung. *Thorax* 30:669–673, 1975

Traystman RJ, Terry PB, Menkes HA: Carbon dioxide—a major determinant of collateral ventilation. *J Appl Physiol* 45:69–74, 1978

Van Allen CM, Jung TS: Postoperative atelectasis and collateral respiration. *J Thorac Surg* 1:13–14, 1931

Van Allen CM, Lindskog GE: Collateral respiration in the lung. *Surg Gynecol Obstet* 53:16–21, 1931

Vraciu JK, Vraciu RA: Effectiveness of breathing exercises in preventing pulmonary complication following open heart surgery. *Phys Ther* 57:1367–1371, 1977

Wagner PD, Dantzker VE, Iacovoni WC, Tomlin WC, West JB: Ventilation-perfusion inequality in asymptomatic asthma. *Am Rev Respir Dis* 118:511–524, 1978

Wagner PD, Saltzman HA, West JB: Measurement of continuous distributions of ventilation-perfusion ratios: Theory. *J Appl Physiol* 36:588–599, 1974

Welply NC, Mathias CJ, Frankel HL: Circulatory reflexes in tetraplegics during artificial ventilation and general anesthesia. *Paraplegia* 13:172–182, 1975

Winning TJ, Brock-Utne JG, Goodwin NM: A simple clinical method of quantitating the effects of chest physiotherapy in mechanically ventilated patients. *Anaesth Intensive Care* 3:237–238, 1975

Zack MB, Pontoppidan H, Kazaim H: The effects of lateral position on gas exchange in pulmonary disease. *Am Rev Respir Dis* 110:49–55, 1979

Zidulka A, Demedts M, Nadler S, Anthonisen NR: Pleural pressure with lobar obstruction in dogs. *Resp Physiol* 26:239-248, 1976

CHAPTER 8

Chest Physiotherapy for Special Patients

Nancy Ciesla, B.S., P.T.

This chapter discusses chest physiotherapy for patients with specific problems predisposing to retention of lung secretions. Acute and chronic diseases are included and individual approaches to treatment are described for each group of patients. The literature appropriate to these groups is reviewed.

PEDIATRIC PATIENTS

Physiotherapy is indicated in pediatric patients with neurological impairment, asthma, cystic fibrosis, or following meconium aspiration (Crane, 1981; 1985; DeCesare, 1985; DeCesare et al., 1982; Parker, 1985). It is also indicated when secretion retention occurs after surgery. As with the adult population, decreased morbidity and duration of fever, and improvement in chest x-ray are not documented in patients with viral pneumonia and acute bronchiolitis receiving chest physiotherapy (Webb et al., 1985; Levine, 1978).

Infants

Full-term infants and adults have anatomical similarities and differences. At birth, all large airways are formed; the trachea and bronchi rapidly increase in length and diameter during the first few months of life (Doershuk et al., 1975). In the neonatal period the trachea is funnel-shaped (upper end wider than the lower end), and becomes cylindrical within the first 5 years of life (Wailoo and Emery, 1982). The respiratory zone of the lung is composed of three generations of respiratory bronchioles and one order of alveolar ducts and sacs. By 2 months of age, four generations of respiratory bronchioles and three of alveolar ducts are present. Because of the lack of smooth muscle development until 3–4 years of age, the bronchiole walls are weak in early childhood. Alveolar surface area is 5% that of the adult (Johnson et al., 1978). Collateral ventilation is acquired after birth. The pores of Kohn appear in the first year of life and increase in size and number with age (Menkes and Traystman, 1977). Channels of Lambert are most likely present by 6 years of age (Macklem, 1977). Alveolar ducts are thought to increase in number until 8 years of age, although the precise age at which alveolar growth stops is unknown (Angus and Thurlbeck, 1972). Alveolar ducts increase in size until adulthood when the chest wall is fully developed. Elastic fibers surrounding the alveoli are not fully mature until adolescence. Therefore, the majority of lung development occurs by 2 years of age with lung growth continuing until adulthood (Fig. 8.1).

The infant and child under 4 years of age have more mucus glands per surface area of bronchi than adults (Lough et al., 1974; Hislop and Reid, 1974). Doershuk et al. (1975) report twice as many glands per unit surface area in children under 4 compared with the adult. Goblet cells may extend beyond the cartilaginous portion of the tracheobronchial tree into the bronchioles and replace ciliated cells in disease (DeCesare, 1985).

The rib cage of an infant is circular in the horizontal plane (Muller and Bryan, 1979) and the diaphragm has a horizontal insertion. Twenty-five percent of the muscle fibers are type I red, slow-twitch, fatigue-resistant muscle fibers compared with 50% in the adult.

The physiological consequences of these anatomical differences between child and adult include reduced compliance of the infant lung with increased chest wall compliance. A decreased number of oxidative muscle fibers in the diaphragm make the infant more susceptible to respiratory muscle fatigue and subsequently respiratory muscle failure (Muller and Bryan). Decreased surfactant leads to alveolar collapse. Premature infants may also have decreased flow rates

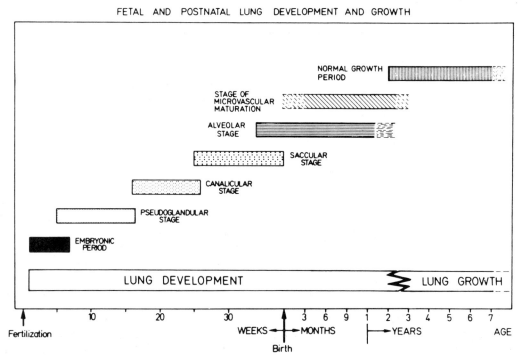

Figure 8.1. Fetal and postnatal lung development from fertilization to age 7. Note that the majority of lung development takes place before age 3; alveolar growth continues until adulthood. (From The postnatal development and growth of the human lung. II. Morphology. B Zeltner and PH Burri: *Respir Physiol* 67:269–282, 1987.)

and increased resistance in the peripheral airways (Stocks and Godfrey, 1976). Children have less pulmonary reserve than adults, probably related to increased resting oxygen consumption in relationship to lung surface area (Doershuk et al.). The small airway diameter, large size, and high density of mucus glands and reduced structural support of the airway may increase the chance of airway occlusion. The sick neonate may be more prone to increased secretion production and therefore retention. Infants who develop bronchopulmonary dysplasia have a high incidence of recurrent pulmonary infection in the first 2 years of life (Johnson et al., 1974). Myers et al. (1986) did not find an increased risk in the frequency of respiratory illness in a comparison of preterm infants with and without respiratory distress syndrome (RDS), although RDS survivors experienced more severe and lower respiratory infections at a younger age. Infants may also have a higher incidence of laryngeal injury following extubation. Fan et al., 1982, documented a 44% incidence of moderate or major laryngeal injury after extubation.

Intubation may also contribute to secretion retention in the neonate. Whitfield and Jones (1980) found that the intubated infant with hyaline membrane disease, weighing less than 1500 gm, had an increased incidence of atelectasis, directly related to the duration of intubation. The right upper lobe is most frequently involved both while the infant is intubated and following extubation. The right lung is more often affected than the left. The primarily right-sided atelectasis may be due to malalignment of the tracheal tube or mucosal damage of the right main stem bronchus resulting from prolonged intubation, suctioning, and saline lavage (Roper et al., 1976; Whitfield and Jones). For this reason, Roper and colleagues recommend vigorous chest physiotherapy primarily to the right upper lobe, commenced as soon as the infant is intubated and continued for several days after removal of the tracheal tube. These authors also recommend that chest physiotherapy should not be performed more frequently than every 3 hr. This minimizes bronchial mucosal damage from suctioning. Pediatric respiratory disease is a risk factor for development of atelectasis and chronic lung disease (Streider, 1974). Long-term residual abnormalities in lung function may occur (Katten, 1979).

Chest physiotherapy does not appear to alter the disease processes of hyaline membrane disease, acute bronchiolitis, and meconium aspiration. In a controlled study evaluating the effects of chest physiotherapy on 90 infants with acute bronchiolitis chest physiotherapy did not decrease the severity or length of the disease process (Webb et al. 1985). Treatment included 3 min of chest percussion in 5 postural drainage positions followed by assisted coughing or oropharyngeal suction. Indications for treatment did not specifically relate to the infant's secretion production or radiological evidence of atelectasis or infiltrate. The primary indications for chest physiotherapy treatment are retained secretions resulting from prolonged intubation and mechanical ventilation, increased mucus production, narrowing and decreased smooth muscle of infant airways, decreased collateral ventilation, and immobility.

Marked variations in technique may account for conflicting results noted in research evaluating chest physiotherapy. In some studies the methods of performing chest physiotherapy are not described, while in others the duration of treatment and the use of hyperinflation, percussion, vibration, or postural drainage differ. One important difference in administering chest physiotherapy to the neonate versus the adult is the infant's response to handling. This may significantly alter both the scheduling and duration of therapy. It is also more difficult to clinically assess lobar or segmental lung pathology. Chest x-ray reports and the secretions obtained during and after treatment may be more important determinants of appropriate positioning and duration of therapy than auscultation and diagnostic percussion. Infants with prolonged respiratory distress are prone to stress fractures of the ribs (Burnard et al., 1965; Parker, 1985). Manual techniques therefore should be carefully performed by experienced health care personnel (pp. 144).

Clinical Assessment

The clinical assessment of the infant is the same as that for the adult (p. 74) with a few exceptions. The therapist should be aware of additional clinical signs of respiratory distress, for example, expiratory grunting, head bobbing, retractions of the rib cage, and stridor. Treatment should be carried out after assessing the specific indications for treatment and the infant's oxygenation. Information gained from chest x-ray, auscultation, the infant's response to handling, position change, and suctioning is utilized to plan appropriate treatment. Tactile stimulation associated with auscultation of the chest should be minimized (Klaus et al., 1979). Positioning may be determined by the quantity or quality of secretions obtained from draining specific lung segments.

Handling/Positioning

Excessive handling of the low-birth-weight infant causes hypoxemia (Long et al., 1980; Speidel, 1978). Yeh and colleagues (1982) documented significant increases in oxygen consumption with intravenous line insertion, heel sticks, and chest percussion. Danford et al. (1983) noted positioning for chest x-rays had the greatest fall in TcPO2, when studying 8 routine ICU procedures. Continuous monitoring of pulse oximetry or transcutaneous oxygen pressure (TcPO2) allows identification of unacceptable oxygenation during routine intensive care unit procedures such as chest physiotherapy, handling, and suctioning (Speidel). For infants whose PO_2 drops during handling, chest physiotherapy should be scheduled around other routine procedures.

Research is inconclusive regarding optimum positioning of infants. Tidal volume and minute ventilation increase and periods of apnea are reduced in the prone compared to supine position; a 25% increase in PaO_2 is also documented (Martin et al., 1979; Dhande et al., 1982). Specific anatomical areas of lung pathology were not described in either study. Dhande and colleagues studied five preterm infants with birth weights of 1030 to 1817 gm. These authors speculated that

the reduced occurrence of apnea in the prone position may result from improved ventilation and oxygenation. Martin and colleagues studied 16 preterm infants with a mean birth weight of 1.53 kg and concluded that placing infants in the prone position may significantly reduce morbidity and mortality. The prone position may stabilize the compliant chest wall of the infant and improve coordination between rib cage, diaphragm, and abdominal movement. As with other patient populations, routine positioning and suctioning may minimize the need for chest physiotherapy treatment (Tudehope and Bagley, 1980).

Arterial Oxygenation

Holloway et al. (1966) found a temporary decrease in arterial oxygenation after chest physiotherapy in eight neonates suffering from tetanus. Oxygenation returned to normal 1 hr after treatment. In 1969, Holloway et al. published similar findings, but noted that the fall in oxygenation could be reversed with lung hyperinflation. This did not alter any long-term decrease in PaO_2. Fox et al. (1978) also found that mean PaO_2 decreased 30 torr in 13 neonates breathing with continuous positive airway pressure. Chest physiotherapy consisted of mechanical chest vibrations and suctioning in the supine position. This fall was thought to be the result of increased right-to-left cardiac shunting due to coughing and suctioning. In 1978, Finer and Boyd noted that PaO_2 rose during chest physiotherapy treatment. Etches and Scott (1978) found that four hourly chest physiotherapy treatments to the lower lobes of six neonates produced greater quantities of secretions than did suctioning alone. During chest physiotherapy and monitoring of transcutaneous oxygen tension (TcPO2) in a crying infant, fell. However, it remained stable when the child was quiet. Ten minutes following the procedure, TcPO2 increased (Gregory, 1980). Tudehope and Bagley (1980) evaluated contact heel percussion, cupping with a Bennett face mask, and vibration using an electric toothbrush applied to 15 consecutively born infants with respiratory distress syndrome (RDS). The infants tolerated chest physiotherapy with the first two techniques very well with a statistically significant increase in PaO_2 (see Chapter 4). Chest physiotherapy given to 7 neonates, which consisted of positioning in the head-up and head-down positions for 60 sec and suctioning, showed no significant improvement in TcPO2 (Raval et al., 1981). Walsh et al. (1987) and Barnes et al. (1981) noted a decrease in TcPO2 during chest physiotherapy although postural drainage was not used in either study. The results of these studies may have been different if longer periods of postural drainage were given to the most involved lung lobes or segments. This in itself would minimize handling and allow more time for secretions to drain from peripheral airways. In view of these results, no definite conclusions can be drawn as to whether chest physiotherapy produces hypoxemia in the neonate, especially since the cardiac effects of chest physiotherapy were not evaluated.

Lung Hyperinflation, Suctioning, Postural Drainage

Chest care for the pediatric intensive care unit (ICU) patient with retained secretions does not vary much from the care provided to a similar adult patient. Hyperinflation with supplemental oxygen before and after suctioning may be critical to reverse hypoxemia and airway closure (see Chapter 5). The literature is inconclusive as to whether bagging with 100% oxygen, which may result in hyperoxemia, is necessary when suctioning neonates. Raval et al. (1980) recommend using 100% O_2 only when the infant's baseline PaO_2 is hypoxemic. Barnes (1981) found decreases in oxygenation associated with suctioning to be minimized when the ventilator rather than bagging was used prior to suctioning. Walsh and associates suggest that controlling supplemental oxygenation without manual bag ventilation is sufficient with a shorter recovery time. Okken et al. (1978) found bag ventilation to be beneficial in quiet infants while PaO_2 significantly decreased in restless infants, yet Simbruner et al. (1981) advocate using ventilators with simultaneous rather than controlled ventilation to minimize decreases in PaO_2 associated with suctioning. Simbruner and colleagues also noted TcPO2 measurements to have a 2 min delayed response when compared to PaO_2. Tracheal stimulation is associated with increased intracranial pressure in brain injured children (Fisher et al., 1982). Preterm infants may be at greater risk of intraventricular hemorrhage after suctioning (Perlman and Volpe, 1983). Suctioning of intubated infants is recommended when secretions are most likely present. Suctioning should be carried out during chest physiotherapy treatment or in conjunction with routine position changes. The child's response to suctioning is observed closely. The nonintubated infant who does not cough spontaneously should have the oropharynx suctioned after postural drainage; this may cause secretions to gravitate to the carina and stimulate a cough. Mild stimulation over the trachea is another beneficial cough stimulation technique that may be used following postural drainage. Head-up, head-down, prone, and supine positions and lying on the right and left sides are encouraged in the patients turning schedule. Mobilization helps prevent stagnation of peripheral secretions in the gravity dependent areas of the lung and minimize the need for chest physiotherapy treatment (Fig. 8.2).

Chest physiotherapy treatments are modified according to secretion production, the incidence of apneic episodes, clinical signs of respiratory distress, changes in vital signs and changes or a fall in TcPO2. Crane (1981) recommends treatment be given for 3–5 min per lung segment. The most involved lung segments are treated first. It is more important to adequately treat involved lung segments than routinely perform treatment to all lung segments. It may be necessary to address different lung segments during each treatment. Children with meconium aspiration should receive chest physiotherapy from birth until they are free of meconium staining. The effect of short sessions (5–10 min) given every hour or two versus longer sessions (15–45 min) given every 4–6 hr requires further investigation. Differences in alveolar number and size, collateral ventilation,

Figure 8.2. An infant with respiratory distress syndrome is positioned prone over a rolled towel to promote drainage of secretions from the posterior segments of the lower lobes.

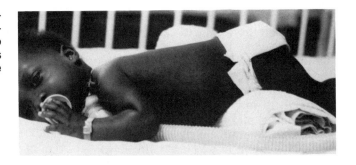

and airway diameter may affect treatment time in the infant compared with procedures used in the adult.

Children with Cystic Fibrosis

The objective of a chest physiotherapy program in the treatment of cystic fibrosis is to prevent or delay irreversible pulmonary fibrotic changes resulting from repeated infections. It is generally accepted that chest physiotherapy is indicated once the diagnosis is made. Physical therapists usually perform treatment during acute exacerbations of the disease that require hospitalization. Parents assume the responsibility at home until the child can perform treatment independently. Compliance is often a problem because of the time and stress placed on the family and psychosocial effects of the disease, particularly during adolescence. Currie et al., 1986, documented only a 46% compliance with postural drainage at home in 50 outpatients with chronic respiratory diseases which included cystic fibrosis. The optimum frequency or duration of chest physiotherapy relative to severity of disease is not yet determined. The effects of cough alone or general physical conditioning influence treatment necessity and frequency. The effects of chest physiotherapy are evaluated by pulmonary function tests, measurements of expectorated sputum volume, and the inhalation of radionucleides. Chest physiotherapy is shown to increase the volume of sputum expectorated (Denton, 1962; Lorin and Denning, 1971; Sutton et al., 1985). Treatment time ranged from 12 to 30 min for bronchial drainage, percussion, and vibration. Denton used mechanical percussion and vibration, Sutton et al. added the forced ex-

piration technique (see Chapter 3). A 25° head-down position improves mucus transport rates in patients with cystic fibrosis (Wong et al., 1977). Whether mucus is primarily mobilized from the central or peripheral airways is currently unknown.

Several studies on patients with cystic fibrosis have tried to document improvement in pulmonary function after chest physiotherapy. The most consistent improvement is in peak expiratory flow rate (PEFR). Tecklin and Holsclaw (1975) found significant increases in forced vital capacity (FVC), PEFR, inspiratory capacity, and expiratory reserve volume 10 min after treatment, which included six postural drainage positions. Motoyama (1973) showed significant improvement in FVC, PEFR, and maximum expiratory flow at 50% and 25% vital capacity (VC) both at 5 and 45 min after chest physiotherapy. Feldman et al. (1979; Feldman 1976) documented improvement in FVC, PEFR, forced vital capacity in 1 min (FEV_1), and V_{max} 50 and V_{max} 25 (maximum expiratory flow rates at 25 and 50% vital capacity) 5, 15, and 45 min after 30 min treatment, which included six postural drainage positions. More recent investigators of cystic fibrosis were unable to reproduce many of these findings. Zapletal and colleagues (1983) did not find significant improvement in any pulmonary function measurements 30 min after treatment; V_{max} 25 deteriorated. A second group of patients with cystic fibrosis was studied at 3-month intervals 20 min and 2 hr after treatment: no significant improvement was noted. Specific airway conduction showed some improvement in 20% of the patients. Kerrebijn et al. (1982) also evaluated changes in pulmonary function 1 and 4 hr after treatment.

The only statistically significant improvement noted was in two patients whose expiratory resistance to flow of the upstream airways improved. Sutton et al. (1985) found no change in pulmonary function when evaluating four different chest physiotherapy regimes. Weller et al. (1980) demonstrated significant improvement in PEFR on days when chest physiotherapy was given versus the control day. FVC and FEV_1 improved on both treatment and control days, most likely as a result of normal physical activity. When Desmond et al. (1983) evaluated pulmonary function in eight children with stable mild to moderate disease, 30 min after treatment, only PEFR improved significantly. Chest physiotherapy was withheld for 3 weeks, resulting in a significant decrease in FVC, FEV_1, forced expiratory flow rate between 25 and 75% vital capacity (FEF25–75), and the maximal expiratory flow rate at 60% of total lung capacity (V_{max}tlc). Reinstituting a single treatment of chest physiotherapy increased FVC and V_{max}tlc 30 min after treatment; the increased airflow limitation completely reversed 3 weeks after resuming treatment. It appears that pulmonary function is not significantly altered as a result of a single chest physiotherapy treatment but may deteriorate if treatment is withheld when assessed by serial pulmonary function tests.

A major area of controversy in the literature is the effect of cough versus chest physiotherapy treatment, and whether either treatment removes secretions from the central versus peripheral airways (see Chapter 5). Rossman et al. (1982) evaluated the removal of radiolabeled serum albumin aerosol from the large airways and concluded that cough was as effective as chest physiotherapy treatment in stable disease. Zinman and DeBoeck (1984) evaluated nine patients with cystic fibrosis in stable condition who had moderate disease. Twenty-five minutes of chest physiotherapy in 11 positions was compared with vigorous coughing 11 times in 10 min. Neither treatment demonstrated improvement in pulmonary function. Comparing supervised coughing to chest physiotherapy in 38 patients Bain et al. (1988) found no dif-

ference in sputum characteristics or pulmonary function. It is interesting to note that Bain and colleagues eliminated subjects under 7 years who did not have an effective cough, or were unreliable with pulmonary function testing. This may be the group of patients most responsive to chest physiotherapy. Pulmonary function and aerosol clearance techniques deposited in the central airway may not be sensitive enough to measure the effect of chest physiotherapy treatment on the intermediate and smaller airways. Krypton scintigraphy is thought by some investigators to provide a more sensitive measure of peripheral airway clearance. DeCesare et al. (1982) demonstrated improvement in ventilation (peripheral airway clearance) in three patients with severe disease, although the results of the study were not statistically significant. The outcome may have been different if the primary areas of lung involvement were determined prior to treatment and therapy directed specifically to diseased lung segments.

The effect of regular exercise on pulmonary function was recently evaluated with the goal of replacing chest physiotherapy treatment with a less time-consuming, more normal activity. Henke and Orenstein (1984) studied 91 stable and hospitalized patients with cystic fibrosis and found the majority to tolerate maximal exercise without significant oxygen desaturation. Oxygen desaturation was not related to severity of the disease. Cropp et al. (1982) found that 20 cystic fibrosis subjects with mild or moderate disease exercised as well as normal subjects. Daily physical exercise may include swimming, hiking, and jogging, and replace chest physiotherapy treatment. Forced vital capacity, FEV_1, FEF25–75, and PEFR improved with these activities (Zach et al., 1981, 1982). Most pulmonary function measurements returned to baseline 8–10 weeks after training. Keens (1977) demonstrated that physical exercise was as effective as ventilatory muscle training (see Chapter 3). Improvement of airway function is thought to depend on physical activity. Orenstein and colleagues (1981) found that 3 months of a jog–walk exercise program significantly increased exercise tolerance and peak oxygen consumption. Parameters used to determine when strenuous exercise can be performed safely, without supervised exercise testing and ear oximetry include a FEV_1 less than 50% vital capacity or pulmonary function score >12 determined from 6 pulmonary function measurements (Cropp et al., 1982; Henke and Orenstein, 1984). Daily physiotherapy may be replaced by frequent swimming or other physical activity, particularly in mild to moderate disease, following further investigation.

In summary, chest physiotherapy is often performed for cystic fibrosis regardless of the severity of disease. This may account for the conflicting evidence regarding the efficacy of chest physiotherapy. Treatment is directed to 4–11 lung segments per treatment lasting 2–30 min. Some authors (Pryor and Webber, 1979) advocate use of the forced expiration technique to enhance sputum expectoration and minimize airway collapse associated with coughing. Currie et al. (1986) believe that percussion and shaking should not be taught to cystic fibrosis patients. They believe these techniques should be replaced by the forced expiration technique (pp. 121–122) and directed cough. The effect of chest physiotherapy treatment compared with cough alone and physical exercises requires further study to determine when each of these therapies is most appropriate. Patients with acute exacerbations of cystic fibrosis continue to require chest physiotherapy treatment. Treatment is emphasized in lung areas where radiological or clinical evidence of disease is present. Frequency of treatment is determined by the patient's activity level and sputum production; duration is judged by the patient's clinical response to treatment.

Neurologically Impaired Children

Children with neurological impairment are prone to respiratory complications requiring treatment in the ICU. Muscular dystrophy, myelomeningocele with paraplegia, and cerebral palsy are just a few of the diseases which may interfere with the respiratory musculature. As a result, the cough mechanism and normal neuromuscular development are impaired. This may lead to secretion retention, orthostatic pneumonia, and recurrent chest infections. A habilitative physiotherapy program for these patients is aimed at facilitating normal motor development. Parental participation is encouraged.

The cerebral palsy child with marked spasticity sufficient to interfere with normal intercostal and diaphragmatic activity may require specific body positioning to minimize spasticity and encourage relaxation (Finnie, 1971). This allows postural drainage and improved costal excursion to occur more easily. Vibration, or any stimulation, may increase extensor spasticity. As a result, treatment may be limited to postural drainage with gentle percussion. Normal active or spontaneous movement is encouraged while the child is in the ICU. Individual child evaluation is essential and beyond the scope of this book.

PATIENTS WITH BRAIN INJURY

Approximately 500,000 Americans sustain brain injury per year, with a mortality ranging from 17 to 70% (Jennett and Teasdale, 1981; Geisler and Salcman, 1987; Seigel, personal communication). Brain injury is estimated to be present in 75% of young people who die from motor vehicle accidents (Auer et al., 1980). The highest mortality is in centers without specialty neurotrauma units (Matjasko and Pitts, 1986). Siegel (personal communication) evaluated 1709 traumatic brain-injured patients with Glasgow Coma Scales (GCS) of 3–14 admitted to a level one trauma center from 1983 to 1986 inclusive. Excluding cardiac arrests on admission the overall mortality was 17.5%. Single system injured patients had a mortality of 11.1% compared to a 21.8% mortality when two or more systems were injured. Three hundred eighty (22.2%) of these patients had chest injury in addition to brain injury and a 27.6% mortality. Lung injury in 187 patients, which included lung contusion, lacerations, pneumothorax, and hemothorax, increased the mortality to 34.2%. Twenty-eight percent of these patients required in-patient rehabilitation. Mackenzie et al. (1979), including patients dead on arrival to the trauma center, documented a higher mortality (49%) in 173 patients with closed head injuries admitted directly from the scene of a motor vehicle accident. Fulton and Jones (1975) reported a 20% incidence of respiratory failure in patients with trauma affecting the central nervous system. These statistics demonstrate the need for intensive pulmonary and rehabilitative care for the brain-injured person, especially with associated extracerebral injuries.

Damage to the central nervous system may result in hypoxemia, noncardiac pulmonary edema, altered patterns of respiration, and aspiration (Baigelman and O'Brien, 1981). Lack of spontaneous cough and immobility following brain injury cause secretion retention and subsequent hypoxemia that may lead to the development of cerebral edema. Patients with head injury, a normal chest x-ray, and normal pulmonary capillary wedge pressure have decreased ventilation and increased perfusion while spontaneously breathing (Schumacker et al., 1979). The altered mental status, inability to protect the airway, and neurological deficits associated with head trauma predispose the patient to aspiration. Hypoxemia associated with secretion retention, atelectasis, and aspiration are indications for chest physiotherapy treatment. Airway suctioning and the position changes associated with routine nursing care and chest physiotherapy treatment may be particularly hazardous to the brain-injured person with elevated intracranial pressure. Therefore, chest physiotherapy treatment should be performed by trained health care personnel familiar with positioning the patient with abnormal muscle tone and acquainted with ICU equipment, particularly intracranial pressure monitoring (ICP) devices.

Raised Intracranial Pressure

Recent studies support giving chest physiotherapy treatment following brain injury utilizing head-down postural drainage positions (Hammon et al., 1981; McQuillan, 1987; Imle et al., 1988). Hammon studied 11 patients, 8 with an initial ICP less than 17 and 3 with an initial ICP greater than 20. Bronchial drainage with percussion in the supine head-down position did not significantly alter cerebral perfusion pressure (CPP). McQuillan studied 20 adult head-injured patients receiving chest physiotherapy treatment either in the side-lying flat or head-down position. ICP was statistically higher in the head-down position but returned to baseline more rapidly than for subjects in the flat position. CPP and mean arterial blood pressure (MABP) remained adequate throughout all treatments and PaO_2 improved only after chest physiotherapy in the head-down position. Imle and associates studied 16 patients following craniocerebral trauma with a GCS of 3–8. Chest physiotherapy was given to the lower lobes, lingula, or right middle lobe for 15 min. Subjects were randomly postured head flat or head down. Positioning was determined by latest chest x-ray and clinical assessment. No significant difference in heart rate, MABP, ICP, end tidal carbon dioxide tension ($P_{et}CO_2$), or CPP was noted in the two positions before and after treatment. ICP was greater in the head-down group but CPP and MABP remained adequate. Brimioulle and colleagues (1988) studied the effects of chest percussion on ICP in 32 brain-injured patients. ICP was not affected by chest percussion but markedly increased while turning patients into the lateral decubitus position. Moraine et al. (1988) evaluated 18 patients with ICP monitoring and noted a significant but transient decrease in ICP with incentive spirometry and deep breathing exercises.

Garradd and Bullock (1986) documented that prolonged manual hyperinflation raises ICP. CPP was not measured in the 20 subjects studied. ICP did not significantly increase in the pharmacologically paralyzed patients. Clinicians in many centers are reluctant to position patients with head injury head down for chest physiotherapy treatments to the lower lobes, lingula, and right middle lobe. However, the lower lobes are the most frequently atelectatic or diseased (see Appendix A1.3). Respiratory dysfunction increases shunt, decreases PaO_2, and may increase mortality in patients with brain injury. It is the authors opinion that chest physiotherapy which includes the manual techniques of percussion and vibration can be safely performed in the head-down position with the precautions described below.

ICP normally rises with coughing, sneezing, straining, or the head-down position. Flexion, rotation, and extension of the head may significantly affect ICP if cerebral spinal fluid is squeezed from the subarachnoid space and trapped in the cranial cavity (Shalit and Umansky, 1977). Spontaneous movements are associated with the greatest increases in ICP in infants (Tomney and Finer, 1980). In the normal brain, ICP elevations may briefly reach 40–50 mm Hg during maneuvers such as coughing but return to baseline levels rapidly because cerebral compliance is high (Schultz and Taylor, 1977). In a patient with low cerebral compliance, elevations in ICP are prolonged, and cerebral perfusion is reduced and can be life threatening. CPP is calculated as the difference between mean arterial pressure and intracranial pressure (CPP = MAP − ICP). When CPP reaches 50 mm Hg total cerebral blood flow is decreased approximately 25%. When CPP is below 40 mm Hg cerebral perfusion is compromised. Reduced CPP results in reflex vasodilation of the cerebral vasculature and increased cerebral blood volume, which leads to elevation of ICP and ultimately decreased cerebral blood flow. Cessation of blood flow, bilateral fatal cerebral infarction, and brain death may occur following severe brain injury. Close monitoring is essential, especially during chest physiotherapy for those patients who are at the elbow of the cerebral pressure/volume curve (Fig. 8.3). It is our opinion that chest physiotherapy can be safely administered when the ICP is less than or equal to 15 mm Hg in the upright position and does not exceed 25 mm Hg in the head-down position. CPP should remain greater than 50 mm Hg. Percussion does not adversely affect ICP in patients with space occupying lesions (Hammon et al; McQuillan; Brimioulle et al.) (Fig. 8.4). An ICP that rises above 25 mm Hg with suctioning or other stimulation and returns to baseline in 30–60 sec indicates high cerebral compliance and should not interfere with chest physiotherapy treatment.

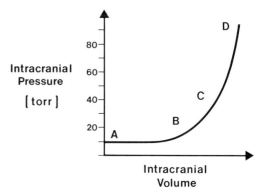

Figure 8.3. Idealized intracranial pressure/volume relationships. It may be necessary to restrict chest physiotherapy only in patients whose cerebral compliance is low, beyond the elbow of the curve between **B** and **C**.

Guidelines for Chest Physiotherapy Treatment

1. Observe ICP and MABP with patient supine in bed, head elevated 30–45°; calculate CPP.
2. If ICP is less than 15 mm Hg and CPP greater than 50 mm Hg, lower the bed into the flat position and turn the patient into the appropriate bronchial drainage position. When an intraventricular catheter is in place, cerebral spinal fluid can be drained prior to treatment to lower ICP.
3. When the head-down position is indicated and ICP is elevated, a modified tilt test may be performed. Observe ICP and CPP while the patient is positioned with the bed horizontal. If ICP exceeds 20 mm Hg and CPP is less than 50 mm Hg the head of the bed is elevated and the patient is repositioned supine. If ICP returns to baseline in a short period of time, the patient has high cerebral compliance. Proceed with the head-down position for treatment. If ICP fails to return to baseline the neurosurgical staff is notified. Therapeutic intervention is indicated to decrease ICP. Barbiturates or fentanyl may be used. Once CPP is adequate, the patient is positioned head-down for treatment of the appropriate lung lobes.
4. Perform manual techniques and suctioning as described in Chapters 4 and

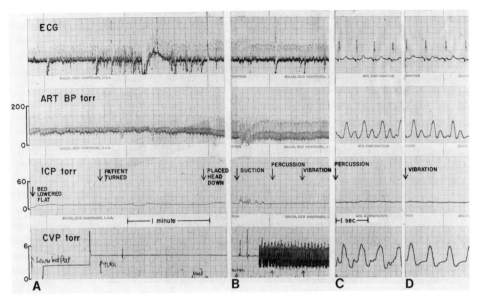

Figure 8.4. The effects of turning and the head-down position on arterial blood pressure (ART BP) and ICP are shown in **A**. The ICP transducer was attached to the patient's head. The effects of suction and chest percussion and vibration on ART BP, ICP, and central venous pressure (CVP) are shown in **B**. Pressure traces during chest percussion (**C**) and vibration (**D**) are shown at a faster paper speed (30 mm/sec). Note in **A** the rise in ICP with flattening of the bed and turning and positioning the patient with the head down. Note in **B**, **C**, and **D** that chest percussion and vibration have no effect on ART BP, ICP, or CVP but that suction caused a decrease in ART BP and a rise in ICP and CVP. (Traces in Figures 8.4 and 8.5 were made and provided by C. F. Mackenzie, M. B., Ch.B., F.F.A.R.C.S.)

5. Hyperventilation via the ventilator or a manual resuscitator bag may be necessary following suctioning if ICP does not rapidly return to baseline.

5. When ICP exceeds 25 mm Hg or CPP is less than 50 mm Hg with the head-down position the neurosurgical staff is notified. The indication for chest physiotherapy and severity of lung pathology and brain injury determines whether medical intervention is indicated to continue treatment.

6. Chest physiotherapy routinely lasts 15 min for patients with ICP monitoring. Chest physiotherapy duration may exceed 15 min when treatment is administered to lung segments not requiring the head-down position for drainage (all upper lobe segments and superior segments of the lower lobes). When copious secretions are mobilized with chest physiotherapy, or a lobar collapse does not improve with a 15-min session in the head-down position treatment time may be extended at

the discretion of the neurosurgeon. Using these guidelines, the authors have found treatments longer than 15 min necessary only for 1–2 sessions.

Measures to Reduce ICP

Suctioning the upper airway increases ICP. Shalit and Umansky noted that in patients where the trachea is blocked by secretions suctioning may have a favorable effect on ICP. This is also the authors clinical impression. Suctioning is necessary and routinely performed on brain-injured persons in the ICU. To prevent spillage of secretions into dependent lung regions, patients should be suctioned during chest physiotherapy and before changing position. White et al. (1982) studied the effects of several drugs used to prevent the acute intracranial hypertension associated with endotracheal suctioning. Intravenous lidocaine and thiopental produced an initial 4–6 mm Hg decrease in ICP but neither drug affected the increase in ICP after endotracheal suctioning. Succinylcholine was effective in abolishing increases in ICP due to suctioning. Fentanyl produced no acute changes in ICP. Cerebral perfusion pressure was not significantly altered by any of the prophylactic medications. For patients requiring sedation prior to treatment drugs such as fentanyl or diazepam may be helpful, although barbiturates that reduce ICP and cerebral O_2 consumption may be more beneficial. Lidocaine in doses of 1.5 mg/kg was found to be as effective as thiopental for rapid (within 66 sec) reduction in ICP (Bedford et al., 1980). Other methods to reduce ICP to allow chest physiotherapy treatment and routine nursing care include venting cerebrospinal fluid through an intraventricular monitoring catheter and administration of diuretics. For patients in barbiturate coma the cough reflex is absent and position changes do not cause such marked increases in ICP. White and colleagues recommend short-term paralysis for patients who develop intracranial hypertension in response to tracheal suctioning; Garradd and Bullock noted that ICP was not elevated during chest physiotherapy when patients were pharmacologically paralyzed. However, the benefit of reducing ICP with neuromuscular blockers must be weighed against the risk of eliminating the cough reflex associated with suctioning. Paralysis may be necessary only when ICP is elevated for prolonged periods which prohibit effective nursing care and chest physiotherapy treatment. Details of cough efficacy and suctioning procedures can be found in Chapter 5.

Patients should be adequately sedated prior to stimulation that increases ICP. Routine turning and positioning for nursing care and chest physiotherapy treatment may be prevented if ICP increases. Position changes may cause the most marked changes in ICP (Fig. 8.4). Although sedation is often beneficial, Shalit and Umansky (1977) found patient positioning more effective than mannitol in reducing ICP (Fig. 8.5). Placement of the head in a neutral position or at times elevated on an i.v. bag (see Chapter 3) is effective in reducing ICP. ICP often appears higher when the patient is positioned with the ICP monitoring device dependent. The stimulation associated with position changes is usually associated with higher transient increases in ICP than lying in the lateral and head-down positions. Multiple interventions that result in increased ICP or decreased CPP should be avoided in the patient with brain injury. CPP may be a more reliable indicator than ICP of the brain-injured patient's ability to tolerate chest physiotherapy treatment.

Routine Chest Care for the Unconscious Patient

For the patient with head injury, a clear chest x-ray, minimal secretions, and low intrapulmonary shunt, routine turning and suctioning are found to be adequate chest care. Positioning the unconscious patient who does not have problems with increased ICP follows the normal postural drainage routine. Restriction of treatment time is unnecessary in this group of patients. In fact, prolonged periods of the head-down position may be indicated in nonintubated unconscious or semiconscious patients who have copious secretions noted clinically but have no spontaneous cough (Fig. 8.6). After postural drainage, secretions may be suctioned from the oropharynx. If suctioning the oropharynx and the other methods of cough stimulation discussed in Chapter 5 are ineffective after postural drainage, tracheal intubation may be necessary. Nasotracheal suctioning should not be performed (see p. 179). This is especially the case in patients with CSF rhinorrhea or facial fractures.

QUADRIPLEGIC PATIENTS

During the first 3 months after acute traumatic quadriplegia, death is most frequently due to pulmonary complications (Cheshire, 1964; Bellamy et al., 1973). Reines and Harris (1987) documented an 18% mortality in 123 consecutive spinal cord injury patients, 49 of whom were quadriplegic. Sixty-three percent of the deaths were attributed to pulmonary complications. Mortality increased to 30% in the quadriplegic patient who developed atelectasis or pneumonia. There-

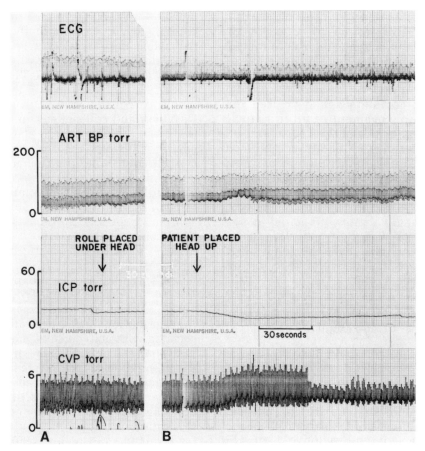

Figure 8.5. Pressure trace changes following placement of a roll under the head of the patient without any changes in bed or patient position are shown in **A**. The effects on arterial blood pressure (ART BP), ICP, and central venous pressure (CVP) of placing the patient with the head up are shown in **B**. Note the fall in ICP shown in **A**, resulting from head elevation after placement of a roll. The ICP transducer was attached to the head and similarily elevated. This technique may be used to reduce ICP once the patient is appropriately positioned for postural drainage. Note the fall in ICP following head elevation, shown in **B**. The rise in ART BP and CVP was an artefact due to constant transducer height. This was rectified 30 sec after the head-up position was assumed.

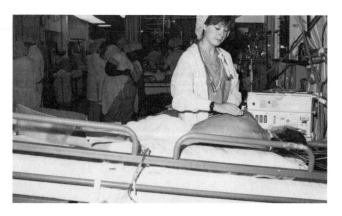

Figure 8.6. This brain-injured patient with facial fractures required 30 min of postural drainage to mobilize secretions to the oropharynx because he was unable to cough spontaneously.

fore, the importance of close observation and intensive respiratory care for the acutely injured quadriplegic cannot be overemphasized. Cough is severely affected by paresis or paralysis of the abdominal muscles. Loss of intercostal muscle innervation and decreased diaphragmatic movement result in reduced lung volumes (Fig. 8.7). Trunk and extremity muscles are paralyzed and sympathetic cardiac innervation is lost. Position changes are more precarious and require assistance of two or three persons for turning and sitting out of bed. Reduced lung volumes, impaired cough, and decreased mobility affecting activities of daily living make the quadriplegic patient extremely susceptible to respiratory problems.

Respiratory Muscle Function/Thoracic Cage Mobility

Several authors have investigated the role of the muscles of respiration and rib cage mobility both in normal and quadriplegic patients. The diaphragm, parasternal intercostal and scalene muscles, sternocleidomastoid, platysma, sternohyoid, trapezii, and mylohyoid muscles may all assist in inspiration after quadriplegia. Specific muscle activity depends on the level of the lesion (Fig. 8.8). The parasternal intercostal muscles are traditionally considered accessory muscles of inspiration. Whether they increase the anterior posterior (AP) or transverse diameter (DeTroyer and Kelly, 1984) of the chest is controversial. These accessory muscles are thought to pull the sternum cranially. The scalenes and sternocleidomastoid muscles also increase the AP chest diameter (Danon et al., 1979; DeTroyer and Kelly, 1984; DeTroyer et al., 1985, 1986). After studying the thoracic mobility in a C1 and C2 quadriplegic, DeTroyer and colleagues concluded that the sternocleidomastoid, platysma, trapezii, mylohyoid, and sternohyoid muscles all contribute to quiet breathing in quadriplegia. The neck inspiratory muscles pull the sternum cranially and the trapezii fix the head to prevent excessive shortening of the sternocleidomastoid. This allows the sternocleidomastoid muscles to work at a greater mechanical advantage.

major may play a role in expiration following quadriplegia (DeTroyer et al., 1986). In 10 subjects, a decrease in upper rib cage motion during expiration was associated with active use of the clavicular portion to the pectoralis major. Changing the orientation of the muscle fibers using shoulder abduction reduced expiratory reserve volume by 60%. Clinically, increasing the strength and endurance of this muscle or upper extremity ergometry (Walker and Cooney, 1987) may improve cough effectiveness.

There is much variability in the literature regarding inspiratory muscle function and the thoracic and abdominal components of respiration both in normal and quadriplegic subjects. In normal subjects, rib cage movement accounts for 33% of vital capacity and the diaphragm contributes to 66% (Campbell et al.,

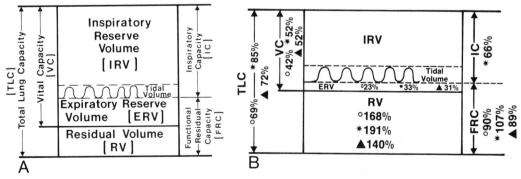

Figure 8.7. Comparison of lung volumes in the normal **(A)** and the quadriplegic **(B)** patient. Note decreased VC, total lung capacity, and ERV in the quadriplegic patient, (▲, Estenne, 1987; ○, Fugl-Meyer, 1971a; *, Haas, 1965).

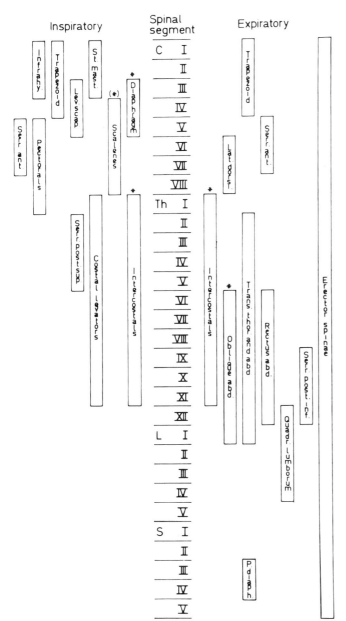

Inspiratory   Spinal segment   Expiratory

Figure 8.8. (left). The respiratory muscles. Inspiratory muscles to the left and expiratory muscles to the right of the spinal segmental indicator. *Primary respiratory muscles (different opinions in the literature on whether these are primary or auxiliary). (From A. R. Fugl-Meyer: *Scandinavia Journal of Rehabilitation Medicine* 3:141–150, 1971a.)

1970). Bake et al. (1972) found that the abdominal contribution to quiet respiration was 31% in normal subjects and 50% in the quadriplegic patient. Therefore, tetraplegic subjects have a smaller rib cage contribution and a greater diaphragmatic contribution to tidal volume than healthy subjects (Fugl-Meyer 1971b; Mortola and Sant'Ambrogio, 1978; Estenne and DeTroyer, 1985, 1987). Accessory muscle activity is variable in quadriplegics; this may affect the thoracic component of ventilation that ranges from 22 to 90% of total ventilation (McKinley et al., 1969). Estenne and DeTroyer (1985) studied 20, C4–C7 quadriplegic patients between 10 days and 312 months after injury with EMG recordings of the parasternal intercostals and scalene muscles. The degree of rib cage motion could not be predicted; there was no relationship between thoracic motion and duration of quadriplegia. Spastic or silent scalene EMG activity was associated with paradoxical upper rib cage AP motion. These authors conclude that quadriplegics have a very complex pattern of muscle activity during inspiration and that coordination of the scalenes and diaphragm may be important. Three forces act upon the rib cage when the diaphragm contracts: a fall in pleural pressure, a rise in abdominal pressure, and a force on the insertion of the diaphragm elevating the lower ribs.

Pulmonary Function

Vital capacity has been shown to double within 3 months of injury and continue to increase spontaneously 4–10 months after quadriplegia (Ledsome and Sharp, 1981; Haas et al., 1986; Axen et al., 1985). Proportional increases in inspiratory capacity and total lung capacity (TLC) and maximum inspiratory pressure (PI_{max}) also occur in the acute stage (McMichan et al., 1980; Haas et al., 1986). During the chronic stage, vital capacity increases and functional residual capacity decreases while TLC remains the same. Absolute improvement in vital capacity cannot be predicted by pulmonary function tests, neurologic examinations, or muscle function evaluations performed in the early stage of recovery (Axen et al.).

Postural Dependence. Pulmonary function varies with body position and the use of abdominal binders in the spontaneously breathing quadriplegic patient. Unlike normal subjects whose vital capacity decreases by 7.5% in the supine position (Allen et al., 1985), patients with cervical cord transection have a decreased vital capacity, tidal volume, and inspiratory capacity, increased residual volume (RV), and decreased ventilation in the lung bases when changing from the supine to seated position (Maloney, 1979; Haas et al., 1965; Fugl-Meyer, 1971a; Bake et al., 1972; McMichan et al., 1980; Estenne and DeTroyer 1987). Vital capacity is increased by the 20° head-down position (Cameron et al., 1955). Total lung capacity is smaller in the supine position (Estenne and DeTroyer, 1987) probably because of a reduction in RV, although inspiratory capacity (IC), VC, and tidal volume increase (Maloney,

1979). Reduced residual volume is thought to be related to the effect of gravity on the abdominal contents and not an abnormal increase in intrathoracic blood volume (Estenne and DeTroyer, 1987). McMichan and colleagues associated the increased lung volumes with shortened diaphragmatic descent and lack of abdominal rebound. Increased paradoxical inward movement of the lateral chest wall is also noted in the supine position when compared to sitting (Moulton and Silver, 1970; Mortola and Sant' Ambrogio, 1978; Estenne and DeTroyer). The reduced lower rib cage expansion in the supine position is thought to be due to the increase in abdominal compliance that occurs with assuming this position (Estenne and DeTroyer).

Cardiac function is also affected by changes in position after cervical cord transection or spine injury. Rapid changes in body position for the acute quadriplegic patient during spinal shock may cause marked changes in cardiac function. Head elevation of greater than 20° may cause a sudden decrease in cardiac filling pressures, a resulting fall in cardiac output, and even cardiac arrest. Similarly, sudden head-down positioning may cause a rise in cardiac filling pressures. Because of loss of sympathetic cardiac innervation associated with lesions above the T1 level, the steep head-down position may precipitate acute myocardial failure with pulmonary edema. Therefore, in the early stages of acute quadriplegia, these movements should be performed with careful monitoring of arterial and venous pressures. Ace wraps around the lower extremities, a G suit, or MASTrousers may be used to minimize orthostatic hypotension until vasomotor control is established.

Abdominal Binders. Abdominal binders are used to align the abdominal contents under the diaphragm, thus improving respiratory function both in the acute and chronic phases of quadriplegia. When comparing eight C5–C7 quadriplegic subjects 1–456 months after injury to five normal subjects, McCool et al. (1986) demonstrated that abdominal binding increased IC, TLC, and decreased FRC in the quadriplegic subjects. FRC and TLC decreased in normal subjects in all three positions tested (supine, seated, and tilted head-down 37°). The greatest improvement in inspiratory capacity for quadriplegic patients was in the seated and tilted positions, because of the normal lengthening of the diaphragm that occurs in the supine position. Maloney studied 15 quadriplegic patients 1 year postinjury. It was found that wearing a corset in the sitting (not supine) position improved IC, VC, and tidal volume. The authors conclude that the increased abdominal pressure associated with binder use improves rib cage expansion. Goldman and colleagues (1986) also demonstrated an increase in transdiaphragmatic pressure and VC with abdominal binding in the sitting position, although VC was not altered in the supine position. Estenne and DeTroyer (1987) noted that abdominal binding abolished the postural dependence of RV in the supine position, the effect on TLC is not mentioned. Imle et al. (1986) studied the affects of abdominal binding on acute quadriplegics and also documented that VC was unchanged with binding in the supine position.

Binder type and placement may be crucial in demonstrating improvement in pulmonary function. Elastic binders wrapped tightly around the abdomen, extending over the iliac crests to the pubis, are preferred (McCool et al., 1986; Goldman et al., 1986). The binder should not be positioned more cranially than the floating ribs because of interference with epigastric rise during inspiration (Alvarez et al., 1981). It is the author's experience that binders placed below the anterior superior iliac spine are more prone to tissue breakdown, particularly in the sitting position. When improperly donned, thoracic mobility may be impaired. Binders with an orthoplast front are not as effective as conventional binders in improving end inspiratory tidal and transdiaphragmatic pressure during maximal sniffs (Goldman, et al.).

The overall benefits of wearing an abdominal binder remain unknown because of the decrease in FRC that may impair gas exchange. Improvement in VC enhances cough ability, yet decreased FRC leads to alveolar collapse. The authors have found binders clinically beneficial for some quadriplegic patients both to decrease respiratory rate and increase VC and tidal volume when used in supine and sitting positions. Pulmonary function testing may be performed when using binders, particularly with supine positioning. Binders are worn until pulmonary function ceases to improve with their use, or breathing fails to appear easier during functional activities.

Chest Physiotherapy Treatment

Reduced VC, restricted deep breathing, and cough, together with an inability to change body position, lead to secretion retention. Quadriplegic patients are, therefore, very susceptible to pulmonary complications (McMichan et al.). In order to improve respiratory management, chest physiotherapy treatment, including breathing exercises and specific active and passive range of motion exercises are necessary (see pp. 163). Chest physiotherapy is reported to be highly successful in reducing pulmonary complications in these patients (McMichan et al.). Treatment is instituted prophylactically and continued, with emphasis on any areas showing radiological involvement. No benefit from the use of bronchodilators for the quadriplegic patient was documented by Fugl-Meyer (1976). It is our opinion that adventitial breath sounds, including wheezing, are often a result of retained secretions, since they clear with chest physiotherapy. Both the mechanically ventilated and spontaneously breathing quadriplegic patient require immediate attention to prevent atelectasis and pneumonia.

Quadriplegic patients should have chest physiotherapy performed during weaning from mechanical ventilation. The authors are in agreement with Wicks and Menter (1986) that IMV is not particularly beneficial for these patients. Retained secretions are removed prior to a weaning session to enhance gas exchange and decrease the work of spontaneous breathing. This is particularly important for the quadriplegic who may lack the necessary intercostal and accessory muscle strength to decrease diaphragmatic muscle fatigue (Lerman and Weiss, 1987). While spontaneously breathing cough assistance and breathing exercises are con-

Figure 8.9. The physical therapist clinically assesses a quadriplegic patient prior to performing percussion over the posterior segments of the lower lobes. The turning frame allows head-down positioning.

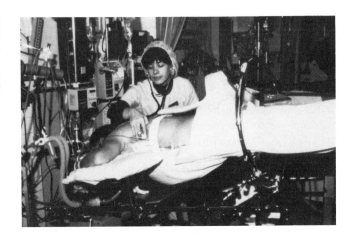

tinued for secretion removal, ventilatory muscle strengthening, and relaxation.

Postural Drainage, Percussion, and Vibration

Both the turning frame and a standard bed permit chest physiotherapy in 7 of the 11 bronchial drainage positions. Percussion and vibration may be performed over appropriate lung segments (Fig. 8.9). Thoracic excursion in varied positions that include more than one plane of motion may prevent cavus deformity and flaring of the lower rib cage, particularly in children (Massery, 1987). Position changes for quadriplegic patients should be made carefully by experienced health care personnel because of their effect on cardiac and pulmonary function. It is our opinion that a standard bed and turning frame are superior to the kinetic bed for care of the quadriplegic patient. Com-

pared to the kinetic bed the turning frame and standard bed allow more optimum postural drainage of the lower and middle lobes and better positioning for exercises to enhance early rehabilitation and prevent contractures. The manufacturers claims of improved pulmonary function and decreased tissue breakdown and contracture formation with the kinetic bed are not substantiated by our clinical practice. Skin breakdown occurs on the heels and buttocks and shoulder contractures may develop when quadriplegic patients are managed on a kinetic bed. See Chapter 3 for details regarding specialty beds and positioning the spinal injury patient. Quadriplegic patients may be taught to cough while lying supine, on their side, and prone (Fig. 8.10). The turning frame may be positioned in the head-up, head-down, prone, and supine positions (Fig. 8.11). Adequate diaphragmatic excursion can be obtained for patients

Figure 8.10. Cough assistance for a quadriplegic patient is achieved by placing a towel over the abdomen and the therapist applying even pressure during expiration.

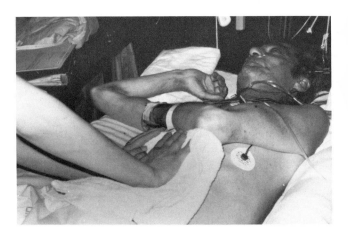

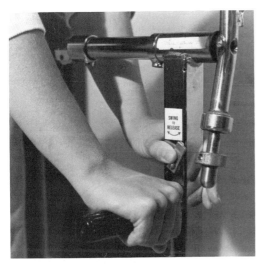

Figure 8.11. One person may raise or lower the head of the Stryker frame.

positioned prone on a turning frame by placing a roll under the iliac crests (Fig. 8.12). Well-padded straps may be used to prevent the patient from slipping and losing traction while in the head-down position (Fig. 8.13). If straps are used they should be released immediately following treatment to prevent tissue breakdown or circulatory occlusion. Cameron et al. (1955) describe padded boots to achieve the same effect. Once adequate traction is assured, both hydraulic and manual frames may be positioned for postural drainage. During rehabilitation, the prone on elbows position may be used on a bed or mat to strengthen neck accessory muscles while limiting and resisting diaphragmatic excursion.

The philosophy of the neurosurgical or orthopedic staff will determine when surgical intervention and use of a vest for spinal stabilization are indicated. A halo vest is preferred to the use of a body cast. Manual chest physiotherapy techniques are more easily performed because the straps can be unfastened and vest opened (Fig. 8.14). The jacket is unfastened on both sides and the back raised to allow percussion over the posterior basal segments of the lower lobes. Padding can be added for patient comfort, two or three staff members are required to position the patient prone in a vest. Jacket straps should be closed prior to changing the patients position. Chest physiotherapy is also performed when a Yale brace is required for spinal stabilization (Fig. 8.15). When body casts are used windows should be cut to expose the chest wall (Fig. 8.16). Casts compromise respiratory function, interfere with chest-ray interpretation, and cause pressure sores. In patients with quadriplegia and copious secretions, prolonged periods of the head-down position may be necessary to assist secretion drainage into the oropharynx. In a minority of patients, 90–120 min of drainage is required for one or two treatments before clinical clearance is noted. This is especially the case in spontaneously breathing patients who do not cough well.

Cough

Due to abdominal and intercostal muscle weakness, cough is often severely impaired in the quadriplegic patient. If the patient is taught to take as large an inspiration as possible, followed by a forceful expiration during which the abdomen is

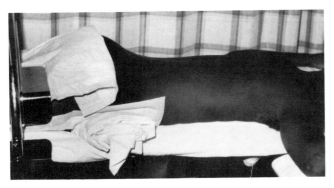

Figure 8.12. A roll under the iliac crests allows anterior diaphragmatic excursion during prone positioning on a turning frame.

Figure 8.13. Kerlex and abdominal dressing pads are easily obtained in the ICU and can be utilized to prevent the patient on a turning frame from slipping when placed head-down.

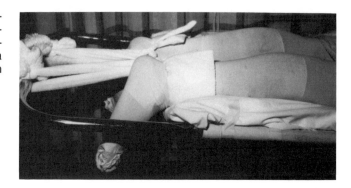

Figure 8.14. A quadriplegic patient is receiving chest percussion over the left lower lobe after the vest used for spinal stabilization is opened and taped to the siderails of the bed. The vest was opened after proper patient positioning.

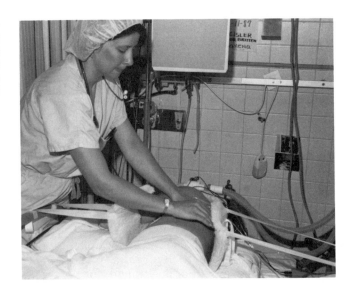

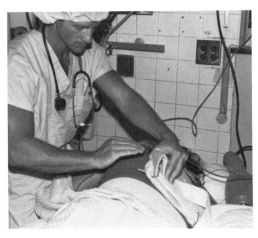

Figure 8.15. When a Yale brace is used for spinal stabilization, the straps may be unfastened to allow chest physiotherapy treatment.

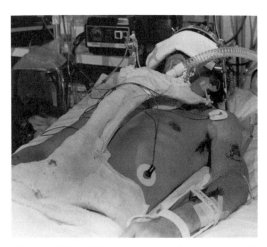

Figure 8.16. When body casts are used for spinal stabilization in the quadriplegic patient, windows must be cut to expose the chest wall.

Table 8.1
Comparison of Air Flow, Duration, and Volume of Cough in Quadriplegic and Normal Subjects

	Peak Air Flow (liters/sec)	Duration of Cough (sec)	Volume of Cough (liters)	Resistance to Air Flow (Peak Flow) (cm H_2O/liters sec)
Normal	7.09	1.09	3.14	12.50
Quadriplegic	4.54	2.3	2.91	2.59

supported, a more effective cough may be achieved (Fig. 8.10). The patient can be taught to perform this maneuver independently. Huffing is also helpful (see p. 162).

Siebens et al. (1964) found abnormal volume and pressure changes during coughing in three male quadriplegic patients with C5 and C6 spinal cord transections (Table 8.1). Flow and resistance were decreased compared to those values in three healthy men.

Breathing Exercises

Breathing exercises to increase tidal volume and assist coughing are advocated for the nonintubated quadriplegic patient. Quadriplegic patients with a vital capacity less than 1,000 ml usually require mechanical ventilation (Wicks and Menter, 1986). Because alternating periods of rest and exercise improve pulmonary function in some patients (Braun et al., 1983), the authors use breathing exercises during periods of spontaneous breathing while weaning from mechanical ventilation. Exercising the intact respiratory muscles such as the diaphragm, sternocleidomastoid, levator scapulae, platysma, and trapezius may increase thoracic and abdominal excursion, therefore increasing tidal volume (Guttmann, 1976; McMichan et al., DeTroyer and Heilporn, 1980; Wetzel et al., 1985). Breathing exercises most often taught to quadriplegic patients include active and resistive diaphragmatic breathing, summed breathing exercises, inspiratory muscle training, and glossopharyngeal breathing. Fifteen chronic quadriplegics improved VC after 7–12 weeks of incentive spirometry and arm ergometry (Walker and Cooney, 1987). Active diaphragmatic breathing exercises and inspiratory muscle training are described in Chapter 3.

Breathing exercises are initially taught to the quadriplegic patient in the supine position because of the associated increase in vital capacity. Resistive diaphragmatic exercises are achieved by placing dish or cuff weights over the epigastric region (Fig. 8.17). Inspiratory capacity and vital capacity are measured to determine the maximum weight used during training while achieving a full epigastric rise. During breathing exercises and pulmonary function testing, nose clips are worn unless the patient is tracheally intubated. In the acute phase, for the spontaneously breathing quadriplegic patient the authors advocate diaphragmatic breathing exercises for 40 repetitions twice daily five days per week or inspiratory muscle training for 15 min twice daily.

Ciesla et al. (1989) compared the effectiveness of abdominal weight training to inspiratory muscle training on 29 acute C4–C7 quadriplegic subjects. FVC, IC, MVV, PEFR, and PI_{max} were measured before and after 3 weeks of training. No significant difference was found between

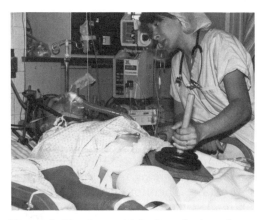

Figure 8.17. A quadriplegic patient performs diaphragmatic progressive resistive exercises with dish weights. Weights are added until the patient's inspiratory capacity is greater than or equal to baseline measurements.

these treatment modalities, although significant improvement ($p < .05$) was noted in both subject groups.

Glossopharyngeal Breathing

Glossopharyngeal breathing (GPB) is recommended for the patient with quadriplegia. The technique can be broken into four steps (Fig. 8.18 A–C). Dail and Affeldt (1955) studied GPB in patients with poliomyelitis. Of 100 patients who were taught GPB, 69 used it to assist normal breathing, and 31 used it to assist speech and stretch the chest to help coughing. Forty-two of these patients found that GPB freed them of the need for respiratory support.

Ardran et al. (1959) found that the GPB rate varied from 60 to 200 times/min in individuals with poliomyelitis. Those patients who could swallow normally were capable of GPB; those with palatal and laryngeal weakness were sometimes capable of GPB if a nose clip was used. It may not, therefore, be necessary to close the larynx for GPB. Affeldt et al. found no relationship between the polio patient's proficiency at GPB and the severity of respiratory muscle paralysis. VC was increased from 0.28 to 2.40 liters, with GPB ranging from 14 to 48 strokes/min, and normal arterial blood gases were maintained. The mean increase of VC ranged from 11 to 50% of the predicted normal, in seven patients. Metcalf (1966) and Montero et al. (1967) specifically studied quadriplegic patients. Metcalf found that vital capacity was increased from 60 to 81% of normal by means of GPB. Montero and colleagues believed that if 700–1,000 ml of air could be added to a patient's VC with 10–20 glossopharyngeal gulps, the technique was then mastered. This volume provides sufficient supplemental air for effective coughing and secretion clearance. Many quadriplegic patients who require respiratory support undergo tracheostomy to reduce the problems associated with long-term translaryngeal intubation. Therefore, GPB is limited to extubated patients or those without an inflated tracheostomy tube cuff (G. T. Spencer, personal communication).

"Summed breathing" may also increase tidal volume. This is carried out by encouraging the patient to take several quick, shallow but cumulative breaths before expiration. The patient can gradually increase the volume of inspired air once this is mastered.

Fugl-Meyer (1971b) devised a manually operated pump and valve system that was used as a passive breathing exercise and increased total lung capacity 14% in quadriplegic patients. Productive coughing was improved. This was most effective with patients in the sitting position.

In summary, prophylactic chest physiotherapy is important for the patient with acute quadriplegia. Emphasis on increasing VC and cough efficacy are essential in the spontaneously breathing patient. Exercising the remaining accessory muscles, performing diaphragmatic, inspiratory resistive, glossopharyngeal, and summed breathing, or the use of a pump and valve system may all improve pulmonary function. In order to maintain rib cage mobility, these exercises are started as soon as possible following injury. Activities of daily living may eventually replace the need for chest physiotherapy and breathing exercises.

PATIENTS WITH CHRONIC LUNG DISEASE

Evidence of the benefits of chest physiotherapy for patients with chronic obstructive lung disease is limited. Anthonisen et al. (1964), Petersen et al. (1967), March (1971), Newton and Bevans (1978), Newton and Stephenson (1978), and Oldenburg et al. (1979) were unable to demonstrate improvement in pulmonary function or sputum clearance with chest physiotherapy. May and Munt (1979) found postural drainage and percussion effective in augmenting the volume of expectorated sputum, but this did not produce significant alterations in air flow or gas exchange. Campbell et al. (1975) found a fall in FEV_1 when percussion was added to postural drainage and coughing.

The patient who is subacutely ill and has chronic lung disease with retained secretions is encouraged to become independent in activities of daily living, as opposed to having a vigorous chest physiotherapy regime implemented. Pulmo-

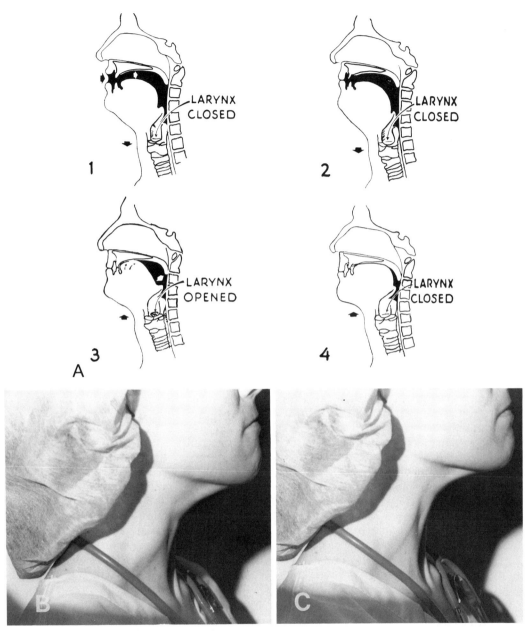

Figure 8.18. **(A)** Steps of GPB: **(1)** The mouth and throat are filled with air; the tongue, jaw and larynx are depressed. **(2)** The lips are closed, and the soft palate is raised to trap air. **(3)** The larynx is opened; the jaw and floor of the mouth and larynx are then raised. With repeated motion of the tongue, air is forced through the opened larynx into the trachea. **(4)** The larynx is closed, and air is trapped in the trachea and lungs. (From C. W. Dail and J. E. Affeldt: *Journal of the American Medical Association* 158:445–449, 1955.) **(B)** GPB steps **1** and **2**: The jaw and larynx are depressed; the soft palate is raised. **(C)** GPB steps **3** and **4**: Air is forced through the opened larynx into the trachea.

nary rehabilitation that includes patient education and exercise testing and training are indicated. Exercise training may include PaO$_2$ measurements during exercise and the use of supplemental oxygen; inspiratory muscle training (IMT) may also be indicated (pp. 122) (Butts, 1981; Stein et al., 1982; Ries et al., 1983). Whether (IMT) alone improves respiratory muscle endurance in patients with chronic lung disease is unknown (Belman and Sieck, 1982). IMT has not been shown to increase exercise tolerance when compared to a pulmonary rehabilitation program (Casaburi and Wasserman, 1986), although Ries et al. (1986) demonstrated improvement in ventilatory muscle endurance and exercise performance when IMT was compared to a walking program. See Chapter 3 for details regarding IMT. The major indications for chest physiotherapy in the patient with chronic lung disease are excess sputum production, exacerbations of the disease resulting in immobility, or major abdominal surgery or trauma. Cochrane et al. (1977) showed reduced air flow obstruction, and Bateman et al. (1979) and Sutton et al. (1982) showed increased clearance of radioactive polystyrene particles from central and peripheral airways following chest physiotherapy in patients producing regular daily sputum. Similarly, Feldman et al. demonstrated increased expiratory air flow in ten patients with chronic bronchitis up to 45 min after postural drainage, percussion, and vibration in six positions.

After surgery, spontaneously breathing and mechanically ventilated patients with chronic sputum-producing lung disease are likely to retain secretions as a result of immobility, pain and the use of dry anesthetic gases. Altered pulmonary function before surgery puts these patients at a greater risk for respiratory complications. Prophylactic chest physiotherapy, which includes the forced expiration technique, is, therefore, indicated. Chronic lung diseased patients may need to be coaxed into the necessary postural drainage positions. If retained secretions interfere with gas exchange, tolerance to treatment usually improves as treatment is continued. The spontaneously breathing patient who becomes more dyspneic with treatment may benefit from relaxation and gentle conditioning exercises in the sitting position. This may aid muscular relaxation and help conserve energy needed for effective deep breathing and coughing. As the patient's shortness of breath improves, postural drainage may then be administered. If low rates of intermittent mandatory ventilation (IMV) are in use, the patient with chronic obstructive lung disease or cardiac disease may become dyspneic when placed in the head-down position. Increasing the mandatory ventilation rate or fractional inspired oxygen concentration, using controlled mechanical ventilation, or pressure support may allow these patients to tolerate better the head-down positions necessary for postural drainage of the middle and lower lobes.

ASTHMATIC PATIENTS

Physiotherapy for patients with asthma consists of breathing retraining exercises, physical conditioning, and postural exercises (Livingstone, 1952; Wood et al., 1970; Mascia, 1976; Landau, 1977). Breathing exercises are often used to reduce anxiety and relieve dyspnea (Freedberg et al., 1987). Singh (1987) studied 12 asthmatics with nocturnal wheeze. In a controlled study statistically significant increases in PEFR were noted following breathing exercises using a "pink city lung exerciser." This device maintained a 1:2 inspiratory–expiratory ratio, similar to that obtained with diaphragmatic breathing exercises (see Chapter 3). Postural drainage with percussion and vibration is only necessary when the asthmatic patient has excess mucus production or secretion retention which is present after physical conditioning, breathing, or postural exercises.

The spontaneously breathing asthmatic with retained bronchial secretions may require breathing exercises or relaxation before postural drainage. The patient is positioned to promote relaxation of the upper chest and shoulder girdle musculature. Relaxation in several positions, such as sitting, lying on the side, and standing, should be incorporated when possible into the treatment. Postural drainage with percussion and vibration often cannot be tolerated unless the patient is relaxed. Chest physiotherapy is directed at the specific areas of segmental atelectasis (Wood et al.; McKaba, 1976). Huber et al. (1974) showed up to a 40% increase in forced expiratory volume, 30 min following percussion and vibration in 11 asthmatic children with mild-to-moderate airway obstruction. This suggests that chest physiotherapy and secretion removal decrease bronchospasm. Patients with asthma, hospitalized for treatment other than asthma, usually tolerate chest physiotherapy. The head-down position may be used when it is indicated. This is exemplified by the following case study.

Case History 8.1. A 15-year-old female was admitted to the trauma center after an auto accident in which she was a backseat passenger.

The patient sustained a fractured right pubis and sacroiliac joint, a ruptured bladder, liver lacerations, a serosal tear of the rectum, and a retroperitoneal hematoma. Her past medical history was noncontributory except for a his-

tory of asthma and shortness of breath on exertion.

Following admission, the patient underwent laparotomy, and a suprapubic cystostomy was performed. After surgery the patient showed radiological evidence of a right upper lobe atelectasis that cleared with chest physiotherapy. The patient was given prophylactic chest physiotherapy every 4 hr because of her history of asthma. This was supplemented in the evening and at night by the nursing staff. There were no turning restrictions, and the patient's chest x-ray remained clear until the fifth day after surgery when, due to concern over the pelvic fracture (Fig. 8.19A), turning was limited to lying on the left side only. Two days later the patient developed atelectasis of the left lower lobe (Fig. 8.19B) and an associated tempera-

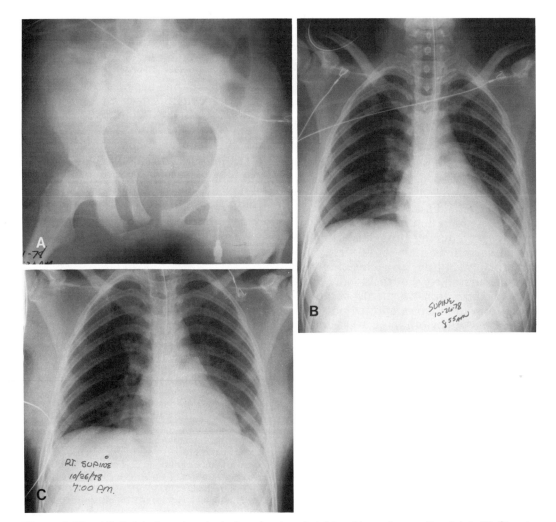

Figure 8.19. **(A)** Pelvic fracutres include a fractured right pubis and sacroiliac joint. **(B)** Chest x-ray showing left lower lobe atelectasis. **(C)** The left lower lobe atelectasis has cleared following 45 min of chest physiotherapy.

ture spike to 102°F. Turning was again permitted, and chest physiotherapy was given. Treatment consisted of postural drainage and vigorous percussion, vibration and assisted coughing with the patient in the head-down position. Side-lying prone and supine positions were included while the patient was in the head-down position. Treatment lasted 45 min, at which time the physiotherapist believed that the lungs were clear on auscultation, except for some wheezing which was apparent since admission.

Repeat chest x-ray revealed complete clearing of the left lower lobe atelectasis (Fig. 8.19C). Temperature decreased to 99°F. A turning frame was subsequently used to manage both the patient's pelvic fracture and her pulmonary condition.

The patient in status asthmaticus does not usually require chest physiotherapy initially (*British Medical Journal* editorial, 1972). However, following medical treatment, breathing control and chest physiotherapy may be instituted to assist secretion removal (Wood et al., Webber, 1973). The intubated asthmatic patient is especially prone to secretion retention as a result of bronchospasm, immobility, decreased ciliary activity, and interference with the normal cough mechanism. Therefore, routine turning and suctioning are performed. In addition, chest physiotherapy treatment of any areas of the lungs with clinical or radiological evidence of secretion retention may be helpful in reducing bronchospasm. Retained secretions may cause airway obstruction resulting in wheezing and should, therefore, be removed. Treatment of the asthmatic should be guided by sputum production and patient tolerance. Chest physiotherapy treatment of the asthmatic patient should follow prescribed bronchodilator administration whenever possible.

SUMMARY

Chest physiotherapy when administered to different patient populations has variable effects. In neonates, chest physiotherapy appears to be more hazardous than in adults, and there is evidence of hypoxemia associated with suctioning, handling, and chest physiotherapy. Conversely, removal of secretions, mobilized

by manual techniques, may be more important in children because of their small airways which are more easily occluded with retained secretions and the increased number of mucus glands. Patients with cystic fibrosis respond favorably to chest physiotherapy, which includes the forced expiration technique, although further research is needed to determine if the effects of therapy vary with the severity of the disease and general physical conditioning. Patients with spinal cord injury and neurological deficit involving intercostal and abdominal muscle activity require prophylactic chest physiotherapy to assist mobilization and expectoration of secretions. In the quadriplegic patient, specific breathing exercises are beneficial to improve coughing and secretion clearance. Abdominal binders may improve vital capacity and cough ability. Unconscious patients with closed head injuries are prone to increased retention and stagnation of secretions because of immobility and poor cough. These patients usually tolerate chest physiotherapy in the head-down position despite transient increases in ICP. The primary indications for chest physiotherapy in patients with obstructive lung disease or asthma occur during acute exacerbations and after surgery or trauma. In chronic stages of these diseases, the benefit of chest physiotherapy is not established.

References

Affeldt JE, Dail CW, Collier CR, Farr AF: Glossopharyngeal breathing: Ventilation studies. *J Appl Physiol* 8:111–113, 1955

Allen SM, Hunt B, Green M. Fall in vital capacity with posture. *Br J Dis Chest* 79:267–272, 1985

Alvarez SE, Peterson M, Lunsford BR: Respiratory treatment of the adult patient with spinal cord injury. *Phys Ther* 61:1737–1745, 1981

Angus E, Thurlbeck W: Number of alveoli in the human lung. *J Appl Physiol* 32(4):483–485, 1972

Anthonisen P, Riis P, Sogaard-Anderson T: The value of lung physiotherapy in the treatment of acute exacerbation in chronic bronchitis. *Acta Med Scand* 175:715–719, 1964

Ardran GM, Kelleher WH, Kemp FH: Cineradiographic studies of glossopharyngeal breathing. *Br J Radio* 32:322–328, 1959

Auer LM, Gell G, Richling B, et al.: Predicting lethal outcome after severe head injury—a computer assisted analysis of neurological symptoms and laboratory values. *Acta Neurochir* 52:225–238, 1980

Axen K, Pineda H, Shunfenthal H, Haas F: Diaphragmatic function following cervical cord injury: Neurally mediated improvement. *Arch Phys Med Rehabil* 66:219–222, 1985

Baigelman W, O'Brien J: Pulmonary effects in head trauma. *Neurosurgery* 9(6):729–740, 1981

Bain J, Bishop J, Olinsky A: Evaluation of directed coughing in cystic fibrosis. *Br J Dis Chest* 82:138–148, 1988

Bake B, Fugl-Meyer AR, Gimby G: Breathing patterns and regional ventilation distribution in tetraplegic patients and in normal subjects. *Clin Sci* 42:117–128, 1972

Barnes CA, Asonye UO, Vidyasaqar DI: The effects of bronchopulmonary hygiene on $P_{tc}O_2$ values in critically ill neonates. *Crit Care Med* 9(12):819–822, 1981

Bateman JRM, Newman SP, Daunt DM, Pavia D, Clarke SW: Regional lung clearance of excessive bronchial secretions during chest physiotherapy in patients with stable chronic airways of obstruction. *Lancet* 1:294–297, 1979

Bedford RF, Persing JA, Pobereskin L, Butler A: Lodocaine or thiopental for rapid control of intracranial hypertension? *Anesth Analg (Cleve)* 59:435–437, 1980

Bellamy R, Pitts FW, Stauffer ES: Respiratory complications in traumatic quadriplegia. *J Neurosurg* 39:596–600, 1973

Belman MJ, Sieck G: The ventilatory muscles, fatigue, endurance and training. *Chest* 82(6):761–766, 1982

Braun NM, Faulkner J, Hughes R, Roussos C, Sahgal V: When should the respiratory muscles be exercised? *Chest* 84(1):76–84, 1983

Brimioulle S, Moraine JJ, Kahn RJ: Passive physical therapy and respiratory therapy effects on intracranial pressure (Abstract). *Crit Care Med* 16(4):449, 1988

British Medical Journal Editorial: Treatment of status asthmaticus. *Br Med J* 4:563–564, 1972

Burnard ED, Grattan-Smith P, et al.: Pulmonary insufficiency in prematurity. *Aust Paediatr J* 1:12–38, 1965

Butts J: Pulmonary rehabilitation through exercise and education. *CVP* 17–61, December–January, 1981

Cameron GC, Scott JW, Jousse AT, Botterell EH: Diaphragmatic respiration in the quadriplegic patient and the effect of position on his vital capacity. *Ann Surg* 141:451–456, 1955

Campbell AH, O'Connell JM, Wilson F: The effect of chest physiotherapy upon the FEV, in chronic bronchitis. *Med J Aust* 1:33–35, 1975

Campbell EJM, Agostoni E, David JN: *The Respiratory Muscles: Mechanics and Neural Control*, p 46. WB Saunders, Philadelphia, 1970

Casaburi R, Wasserman K: Exercise training in pulmonary rehabilitation. *N Engl J Med* 314:1509–1511, 1986

Cheshire DJE: Respiratory management in acute traumatic tetraplegia. *Paraplegia* 1:252–261, 1964

Ciesla N, Simpson N, Derrickson J, Salmon M: A comparison of two different breathing exercises for quadriplegic patients (abstract). *Phys Ther* 69:393, 1989

Cochrane M, Webber BA, Clarke SW: Effects of sputum on pulmonary function. *Br Med J* 2:1181–1183, 1977

Crane L: Physical Therapy in neonates with respiratory dysfunction. *Phys Ther* 61(12):1764–1773, 1981

Crane L: Physical Therapy for the neonate with respiratory disease. In *Cardiopulmonary Physical Therapy*, edited by S Irwin and J Tecklin, pp. 305–310. Mosby, St. Louis, 1985

Cropp GJ, Pullano TP, Cerny FJ, Nathanson IT: Exercise tolerance and cardiorespiratory adjustments at Peak Work Capacity in Cystic Fibrosis. *Am Rev Respir Dis* 126:211–216, 1982

Currie DC, Munro C, Gaskell D, Cole J: Practice, problems and compliance with postural drainage: A survey of chronic sputum producers. *Br J Dis Chest* 80:249–253, 1986

Dail CW, Affeldt JE: Clinical aspects of glossopharyngeal breathing. *JAMA* 158:445–449, 1955

Danford D, Miske S, Headley J, Nelson RM: Effects of routine care procedures on transcutaneous oxygen in neonates: A quantitative approach. *Arch Dis Childhood* 58:20–23, 1983

Danon J, Druz WS, Goldberg NB, Sharp JT: Function of the isolated paced diaphragm and the cervical accessory muscles in CI quadriplegics. *Am Rev Respir Dis* 119:909–919, 1979

DeCesare J: Physical therapy for the child with respiratory dysfunction. In *Cardiopulmonary Physical Therapy*, edited by S Irwin and J Tecklin, pp. 334–338, Mosby, St. Louis, 1985

DeCesare J, Babchyck BM, Colten HR, Treves S: Radionuclide assessment of the effects of chest physical therapy on ventilation in cystic fibrosis. *Phys Ther* 62(6):820–825, 1982

Denton R: Bronchial secretions in cystic fibrosis: The effects of treatment with mechanical percussion vibration. *Am Rev Respir Dis* 86:41–46, 1962

Desmond KJ, Schwenk WF, Thomas E, Beaudry PH, Coates AL: Immediate and long-term effects of chest physiotherapy in patients with cystic fibrosis. *J Pediatr* 103:538–542, 1983

DeTroyer A, Heilporn A: Respiratory mechanics in quadriplegia: The respiratory function of the intercostal muscles. *Am Rev Respir Dis* 122:591–599, 1980

DeTroyer A, Kelly S: Action of neck accessory muscles on rib cage in dogs. *J Appl Physiol* 56:326–332, 1984

DeTroyer A, Estenne M, Ninane V: Rib cage mechanics in simulated diaphragmatic paralysis. *Am Rev Respir Dis* 132:793–799, 1985

DeTroyer A, Estenne M, Heilporn A: Mechanism of active expiration in tetraplegic subjects. *N Engl J Med* 314:740–744, 1986

Dhande VG, Kattwinkel J, Darnall RA: Prone position reduces apnea in preterm infants. *Pediatr Res* 16(2):285, 1982

Doershuk CF, Fisher BJ, Matthews LW: Pulmonary physiology of the young child. In *Pulmonary Physiology of the Fetus Newborn and Child*, edited by EM Scarpelli, pp. 167–169. Lea & Febiger, Philadelphia, 1975

Estenne M, DeTroyer A: Relationship between respiratory muscle electromyogram and rib cage motion in tetraplegia. *Am Rev Respir Dis* 132:53–59, 1985

Estenne M, DeTroyer A: Mechanism of the postural dependence of vital capacity in tetraplegic subjects. *Am Rev Respir Dis* 135:367–371, 1987

Etches MB, Scott B: Chest physiotherapy in the

newborn: Effect on secretions removed. *Pediatrics* 62:713–715, 1978

Fan LL, Flynn JW, Pathak DR, Madden WA: Predictive value of stridor in detecting laryngeal injury in extubated neonates. *Crit Care Med* 10(7):453–455, 1982

Feldman J. Changes in maximal expiratory flow volume curves after postural drainage in patients with cystic fibrosis or chronic bronchitis (abstract). *Am Rev Respir Dis* 113:272, 1976

Feldman J, Traver GA, Taussig LM: Maximal expiratory flows after postural drainage. *Am Rev Respir Dis* 119, 239–245, 1979

Finer NN, Boyd J: Chest physiotherapy in the neonate: A controlled study. *Pediatrics* 61:282–285, 1978

Finnie NR: *Handling the Young Cerebral Palsied Child at Home*, pp 24–28. William Heinemann Medical Books, London, 1971

Fisher D, Frewen T, Swedlow DB: Increase in intracranial pressure during suctioning-stimulation vs. rise in PaCO$_2$. *Anesthesiology* 57:416–417, 1982

Fox WW, Schwartz JG, Shaffer TH: Pulmonary physiotherapy in neonates: Physiological changes and respiratory management. *Pediatrics* 92:977–981, 1978

Freedberg PD, Hoffman LA, Light WC, Kreps M: Effect of progressive muscle relaxation on the objective symptoms and subjective responses associated with asthma. *Heart Lung* 16:24–30, 1987

Fugl-Meyer AR: Effects of respiratory muscle paralysis in tetraplegic and paraplegic patients. *Scand J Rehabil Med* 3:141–150, 1971a

Fugl-Meyer AR: A model for treatment of impaired ventilatory function in tetraplegic patients. *Scand J Rehabil Med* 3:168–177, 1971b

Fugl-Meyer AR: *Handbook of Clincal Neurology, Injuries of the Spine and Spinal Cord*, Chap 19, The Respiratory System, pp. 335–349. American Elsevier Publishing, New York, 1976

Fulton RL, Jones CE: The course of post-traumatic pulmonary insufficiency in man. *Surg Gynecol* 140:179–186, 1975

Garradd J, Bullock M: The effect of respiratory therapy on intracranial pressure in ventilated neurosurgical patients. *Aust J Physiol* 32(2):107–111, 1986

Geisler FH, Salcman M: The head injury patient. In *Emergency Surgery and Critical Care*, edited by JH Siegel, pp. 919–946. Churchill Livingstone, New York, 1987

Goldman JM, Rose LS, Williams SJ, Silver JR, Denison DM: Effect of abdominal binders on breathing in tetraplegic patients. *Thorax* 41:940–945, 1986

Gregory GA: Respiratory care of the child. *Crit Care Med* 8:582–586, 1980

Guttmann L: *Spinal Cord Injuries, Comprehensive Management and Research*, 2nd ed, pp. 209–215, 575. Blackwell Scientific Publications, London, 1976

Haas A, Lowan EW, Bergofsky EH: Impairment of respiration after spinal cord injury. *Arch Phys Med Rehabil* 46:399–405, 1965

Haas F, Axen K, Pineda H, Gandino D, Haas A: Temporal pulmonary function changes in cervical cord injury. *Arch Phys Med Rehabil* 66:139–144, 1986

Hammon WE, Kirmeyer PC, Connors AF, McCaffee DR, Kaplan RJ: Effect of bronchial drainage on intracranial pressure in acute neurological injuries (abstract). *Phys Ther* 61(5):735, 1981

Henke KG, Orenstein DM; Oxygen saturation during exercise in cystic fibrosis. *Am Rev Respir Dis* 129:708–711, 1984

Hislop A, Reid L: Growth and development of the respiratory system—anatomical development. In *Scientific Foundations of Pediatrics*, edited by JA Davis and J Dobbing, p. 221. WB Saunders, Philadelphia, 1974

Holloway R, Adam EB, Desai SD, Thabiran AK: Effect of chest physiotherapy on blood gases of neonates treated by intermittent positive pressure respiration. *Thorax* 24:421–426, 1969

Holloway R, Desai MB, Kelly SD, Thambiran AK, Strydom SE, Adams EB: The effect of chest physiotherapy on arterial oxygenation of neonates during treatment of tetanus by intermitten positive pressure respiration. *S Afr Med J* 40:445–447, 1966

Huber AL, Eggleston PA, Morgan J: Effect of chest physiotherapy on asthmatic children (abstract). *J Allergy Clin Immunol* 111:109–110, 1974

Imle PC, Anderson PA, Ciesla ND: The effect of wearing an abdominal binder during the acute phase following quadriplegia (abstract). *Arch Phys Med Rehabil* 67:656, 1986

Imle PC, Mars MP, Eppinghaus CE, Anderson P, Ciesla N: Effect of chest physiotherapy positioning on intracranial and cerebral perfusion pressure (abstract). *Crit Care Med* 16(4):449, 1988

Jennett B, Teasdale G: *Management of Head Injuries*. Davis, Philadelphia, 1981

Johnson JD, Malachowski NC, Grobstein R, et al.: Prognosis of children surviving with the aid of mechanical ventilation in the newborn period. *J Pediat* 84:272, 1974

Johnson TK, Moore EM, Jeffries JE editors: *Children Are Different: Developmental Physiology*, 2nd ed. Ross Laboratories, Columbus, 1978

Kattan M: Long term sequelae of respiratory illness in infancy and childhood. *Pediatr Clin North Am* 26(3):525–535, 1979

Keens TG, Krastins IRB, Wannamaker EM, Livison H, Crozier DN, Bryan AC: Ventilatory muscle endurance training in normal subjects and patients with cystic fibrosis. *Am Rev Respir Dis* 116:853–860, 1977

Kerrebijn KF, Veentzer R, Bonzet E, Water VD: The immediate effect of physiotherapy and aerosol treatment on pulmonary function in children with cystic fibrosis. *Eur J Respir Dis* 63:35–42, 1982

Klaus M, Fanaroff A, Martin R: Respiratory problems. In *Care of the High Risk Neonate*, edited by M Klaus and A Fanaroff, p. 190. Saunders, Philadelphia, 1979

Landau LI: Management of a child with asthma. *Med J Aust* 1:340–344, 1977

Ledsome JR, Sharp JM: Pulmonary function in acute cervical cord injury. *Am Rev Respir Dis* 124:41–44, 1981

Lerman RM, Weiss MS: Progressive resistive exercise in weaning high quadriplegics from the ventilator. *Paraplegia* 25:130–135, 1987

Levine AL: Chest physical therapy for children with pneumonia. *JAOA* 78:122–125, 1978

Livingstone JL: Physical treatment in asthma. *Br J Phys Med* 15:136–139, 1952

Long JG, Philip AGS, Lucey JF: Excessive handling as a cause of hypoxemia. *Pediatrics* 65(2):203–207, 1980

Lorin MI, Denning ER: Evaluation of postural drainage by measurement of sputum volume and consistency. *Am J Phys Med* 50:215–219, 1971

Lough MD, Doershuk CF, Stern RC: *Pediatric Respiratory Therapy*, p. 9. Year Book Medical Publishers, Chicago, 1974

Mackenzie CF, Shin B, Fisher R, Cowley RA: Two-year mortality in 760 patients transported by helicopter direct from the road accident scene. *Am Surg* 45:101–108, 1979

Macklem PT: Airway obstruction and collateral ventilation. *Am Rev Respir Dis* 116:287–289, 1977

Maloney FP: Pulmonary function in quadriplegia. Effects of a corset. *Arch Phys Med Rehabil* 60:261–265, 1979

March H: Appraisal of postural drainage for chronic obstructive pulmonary disease. *Arch Phys Med Rehabil* 11:528–530, 1971

Martin RL, Herrell N, Rubin D, Fanaroll A: Effect of supine and prone positions on arterial oxygen tension in the preterm infant. *Pediatrics* 63(4):528–531, 1979

Mascia AV: Manual on the standardization of care of the severely asthmatic child. *J Asthma Res* 13:115–127, 1976

Massery M: Respiratory rehabilitation secondary to neurological deficits: understanding the deficits. In *Chest Physical Therapy and Pulmonary Rehabilitation*, edited by D Frownfelter, pp. 501, 541, 2nd ed. Year Book, Chicago, 1987

Matjasko J, Pitts L: Controversies in severe head injury management. In *Clinical Controversies in Neuroanesthesia and Neurosurgery*, edited by J Matjasko and J Katz, pp. 181–231 Grune & Stratton, New York, 1986

May DB, Munt PW: Physiologic effects of chest percussion and postural drainage in patients with stable chronic bronchitis. *Chest* 75:29–32, 1979

McCool FD, Pichurko BM, Slutsky AS, Sarkarati M, Rossier A, Brown R: Changes in lung volume and rib cage configuration with abdominal binding in quadriplegia. *J Appl Physiol* 60(4):1198–1202, 1986

McKaba PG: Treatment of asthma in adults. *Cutis* 17:1115–1119, 1976

McKinley CA, Auchincloss JH, Gilbert R, Nicholas J: Pulmonary function, ventilatory control, and respiratory complications in quadriplegic subjects, *Am Rev Respir Dis* 100:526–532, 1969

McMichan JC, Michel L, Westbrook PR: Pulmonary dysfunction following traumatic quadriplegia. *JAMA* 243:528–531, 1980

McQuillan KA: The effects of the trendelenberg position for postural drainage on cerebrovascular status in head-injured patients. *Heart Lung* 16:327, 1987

Menkes HA, Traystman RJ: Collateral ventilation. *Am Rev Respir Dis* 116:287–289, 1977

Metcalf VA: Vital capacity and glossopharyngeal breathing in traumatic quadriplegia. *Phys Ther* 46:835–838, 1966

Montero JC, Feldman DJ, Montero D: Effects of glossopharyngeal breathing on respiratory function after cervical cord transection. *Arch Phys Med Rehabil* 48:650–653, 1967

Morraine JJ, Brimioulle S, Kahn R: Active physical therapy and respiratory therapy effects on intracranial pressure (Abstract). *Crit Care Med* 16(4):450, 1988

Mortola JP, Sant'Ambrogio G: Motion of the rib cage and the abdomen in tetraplegic patients. *Clin Sci Mol Med* 54:25–32, 1978

Motoyama EK: Lower airway obstruction. In *Fundamental Problems of Cystic Fibrosis and Related Diseases*, edited by JA Mangos and RC Talamo, pp 335–343. Stratton Intercontinental Medical Book Corporation, New York, 1973

Moulton A, Silver JR: Chest movements in patients with traumatic injuries of the cervical cord. *Clin Sci* 39:407–422, 1970

Muller NL, Bryan AC: Chest wall mechanics and respiratory muscles in infants. *Pediatr Clin North Am* 26(3):503–516, 1979

Myers MG, Mcguiness GA, Lachenbrunch PA, Koontz FP, Hollingshead R, Olson DB: Respiratory illness in survivors of infant respiratory distress syndrome. *Am Rev Respir Dis* 133:1011–1018, 1986

Newton DAG, Bevans HG: Physiotheray and intermittent positive-pressure ventilation of chronic bronchitis. *Br Med J* 2:1525–1528, 1978

Newton DAG, Stephenson A: Effect of physiotherapy on pulmonary function. *Lancet* 2:228–230, 1978

Okken A, Rubin IL, Martin RJ: Intermittent bag ventilation of preterm infants on continuous positive airway pressure. The effect on transcutaneous PO_2. *J Pediatric* 93(2):279–282, 1978

Oldenburg FA, Dolovich MB, Montgomery JM, Newhouse MT: Effects of postural drainage, exercise and cough on mucous clearance in chronic bronchitis. *Am Rev Respir Dis* 20:739–746, 1979

Orenstein DM, Franklin BA, Doershuk C, Hellerstein HK, Germann KJ, Horowitz JG, Stern RC: Exercise conditioning and cardiopulmonary fitness in cystic fibrosis. *Chest* 80(4):392–397, 1981

Parker AE: Chest physiotherapy in the neonatal intensive care unit. *Physiotherapy* 71(2):63–65, 1985

Perlman J, Volpe J: Suctioning the preterm infant: Effects on cerebral blood flow velocity, intracranial pressure, and arterial blood pressure. *Pediatrics* 72(3):329–334, 1983

Petersen ES, Esmann V, Honcke P, Munkner C: Effect of treatment on chronic bronchitis. *Acta Med Scand* 182:295–303, 1967

Pryor JA, Webber BA: An evaluation of the forced expiration technique as an adjunct to postural drainage. *Physiotherapy* 65:304–307, 1979

Purohit DM, Caldwell C, Levkoff AH: Clinical memorandum, multiple rib fractures due to physiotherapy in a neonate with hyaline membrane disease. *Am J Dis Child* 129:1103–1104, 1975

Rava P, Yeh TF, Mora A, Pildes RS: Changes in transcutaneous PO_2 during tracheobronchial hygiene in neonates. *Perinatology-Neonatology* 4:41–45, 1980

Reines AD, Harris RC: Pulmonary complications of acute spinal cord injuries. *Neurosurgery* 21(2):193–196, 1987

Ries AL, Fedullo PF, Clausen JL: Rapid changes in arterial blood gas levels after exercise in pulmonary patients. *Chest* 83(3):454–456, 1983

Ries AL, Moser K: Comparison of isocapnic hyperventilation and walking exercise training at home in pulmonary rehabilitation. *Chest* 90(2):285–289, 1986

Roper PC, Vonwiller JB, Fisk GC, Gupta JM: Lobar atelectasis after nasotracheal intubation in newborn infants. *Aust Paediatr J* 12:272–275, 1976

Rossman CM, Waldes R, Sampson D, Newhouse MT: Effect of chest physiotherapy on the removal of mucus in patients with cystic fibrosis. *Am Rev Respir Dis* 126:131–135, 1982

Schumacker PT, Rhodes GR, Newell JC, Dutton RE, Shah DM, Scovill WA, Powers SR: Ventilation-perfusion imbalance after head trauma. *Am Rev Respir Dis* 119:33–43, 1979

Schultz H, Taylor FA: Intracranial pressure and cerebral blood flow monitoring in head injuries. *Can Med Assoc J* 116:609–613, 1977

Shalit MN, Umansky F: Effect of routine bedside procedures on intracranial pressure. *Israel J Med Sci* 13(9):881–886, 1977

Siebens AA, Kirby NA, Poulos DA: Cough following transection of spinal cord at C-6. *Arch Phys Med Rehabil* 45:1–8, 1964

Simbruner G, Coradello H, Fodor M, Havelec L, Lubec G, Pollak A: Effect of tracheal suction on oxygenation, circulation, and lung mechanics in newborn infants. *Arch Dis Child* 56:326–330, 1981

Singh V: Effect of respiratory exercises on asthma—the pink city lung exerciser. *J Asthma* 24(6):355–359, 1987

Speidel BD: Adverse effects of routine procedures on preterm infants. *Lancet* 1:864–866, 1978

Stein DA, Bradlwy BL, Miller WC: Mechanisms of oxygen effects on exercise in patients with chronic obstructive pulmonary disease. *Chest* 81:6–10, 1982

Sutton PP, Pavia D, Bateman JRM, Clarke SW: Chest physiotherapy: A review. *Eur J Respir Dis* 63:188–201, 1982

Sutton PP, Lopez-Vidriero MT, Pavia D, Newman SP, Clay MM, Webber B, Parker A, Clarke SW: Assessment of percussion, vibratory shaking, and breathing exercises in chest physiotherapy. *Eur J Respir Dis* 66:147–152, 1985

Stocks J, Godfrey S: The role of artificial ventilation, oxygen and CPAP in the pathogenesis of lung damage in neonates. Assessment by serial measurements of lung function. *Pediatrics* 57:352–357, 1976

Streider DJ: Pediatric origins of chronic obstructive lung disease. *Bull Physiopathol Respir* 11:273, 1974

Tecklin JS, Holsclaw DS: Bronchial drainage in patients with cystic fibrosis. *Phys Ther* 55:1081–1084, 1975

Tomney PM, Finer NN: A controlled evaluation of muscle relaxation in ventilated neonates (abstract). *Crit Care Med* 8:228, 1980

Tudehope DI, Bagley C: Techniques of physiotherapy in intubated babies with the respiratory distress syndrome. *Aust Paediatr J* 16:226–228, 1980

Wailoo MP, Emery JL: Normal growth and development of the trachea. *Thorax* 37:584–587, 1982

Walker J, Cooney M: Improved respiratory function in quadriplegics after pulmonary therapy and arm ergometry. *N Engl J Med* 316(8):485–487, 1987

Walsh CM, Bada H, Korones SB, Carter M, Wong SP, Arheart K: Controlled supplemental oxygenation during tracheobronchial hygiene. *Nurs Res* 36(4):211–215, 1987

Webb MSC, Martin JA, Cartlidge PH; NGYK, Wright NA: Chest physiotherapy in acute bronchiolitis. *Arch Dis Child* 60:1078–1079, 1985

Webber BA: Current trends in the treatment of asthma. *Physiotherapy* 59:388–390, 1973

Weller PH, Bush E, Preece MA, Matthew DJ: Short term effects of chest physiotherapy on pulmonary function in children with cystic fibrosis. *Respiration* 40:53–56, 1980

Wetzel J, Lunsford BR, Peterson MJ, Alvarez SE: Respiratory rehabilitation of the patient with a spinal cord injury. In *Cardiopulmonary Physical Therapy*, edited by S Irwin and J Tecklin, pp. 395–411. Mosby, St. Louis, 1985

White PF, Schlobohm RM, Pitts LH, Lindauer JM: A randomized study of drugs for preventing increases in intracranial pressure during endotracheal suctioning. *Anesthesiology* 57:242–244, 1982

Whitfield JM, Jones MD: Atelectasis associated with mechanical ventilation for hyaline membrane disease. *Crit Care Med* 8:719–732, 1980

Wicks AB, Menter RR: Long-term outlook in quadriplegic patients with initial ventilator dependency. *Chest* 90(3):406–410, 1986

Wong JW, Keens TG, Wannamaker EM, Crozier DN, Levison H, Aspin N: Effects of gravity on tracheal mucus transport rates in normal subjects and in patients with cystic fibrosis. *Pediatrics* 60:146–151, 1977

Wood DW, Kravis LP, Lecks HI: Physical therapy for children with intractable asthma. *J Asthma Res* 7:177–182, 1970

Yeh TF, Leu ST, Pyati S, Pildes RS: Changes in O_2 consumption in response to NICU care procedures in premature infants. *Pediatr Res* 16(2):315, 1982

Zach M, Oberwalder B, Hansler F: Cystic fibrosis: Physical exercise versus chest physiotherapy. *Arch Dis Child* 57:587–589, 1982

Zach M, Purrer B, Oberwaldner B: Effect of swimming on forced expiration and sputum clearance in cystic fibrosis. *Lancet* I:1201–1203, 1981

Zapletal A, Stefanova J, Horak J, Vavrova V, Samanek M: Chest physiotherapy and airway obstruction in patients with cystic fibrosis—a negative report. *Eur J Respir Dis* 64:426–433, 1983

Zinman R, DeBoeck C: Cough versus chest physiotherapy: A comparison of the acute effects on pulmonary function in patients with cystic fibrosis. *Am Rev Respir Dis* 129:182–184, 1984

CHAPTER 9

Adjuncts to Chest Physiotherapy

P. Cristina Imle, M.S., P.T.

Often the therapy given to patients requiring intensive respiratory care affects both the airways and the types of secretions they produce. As a result, there is much investigation into techniques for improving secretion clearance. Supplemental humidity is routinely given to most intensive care unit (ICU) patients; other methods advocated to clear pulmonary secretions include intermittent positive pressure breathing (IPPB), aerosols, incentive spirometry (IS), continuous positive airway pressure (CPAP), positive expiratory pressure (PEP), blow bottles, and bronchoscopy. This chapter discusses some of the indications, effectiveness, and complications of these techniques.

HUMIDITY

Normal and Supplemental Humidity

Adequate humidity is necessary for proper respiratory function. Studies on the humidification of inspired air show that by the time the gas reaches the subglottic region of the trachea, it not only is warmed to 37°C but also is fully saturated with water vapor (Robinson, 1974). It is well documented that ciliary activity is dependent on humidification levels (Dalhamn, 1956; Toremalm, 1961; Kilburn, 1967; Graff and Benson, 1969; Asmundsson and Kilburn, 1970). Cilia extend from the respiratory bronchioles to the larynx (Hilding, 1957), and ciliary action is considered the most efficient and physiological means of cleansing the respiratory tract (Graff and Benson). Therefore, it can be concluded that normal clearance of secretions from the lungs is also dependent upon proper humidification. Both Dalhamn and Forbes (1973) found significant reductions or cessation of mucus flow at 50% relative humidity (RH)* levels in animals.

Based on these findings, Graff and Benson, along with many others, believe that all inspired gases must be humidified, if not by the nose and pharynx, then by artificial means—hence the use of humidifiers. Various types of humidifiers are available. In the literature, addition of humidity is specifically recommended for patients who are intubated, ventilated, anesthetized, or receiving supplemental oxygen; for the newborn; and for those with severe chest injury, chronic obstructive pulmonary disease (COPD), asthma, pneumonia, atelectasis, respiratory burns, or innumerable other clinical conditions (Sara, 1965; Egan, 1967; Rashed et al., 1967; Chamney, 1969; Graff and Benson; Forbes; Downie, 1979; and others). In short, it seems widely agreed that anyone breathing dry gases, having an artificial airway, or having abnormally thick secretions should receive supplemental humidity. There are two classifications of humidifiers, controlled environment and controlled inspired atmosphere.

Controlled Environment

Controlled environment systems are applicable to spontaneously breathing patients but not necessarily those whose upper respiratory tracts are bypassed. They consist of such devices as fog rooms, steam or mist tents, and incubators. These systems are all constructed so that the patient is contained and cared for in the humidified environment. They suffer the same complication as con-

*Relative humidity is the vapor content of a gas expressed as a percentage of that gas at full saturation at the same temperature. Another way of describing water content is in milligrams per liter. At 37°C, fully saturated water content can be expressed as 44 mg/liter or 100% relative humidity.

trolled inspired atmosphere systems in that they are susceptible to infection transmission, which is primarily bacterial. Controlled environment devices are more expensive and limited in their mobility, especially compared with most controlled inspired atmosphere equipment (Chamney).

Controlled Inspired Atmosphere

Controlled inspired atmosphere systems alter the inspired gases of a patient but not the entire environment. They can be divided into four main groups, which are discussed in greater detail below: (1) heat and moisture exchangers or condensers, (2) instillation or infusion methods, (3) nebulizers, both pneumatically driven and mechanically or ultrasonically activated, and (4) water bath humidifiers.

Heat and Moisture Exchangers/ Condensers

Heat and moisture exchangers/condensers minimize heat and humidity loss from the upper respiratory tract and are commonly referred to as "artificial noses" (Walley, 1956; Toremalm; Mapleson et al., 1963; Siemens-Elema, 1979; Weeks and Ramsey, 1983). They function as follows: Humidified expired gases pass through a sponge, paper, metal, or gauze mesh, which causes condensation of moisture and heat retention. Most currently used condensers are composed of a synthetic felt and cellulose sponge. The retained heat and moisture are then added to the inspired gases. Heat and moisture exchangers can be used during spontaneous or artificially controlled ventilation. Over the past decade, there has been increased emphasis on airway humidification during anesthesia as well as for postoperative management. When added to inhaled anesthetic systems, the newer condensers have been shown effective in conserving some of the heat and moisture loss that would otherwise occur. They are also easy to use and require no supplemental power source.

The role of condensers for patients in the ICU or requiring mechanical ventilation for longer than 24 hr is more controversial. Primiano and associates (1984) found that adding a condenser (compared with using no supplemental humidity source) improved the RH to 69.2% at body temperature in six ICU patients. MacIntyre and co-workers (1983) reported no significant difference in airway pressure, compliance, resistance, or arterial blood gases in 26 ICU patients when conventional cascade humidification was compared to a condenser for 24 hr. The authors also estimated sputum volume (over 4 hr) and radioaerosol clearance (over 1 hr) to be similar with both types of humidifiers. The temperature settings used during cascade humidification in this study were not specified. Others question the use of condensers when longer periods of mechanical ventilation are needed (Hay and Miller, 1982; Kahn, 1983; Perch and Realey, 1984; Cohen et al., 1988). Significant increases in endotracheal tube occlusion (within 12 hr), pneumonia, atelectasis, and bronchial cast formation have been associated with condenser use compared with cascade humidification (Perch and Realey; Cohen et al.). Microscopic studies on the effects of condenser humidification (less than 100% RH at body temperature) are limited. When inspired air is only 60–70% saturated, there is evidence that the lower airways can supply additional heat and moisture for up to 3 hr. It is not known what happens to the subcarinal airways of humans during prolonged periods of reduced RH (Kahn) or reduced systemic hydration. Histologic damage to the tracheal epithelium of dogs exposed to desiccation and then rehumidification did not correspond with the noted changes in mucus velocity that rapidly improved (Hirsh et al., 1975). Our clinical experience is similar to Cohen and associates. We believe that condenser humidifiers are not adequate for all ICU patients. Particular attention should be given to patients with thick secretions or respiratory muscle weakness and those who are spontaneously breathing, require delivered minute volumes of >10 liters/min, or a $FIO_2 > 0.4$. When condensers are used, they should be replaced with conventional humidifiers if sputum becomes tenacious or if difficulty occurs with suctioning.

Although there is some debate as to the minimal acceptable levels of supplemental humidity, the American National Standards Institute (1979) suggests a minimum output of 30 mg H_2O/liter gas while the Emergency Care Research Institute (1983) recommends a minimum output of 21–24 mg H_2O/liter gas. Not all condensers provide acceptable humidification, particularly at increasing flow rates, tidal volume, or oxygenation. The overall effectiveness of condensers depends on the heat and humidity already present in the gas before exposure to the exchanger system. Mapleson et al. reported that from 40 to 90% of the moisture that might otherwise be lost may be retained by this method. Unlike the nasopharynx, which increases heat and moisture retention under colder and drier conditions, full saturation of dry gases is not possible with a condenser (Robinson, 1974). The condenser's ability to humidify is inversely related to volume and FIO_2 delivery (Hay and Miller; Weeks and Ramsey; Perch and Realey; Cohen et al.). Heat and moisture exchangers also cause an increase in resistance and dead space which should be considered during use with children and "borderline" patients during spontaneous breathing (Siemens-Elema; Weeks; Hay and Miller; Branson et al., 1986). In weak or critically ill patients the added breathing load imposed by the condenser may cause respiratory muscle fatigue and interfere with weaning from the ventilator (Ploysonsang et al., 1988). Gas leakage around the condenser is another concern, particularly with neonates; however, condenser humidification may be successfully used in this patient population (Gedeon et al., 1987).

The earlier model condensers were found most effective when the gauze or mesh was kept reasonably dry. Frequent changing was thought to minimize bacterial contamination. There is some evidence that the new type of heat and moisture exchangers may reduce ventilator contamination by trapping exhaled bacteria in the inner core of the humidifier (Stange and Bygdeman, 1980). This has not been associated with an increased risk of airborne inhaled bacteria during mechanical ventilation (Powner et al., 1986). However, when mucus is trapped in the condenser, the system should be changed due to the increased airway resistance or obstruction (Robinson; Sykes et al., 1976; Weeks); otherwise, changing the heat and moisture exchanger every 24 hr is recommended (Siemens-Elema).

Instillation/Infusion

Instillation/infusion is a simple yet controversial method of humidifying inspired gases. It consists of instilling a fluid, usually physiological saline or a mucolytic agent, at a set rate into the inspiratory limb of the ventilator tubing or directly into the tracheal tube. Though this method is easy to perform, the effect is probably no different from instilling fluid directly into the trachea (see p. 180). Hayes and Robinson (1970) found that humidity levels decreased sharply when this method of humidification was used in comparison to a hot water bath humidifier or a nebulizer. Instillation can also lead to increased airway resistance (Sykes et al.). Another hazard of instillation is the uncontrolled or improperly controlled rate of infusion, which could lead to drowning. At best, this intermittent flooding of the respiratory mucosa is unlikely to be an acceptable physiological substitute for normal conditions and may have serious consequences, especially if large amounts of fluid are absorbed through the lungs (Huber and Finley, 1965; Chamney). It is doubtful that instillation of fluid into the artificial airway has any effect on humidifying distal airways. Although it may be helpful in compensating for humidity loss from the upper airways of an intubated patient, it is considered an unsatisfactory method of humidification during mechanical or spontaneous respiration (Hayes and Robinson).

Supplemental saline or water is often added during high frequency ventilation (HFV) where adequate airway humidification has emerged as a problem (Berman et al., 1984; Ophoven et al., 1984). Two gas sources, entrained and injected, must be considered during this mode of ventilation. Moisture may be added to en-

trained gases with a nebulizer or water bath humidifier, while some method of instillation/infusion is commonly used to humidify the injected gas (Berman et al., Doyle et al., 1984; Ophoven et al.). For paitents with adequate lung compliance and no significant lung pathology, the ratio of entrained-to-injected gas is high. Therefore, entrained gas that is optimally humidified may partially compensate for the effect of the dry injected gas. Problems with tracheal mucosa damage arise when the proportion of entrained gas decreases, as occurs in patients with pulmonary pathology or poor compliance, who may require HFV. When instillation/infusion of injected gas is used without humidified entrained gas, mucus transport is markedly reduced (Klain et al., 1982). Warming the instillate or the injected gas does not prevent heat loss since rapid cooling occurs during the aerosolization of the infused water or saline. These factors are thought to be partially responsible for the increase in inspissated secretions and tracheal damage seen with HFV (Berman et al.; Doyle et al.; Ophoven et al.).

Nebulizers

There are two basic types of nebulizers, the pneumatically powered and the mechanically or ultrasonically activated. Both can be used on spontaneously breathing patients as well as those requiring intubation or mechanical ventilation. However, nebulizers are reported to interfere with mechanical ventilation (Sara and Clifton, 1962; Glover, 1965; Bosomworth and Spencer, 1965; Hayes and Robinson; Klein et al., 1973). If the gas flow delivered to the patient by the ventilator also operates the nebulizer, inadequate humidity can result, especially at low flow rates (Hayes and Robinson; Klein et al.). Alternatively, if the nebulizer is driven by an auxiliary oxygen supply, humidification may improve, but the concentration of delivered oxygen can also increase significantly (Bosomworth and Spencer).

Pneumatically Powered Nebulizer. The pneumatic-powered humidifier works on the Bernoulli principle. A narrow jet of high-pressure gas is blown across a water reservoir. Both water vapor and droplets are formed and blown against an anvil or system of baffles, which usually filters out the larger water particles. The gas entering the patient's delivery tube still contains a visible mist of both water vapor and droplets ranging from 5 to 20 μ (Robinson). This dense mist does not necessarily imply complete gas saturation with humidity, since visible mists with relative humidities of less than 78% are possible (Robinson). Klein and associates found that no correlation could be made between the visible mist and the water content of a gas. Heated and unheated pneumatic-powered humidifiers are available commercially. Studies show that humidities of only up to 29 mg/liter (at the patient's end of the delivery tube) are possible with unheated nebulizers, while up to 50 mg/liter can be achieved using heated types (Sara and Curie, 1965; Sara; Bosomworth and Spencer). More recently, some unheated pneumatically driven nebulizers are reported to deliver nearly 100% relative humidity (Klein et al.).

Marked condensation along the delivery tube is a problem, particularly with heated pneumatic-powered humidifiers. In fact, this system should not be used with narrow-gauge delivery tubing, since condensation can effectively block both gas and humidity flow to the patient. Jones and co-workers (1969) demonstrated how a fluid-lined tube could increase resistance to gas flow. Much as a fluid-lined delivery tube can increase resistance or block air flow, the inhalation of high-density mists can increase the fluid lining of the respiratory tract, causing greater airway resistance (Robinson). Due to the small water particle size delivered to the airways, the problem of transmitting bacterial infections is also great. Therefore, cleaning and sterilization are extremely important. Despite these complications, the pneumatically driven humidifiers are more effective than those previously described, especially when used on the spontaneously breathing patient.

Mechanically or Ultrasonically Activated Nebulizer. The small particle size of ultrasonically or mechanically activated nebulizers is achieved by dropping water onto a disc rotating at high speeds or onto a crystal vibrating at very high frequencies (Chamney). These methods are reported to produce varying levels of humidification ranging from 30 to 200 mg/liter (Smith, 1966; Robinson). The potentially large amount of humidity delivered by this method, though thought to be effective in loosening thick secretions by acting as a solvent, has also led to much criticism (Robinson; Downie). Because of the lack of output control on ultrasonic nebulizers, fluid gain, increased airway resistance and water intoxication were reported to occur, especially in infants (Glover; Harris and Riley, 1967; Modell et al., 1967; Cheney and Butler, 1968; Pflug et al., 1970; Malik and Jenkins, 1972). Modell and associates studied the effects of continuous ultrasonic nebulization on dogs. Pathological changes compatible with bronchopneumonia were seen in all eight dogs exposed to a physiological saline aerosol. This effect was only seen in two of the eight dogs receiving nebulized distilled water, yet five of the eight demonstrated mild to moderate focal atelectasis.

Other authors investigating the effects of short-term use of ultrasonic nebulization reported excessive coughing and wheezing in patients with chronic lung disease and in normal subjects (Cheney and Butler; Pflug et al; Malik and Jenkins). Cheney and Butler found increased airway resistance in patients and normal subjects using ultrasonic nebulizers. This repsonse was not seen with other forms of nebulizers. In patients with chronic bronchitis, Pflug and co-workers reported significant decreases in forced expiratory volume in 1 sec (FEV_1) and vital capacity following ultrasonically delivered aerosols. Similarly, increased airway resistance was noted by Malik and Jenkins, who reported that these physiological alterations were most marked when a 5% saline solution was nebulized, as opposed to distilled water or normal saline. The results of these studies provide evidence that a seemingly innocuous procedure, such as ultrasonic nebulization of water or saline, produces definite side effects that may be disastrous, particularly in patients with chronic airway disease (Cheney, 1972).

Ultrasonic nebulization can deliver water particles of 1–5 μ in size. In fact, 97% of ultrasonically nebulized humidity, but only 55% of the pneumatically nebulized humidity, are delivered in particles within this range (Moffet et al., 1967). A droplet-size spectrum of 2–10 μ is recommended for water deposition throughout the airways, since alveolar sacs and ducts may be theoretically reached by 1- to 3-μ droplets, bronchioles by around 6-μ droplets, and bronchi and upper airways, by 10-μ droplets (Robinson). However, Sawyer (1963) states that in the spontaneously breathing patient, approximately 50% of particles 1–5 μ in size are retained in the nasopharynx, while only 10–40% are deposited in the depths of the lungs. The pharynx and upper trachea are bypassed in tracheally intubated patients. As a result, droplet delivery to the smaller airways may be altered. Aerosol deposition is dependent on many variables and is not well understood.

The complication of transmitted infection is a greater hazard with ultrasonic and mechanical nebulization due to the higher percentage of minute-sized water particles. The smaller size potentially allows particles to reach the distal airways where pulmonary clearance mechanisms may not be as efficient. This is compounded by the fact that these same particles can carry a signficant number of viable bacteria (Reinarz et al., 1965; Edmondson et al., 1966; Ringrose et al., 1968). The small droplet size also allows some particles to leave the lungs during expiration and to remain airborne, thereby providing a vehicle of transmission from one patient to another.

Generally, pneumatic and ultrasonic nebulizers have four disadvantages: (1) There is poor control over the upper level of humidity delivered; (2) delivery tubes require frequent checking to prevent obstruction by condensation; (3) lengthy warm-up periods may be necessary to achieve steady outputs in some heated models; and (4) nebulizers can introduce massive doses of bacteria to the

respiratory tract. This has a potentially great impact because bacteria carried by small water particles may be delivered to the distal airways (Chamney; Klein et al.; Sykes et al.).

Water Bath

In water bath humidifiers, inspired gas is either blown over or bubbled through water. This may allow full saturation for a given temperature. The humidified gas then passes through a delivery tube to the patient. Both heated and unheated water bath models are available. The unheated models are capable of saturating a gas only at ambient temperature and, therefore, do not allow full saturation at body temperature. Consequently, only inadequate humidities of 7–22 mg/liter are possible (Wells et al., 1963; Bosomworth and Spencer; Darin et al., 1982). Heated water bath humidifiers lead to heavy condensation in the delivery tubes. This results from heating and saturating the air at above body temperature, therefore increasing the water vapor-carrying capacity, and then allowing the air to cool while in the delivery tubes. Heated models can provide up to 42 mg/liter at 35°C (Wells et al.; Chamney). Humidifiers with a thermostat on the inspiratory limb of the ventilator tubing can deliver up to 44 mg H_2O/liter at 37°C (Robinson).

Because of the amount of condensation, water bath humidifiers should always be kept lower than the patient to prevent accidental spillage into the patient's airway. Excess condensation also often calls for frequent delivery tube drainage or moisture traps. If the temperature at the patient's end of the delivery tube is controlled, condensation can be minimized (Chamney). Problems of bacterial infection from water bath humidifiers are reported low, nearing that of ambient air (Reinarz et al.; Edmondson et al.; Moffet et al., 1967; Schulze et al., 1967). This is possible because water bath systems deliver humidity in vapor form, which does not carry bacteria (Chamney). Although condensate is frequently contaminated during 24 hr of mechanical ventilation, the patient's secretions are reported as the primary source of colonization. Nonetheless, care should be taken to prevent inadvertent lavage with the condensate (Craven et al., 1984). Also, water bath humidifiers can be used on both ventilated and spontaneously breathing patients, since their humidity production tends to be less susceptible to changes in flow or tidal volume (Hayes and Robinson).

Summary

There is a wide range in the effectiveness of commercially available humidifiers. The optimal amount of water content that should be added to inspired gases is still a matter of controversy. It is generally agreed that humidification should approach 44 mg H_2O/liter. The three acceptable methods of humidifying gases use a heat and moisture exchanger or condenser, a nebulizer, or a water bath system (Robinson). Instillation of infusion is of no proven benefit except possibly with HFV, where appropriate airway humidification remains a problem. The new types of condensers are able to retain most of the heat and moisture that would otherwise be lost, but they are less effective when increased oxygenation or volume delivery is necessary. Condensers increase resistance and their use with patients requiring mechanical ventilation for longer than 24 hr remains under scrutiny. When used, condensers should be replaced with conventional humidifiers if complications occur with inspissated secretions or during spontaneous ventilation.

Both water baths and nebulizers cause condensation in the delivery tubing; they should be frequently checked to prevent blockage or inadvertent patient lavage. By controlling the temperature of the patient's inspired air, condensation produced by water bath humidifiers can be markedly decreased. Ideally, all heated humidifiers should contain a temperature control alarm to warn of potential overheating. Though both types of nebulizers may provide adequate humidification, in comparing the two, the heated, pneumatically driven type is preferable. It is up to one-sixth the cost, and its drop-

let size is theoretically of greater benefit than that of the ultrasonic nebulizer (Robinson). There are fewer complications of overhumidification and increased airway resistance associated with pneumatic nebulizers. Both methods of nebulization interfere with mechanical ventilation. However, heated water bath humidifiers are surprisingly efficient and, when incorporated in a ventilator circuit, create less interference with ventilation (Chamney; Hayes and Robinson; Robinson). They probably represent the best method of providing humidity for the majority of patients (Sykes et al.). Water bath humidifiers are also less prone to bacterial contamination than the nebulizers. Although often referred to as "old fashioned," water bath humidifiers are recommended for the patient in the ICU who requires mechanical ventilation for more than 24 hr. As with all types of heated humidifiers, care must be taken to prevent overheating.

IPPB

The effects of IPPB have been studied since its introduction over 40 years ago (Motley et al., 1948). During this time, it has been prescribed for use both before and after surgery and in the treatment of COPD, asthma, emphysema, and cystic fibrosis. Because of this wide spectrum, it is hard to compare the results found in one group of patients with those in another. Much of the original information on IPPB was based on studies of patients with chronic lung disease. These findings were often extrapolated and claimed to be valid for surgical patients with acute secretion retention. The most commonly cited benefits of IPPB include improved aerosol delivery, reduced work of breathing, improved respiratory function in patients with chronically diseased lungs, psychological support, and prevention of pulmonary complications in the surgical patient. Currently, there is little scientific support for IPPB as a therapeutic modality (Gold, 1982; American Thoracic Society; 1987). This section addresses the claimed benefits and complications of IPPB, including its uncontrolled growth and cost.

Aerosol Delivery

IPPB is commonly used to deliver aerosols. There is little controversy in the literature about its efficacy in this area. Many authors report that IPBB is useful in delivering bronchodilating aerosols, though IPPB is not known to have any bronchodilatory effect of its own (Goldberg and Cherniack, 1965; Chang and Levison, 1972; Smeltzer and Barnett, 1973; Cherniack, 1974; Loren et al., 1977; Sackner, 1978). In fact, significant increases in airway resistance, air trapping, and dead space, as well as reductions in expiratory flow rates and alveolar ventilation, were found following IPPB when no bronchodilator was used (Wu et al., 1955; Kamat et al., 1962; Moore et al., 1972; Ziment, 1973; Fouts and Brashear, 1976). Increased sputum production without corresponding improvement in vital capacity or FEV_1 was also reported following IPPB, implying that mucus production may be stimulated by IPPB itself (Shim et al., 1978).

The real question is not whether IPPB is effective in delivering aerosols but, rather, whether IPPB is the *most* effective method of delivery. The research done in this field is extensive, though Petty (1974) states that no well-designed study has shown convincingly that a bronchodilator, or any other drug delivered by IPPB, is more effective than inhalation of the same aerosol delivered by a powered or hand-held nebulizer. Numerous studies support Petty's claims (Froeb, 1960; Goldberg and Cherniack; Smeltzer and Barnett; Cherniack; Cherniack and Svanhill, 1976; Loren et al.; Shim et al.). Chang and Levison found no difference in delivering isoproterenol by means of IPPB or a powered nebulizer, except that the latter produces the same results at much lower dosages (5 mg compared to 0.225 mg). Goldberg and Cherniack and Wu and associates suggest that IPPB may be of added benefit for the patient who is unable to take a deep breath or coordinate breathing with a hand-held nebulizer. However, Murray (1974) states that the inability to teach patients how to use a hand-held or compressor-driven nebulizer constitutes a failure of instruction, not an indication for IPPB. If a patient is able to breathe, a simple aerosol generator can be used just as effectively as IPPB and possibly better (O'Donohue, 1982). Aerosol deposition to the larger or smaller airways is not enhanced by IPPB compared with quiet breathing (Newhouse and Ruffin, 1978).

Ziment (1973) delineates four disadvantages of aerosol delivery with IPPB: (1) Because gas flow follows the pathway of least resistance, aerosols are preferentially delivered to the compliant airways. Therefore, less is delivered to the more spastic airways that may benefit most from bronchodilator therapy. (2) Controlled dosages of medication delivery are not possible with IPPB. Aerosol dosages may be 10–20 times greater than those used subcutaneously or intravenously, yet only 5–15% of a total dosage is normally retained in the lungs. If, however, IPPB is connected directly to an artificial airway and no dosage reduction is made, considerably larger quantities may be retained in the body. Systemic effects are not eliminated with aerosol delivery, since variable amounts of the medication may be retained in the mouth, esophagus, stomach, duodenum, and trachea as well as the lungs. (3) Some inhaled bronchodilators that are beta stimulators, such as isoproterenol, result in pulmonary vascular vasodilation. This can cause increased ventilation/perfusion mismatch, particularly in the presence of severe bronchospasm (Pierson and Grieco, 1969). (4) IPPB is more expensive yet no more effective in delivering bronchodilators and mucolytic agents than are hand-held or compressor-driven nebulizers. Water or humidification is believed to be the best mucus-softening agent and is without the side effects of currently used medications.

Work of Breathing

The ability of IPPB to affect the work of breathing has caused much debate in the literature. Sukumalchantra and co-workers (1965) found that IPPB increased the work of breathing in some patients but reduced it in others. Sinha and Bergofsky (1972) reported that IPPB at large inflation pressures (average, 22 cm H_2O) may be beneficial in patients with kyphoscoliosis and chronically decreased lung compliance. In six patients this parameter was found to increase 70%, for up to 3 hr, and was accompanied by decreases in the work of breathing. Recent studies on patients with neuromuscular disease do not substantiate these findings. Patients with muscular dystrophy and quadriplegia demonstrated no improvement in respiratory system compliance (neither chest wall nor static lung compliance) following IPPB treatment that delivered volumes up to three times resting tidal volumes (DeTroyer and Deisser, 1981; McCool et al., 1986).

In part, the ability of IPPB to alter the work of breathing appears to depend on the degree of patient cooperation and relaxation (Ayres et al., 1963; Sukumalchantra et al.). Bader and Bader (1969) noted that increased respiratory work was associated with high flow rates. Similar findings were reported by Ayres and associates, when patients actively led the IPPB apparatus. Increases in airway collapse, expiratory resistance, and air trapping, which are associated with IPPB, may also result in a rise in the work of breathing (Jones et al., 1960; Kamat et al.; Sukumalchantra et al.; O'Donohue, 1982). Alterations in the work of breathing, that may accompany IPPB, were not found to change the overall metabolic rate. The fraction of total body metabolism expended on ventilation is normally small. As a result, if a decrease in respiratory work is accompanied by increased nonrespiratory work, such as agitation or discomfort (also attributed to IPPB), the desired effect may be neutralized (Sukumalchantra et al.). The data generated on the work of breathing associated with IPPB must also be viewed in light of the difficulty in making accurate and reproducible measurements of this parameter, especially in spontaneously breathing patients.

Pulmonary Function

Tidal Volume

IPPB is often prescribed because it is felt to increase tidal volume and, therefore, prevent small airway collapse. Cullen and co-workers (1957) concluded that IPPB did cause an increase in tidal volume in normal subjects but not in patients with emphysema. A study on similar patients reported significant increases in tidal volume with mechanical chest percussion, IPPB, manual chest percussion and voluntary deep breathing (Petty and Guthrie, 1971). Other researchers claimed that the effects of IPPB on gas distribution and tidal volume were similar to those of voluntary hyperventilation (Torres et al., 1960; Emmanuel et al., 1966; Wohl, 1968; McConnell et al., 1974). For persons who are unable to increase their tidal volume voluntarily, Torres and associates suggested IPPB as a way of improving pulmonary gas distribution.

Petty and Guthrie noted that increased dead space ventilation was associated with deep breathing but not with IPPB. Other researchers reported the opposite. Sukumalchantra and co-workers found that the majority (mean, 56%) of the tidal volume increase achieved by IPPB resulted in increased dead space. Voluntary hyperinflation by the same patients caused marked improvement in alveolar ventilation, and only a small portion (mean, 17%) of the tidal volume increase was dead space. This suggests that IPPB, in comparison to voluntary hyperinflation, overventilates alveoli that are already well ventilated. Consequently, its effect is wasted. In order to improve alveolar ventilation, increased driving pressures were suggested. However, this can cause increased alveolar pressure that may result in pulmonary vasculature compression (Riley, 1962; Daly et al., 1963). Therefore, increasing inspiratory flow or pressure may decrease perfusion, creating an even greater ventilation/perfusion mismatch.

In eight supine subjects, Bynum and associates (1976) studied the effects of IPPB and spontaneous breathing at tidal volume and large lung volumes (greater than twice the tidal volume). The effect of these maneuvers on the distribution of ventilation, perfusion, and ventilation/perfusion ratios was measured by using radioactive gas techniques. During tidal volume breathing, ventilation and perfusion were diminished in the lung bases (areas adjacent to the diaphragm) as compared to other areas. However, this decrease was greater in the subjects receiving IPPB, despite the fact that the volume of air, inspiratory flow, and frequency of breathing were the same for both groups. Both voluntary and IPPB-induced hyperinflation caused improved basilar ventilation and perfusion; yet, the spontaneously increased volume resulted in significantly higher ventilation/perfusion ratios than were found with IPPB. Bynum et al. concluded that at similar lung volumes, IPPB was inferior to spontaneous breathing in ventilating and perfusing the lung bases. As a result, voluntary hyperinflations may be more effective in preventing atelectasis than IPPB. IPPB should not be considered as an alternative to deep breathing unless an increase in volume of at least 25% of that obtained by voluntary deep breathing is obtained. It is generally accepted that IPPB has no benefit over volitional hyperinflation, in part because it emphasizes the least appropriate component of inspiration, pressure rather than volume (George and O'Donohue, 1980 and 1982; Gold, 1982; American Thoracic Society, 1987).

Arterial Blood Gases

Blood gas changes that occur after IPPB treatment were found both to improve and to worsen. Following IPPB, reduced arterial carbon dioxide levels were reported in some patients and normal subjects (Cullen et al.; Sukumalchantra et al.; Petty and Guthrie). However, significant decreases in $PaCO_2$ were also demonstrated following mechanical and manual chest compression on patients with obstructive lung disease (Petty and Guthrie). The reported changes in arterial blood gases following IPPB were of short duration. Ziment (1973) emphasized that these fluctuations may be harmful, since short-lived decreases in $PaCO_2$ or increases in PaO_2 following IPPB may diminish respiratory drive and result in hypoventilation. Reduced respiratory rates were also noted by Cullen and associates (1957).

In general, it appears that IPPB may increase tidal volume. However, the same or more beneficial effects are usually seen with voluntary hyperventilation. When IPPB does increase tidal volume, it is not clear in the literature if this correlates with either increased alveolar ventilation or improved arterial blood gases. None of these changes is reported to be of any long-term significance (Bader and Bader; Morris et al., 1970; Ziment, 1973; Leith, 1974; Scheffler and Delaney, 1981). Murray concludes that neither hypoxemia nor CO_2 retention is an indication for IPPB, since any change is only transient. Instead, significant CO_2 retention, hypoxemia, and acute ventilatory failure are more often indications for mechanical ventilation. Maneuvers that attempt to treat the symptoms and provide transient improvement in gas exchange are doomed to certain failure unless the precipitating cause of respiratory failure is removed.

Psychological Effect

Whether IPPB is of psychological benefit is controversial. The claim by the patient of "I feel better" after receiving IPPB should not be ignored. This, in itself, may be an important finding, despite the fact that laboratory tests failed to substantiate any measurable changes (Murray; Thornton et al., 1974). Particularly in the COPD patient, improvement in activities of daily living or quality of life following intensive rehabilitation are documented, while no significant changes in pulmonary function tests or corresponding signs of disease reversal may be noted. However, subjective claims of improvement following IPPB treatment may be unreliable for the following reasons: (1) Some patients may not wish to disappoint their physician or therapist and therefore, claim improvement. (2) Transitory improvement of symptoms is common when initiating a new treatment program, especially in patients with chronic diseases. Improvement is also noted when the person performing the treatment is highly motivated or enthusiastic. (3) The mystique surrounding an expensive and complicated-looking machine that makes hissing noises and emits clouds of vapor can undoubtedly serve to persuade some patients that dramatic relief is imminent (Murray). The problem of psychological dependence, with IPPB serving as a security blanket, is most often described in reference to long-term users, such as COPD patients. Murray states that the machine prescribed to alleviate symptoms of pulmonary disease has developed into a complication that is more debilitating than the disease for which it was prescribed. There is no evidence that IPPB is helpful or desirable for home use (IPPB trial group, 1983).

Prevention of Pulmonary Complications Associated with Surgery

IPPB is believed by some to prevent, as well as treat, atelectasis after surgery by dilating collapsed bronchi and expanding underventilated atelectatic alveoli. To quote McConnell and his associates, it seems that "since Elisha (II Kings 4:34) first used positive pressure breathing to resuscitate a Shunammite child, this method has found great favor with the medical profession." Because pulmonary complications account for 6–70% of problems seen following upper abdominal surgery (Pontoppidan, 1980), it is no wonder that all posssible methods of reducing this morbidity were tried. The overwhelming acceptance of IPPB, as judged by its widespread use, would lead one to believe it is beneficial; yet, the routine use of IPPB prior to surgery is of unproven value in preventing atelectasis following surgery (Ziment, 1974; Gold, 1982). Similarly, its efficacy in preventing complications, such as atelectasis and pneumonia following surgery, has not been proven in any study of acceptable design (Petty).

IPPB is most commonly administered with the patient in the head-up position. This may aid the flow of secretions to the dependent lung zones. Postoperative pulmonary complications most commonly occur in the lower lobes of adult patients (Jaworski et al., 1988; Appendix 1.3). Therefore, the sitting postion is the most unfavorable for postural drainage in this patient population. IPPB also delivers an inspiratory pressure that may impede normal mucus flow. Based on these findings, Ziment (1973) feels that physiother-

apy (including postural drainage, percussion and supervised coughing) should be given after IPPB or the patient may well be harmed by the IPPB treatment.

In 15 patients following surgery, Jones (1968) found that voluntary deep breathing was more effective in increasing tidal volume than IPPB at conventional pressures (15 cm H_2O). When pressures of 25 cm H_2O were used, IPPB was superior. It must be emphasized that this study did not attempt to establish whether IPPB at 25 cm H_2O was beneficial in preventing complications following surgery (Ziment, 1974). It was merely concerned with methods to improve tidal volume. Sequencing of the various therapies studied was not altered, and rest periods of only 10 min existed between trials. Consequently, there may have been an additive effect, since the values may not have returned to normal between therapies. Also, no follow-up was documented as to the long-term effect of these maneuvers in preventing airway collapse.

In contrast, O'Donohue (1979) reported that IPPB was effective in the management of pulmonary atelectasis in four case reports (only one involved a surgical patient). Changes in arterial blood gases and chest x-rays were the criteria for improvement. Inspiratory pressures between 35 and 45 cm H_2O were used. These values are in excess of the normal pressures prescribed during IPPB, yet complications of mediastinal emphysema (reported following conventional pressures) were not noted. Although chest physiotherapy, incentive spirometry, broncho-dilators, antibiotics, and fiberoptic bronchoscopy were initially found ineffective in clearing the atelectasis in these patients, some of these treatments were continued along with maximal volume IPPB therapy. IPPB treatments were performed every 2 hr and repeated for 36–72 hr. Because the degree of patient mobilization was not specified, it is possible that some of the pulmonary improvement was due to increased patient activity (see Case Histories 6.1 and 6.2). Similarly, since other therapies were given simultaneously, it is difficult to conclude that any changes in atelectasis or arterial blood gases were due to the effect of IPPB alone.

Meyers et al. (1975) studied the effects of IPPB on functional residual capacity (FRC) in 10 patients following abdominal surgery. This parameter was chosen because it was believed to most accurately reflect alterations in alveolar ventilation or collapse. IPPB was found to have no influence on changes in FRC. Browner and Powers (1975) also investigated the effects of IPPB on FRC in patients following surgery. Of those having normal or reduced FRC prior to treatment, they found that IPPB caused a significant fall (416 ml) in this value. They also reported significant decreases in PaO_2 and oxygen saturation. Therefore, they suggest that administering IPPB to patients after surgery may not only be of questionable benefit but may be potentially harmful.

Numerous studies were undertaken to evaluate IPPB and its effectiveness in preventing or treating pulmonary complications after surgery. Baxter and Levine (1969) studied 200 patients. Comparing radiological and clinical findings before and after surgery, they concluded that IPPB was not effective in reducing the incidence of pulmonary complications. Becker et al. (1960) studied 100 patients after upper abdominal surgery and concluded that routine IPPB (2–3 times/day for 3 days) did not prevent or clear atelectasis, when compared with a control group. Cottrell and Siker (1973) reached the same conclusion in studying 60 patients treated before and after surgery. Although pulmonary function tests were found to improve in the patients with COPD who received IPPB before their operation, findings following surgery were not affected.

In evaluating the effectiveness of IPPB for patients following thoracic surgery, McConnell and colleagues concluded that although the depth of respiration was increased with IPPB, verbal encouragement of the patient to breathe deeply was just as effective. Sands and co-workers (1961) studied 84 patients receiving IPPB after upper abdominal surgery and found results in agreement with those described above. They also noted that the patients treated with IPPB complained of "more mucus" than did the control group, but that this did not lead to increased cough stimulation or subsequent expectoration. In addition, IPPB was not found to reduce discomfort after surgery, to result in earlier patient ambulation, or to result in decreased hospital stay, as was expected.

On the other hand, Anderson et al. (1963) found that pulmonary complications were markedly decreased when IPPB was used following surgery. Baxter and Levine commented on this study as involving a far more heterogeneous group of patients and attributed the low pulmonary complication rate to the diligence of the therapist rather than the IPPB apparatus. Fouts and Brashear state that Anderson and co-workers' conclusions are difficult to accept because of the disparity in numbers (160 control patients and 42 treated), and the lack of information about the respiratory care given to the controls. Noehren and associates (1958) may have a better explanation:

Most suggestions for the improvement of postoperative management of patients have demonstrated improvement in results, and the common denominator for each of these appears to be closer attention to the patient postoperatively. This factor alone will often be sufficient without any additions, mechanical or otherwise. Perhaps the success with intermittent positive pressure breathing on inspiration has been on the same basis.

Studies in the last decade tend to support this statement. In 1980, Schuppisser et al. found IPPB of no benefit over chest physiotherapy in altering ventilatory function or the incidence of pulmonary complications following upper abdominal surgery. Although both types of therapy were equally effective, the authors recommend physiotherapy because of the added complications and cost associated with IPPB. The specific treatment referred to as "chest physiotherapy" is not defined in this study. Ali and co-workers (1984) compared the added effect of IPPB with chest physiotherapy alone in 30 patients undergoing cholecystectomy. Physiotherapy was described as deep breathing, coughing, turning, leg exercises, and early ambulation. The only statistical difference between the two groups was a severely depressed postoperative vital capacity in patients during IPPB treatment. The authors conclude that IPPB is very costly and not beneficial to patients receiving physiotherapy after surgery. Although both studies reached similar conclusions, neither compared IPPB and chest physiotherapy with a control group, in part for ethical reasons.

A few studies have compared the effect of IPPB with incentive spirometry (IS) for reducing pulmonary complications after surgery and have failed to show an advantage of either therapy (Gale and Sanders, 1980; Jung et al., 1980; Alexander et al., 1981). Similarly, Indihar and Associates (1982) found IPPB, IS, and turning with deep breathing and coughing to be equally effective in reducing pulmonary complications in 300 surgical patients. The variety of operative sites may have masked any possible benefit since extremity and lower abdominal surgery are less likely to cause pulmonary problems from secretion retention. Celli and co-workers (1984) are one of the few investigators to use a control group when comparing the effect of IPPB, IS, and deep breathing exercises on preventing pulmonary complications after abdominal surgery. They found all three methods to be significantly better than no treatment at reducing postoperative lung pathology; undesirable side effects were observed only in the 18% of patients receiving IPPB.

Complications Associated with IPPB

The complications associated with IPPB are shown in Table 9.1. Most are not life-threatening and were discussed earlier in this chapter. Others have more serious sequelae and require further discussion.

IPPB is reported to cause bronchospasm which may produce increased airway obstruction and air trapping (Ziment, 1973; Petty; Moore et al.; Shapiro et al., 1982). Karetzky (1975) reported acute pneumothorax associated with IPPB resulting in fatality. These complications are believed to be particularly important when IPPB is used in the treatment of patients with acute asthma. Though pressures commonly used during IPPB range between 10 and 15 cm H_2O, this limit is

Table 9.1
Reported Complications and Hazards of IPPB[a]

1. Bronchospasm, distension of cysts and bullae, air trapping, pneumothorax
2. Gastric distension and ileus
3. Overdosage or adverse reactions of nebulized drugs
4. Acquired infection from contaminated equipment
5. Reduction of venous return causing hypotension
6. Reduction of respiratory drive in patients with chronic respiratory failure
7. Further impaction of mucus in patients unable or unwilling to expectorate following IPPB treatment
8. Exhaustion of patients who do not participate with treatment effectively
9. Complications of malfunctioning equipment
10. Psychological dependence

[a]Adapted from Ziment (1973), Karetsky (1975), and Shapiro et al. (1982).

often exceeded both intentionally and unintentionally. This occurs when patients exhibit air trapping or are out of phase with the machine. Macklin and Macklin (1944) reported that intraalveolar and pulmonary vascular pressure gradients need not exceed 40 cm H_2O before air can escape from the alveoli into the vascular sheaths. Since 1960, extrapulmonary air has been reported with increasing frequency in children with acute asthma (McGovern et al., 1961; Jorgensen et al., 1963; Bierman, 1967). This complication parallels the increased use of IPPB therapy in the treatment of childhood asthma. The pressurized flow of gas from the IPPB machine was also noted to cause gastric insufflation in patients. Reportedly, this can lead to colonic ileus and cecal perforation but more often resulted in patient discomfort (Ruben et al., 1961; Golden and Chandler, 1975; Gold, 1976).

Humidification and medications are delivered in aerosol form by IPPB. However, IPPB offers no advantages over other less expensive methods of delivering humidity or aerosols (Gold, 1975; O'Donohue, 1982; American Thoracic Society). As with all nebulizers, IPPB nebulization is a source of bacterial contamination, and careful sterilization of the apparatus is mandatory. Based on the spread of infection attributed to IPPB, both Browner and Powers and Gold (1976) recommend abandoning such treatment for surgical patients. Because IPPB is most often prescribed for persons prone to pulmonary complications, its ability to spread infection is significant. Sanders et al. (1970) reported an outbreak of nosocomial infection with *Serratia marcescens* that was traced to contaminated medications delivered by IPPB. The number of patients with *Serratia* isolated from their sputum was proportional to the total number of IPPB treatments administered. Mertz and co-workers (1967) described an outbreak of *Klebsiella* pneumonia (resulting in five deaths in 1 month). All patients involved in the outbreak received IPPB with bronchodilator treatments. The spread of this hospital-acquired infection was attributed to a contaminated stock bottle of bronchodilator solution. Contamination with gram-negative bacilli was reported as high as 91% in IPPB machines with reservoir nebulizers (Reinarz et al.).

The Cost of IPPB

IPPB is primarily used on surgical patients and those with COPD. The average number of treatments performed, average cost of treatment, and the types of patients receiving treatment differ from facility to facility. In 1974, McConnell and associates found the incidence of IPPB treatment at UCLA Hospital (700 beds) to be 7,000/year at a patient cost of $370,000/year. If these findings are extrapolated to acute general hospital usage nationwide, an amount in excess of $400 million is figured. This sum, presumably, does not include amounts spent on outpatient, extended care, or home care treatments and is based on 1974 costs. For the same year, Leith states that $2 billion/year was collected from the public for IPPB treatments.

In sampling both university and community hospitals, Baker (1974) found that a wide variation existed in IPPB usage (0.9–9% of all hospital admissions). Similarly, in surveying the 43 Washington, D.C. hospitals that provide respiratory therapy, Scheffler and Delaney reported the average number of patients receiving IPPB per number of patient admissions to be 6% (range, 3–12%). Baker reported that generally, a greater number of treatments were performed at hospitals associated with schools of inhalation therapy and university hospitals showed a greater use of chest physiotherapy, suggesting the application of alternative methods to IPPB treatments. Of interest, Scheffler and Delaney also found that teaching hospitals showed a dramatic reduction (70%) in the number of IPPB treatments per 100 admissions between 1976 and 1979. Between 1971 and 1979, the monthly number of IPPB treatments at Massachusetts General Hospital fell from a high of nearly 17,000 (1972) to a low of 500 (1979), while the number of chest physiotherapy treatments remained unchanged over this period (Pontoppidan). Braun et al. (1981) also reported a significant decrease in IPPB use by two Wisconsin hospitals between 1971 and 1979. The hospital (university) having a larger critical care population and generally more seriously ill patients showed a concurrent increase in the use of chest physiotherapy. The other hospital (a smaller private hospital) demonstrated a trend of substituting incentive spirometry treatment for IPPB therapy. Pontoppidan attributes the rapid decline in IPPB therapy over the past years to increased challenges as to its cost effectiveness, efficacy and scientific basis for use in both surgical and medical patients.

In 1974, both usage and charges for IPPB showed wide variations that were not necessarily geographical in nature. The costs ranged from $3.75 to $7.50/treatment; daily maximums ranged between $15 and $96 within the same city (Baker). In 1980, Hughes sampled five Chicago hospitals and found that initial treatment costs for IPPB ranged from $8.33 to $18. For all hospitals studied by Scheffler and Delaney, an average of 60 treatments were given for every 100 patient admissions. However, large discrepancies were noted between "for profit" hospitals, which averaged 190 treatments/100 admissions, and federal hospitals, where an average of 11 treatments/100 admissions was performed

Likewise, the hospital bed number was found to be inversely related to the proportion of patients receiving IPPB. These findings are mostly supported by O'Donohue (1985), who found significantly less use of IPPB for treating postoperative atelectasis in hospitals with more than 400 beds, compared to smaller facilities. He also reported a significantly lower use of chest physiotherapy in hospitals with 200 beds or less. Although IPPB appears to be more selectively prescribed from this study than in the past (Baker), it is still reportedly used in 82% of all hospitals to treat postoperative atelectasis. This seems incongruous with the fact that studies have not proven that IPPB benefits surgical patients postoperatively (Gold, 1982).

Another complication associated with IPPB is the use of contract services to provide it. To quote Petty, the use of this "practice is deplorable and offers the greatest chance of harm because the overuse and misuse of IPPB is very likely when there is no medical director as an established member of the hospital staff where the 'service' is provided." The controls surrounding "big business" are a poor means of managing therapeutic treatment and do not lend themselves to minimizing patient costs. Respiratory therapy departments are reported to depend on IPPB income for greater than 75% of their billing (Kittredge, 1973). A recent study in New England demonstrates that IPPB usage can be reduced by greater than 92% without any change in mortality or morbidity (Zibrak et al., 1986). Considering the investments in machinery, equipment, and payroll of contract companies, it is easy to imagine how IPPB became economically oriented rather than a carefully controlled aspect of patient care.

Summary

It is hard to conclude much that is therapeutic about IPPB. Though it is an effective method of aerosol delivery, IPPB is more expensive yet no more effective than simple mechanically powered or hand-held nebulizers. Substantial controversy exists over the ability of IPPB to improve alveolar ventilation, tidal volume, and arterial blood gases. At best, any improvements in pulmonary function accredited to IPPB are short-lived, since most treatment times are 20 min or less and are commonly given only 2–4 times/day. The psychological aspect of this treatment seems to vary considerably and often depends on what other therapies are concurrently employed. IPPB is not an effective means of decreasing or preventing pulmonary complications in surgical patients. Though the hazards associated with IPPB are relatively small, the cost of IPPB is astronomical. In addition, the relationship between contract services and both the quality and cost of their "service" should not be ignored. The ineffectiveness of IPPB may, in part, be attributed to the absence of uniform treatment indications and expectations. There must be clear rationale for implementing IPPB, along with a clear understanding of its indications, contraindications, risks, cost, and cost effectiveness (Petty). This has not occurred in the past. The burden of proof of efficacy and economic justification lies in the hands of those who order and perform such treatment (Gold, 1975). The authors do not recommend IPPB for prophylactic use or for the management of postoperative pulmonary complications.

BRONCHODILATING AND MUCOLYTIC AEROSOLS

A symposium of those that advocate the use of theophylline in the management of COPD patients was published as a supplement to Chest (Vol. 92, 1S–43S, 1987). Ziment (1987) analyzes evidence for the effects of theophylline on mucociliary clearance and suggests the drug may directly and indirectly improve mucociliary clearance. Theophylline increases the secretory output of bronchial glands. The transepithelial secretion of fluid into the respiratory tract is increased. Theophylline stimulates the chloride pump that is controlled by cyclic AMP. Ciliary motility is also stimulated by theophylline. The major effects of theophylline that are likely to be beneficial in the COPD patient occur probably due to bronchodilation and because theophylline improves diaphragm contractility and reverses diaphragm fatigue (Aubier, 1987). Whether the bronchodilating effects of theophylline occur by aerosol inhalation alone or are improved by intravenous administration and addition of β_2-agonists such as salbutamol remains controversial (Brain, 1984; Jenne, 1987a). There is no evidence that theophylline is beneficial in the patient with acute lung disease.

Benefit from use of aerosol-delivered mucolytic agents is poorly substantiated, with the possible exception of its use in children with cystic fibrosis (Brain, 1984). There are no data to substantiate the use of mucolytic agents to assist removal of secretions in acute lung disease. In our clinical experience, neither bronchodilators or mucolytic agents delivered by aerosol appeared to be of benefit in patients with acute lung disease receiving chest physiotherapy. Intuitively it seems that benefit for acutely atelectatic lung is likely to be minimal since nonventilated areas of lung do not directly receive any aerosolized drugs. Intravenously administered bronchodilators, given by continuous infusion after a loading dose and monitored by blood levels, appear beneficial in reversing severe bronchoconstriction. Mild bronchospasm is frequently found to reverse following the removal of retained secretions, which is assisted by adequate systemic hydration of the patient, inhaled humidity and chest physiotherapy.

However, the use of aerosol-delivered mucolytic agents and bronchodilators is widespread in the management of patients with acute chest disorders. It appears that these therapies are inappropriately and, often, reflexly prescribed. A review of the literature does not provide many concrete facts about the indications for and clinical effectiveness of these aerosols (Brain and Valberg, 1979).

Bronchodilators

There is evidence that some bronchodilating aerosols are useful in certain patients with chronic pulmonary disease, particularly asthma and cystic fibrosis. Beta-adrenergic aerosols tend to have a rapid and predictable onset with peak effects detected in minutes, but the efficacy of aerosol compared to intravenous use of bronchodilators needs to be determined (Brain, 1980; Jenne, 1987a). The indications for use and toxicity of bronchodilators in young children, in the presence of cardiovascular impairment, and in the long-term therapy of such diseases as COPD, asthma, and cystic fibrosis need to be determined (Featherby et al., 1970; Brain, 1980; Jenne, 1987b). The significance of the nonbronchodilator pharmacological effects of these medications also requires further investigation (Brain, 1980). The benefits of using bronchodilators in patients with acute lung pathology including lung contusion and flail chest are not established. In this patient population, some clinical signs of bronchospasm, such as wheezing, may be relieved by removing excess secretions.

Mucolytic Agents

Mucolytic agents are ineffective in improving airway clearance, with the possible exception of patients with cystic fibrosis (Thomson et al., 1975; Brain and Valberg; Brain, 1980, 1984). Although aerosols of these drugs can alter mucus characteristics in vitro and probably in vivo, it is not known if the changes enhance mucociliary activity and the cough mechanism (Brain and Valberg). Adequate humidification (100% relative humidity) is probably the best means of liquifying secretions and is without the side effects associated with mucolytic agents (Wanner and Rao, 1980). Bland aerosols including distilled water, saline, and half normal saline have no substantiated benefits in treating lower airway disease. Moreover such aerosols may elicit bronchoconstriction in adults and children (Brain, 1984).

Present understanding of aerosol deposition and location of airway receptors for various drugs is inadequate (Newhouse and Ruffin, 1978). For aerosol delivery to be effective, particle size must be tailored to the delivery system and site of receptors as well as coordinated with specific breathing maneuvers. Positive pressure breathing of aerosols does not produce a more uniform or more peripheral distribution of aerosols than quiet breathing (Newhouse and Ruffin, 1978).

Complications

It is difficult to measure the received dose of a drug given by aerosol (Brain and Valberg). Even if the principles governing aerosol deposition, retention, and clearance are understood, the amount of medication reaching a specific area of the lungs is only an estimate (Brain, 1980). Although the small particles produced by some nebulizers are capable of reaching the terminal airways, the percentage of the drug delivered to these areas also depends upon the tidal volume, breathing frequency, expiratory reserve volume and length of breath holding of the patient, the presence of an artificial airway, and the length of delivery tubing from the source to the patient (Brain and Valberg; Swift, 1980). Nose breathing compared with mouth breathing effects particle deposition and can markedly increase the quantity of medication retained by the nasal mucosa and pharynx (Brain and Valberg). This, in turn, may be swallowed and systemically absorbed, resulting in general effects as opposed to local changes. The efficacy of a bronchodilator or mucolytic agent on the lungs depends on successful delivery to the affected area. In the presence of pulmonary collapse, obstruction, or constriction, airflow and, therefore, aerosol flow are impeded. Nonventilated areas of the lung do not directly receive any benefit from inhaled medications (Brain, 1980). Many aerosol devices used by patients with chronic lung diseases require intelligent use by the patient and they are frequently misused (Brain, 1984).

The possibility of infection through contamination by aerosol-generating equipment is well documented in the literature and is discussed on pp. 284 and 293. Because aerosols can be deposited in the most distal airways and are most often used on patients already suffering from pulmonary complications, the added insult of iatrogenic infection can be significant and should be avoided by proper sterilization.

In mechanically ventilated patients receiving chest physiotherapy, nebulization of N-acteylcysteine (a mucolytic agent) rendered subsequent physiotherapy treatments less effective in increasing pulmonary compliance (Winning et al., 1975). N-Acetylcysteine is also reported to cause bronchoconstriction in patients with asthma and chronic airway disease (Bernstein and Ausdenmore, 1964; Rao et al., 1970) and in normal intubated subjects (Waltemath and Bergman, 1973).

It appears that based on the cost and potential hazards of mucolytic agents and bronchodilators, use should be restricted to those aerosols whose clinical value is documented. The currently prescribed mucolytic aerosols do not meet this requirement (Wanner and Rao, 1980). The indications, complications, and benefits of aerosol-delivered bronchodilators in patients suffering acute lung pathology are not established (Brain, 1980). The minimal effective dose, optimal method of delivery, and type of patient who can most benefit from short-term and continued bronchodilator treatment still need to be determined (Brain, 1980).

MECHANICAL DEVICES USED TO ENCOURAGE LUNG EXPANSION FOLLOWING SURGERY

For many years, mechanical aids to lung expansion enjoyed tremendous popularity without critical analysis of either their rationale or usefulness (Pontoppidan). A wide array of maneuvers and devices were suggested in attempts to prevent pulmonary complications after surgery. Transtracheal aspiration and deep breathing were proposed, and these are discussed elsewhere (see pp. 164 and 119). Inhaling carbon dioxide, once believed to be of benefit (Alder, 1967; Jones, 1968), is no longer used. Aside from IPPB and breathing exercises, the methods most in vogue appear to be forms of incentive spirometry (IS), continuous positive airway pressure (CPAP), and positive expiratory pressure (PEP). Blow bottles represent a type of expiratory IS, while most currently used IS emphasize the inspiratory phase of respiration. For clarity, the term IS refers only to the inspiratory devices in this text. Both CPAP and PEP primarily affect expiration. The use of these techniques is based on research by Anderes et al. (1979), who found improved lung reexpansion through collateral airway channels when CPAP was applied.

Blow Bottles

In eight patients, Colgan et al. (1970) studied the effects of resistance breathing on FRC, using blow bottles and sustained hyperinflations with the Elder demand valve resuscitator. Both methods were found to produce marked increases in airway pressure similar to that seen during a Valsalva maneuver, and neither was found to be beneficial in treating atelectasis following surgery. Significant increases in FRC were reported after blow bottle use, but this was believed to be the result of the sustained deep breath performed prior to treatment. O'Connor (1975) also examined blow bottles, but he compared them to a device that added increased dead space and expiratory pressure. In the 23 patients studied following laparotomy, a significantly greater increase in vital capacity was reported in those using the dead space, expiratory pressure device. Based on these findings, O'Connor suggested that this device may result in a decreased incidence of respiratory complications after surgery. Further information on this device is not available. Heisterberg et al. (1979) compared the effect of using blow bottles (for 10 min every 4 hr) with chest physiotherapy (breathing exercises, postural drainage, and coughing, two times per day) in 98 patients undergoing elective gastric or biliary tract surgery. They found the incidence of radiological pulmonary changes to be the same in both groups and concluded that blow bottles are preferable to chest physiotherapy because they are less time consuming. There are no documented complications of blow bottle use; theoretical concerns include hyperventilation, increased atelectasis, barotrauma, and cost (Shapiro et al., 1982). Based on the existing literature, blow bottles have not been found more effective than other techniques and have

not been shown to decrease pulmonary complications postoperatively. Adjuncts emphasizing inspiration, not expiration, are thought to be better at improving respiratory function after surgery.

Incentive Spirometry

Many authors compared IS to IPPB as a means of reducing respiratory complications after surgery (see p. 293). Both of these devices emphasize inspiration; IPPB is performed passively, while incentive spirometry involves an active maneuver toward maximal inspiration. Van de Water and associates (1972) studied 30 consecutive women following adrenalectomy; 15 of them received IS and the rest IPPB. Both groups were able to be treated with other therapies, which included blow bottles, rebreather tubes, and thoracic physiotherapy. Only three patients in the IS group developed pyrexia (at least 38.5°C) and clinical findings indicative of pulmonary complications, compared with six of the patients who received IPPB. The average hospital stay was 9 days for those treated with IS and 11 days for IPPB-treated patients. The authors claim good patient acceptance of IS at one-tenth the cost of IPPB. Due to the variety of therapies used in each group, it is not possible to tell which therapy, if any, actually altered the morbidity.

Iverson and co-workers (1978) evaluated three methods commonly used after surgery to reduce pulmonary complications. Of the 145 patients in their study, 42 received IPPB, 45 used blow bottles, and 58 received IS. The incidence of pulmonary complications, evaluated by chest x-ray interpretation, clinical findings, and arterial blood gas results, was 30% with IPPB, 8% with blow bottles, and 15% with IS. Also associated with IPPB was a significant increase in gastrointestinal complications. Dohi and Gold (1978) studied 64 patients: 30 received IPPB and the rest received IS. All patients were treated for 5 days after surgery and were observed for pulmonary complications by chest x-ray and clinical examination. Because the data favoring IS over IPPB were statistically slim, the authors claimed no conclusive difference between the two therapies. Based on these findings, they also stated that the use of IS rather than IPPB may be justified, since the former is much cheaper. Another study comparing the postoperative use of IS and IPPB did not find a change in the incidence of pulmonary dysfunction with the two modes of therapy (Gale and Sanders, 1980).

The previous authors failed to compare either IPPB or IS with deep breathing. However, McConnell et al. contrasted the effects of voluntary deep breathing, IPPB, and IS on transpulmonary pressure gradients in 11 thoracotomy patients and 6 normal subjects. Deep breathing produced an average gradient of 24.6 cm H_2O, IPPB of 21.7 cm H_2O, and IS of 29.4 cm H_2O. The authors state that increased transpulmonary pressure gradients are a principal determinant of alveolar and bronchial expansion. Therefore, they claim that IS is more convenient and less costly than IPPB in achieving alveolar and bronchial expansion. The fact that deep breathing is even less expensive and requires no more instruction than the other two methods was not addressed. Alexander and co-workers (1981) failed to show a decrease in pulmonary complications when IS (up to 80% of the preoperative maximal inspiratory volume), IPPB (3 times per day), or IS with IPPB was compared to a control group (encouraged to breathe deeply and ambulate). Similarly, Indihar et al. (1982) found no benefit of IS or IPPB over turning, coughing and deep breathing in 100 surgical patients. Two studies compared the effects of IS and continuous positive airway pressure (CPAP). One evaluated CPAP, IS, and coughing and deep breathing in 65 adults. Patients received their assigned treatment for 15 min, every 2 hr (while awake), for 3 days after abdominal surgery (Stock et al., 1985). The authors concluded that IS offered no advantage over coughing and deep breathing. Ricksten et al. (1986) studied 43 similar patients but compared IS to CPAP and PEP. They found both CPAP and PEP superior to IS in improving gas exchange, lung volumes, and radiological clearing after upper abdominal surgery.

A study comparing three types of IS used following upper abdominal surgery was undertaken in 79 patients (Lederer et al., 1980). Instruction in how to use the assigned device was given prior to surgery. Though only monitored once daily afterwards, all patients were encouraged to use their assigned IS 10 times every waking hour. On each day following surgery, a substantial number of patients in each group did not use their device at all. Other types of therapy, including ultrasonic nebulization, chest percussion, postural drainage, or any combination of these, were given to some patients in each group. There was little statistical difference between the three types of IS in terms of the patient's pulmonary function, vital signs, and white blood cell count, and there was no difference in the length of hospital stay. It would be more interesting if the three groups were compared to both a control group and a group performing voluntary deep breathing. Because of the lack of a control group, it is still not known whether any device at all was of benefit to these patients (Hughes, 1980).

A few studies evaluating the use of IS were performed on patients requiring cardiac surgery. Krastins et al. (1982) studied 17 children and found that when IS (every 2 hr for 12 hr a day) was used in conjunction with chest physiotherapy, a dramatic decrease in atelectasis resulted. However, there was no difference between the postoperative pulmonary function tests (PFT) of children receiving IS with physiotherapy (study group) and those receiving chest physiotherapy (control group). The incidence of atelectasis in this study was higher than that reported by others (88%); also pleural effusion occurred in all control and two study patients. In 25 adults undergoing coronary artery surgery, the efficacy of two different IS techniques was compared with chest physiotherapy (cough, deep breathing, postural drainage, percussion, and vibration) (Oulton et al., 1981). No added benefit was found when one type of IS (Triflow) was performed in addition to chest physiotherapy; however, when the other IS (Spirocare) was used, fever, and less severe pulmonary complications were noted on chest x-ray. The investigators attributed the difference between IS modalities to the fact that Triflow is more flow dependent while Spirocare is more volume sensitive. These conclusions are in conflict with those of Lederer et al. who found no significant difference between the two IS studied by Oulton et al. or another IS (Bartlett-Edwards) that is also volume dependent. Additionally, the Spirocare unit is more expensive than other IS, is not disposable, and requires an electrical power source (Van de Water, 1980).

Vraciu and Vraciu (1977) studied the effects of physical therapist-assisted breathing exercises that included lateral and posterior basal expansion, diaphragmatic breathing, and coughing on 40 patients following open heart surgery. The patients who performed breathing exercises had statistically fewer pulmonary complications (3 of 19) than the controls (8 of 21), even though both groups received IS every 2 hr. The control patients were also turned hourly and assisted in deep breathing and coughing by the nursing staff. Pulmonary complications were defined by the presence of a temperature greater than 38.5°C, radiological evidence of atelectasis, and abnormal breath sounds.

In 1983, Dull and Dull compared the effects of early mobilization to deep breathing and IS in 49 patients after cardiopulmonary bypass surgery. Mobilization consisted of extremity exercises, coughing, and assistance with turning, sitting, or standing. Because IS could not be performed during mechanical ventilation, the patients began their assigned exercise regimen within 4 hr of extubation. The incidence of pulmonary complications was high in this study and was defined as a temperature increase of 4°F above baseline or 2–3°F increase in temperature along with rales, rhonchi, absent breath sounds, or purulent sputum. The authors conclude that neither IS nor deep breathing offers any therapeutic advantage over patient mobilzation in preventing pulmonary complications after cardiopulmonary bypass surgery.

Craven et al. (1974) compared the effects of chest physiotherapy (including postural drainage, percussion, breathing exercises, and assisted coughing) to IS in 70 patients after surgery. Increased pulmonary complications were found in both groups of patients having prior chronic respiratory disease, although patients receiving IS showed significantly fewer complications than those receiving chest physiotherapy. The authors concluded that though there is a need for chest physiotherapy in treating major pulmonary collapse, IS may be a more effective means of prophylaxis.

Work by other investigators (Vraciu and Vraciu, 1977; Lyager et al., 1979; Van de Water, 1980) appears to conflict with that of Craven et al. (1974). Lyager and associates studied the added effect of IS (every waking hour) on patients already receiving instruction by physical therapists. On the basis of random selection, 34 upper abdominal surgical patients were given physical therapist-assisted breathing exercises and coughing, and 49 received IS in addition to this treatment. Radiological and clinical findings (including coughing, expectoration, dyspnea, auscultation, temperature, and respiratory rate) and arterial blood gas analysis revealed no differences between the two groups. The incidence of pulmonary complications after surgery was also the same, even in the subgroup of patients who used their IS on the average of 10 times every hour. The results of this study suggest that no further benefit is gained by adding IS to aggressive pulmonary physiotherapy. Although the results are of doubtful clinical significance, Hedstrand and associates (1978) also found that physical therapist-encouraged techniques of deep breathing were superior to voluntary or device-assisted deep breathing in raising arterial oxygenation. A controlled study was undertaken to assess whether bedside coaching to breathe deeply was as effective as IS in preventing postoperative atelectasis (Van de Water, 1980). Encouragement by the nursing staff was superior to IS in returning pulmonary function to preoperative values. The authors conclude that frequent patient contact appears to be an important component. This human element opens up an area of subjective differences. The rapport between an individual therapist or nurse and patient may well make a difference in patient performance. Likewise, the emphasis placed by a therapist on a maneuver or treatment may also influence its effectiveness.

In 1986, Schwieger et al. performed a well-designed, controlled study on 40 patients to assess the effect of IS following cholecystectomy. IS use was supervised and consisted of a slow, deep inspiratory effort with a volume oriented device. IS was performed for 5 min, hourly, at least 12 times a day, for 3 days after operation. All patients were mobilized on the day of surgery. Subjective and objective clinical data (oxygenation, temperature, PFT, white blood cell count, chest x-ray, and auscultation) were evaluated to establish the incidence of pulmonary complications. There were no significant differences in any of the measured parameters between the two groups, although chest radiograph changes indicating lung pathology occurred in 40% of the IS patients compared with 30% of the controls. None of the study subjects was classified as high risk for developing postoperative respiratory problems. This study does not support the theory of some investigators who attribute the lack of benefit from IS in controlled studies to inadequate supervision, coaching, or patient use.

Although compelling support for prophylactic or paliative IS therapy is not available, few complications are associated with its use. Theoretical problems include hyperventilation and barotrauma (Shapiro et al.). Cost is also an issue, especially when more expensive or nondisposable types of IS are recommended. IS is reportedly used in 95% of the hospitals surveyed in the United States as a prophylactic maneuver to improve lung expansion and in the treatment of postoperative atelectasis (O'Donohue, 1985). This compares with a use of 44% in the United Kingdom (in high-risk, postoperative coronary artery bypass patients) (Jenkins and Soutar, 1986). Cost and questionable efficacy were the major reasons for the much lower use of IS in Great Britain. Even a relatively small cost becomes significant when multiplied by 95% of hospitalized patients receiving surgery in the United States. It is the authors conclusion that

after surgery, early mobilization and volitional deep breathing offer more cost-effective treatment than IS for the spontaneously breathing patient at risk for postoperative pulmonary complications.

Continuous Positive Airway Pressure and Positive Expiratory Pressure

Although originally used with neonates, face-mask CPAP is recommended by some as a means to reduce or reverse the incidence of postoperative respiratory complications in adults. The use of PEP, a modification of CPAP, has also been studied. In 1979, Anderes and coworkers evaluated the effect of CPAP and positive and expiratory pressure (PEEP) on 30 adults undergoing elective upper abdominal surgery. Half of the patients (Group A) were ventilated without PEEP during surgery, were extubated, and breathed spontaneously afterward. The others (Group B) received PEEP (10 cm H_2O) during anesthesia and CPAP (3 cm H_2O) while intubated for 3 hr before extubation. The author reported significant deterioration in PaO_2 and right to left shunt (Q_s/Q_T) and adverse radiological findings in Group A compared with Group B. These changes occurred over 3 days after surgery although PEEP was given only during, and CPAP was given once, only immediately after surgery. It is difficult to separate the effects of CPAP from PEEP in this study. Carlsson and associates (1981) studied 24 patients undergoing elective cholecystectomy. Face-mask CPAP (about 5–10 cm H_2O) was given to 13 patients for 4 hr after surgery; the other patients wore a face mask but did not receive CPAP. PEEP was not used. All subjects were evaluated during treatment and for 24 hr postoperatively. No significant difference between groups was found in chest x-ray findings or spirometry or blood gas measurements. The results of these two investigations are different although similar patients were studied. Information on other types of pulmonary therapy, including patient mobilization, was not addressed but may be responsible for the different findings.

Anderson et al. (1980) evaluated the effect of face-mask CPAP in reversing atelectasis in a variety of surgical patients during the first 24 hr after operation. Twelve subjects received conventional therapy (including posteral drainage, deep breathing, and suctioning three times a day) and 12 patients additionally received CPAP (at about 15 cm H_2O for 25–35 respirations, hourly while awake and twice at night). Treatment was considered successful if PaO_2 increased by 15% of predicted value or if chest x-ray findings improved by 50%. CPAP was found to significantly improve atelectasis resolution; augmented collateral ventilation was thought to be the mechanism responsible for the change. This is one of the few studies that used a modality to reverse, rather than prevent, chest pathology.

Two studies compared the effects of IS and CPAP in preventing postoperative pulmonary complications. In 65 adults undergoing elective upper abdominal surgery, Stock and associates (1985) evaluated the use of face-mask CPAP, IS, and coughing with deep breathing. All treatments were given for 15 min, every 3 hr while awake for 3 postoperative days. Very few differences were found between treatment groups; a more rapid increase in FRC occurred in patients who received CPAP, but x-ray changes and fever were not significantly different between groups. In 50 patients undergoing similar surgery, Ricksten et al. (1986) compared IS, CPAP (10–15 cm H_2O), and PEP (10–15 cm H_2O). Each treatment was applied for 30 breaths, every waking hour, for 3 days after operation. The authors reported that both CPAP and PEP were superior to IS with respect to improving gas exchange, preserving lung volumes, and resolving atelectasis after upper abdominal surgery. They advocate using the simple PEP mask since it was as effective and less complicated than face-mask CPAP.

Conflicting results are also found on the effect of PEP on patients with cystic fibrosis. Falk et al. (1984) reported that PEP increased skin oxygen tension and sputum production over that obtained from posteral drainage with percussion and vibration or forced expiratory technique (FET). No radiographic changes were observed in any study situations. Contrary findings are reported by Hofmeyr and co-workers (1986), who found that oxygen saturation was unchanged and that sputum clearance was less effective when PEP (12–17 cm H_2O) was incorporated in a regimen of breathing exercises, postural drainage, and FET.

Two studies have looked at whether intermittent PEP augments the effects of chest physiotherapy in the management of postoperative pulmonary complications. Campbell and associates (1986) randomly assigned 71 patients to receive chest physiotherapy (control) or chest physiotherapy plus PEP (study group) after abdominal surgery. Chest physiotherapy in both groups consisted of breathing exercises, huffing, and coughing, while sitting, every 2 hr. Postural drainage was used if indicated. The study group also received PEP for 10 breaths every 2 hr. Thirty-one percent of the control patients developed respiratory complications compared to 22% of the study patients. This difference corresponded to the larger number of smokers in the control group. The effect of PEP in addition to chest physiotherapy was studied in 56 patients after thoracotomy (Frolund and Madsen, 1986). Chest physiotherapy was given two times a day and consisted of early mobilization, arm exercises, deep breathing, and coughing. Patients were encouraged to use face-mask PEP (about 10 cm H_2O) at least 10 min each waking hour and were supervised in its use two times a day. All patients were evaluated for 3 days after surgery. The authors conclude that PEP offered no benefit over conventional physiotherapy in preventing atelectasis or improving arterial oxygenation.

Although research on the effects of postoperative PEP or CPAP is conflicting, complications are not associated with its use. The added expense of this modality is a concern, but research on the cost of PEP or CPAP is scarce. In the treatment of postoperative atelectasis, CPAP is reportedly used in 25% of hospitals in the United States and use is dramatically greater in hospitals with more than 200 beds (O'Donohue, 1985).

Summary

Few conclusions can be drawn from all the research on the mechanical aids to lung expansion discussed in this section. Differing durations and frequencies are recommended for the same device, and few authors compared similar techniques, other than contrasting IPPB to IS. It is no surprise that the results are so inconsistent. Only the finding that IPPB is more costly and less effective than the other methods mentioned appears with regularity. The benefit (or lack of it) obtained from using blow bottles is no more substantiated than the outdated method of having a patient inflate a rubber surgical glove (Hughes). Similarly, there is no supporting evidence that blow bottles decrease the incidence of pulmonary complications following surgery (Pontoppidan). Though forced expiration against resistance is encouraged by those recommending and ordering blow bottles (or inflatable surgical gloves), forced expiration alone is reported to produce atelectasis and hypoxemia (Nunn et al., 1965). Pontoppidan notes that improper use of blow bottles may decrease both end-expiratory volume (if the patient exhales too forcefully) and cardiac output due to the increased airway pressure.

While in agreement with Kasik and Schilling (1981) that little is gained by replacing IPPB with yet another form of therapy (such as IS, CPAP, PEP, or chest physiotherapy techniques) that is still under investigation, the ethical issue of withholding a treatment that has been shown to be beneficial by some, cannot be ignored. Methods that encourage maximal inspiration, such as IS and deep breathing, may, in theory, be more beneficial than blow bottles. However, the available research has not proved IS superior in terms of cost and effectiveness to deep breathing and the other aspects of chest physiotherapy. The principle that CPAP improves collateral ventilation and therefore lung reexpansion is exciting. However, studies on the efficacy of CPAP or PEP to reduce postoperative pulmonary complications are conflicting. These modalities appear to be of little added benefit to a regimen of chest physiotherapy including patient mobilization. It is important to note that CPAP, PEP, IS, blow bottles, and IPPB are of limited value in the ICU, since they cannot be used on patients requiring mechanical ventilation. Chest physiotherapy does not have this limitation.

Despite the huge cost and widespread use of mechanical aids following surgery, the incidence of respiratory complications has not significantly changed with any single or combination of treatments. It appears that the type of patient who could *perhaps* benefit from IS, CPAP, or PEP still needs to be defined. Alternately, it may mean that none of the described modalities represents an optimal method of preventing pulmonary complications. Ford and Guenter (1984) suggest research into specific diaphragm function during the early postoperative phase (see p. 15).

BRONCHOSCOPY

Bronchoscopy is used both therapeutically and diagnostically. The indications for therapeutic bronchoscopy include aspiration, secretion retention, atelectasis, lung contusion, and lung abscess (Wanner et al., 1973; Lindholm et al., 1974; Sackner, 1975; de Kock, 1977; Barrett, 1978; Dreisin et al., 1978). Bronchoscopy is often used as an adjunct to chest physiotherapy. However, since chest physiotherapy was introduced to our facility in mid-1973, the need for therapeutic bronchoscopy has diminished markedly (Table 1.2). Complications, restrictions, and precautions of therapeutic bronchoscopy are discussed and compared to chest physiotherapy.

Complications and Precautions

Suratt and co-workers (1976) reported a 0.022% death rate and a 2.92% incidence of serious-to-life-threatening complications associated with fiberoptic bronchoscopy. In reviewing 24,521 fiberoptic bronchoscopic procedures, Credle et al. (1973) reported a low incidence of major complications (<1%) and a mortality of 0.01%. In prospective studies, Dreisin et al. and Pereira et al. (1978)

found the overall complication rate to be 11% and 8%, repectively (Table 9.2). None of the authors reported the mortality or morbidity resulting solely from use of fiberoptic bronchoscopy in the treatment of retained secretions, and a wide spectrum of patients ranging from those in the ICU to the office outpatient were included in these studies. Pneumonia, bronchospasm and laryngospasm, pneumothorax, hypoxemia, hemodynamic changes, cardiac dysrhythmia, respiratory arrest, and hemorrhage of sufficient quantity to compromise the airway are among the serious complications associated with bronchoscopy (Credle et al.; Dubrawsky et al., 1973; Harrell et al., 1973; Britton and Nelson, 1974; Albertini et al., 1974; Karetzky et al., 1974; Salisbury et al., 1975; Feldman and Huber, 1976; Sahn and Scoggin, 1976; Suratt et

al.; de Kock; Dreisin et al.; Periera et al., 1978; Shrader and Lakshminarayan, 1978; Lundgren et al., 1982).

In addition to pneumonia, febrile reactions and bacteremia are noted following both rigid and fiberoptic bronchoscopy (Burman, 1960; Pereira et al., 1974, 1978; Timms and Harrell, 1975; Dreisin et al.). Patients over 60 years of age or those with a history of cardiovascular disease or immunoincompetence appear to be at increased risk of developing these complications. In patients with bronchial asthma, life-threatening laryngospasm and bronchospasm from fiberoptic bronchoscopy are reported despite prior premedication, application of topical anesthetics, and supplemental oxygen delivery (Sahn and Scoggin; Dreisin et al.; Pereira et al., 1978). As a result, fiberoptic bronchoscopy should be performed with

Table 9.2
Reported Complications Within 24 hr of Fiberoptic Bronchoscopy (Prospective Studies)[a]

Complications	Dreisin et al. (205 Procedures)	Pereira et al. (908 Procedures)
Major		
Pneumonia	—[b]	5
Bronchospasm/laryngospasm or airway obstruction	4(1[c])	4
Pneumothorax requiring chest tube	2	4
Hemoptysis (40 ml in 15 min or 200 ml in 24 hr)	4	—
Respiratory arrest	—	2(1[c])
Total	10	15
Minor		
Vasovagal reactions	—	22
Fever	—	11
Cardiac dysrhythmias	[d]	8[e]
Bleeding (nosebleed)	(2)	6
Obstruction of airways	—	4
Infiltrates without fever	4	—
Nausea and vomiting	—	2
Pneumothorax	—	2
Dyspnea	2	—
Subcutaneous emphysema	2	—
Electrocardiogram abnormality	[d]	2[e]
Acute maxillary sinusitis	1	—
Psychotic/hysterical reaction	1	1
Aphonia	—	1
Total	12	59

[a]Adapted from Dreisin et al. (1978) and Pereira et al. (1978).
[b]—Information not given.
[c]Denotes mortality.
[d]Apparently not routinely monitored.
[e]Only 24% of all patients received cardiac monitoring.

great caution and only when absolute indications are present in this patient population.

Hypoxemia and Cardiac Dysrhythmia

Decreases in arterial oxygenation resulting from fiberoptic bronchoscopy are due to the combined effects of (1) mechanical obstruction of the airways, (2) alveolar filling with lavage or anesthetic solutions, and (3) the effects of suctioning (Khan, 1978). Changes in PaO_2 are noted by many authors, as shown in Table 9.3. Hypoxemia is reported not only during bronchoscopy itself but also following the procedure (Harrell et al., Albertini et al.; Lundgren et al.). Harrell and co-workers found that the magnitude of the fall in PaO_2 was related to the duration of the bronchoscopic examination. However, Albertini and associates found no correlation between decreases in PaO_2 and either the duration of the procedure or the amount of anesthetic or lavage fluid left in the lungs. Lundgren et al. found the greatest fall in PaO_2 occurred during the suctioning phase of bronchoscopy and continued for up to 15 min after the procedure was completed.

The cardiac dysrhythmias reported during and following bronchoscopy may be related to hypoxemia. Shrader and Lakshminarayan studied 70 patients undergoing fiberoptic bronchoscopy; all patients were spontaneously breathing, receiving supplemental oxygen, and predisposed to cardiac dysrhythmias due to chronic cardiac or pulmonary pathology. Arterial blood gases and cardiac rhythm were monitored for an hour preceding, during, and after bronchoscopy. Thirty-nine patients demonstrated dysrhythmias during the control period. Forty-nine patients had dysrhythmias during bronchoscopy; of these, 8 (11%) were considered major or having the potential to cause hemodynamic compromise. Hypoxemia (mean PaO_2, 53 mm Hg) following bronchoscopy was seen in 12 patients and correlated significantly with the development of dysrhythmias. Khan (1978) suggested that patients with poor oxygenation initially, further aggravated by bronchoscopy, may demonstrate enhanced myocardial sensitivity to circulating catecholamines. Although sinus tachycardia is observed during bronchoscopy, it is of doubtful clinical significance (Lindholm et al.; Credle et al.; Khan, 1978; Luck et al., 1978). Cardiac dysrhythmias, including bradycardia, ventricular ectopic beats, ventricular tachycardia and "cardiac arrest," are reported to occur during and following bronchoscopy (Credle et al.; Suratt et al.). The low incidence of cardiac dysrhythmias shown in Table 9.2 is probably a result of the limited number of patients that were monitored with electrocardiography.

Pereira et al. (1978) and Zavala (1978) maintain that the incidence of cardiac complications associated with bronchoscopy cannot be predicted by evidence of prior heart disease alone. However, if cardiac compromise is the result of hypoxemia, complications may be minimized by either increasing the fractional inspired oxygen, flow rate or tidal volume (in mechanically ventilated patients) (Dubrawsky et al.; Albertini et al.; Pierson et al., 1974; Karetzky et al., 1974; Perry, 1978; Shrader and Lakshminarayan). Lundgren et al. suggest that reflex sympathetic discharge from mechanical stimulation may be a major cause of the hemodynamic changes that occur during bronchoscopy. In addition, patients having low lung compliance or high intrapulmonary shunt may require mechanical ventilation and PEEP to prevent hypoxemia. Since sudden and prolonged decreases in PEEP or inspired volume may occur with bronchoscopy, attempts to minimize these effects are necessary. In our experience, a disposable adaptor (by Portex) appears to be an effective means of reducing both PEEP and volume loss. Care should be taken to ensure that ventilator volume delivery exceeds the volume evacuated while suctioning during bronchoscopy.

Lavage

Because the outer diameter of fiberoptic bronchoscopes is small, the suction port is correspondingly diminished or absent (Table 9.4). Khan et al. (1976) and Sanderson and McDougall (1978) note dif-

Table 9.3
Reported Changes in Arterial Blood Gases from Fiberoptic Bronchoscopy[a]

Author	Number and Type of Patient (A and B Denote Subgroups)	Reported Changes (Before to After, Unless Stated)	Comments
Dubrawsky et al. (1973)	49, SB A. 30, room air B. 19, supplemental O_2	$PaCO_2$ and pH unchanged A. $PaO_2 \downarrow$ 22.4 mm Hg ($p < 0.0005$) after insertion $PaO_2 \downarrow$ 18.8 mm Hg ($p < 0.0005$) after lavage and suctioning B. PaO_2 unchanged	60 to 80 ml of lavage used Bronchial lavage results in hypoxemia Initially hypoxemic and normal patients showed similar $PaO_2 \downarrow$ after procedure
Harrell et al. (1973)	15, SB	$PaO_2 \downarrow$ >10 mm Hg (in 2 patients) $PaCO_2 \uparrow \geq 5$ mm Hg	Degree of hypoxemia did not correlate with extent of lavage or preprocedural PaO_2 levels Degree of hypoxemia did relate to procedure time and amount of suctioning $\uparrow PaCO_2$ was related to bronchospasm
Kleinholz et al. (1973)	10, SB	6 patients, $PaO_2 \downarrow \geq 9$ mm Hg; 3 patients, PaO_2 unchanged; 1 patient, $PaO_2 \uparrow$ from hyperventilation	No supplemental O_2 given
Albertini et al. (1974)	18, SB A. 16, SB B. 15, SB ($FIO_2 = 1.0$)	A. $PaO_2 \downarrow$ 20 mm Hg (range, 4–38) B. $A\text{-}aDO_2 \uparrow$ 56 mm Hg (range, 2–188)	$\downarrow PaO_2$ did not correlate with amount of anesthetic or lavage material used or duration of treatment PaO_2 remained $\downarrow$ from <1 hr to >4 hr; most returned to values obtained before procedure by 2 hr
Karetzky et al. (1974)	14, SB	$PaO_2 \downarrow$ 12 mm Hg during (range, −2−−21) $PaO_2 \downarrow$ 5 mm Hg after (range, +3−−19)	
Pierson et al. (1974)	10 MV	$PaO_2 \uparrow$ 10 mm Hg during (range, +100−−132) $PaCO_2 \uparrow$ 5.2 mm Hg during (range, −4−+14) pH $\downarrow$ 0.06 during $PaO_2 \uparrow$ 14.3 mm Hg after (range, +75−−39)	All patients had retained secretions or atelectasis $FIO_2 \uparrow$ to 1.0, 20 min prior to procedure in most instances

Reference	Sample	Results	Comments
Salisbury et al. (1975)	23, SB A. 10 controls, SB B. 18 COPD, SB	A. $PaO_2 \downarrow 12 \pm 3$ mm Hg; B. $PaO_2 \downarrow 10 \pm 3$ mm Hg; $PaCO_2$ and pH unchanged	3 controls had $PaO_2 \downarrow >15$ mm Hg 2 patients had $PaO_2 \downarrow >22$ mm Hg PaO_2 did not $\downarrow$ significantly with $\uparrow$ treatment time (average, 25 min) PaO_2 returned to initial level 15–30 min after procedure No patients had significant amounts of secretions
Brach et al. (1976)	16, SB A. 6 with $\downarrow \uparrow \dot{V}/Q$ mismatch B. 10 with $\uparrow$ or no change in $\dot{V}/Q$ mismatch	$PaCO_2$ unchanged A. $PaO_2 \uparrow 7.0 \pm 8.4$ mm Hg (SD); $A\text{-}aDO_2 \downarrow 7.7 \pm 2.4$ mm Hg (SD) B. $PaO_2 \downarrow 6.8 \pm 5.4$ mm Hg (SD); $A\text{-}aDO_2 \uparrow 7.7 \pm 5.5$ mm Hg (SD)	Mucus plugs or thick secretions noted in 4 of 6 patients in A No excessive secretions noted in B One patient receiving 250 ml of lavage showed $\uparrow \dot{V}/Q$ mismatch and $\uparrow$ A-aDO_2.
de Kock (1977)	9	$PaO_2 \downarrow 12.4$ mm Hg (range, $+3--23$)	Supplemental O_2 given during procedure
Shrader and Lakshminarayan (1978)	70, SB	$PaO_2 \downarrow 30$ mm Hg (range, $+9--78$)	Supplemental O_2 given during procedure Duration of procedure averaged 30 min
Marini et al. (1979)	16, SB and MV	$A\text{-}aDO_2 \uparrow 8.4\%$	
Lundgren et al. (1982)	10, SB with pulmonary fibrosis	MAP $\uparrow$ during and for 7 min after ($p < 0.05$) HR $\uparrow$ during and for 15 min after ($p < 0.05$) MPAOP $\uparrow$ during insertion, suctioning, and after ($p < 0.05$) CI $\uparrow$ during and for 7 min after ($p < 0.05$) $PaO_2 \downarrow$ during suctioning and for 15 min after ($p < 0.05$) 3 patients showed ST-T segment depression ($p < 0.05$) $PaCO_2$ unchanged	50 ml of warmed lavage was used Laryngeal and bronchial stimulation responsible for most hemodynamic changes

[a] SB, spontaneously breathing; MV, mechanically ventilated; FIO_2, fractional inspired oxygen; A-aDO_2, alveolar-arterial oxygen difference; $\dot{V}/Q$, ventilation/perfusion ratio; MAP, mean arterial pressure; HR, heart rate; MPAOP, mean pulmonary arteriolar occlusion pressure; CI, cardiac index; $\uparrow$, increase; $\downarrow$, decrease.

Table 9.4
Diameters of Fiberoptic Bronchoscopes

Model	Outside Diameter (mm)	Suction Channel Diameter (mm)
Olympus BF-B	6.0[a]	2.0[a]
Olympus BF-3A	3.0[a]	None[a]
Olympus BF-4B	4.0[a]	0.8[a]
Olympus BF-5B	5.0[b]	1.5[b],1.4[a]
Olympus BF-FB2	5.2[c]	2.0[c]
Olympus BF-5B2	5.8[b],6.0[a]	2.0[b],1.9[a]
Olympus BF-3C4	35[d]	1.2[d]
Manchida FBS-4	4.0[a]	0.8[a]
Manchida FBS-5	5.0[a]	1.4[a]
Manchida FBS-6	6.0[a]	2.2[a]
Manchida FBS-6T	5.8[b]	2.2[b]
Manchida FBS-6TL	5.8[b]	2.6[b]
Manchida FBS-6TL-W	5.8[b]	2.6[b]

[a]Adapted from Sackner (1975).
[b]Adapted from Barrett (1974).
[c]Adapted from Feldman and Huber (1976).
[d]Adapted from Nussbaum (1982).

ficulty in removing bloody or excessive secretions through the small suction channel, thus lengthy periods of suctioning may be necessary. Feldman and Huber report plugging of the suction channel with thick secretions. Therefore, some authors recommend using the rigid, rather than fiberoptic, bronchoscope when copious or viscous secretions are present (Ayella, 1978; Landa, 1978). Others advocate using lavage in conjunction with fiberoptic bronchoscopy to assist the removal of tenacious secretions. Aliquots of 5–20 ml, totaling up to 200 ml of lavage, are suggested in the literature (Sackner et al., 1972; Wanner et al.; Milledge, 1976; de Kock; Barrett; Mahajan et al., 1978; Marini et al., 1979; Lundgren et al.). However, Sackner et al. and Wanner et al. report deterioration in chest x-ray appearance when large quantities of lavage are used. It appears that limiting both the quantity of lavage and the duration of suctioning may decrease the hazards associated with fiberoptic bronchoscopy.

Restrictions

The use of fiberoptic bronchoscopy is restricted in certain patients requiring artificial airways. Nasotracheal intubation, which may be used because of oral lacerations, oral fractures, or out of preference, can restrict tracheal tube size. As a result, the ability to pass a bronchoscope may also be limited (Sackner, 1975). Perry states that tracheal tubes at least 8.5 mm in internal diameter (ID) are necessary to allow adequate gas exchange around a fiberoptic bronchoscope. Other researchers conclude that bronchoscopy should be cautiously performed through a cuffed airway of no less than 8 mm (ID); smaller tracheal tubes may compromise air flow and reduce tidal volume even during mechanical ventilation (Rauscher, 1972; Grossman and Jacobi, 1974; Pierson et al.; Baier et al., 1976; Feldman and Huber; Barrett). Baier and co-workers report increased airway pressures (up to 70 cm H_2O), a 50% reduction in flow rate, and an 20% decrease in delivered tidal volume when a fiberoptic bronchoscope is introduced through a 7.5-mm (ID) tracheal tube. Similarly, critical increases in air flow resistance are noted when larger caliber bronchoscopes are used (Fig. 9.1).

Despite some favorable reports (Nussbaum, 1982) fiberoptic bronchoscopy is generally of limited use in the pediatric patient (Sackner, 1975; Berci, 1978; Wood and Fink, 1978). The decreased airway diameters of children necessitate the use of smaller caliber bronchoscopes. These lack or have limited suction ports that are not effective in removing retained secretions (Table 9.4) (Sackner, 1975; Wood and Fink). In order to avoid further

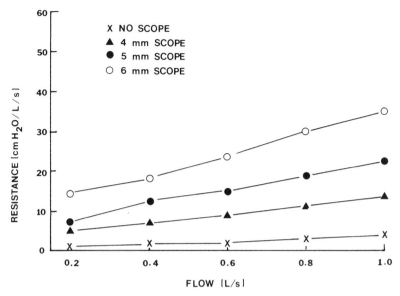

Figure 9.1. Resistance to air flow through 8.5-mm-ID endotracheal tube with fiberoptic broncho-scope inserted. Adapted from L. B. Perry (1978).

trauma or infection, nonintubated patients with nasal or facial fractures or a CSF leak should not receive transnasal bronchoscopy. Attempts at oral fiberoptic bronchoscopy may prove to be very expensive if the patient bites the bronchoscope.

Comparison with Chest Physiotherapy

The literature comparing the advantages and effectiveness of bronchoscopy to chest physiotherapy for acute secretion retention is limited. Mackenzie et al. (1978) reported that a single chest physiotherapy treatment resulted in clinical and radiological improvement in 68% of the 47 patients studied. The 27 patients having unilobar densities demonstrated a 74% improvement. These findings are similar to those of Lindholm et al. who reported a 67% (17 of 70) improvement in chest x-rays after fiberoptic bronchoscopy in patients previously unresponsive to routine respiratory therapy.

In 51 patients with a variety of diagnoses, therapeutic bronchoscopy (rigid or fiberoptic) was 47–85% successful in clearing atelectasis, depending on the location of the pathology (Perruchoud et al., 1980). Thirty-one of the patients were receiving mechanical ventilation. Nine additional patients received intubation

and were ventilated during this study. Because the atelectasis reexpansion rate was lower and the relapse rate higher in patients with segmental rather than lobar atelectasis, the authors reported that peripheral secretions could not be removed as effectively as those that were more centrally located. Harada and associates (1983) reported successful bronchoscopic clearing in 14 or 15 patients with atelectasis and a recurrence rate of 43%. Neither paper reported trying chest physiotherapy prior to bronchoscopy. Because of the recurrence rate in both studies and the reduced efficacy when segmental atelectasis was present, chest physiotherapy appears to have advantages over bronchoscopy. It is cheaper, easily repeated, associated with fewer complications, and may be better able to clear peripheral secretions (Marini et al., 1984; Mackenzie and Shin, 1986).

Marini et al. (1979) compared the effectiveness of fiberoptic bronchoscopy and chest physiotherapy in 31 patients with acute lobar atelectasis. The bronchoscopy procedure included cannulation of every segmental and most subsegmental bronchi, accompanied by suction and saline lavage. Chest physiotherapy (performed every 4 hr) consisted of IS for 3 min (or multiple 1–2 liter inflations if the patient was intubated), coughing and tracheal suctioning, nebulized isoetharine, and postural drainage with chest percussion to each involved area for 5 min. Chest x-rays were compared immediately following and 24 and 48 hr after these procedures. All patients who did not demonstrate at least 50% improvement immediately following chest physiotherapy underwent bronchoscopy. It was concluded that in acute atelectasis, no demonstrable benefit was obtained by using routine bronchoscopy in addition to chest physiotherapy. In fact, improvement following fiberoptic bronchoscopy was nearly identical to that demonstrated following a single treatment with chest physiotherapy.

Jaworski et al. (1988) evaluated the effect of fiberoptic bronchoscopy in 20 patients after lobectomy. All subjects received chest physiotherapy while 10 also underwent postoperative bronchoscopy. The incidence of atelectasis was similar for both groups. Of the 5 patients who developed atelectasis, 60% responded favorably to chest physiotherapy alone; 2 patients underwent bronchoscopy, which was palliative in 1 case. The authors conclude that routine postlobectomy bronchoscopy offers no advantage over usual physiotherapy in preventing postoperative atelectasis.

Marini and associates (1984) believe that there are few appropriate indications for therapeutic bronchoscopy. Whenever possible, they recommend chest physiotherapy. Only when an important diagnostic question coexists or when a massive collapse is unresponsive (within 24 hr) to respiratory therapy and the patient remains intolerably symptomatic is fiberoptic bronchoscopy considered. They regard the presence of an air bronchogram as a contraindication to bronchoscopy. This approach avoids the expense, discomfort, and potential complications of an unnecessary bronchoscopy. Similarly, O'Donnell (1975) states that bronchoscopy should not be used as a substitute for chest physiotherapy in treating secretion retention; rather, it should be reserved for cases with persistent radiological findings. The authors support these statements and consider chest physiotherapy the treatment of choice in clearing retained secretions at our facility. Bronchoscopy is performed only when improvement is not noted following physiotherapy (usually 1–3 treatments). Depending on the preference of the physician, either rigid or fiberoptic bronchoscopy is utilized. Over a 6–7 year period after the introduction of chest physiotherapy in 1973, fewer than 20 patients/year required therapeutic bronchoscopy (Table 1.2). Between 1973 and 1987, 7,123 patients were treated with chest physiotherapy (see Appendix AI.1). In 1979, 18 therapeutic bronchoscopies were performed on 14 patients; only three procedures resulted in radiological evidence of improvement. Although earlier bronchoscopy may have been more successful, it appears that little benefit is gained by performing bronchoscopy in addition to aggressive chest physiotherapy. It is the authors' experience that chest physiotherapy is frequently more effective than therapeutic bronchoscopy in the ICU. The following two case histories demonstrate that chest physiotherapy improved oxygenation and radiological appearance of the chest when bronchoscopy was unsuccessful.

Case History 9.1. During a motor vehicle accident a 36-year-old white male was thrown through the windshield and sustained multiple severe facial lacerations. No loss of consciousness was reported prior to admission to the trauma center. After admission, the patient became bradycardic, hypotensive, and his level of consciousness deteriorated. The patient was intubated, ventilated, and resuscitated with fluids. Admitting chest x-ray showed no cardiac, lung, pleural, or skeletal pathology. Two hours after admission, repeat chest x-ray demonstrated a right upper lobe atelectasis (Fig. 9.2A). A bronchoscopy was performed and thick mucus was suctioned from the right upper lobe bronchus. Repeat chest x-ray showed worsening of the right upper lobe atelectasis (Fig. 9.2B). A second bronchoscopy was performed, after which a repeat chest x-ray showed complete atelectasis of the right upper lobe (Fig. 9.2C). Three hours after the second bronchoscopy a 60-min chest physiotherapy treatment was given to the area of lung pathology. Treatment consisted of segmental postural drainage to the anterior, apical, and posterior segments of the right upper lobe, manual percussion, and suctioning. Copious secretions were suctioned from the endotracheal tube. Repeat chest x-ray demonstrated considerable improvement of the right upper lobe atelectasis (Fig. 9.2D). Chest physiother-

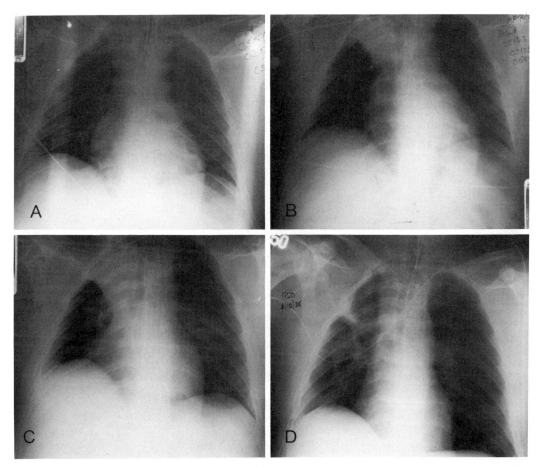

Figure 9.2. (**A**) A chest x-ray taken 2 hr after admission shows a right upper lobe atelectasis. The tracheal tube is correctly positioned. (**B**) The right upper lobe atelectasis persists following the first bronchoscopy. (**C**) After a second bronchoscopy, the right upper lobe atelectasis is still evident on chest x-ray. (**D**) Improved aeration is evident in the right upper lobe after chest physiotherapy

apy cleared an atelectasis that did not respond favorably to bronchoscopy and significantly improved oxygenation (Table 9.5). The FIO_2 was decreased from 1.0 to 0.6 after this treatment and the patient was extubated 12 hr later. Total hospital stay was 3 days.

This case study demonstrates that chest physiotherapy treatment improved oxygenation and removed retained secretions from airways that were inaccessible to the bronchoscope. Bronchoscopy, which requires physician and nurse participation, failed to produce beneficial effects.

Case History 9.2. A 37-year-old white male was transferred to the trauma center from an-

Table 9.5
Arterial Blood Gases

	03:35	BR[a]	0:530	0:655	BR	10:00	13:00	CPT[a]	14:45	15:45
					Intervention Time					
FIO_2	1.00		1.00	1.00		1.00	1.00		1.00	0.6
PEEP	8		8	10		10	10		10	12
PaO_2	340		155	125		156	192		409	117
pH	7.38		7.33	7.25		7.36	7.39		7.35	7.40
$PaCO_2$	28		35	47		40	37		42	40

[a]BR, bronchoscopy; CPT, chest physiotherapy.

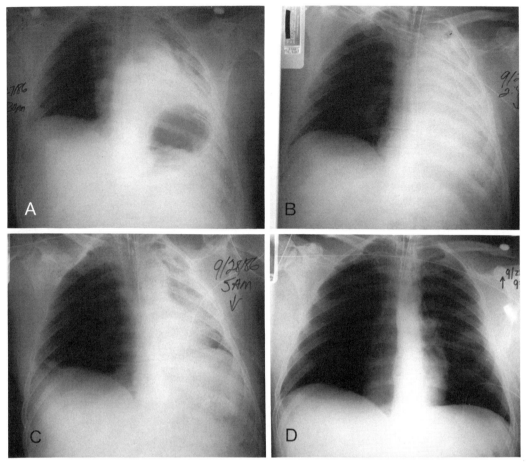

Figure 9.3. (**A**) A left lower lobe atelectasis is shown. (**B**) After bronchoscopy the left lung appears atelectatic and subsegmental atelectasis is present in the right lower lobe. (**C**) After chest physiotherapy by a nurse there is some improved aeration in the left lung. (**D**) Complete reexpansion of both lungs occurs after treatment by a physical therapist.

other medical institution after a fall from a three-story building the previous day. Admitting diagnoses included a left pelvic fracture, left hemothorax, and fractured left eighth and ninth ribs. The patient underwent an exploratory laporotomy for a suspected diaphragm rupture and a splenic tear. The patient was intubated and mechanically ventilated due to deteriorating arterial blood gases and a left lower lobe atelectasis (Fig. 9.3A). Bronchoscopy was performed after which a repeat chest x-ray revealed complete opacification of the left hemithorax with mediastinal shift to the left and minimal subsegmental atelectasis in the right lung base (Fig. 9.3B.) After two chest physiotherapy treatments by the nursing staff, the left lung was partially reaerated but the subsegmental atelectasis in the right lung base was unchanged (Fig. 9.3C). Arterial blood gases improved after the first nursing treatment (Table 9.6). Three hours after the second nursing treatment a physical therapist gave an inten-

sive chest physiotherapy treatment consisting of postural drainage, manual percussion, and vibration to the left lower lobe, followed by tracheal suction. Copious yellow secretions were obtained and arterial oxygenation markedly improved (Table 9.6). Follow-up chest x-ray showed clearing of the left lower lobe and right lower lobe atelectasis (Fig. 9.3D). The FIO_2 was reduced from 0.8 to 0.5 10 hr later. The patient was extubated in 5 days and discharged 13 days after admission.

Chest physiotherapy treatment performed by both the nursing and physical therapy staff was more effective than bronchoscopy in treating a left lung atelectasis. The treatment by the physical therapist resulted in a longer lasting and greater improvement in PaO_2, oxygen saturation, and chest x-ray than that by the nurse. This may be related to the

Table 9.6
Arterial Blood Gases and Nursing Treatment

Time	0105	a	0315	NCPT[b]	0415	NCPT	0530	0705	0810	PT CPT	1020	2000
F102	100		100		100		60	80	80		80	50
PEEP	5		10		10		10	12	15		15	15
PaO2	168		95		158		53	56	65		267	173
pH	7.39		7.29		7.44		7.35	7.35	7.4		7.44	7.49
PaCO2	42		50		35		35	42	41		35	33
O$_2$ sat	99		96		99		85	87	92		99	99

[a]Bronchoscopy.
[b]NCPT, nursing chest physiotherapy; PT CPT, physical therapy chest physiotherapy.

longer treatment time and segmental postural drainage that is not routinely performed by the nursing staff.

Visualization of the respiratory tract is a frequently stated advantage of performing bronchoscopy rather than chest physiotherapy in the presence of retained secretions. Rigid bronchoscopy is reported to allow observation 0.5–1 cm distal to the lobar orifices (Sackner, 1975). Using fiberoptic bronchoscopy, Ikeda (1970) noted that visualization was limited to just beyond the segmental bifurcation. During diagnostic bronchoscopy (mean duration of 72 minutes), Kovnat and coworkers (1974) reported examining all fourth-order and most fifth- and sixth-order bronchi. However, the diameters of adult airways are relatively small, as shown in Table 9.7. Based on these findings, it is apparent that the majority of fiberoptic bronchoscopes in Table 9.4 are physically unable to enter the average adult segmental bronchus, even during three fourths maximal lung inflation. With current technology, visualizing the infant or small child's airway beyond the lobar bronchi is not practical. Bronchoscopy is often accompanied by bronchospasm, coughing, and reduced tidal volume delivery. These result in greater airway narrowing, making bronchial cannulation even more difficult. Bronchoscopes of small caliber, allowing maximal visualization of the airways, have a reduced suction port size, that decreases their therapeutic value in removing retained secretions.

The added dimension of pulmonary visualization is sometimes considered of particular benefit in removing mucus plugs. Yet, the absence of secretions or mucus plugs within the range of the fiberoptic bronchoscope is reported despite radiological confirmation of collapse (Wanner et al.; Bowen et al., 1974; Lindholm et al.; Brach et al., 1976; de Kock; Marini et al., 1979). When mucus plugs are present, large amounts of lavage are often needed to loosen and break up the obstruction so it can be aspirated through the small suction port. Lindholm and co-workers found no bronchoscopic evidence of mucus plugs or bronchial obstruction in 18 (26%) patients demonstrating x-ray evidence of atelectasis. This suggests that the pulmonary collapse was not a result of more central obstruction or plugging; rather, more peripheral secretions were probably present, beyond the field of the fiberoptic bronchoscope. Mucus plugs are frequently the result of inadequate airway humidification. In our clinical experience, mucus plugging and tenatious secretions can be minimized or eliminated by providing patients with optimal sys-

Table 9.7
Average Adult Airway Diameters at Three-Fourths Maximal Inflation

Anatomical Description	Generation	Diameter (mm)[a]
Trachea	0	18
Main stem bronchus	1	12.2
Lobar bronchus	2	8.3
Segmental bronchus	3	5.6
First subsegmental bronchus	4	4.5
Second subsegmental bronchus	5	3.5

[a]Adapted from Wiebel (1963).

temic hydration and supplemental inhaled humidity.

When air bronchograms accompany pulmonary collapse, neither fiberoptic bronchoscopy nor chest physiotherapy is reported of benefit (Marini et al., 1979 and 1984). It is not surprising that bronchoscopy is ineffective because air bronchograms (extending more peripherally) represent patent larger airways surrounded by areas of atelectasis. The short duration of physiotherapy treatment described by Marini and associates may account for their lack of benefit from this therapy when air bronchograms are present. It is our experience that longer treatment times are necessary to clear more peripheral, as opposed to central, secretions.

Chest physiotherapy has certain advantages over therapeutic bronchoscopy. Chest physiotherapy does not require physician participation or the purchase and maintenance of expensive equipment. It is less costly for the patient and can be easily repeated, if necessary. Bronchoscopy is more invasive, and multiple treatments can cause airway trauma. Physiotherapy treatments are not limited by tracheal tube size, and usually no additional sedation is needed (beyond that normally used to provide relief for discomfort following surgery).

Summary

The reported side effects of bronchoscopy outlined in Table 9.2 appear to be more severe than those experienced with chest physiotherapy. The patient with preexisting hypoxemia, low lung compliance, or high intrapulmonary shunt, requiring mechanical ventilation and PEEP (≥ 15 cm H_2O), is a particularly poor candidate for bronchoscopy (Mackenzie and Shin, 1986). Yet, this same patient can frequently tolerate chest physiotherapy without cardiorespiratory disturbance. In our experience, and that of others (Marini et al., 1979, 1984; Jaworski et al.; M. A. Branthwaite, personal communication), bronchoscopy offers no therapeutic advantage over chest physiotherapy in the management of acute secretion retention.

References

Albertini, RE, Harrell JH, Kurihara N, Moser KM: Arterial hypoxemia induced by fiberoptic bronchoscopy. JAMA 230:1666–1667, 1974

Alder RA: A rebreather for prophylaxis and treatment of postoperative respiratory complications. Dis Chest 52:640–647, 1967

Alexander GD, Schreiner RJ, Smiler BJ, Brown EM: Maximal inspiratory volume and postoperative pulmonary complications. Surg Gynecol Obstet 152:601–603, 1981

Ali J, Serrette C, Wood LDH, Anthonisen NR: Effect of postoperative intermittent positive pressure breathing on lung function. Chest 85:192–196, 1984

American National Standards Institute (ANSI). American national standard for humidifiers and nebulizers for medical use. ANSI Z79.9, 1979

American Thoracic Society: Standards for the diagnosis and care of patients with chronic obstructive pulmonary disease (COPD) and asthma. Am Lung Assoc, 1987

Anderes C, Anderes U, Gasser D, Dittmann M, Turner J, Brennwald J, Keller R, Ferstl A, Wolff G: Postoperative spontaneous breathing with CPAP to normalize late postoperative oxygenation. Intensive Care Med 5:15–21, 1979

Andersen JB, Olesen KP, Eikard B, Jansen E, Qvist J: Periodic continuous positive airway pressure, CPAP, by mask in the treatment of atelectasis. Eur J Respir Dis 61:20–25, 1980

Andersen JB, Qvist J, Kann T: Recruiting collapsed lung through collateral channels with positive end expiratory pressure. Scand J Respir Dis 60:260–266, 1979

Anderson WH, Dossett BE, Hamilton GL: Prevention of postoperative pulmonary complications. JAMA 186:763–766, 1963

Asmundsson T, Kilburn KH: Mucociliary clearance rates at various levels in dog lungs. Am Rev Respir Dis 102:388–397, 1970

Aubier M: Effect of theophylline on diaphragmatic muscle function. Chest 92:27S–31S, 1987

Ayella RJ: Radiologic Management of the Massively Traumatized Patient, p 114. Williams & Wilkins, Baltimore, 1978

Ayres SM, Kozam RL, Lukas DS: The effects of intermittent positive pressure breathing on the intrathoracic pressure, pulmonary mechanics, and work of breathing. Am Rev Respir Dis 87:370–379, 1963

Bader ME, Bader RA: Intermittent positive pressure breathing. Adv Cardiopul Dis 4:271–284, 1969

Baier H, Begin R, Sackner MA: Effect of airway diameter, suction catheters, and bronchofiberscope on airflow in endotracheal and tracheostomy tubes. Heart Lung 5:235–238, 1976

Baker JP: Magnitude of usage of intermittent positive pressure breathing. Am Rev Respir Dis 110:170–178, 1974

Barrett CR: Flexible fiberoptic bronchoscopy in the critically ill patient. Chest [Suppl] 73:746–749, 1978

Baxter WD, Levine RS: An evaluation of intermittent positive pressure breathing in the prevention of postoperative pulmonary complications. Arch Surg 98:795–798, 1969

Becker A, Barak S, Braun E, Meyers MP: The treatment of postoperative pulmonary atelectasis with intermittent positive pressure breathing. Surg Gynecol Obstet 111:517–522, 1960

Berci G: Flexible fiber and rigid (pediatric) bronchoscopic instrumentation and documentation. Chest [Suppl] 73:768–775, 1978

Berman LS, Heard SO, Banner MJ: Humidification techniques for high frequency jet ventilation (abstract). Crit Care Med 12:284, 1984

Bernstein IL, Ausdenmoore RW: Iatrogenic bronchospasm occurring during clinical trials of a new mucolytic agent, acetylcysteine. Dis Chest 46:469–473, 1964

Bierman CW: Pneumomediastinum and pneumothorax complicating asthma in children. Am J Dis Child 114:42–50, 1967

Bosomworth PP, Spencer FC: Prolonged mechanical ventilation. I. Factors affecting delivered oxygen concentrations and relative humidity. Am Surg 31:377–381, 1965

Bowen TE, Fishback ME, Green DC: Treatment of refractory atelectasis. Ann Thorac Surg 18:584–589, 1974

Brach BB, Escano GG, Harrell JH, Moser KM: Ventilation-perfusion alterations induced by fiberoptic bronchoscopy. Chest 69:335–337, 1976

Brain J: Aerosol and humidity therapy. Am Rev Respir Dis 122(2):17–21, 1980

Brain JD: Aerosol and humidity therapy. In Current Advances in Respiratory Care, edited by WJ O'Donohue, Chap 5, pp 72–85. American College Chest Physicians, Park Ridge IL, 1984

Brain JD, Valberg PA: State of the art, deposition of aerosol in the respiratory tract. Am Rev Respir Dis 120:1325–1373, 1979

Branson RD, Ploysongsang Y, Hurst J, Rushkin MC: Flow resistance characteristics of commonly used hygroscopic condensers humidifiers (abstract). Crit Care Med 14:368, 1986

Braun SR, Smith FR, McCarthy TM, Minsloff M: Evaluating the changing role of respiratory therapy services at two hospitals. JAMA 245:2033–2037, 1981

Britton RM, Nelson KG: Improper oxygenation during bronchofiberoscopy. Anesthesiology 40:87–89, 1974

Browner B, Powers SR: Effect of IPPB on functional residual capacity and blood gases in postoperative patients. Surg Forum 26:96–98, 1975

Burman SO: Bronchoscopy and bacteremia. J Thorac Cardiovasc Surg 40:635–639, 1960

Bynum LJ, Wilson JE, Pierce AK: Comparison of spontaneous and positive-pressure breathing in supine normal subjects. J Appl Physiol 41:341–347, 1976

Campbell T, Ferguson N, McKinlay RGC: The use of a simple self-administered method of positive expiratory pressure (PEP) in chest physiotherapy after abdominal surgery. Physiother 72:498–500, 1986

Carlsson C, Sonden B, Thylen U: Can postoperative continuous positive airway pressure (CPAP) prevent pulmonary complications after abdominal surgery? Intensive Care Med 7:225–229, 1981

Celli BR, Rodriguez KS, Snider GL: A controlled trial of intermittent positive pressure breathing, incentive spirometry, and deep breathing exercises in preventing pulmonary complications after abdominal surgery. Am Rev Respir Dis 130:12–15, 1984

Chamney AR: Humidification requirements and techniques: Including a review of the performance of equipment in current use. Anaesthesia 24:602–617, 1969

Chang N, Levison H: The effect of a nebulized bronchodilator administered with or without intermittent positive pressure breathing on ventilatory function in children with cystic fibrosis and asthma. Am Rev Respir Dis 106:867–872, 1972

Cheney FW: Editorial expression. Chest 62:664, 1972

Cheney FW, Butler J: The effect of ultrasonically-produced aerosols on airway resistance in man. Anesthesiology 29:1099–1106, 1968

Cherniack RM: Intermittent positive pressure breathing in management of chronic obstructive pulmonary disease: Current state of the art. Am Rev Respir Dis 110:188–192, 1974

Cherniack RM, Svanhill E: Long-term use of intermittent positive-pressure breathing (IPPB) in chronic obstructive pulmonary disease. Am Rev Respir Dis 113:721–728, 1976

Cohen IL, Weinberg PF, Fein A, Rowinski GS: Endotracheal tube occlusion associated with the use of heat and moisture exchangers in the intensive care unit. Crit Care Med 16:277–279, 1988

Colgan FJ, Mahoney PD, Fanning GL: Resistance breathing (blow bottles) and sustained hyperinflations in the treatment of atelectasis. Anesthesiology 32:543–550, 1970

Cottrell JE, Siker ES: Preoperative intermittent positive pressure breathing therapy in patients with chronic obstructive lung disease: Effects on postoperative pulmonary complications. Anesth Analg (Cleve) 52:258–262, 1973

Craven JL, Evans GA, Davenport PJ, Williams HP: The evaluation of the incentive spirometer in the management of postoperative pulmonary complications. Br J Surg 61:793–797, 1974

Craven DE, Goularte, TA, Make BJ: Contaminated condensate in mechanical ventilation circuits. Am Rev Respir Dis 129:625–628, 1984

Credle WF, Smiddy JF, Elliott RC: Complications of fiberoptic bronchoscopy (abstract). Am Rev Respir Dis 107:1091, 1973

Cullen JH, Brum VC, Reidt WU: An evaluation of the ability of intermittent positive pressure breathing to produce effective hyperventilation in severe pulmonary emphysema. Am Rev Tuberc Pulm Dis 76:33–46, 1957

Dalhamn T: Mucous flow and ciliary activity in the trachea of healthy rats, and rats exposed to respiratory irritant gases. Acta Physiol Scand [Suppl 123] 36:1–161, 1956

Daly WJ, Ross JC, and Behnke RH: The effect of changes in pulmonary vascular bed produced by atropine, pulmonary engorgement and positive pressure breathing on diffusion and mechanical properties of the lung. J Clin Invest 42:1083–1094, 1963

Darin J, Broadwell J, MacDonell R: An evaluation of water-vapor output from four brands of unheated, prefilled bubble humidifiers. Respir Care 27:41–50, 1982 de Kock MA: *Dynamic Bronchoscopy*, pp 32–34. Springer-Verlag, New York, 1977

DeTroyer A, Deisser P: The effects of intermittent positive pressure breathing on patients with respiratory muscle weakness. *Am Rev Respir Dis* 124:132–137, 1981

Dohi S, Gold MI: Comparison of two methods of postoperative respiratory care. *Chest* 73:592–595, 1978

Downie PA (ed): *Cash's Textbook of Chest, Heart and Vascular Disorders for Physiotherapists*, pp 87–93. JB Lippincott, Philadelphia, 1979.

Doyle HJ, Napolitano AE, Lippman HR, Cooper KR, Duncan JS, Eakins K, Glauser FL: Different humidification systems for high-frequency jet ventilation. *Crit Care Med* 12:815–819, 1984

Dreisin RB, Albert RK, Talley PA, Kryger MH, Scoggin CH, Zwillich CW: Flexible fiberoptic bronchoscopy in the teaching hospital, yield and complications. *Chest* 74:144–149, 1978

Dubrawsky C, Awe RJ, Jenkins DE: Effect of fiberoptic bronchoscopy on oxygenation of arterial blood (abstract). *Chest* 64:393, 1973

Dull JL, Dull WL: Are maximal inspiratory breathing exercises or incentive spirometry better than early mobilization after cardiopulmonary bypass? *Phy Ther* 63:655–659, 1983

Edmondson EB, Reinarz JA, Pierce AK, Sanford JP: Nebulization equipment: A potential source of infection in gram-negative pneumonias. *Am J Dis Child* 111:357–360, 1966

Egan DF: Humidity and water aerosol therapy. *Conn Med* 31:353–355, 1967

Emergency Care Research Institute. Heat and moisture exchangers. *Health Devices* 12:155–167, 1983

Emmanuel GE, Smith WM, Briscoe WA: The effect of intermittent positive pressure breathing and voluntary hyperventilation upon the distribution of ventilation and pulmonary blood flow to the lung in chronic obstructive lung disease. *J Clin Invest* 45:1221–1233, 1966

Falk M, Kelstrup M, Andersen JB, Kinoshita T, Falk P, Stovring S, Gothgen I: Improving the ketchup bottle method with positive expiratory pressure, PEP, in cystic fibrosis. *Eur J Respir Dis* 65:423–432, 1984

Featherby EA, Weng TR, Levison H: The effect of isoproterenol on airway obstruction in cystic fibrosis. *Can Med Assoc J* 102:835–838, 1970

Feldman NT, Huber GL: Fiberoptic bronchoscopy in the intensive care unit. *Int Anesthesiol Clin* 14:31–42, 1976

Forbes AR: Humidification and mucus flow in the intubated trachea. *Br J Anaesth* 45:874–878, 1973

Ford GT, Guenter CA: Toward prevention of postoperative pulmonary complications. *Am Rev Respir Dis* 130:4–5, 1984

Fouts JB, Brashear RE: Intermittent positive-pressure breathing, a critical appraisal. *Postgrad Med* 59:103–107, 1976

Froeb HF: On relief of bronchospasm and the induction of alveolar ventilation: A comparative study of nebulized bronchodilators by deep breathing and intermittent positive pressure. *Dis Chest* 38:483–489, 1960

Frolund L, Madsen F: Self-administered prophylactic postoperative positive expiratory pressure in thoracic surgery. *Acta Anaesthesiol Scand* 30:381–385, 1986

Gale GD, Sanders DE: Incentive spirometry: Its value after cardiac surgery. *Can Anaesth Soc J* 27:475–480, 1980

Gedeon A, Mebius C, Palmer K: Neonatal hygroscopic condenser humidifier. *Crit Care Med* 15:51–54, 1987

George RB, O'Donohue WJ: Guidelines for the use of intermittent positive pressure breathing (IPPB). *Respir Care* 25:365–370, 1980

Glover WJ: Mechanical ventilation in respiratory insufficiency in infants. *Proc R Soc Med* 58:902–904, 1965

Gold MI: The present status of IPPB therapy. *Chest* 67:469–471, 1975

Gold MI: Is intermittent positive-pressure breathing therapy (IPPB RX) necessary in the surgical patient? (editorial) *Ann Surg* 184:122–123, 1976

Gold MI: IPPB therapy, a current overview. *Respir Care* 27:586–587, 1982

Goldberg I, Cherniak RM: The effect of nebulized bronchodilator delivered with and without IPPB on ventilatory function in chronic obstructive emphysema. *Am Rev Respir Dis* 91:13–20, 1965

Golden GT, Chandler JG: Colonic ileus nad cecal perforation in patients requiring mechanical ventilatory support. *Chest* 68:661–664, 1975

Graff TD, Benson DW: Systemic and pulmonary changes with inhaled humid atmospheres: Clinical application. *Anesthesiology* 30:199–207, 1969

Grossman E, Jacobi AM: Minimal optimal endotracheal tube size for fiberoptic bronchoscopy. *Anesth Analg (Cleve)* 53:475–476, 1974

Harada K, Mutsuda T, Saoyama N, Taniki T, Kimura H: Re-expansion of refractory atelectasis using a bronchofiberscope with a balloon cuff. *Chest* 84:725–728, 1983

Harrell JH, Albertini RE, Kurihara N, Moser KM: Gas exchange abnormalities induced during fiberoptic bronchoscopy (abstract). *Am Rev Respir Dis* 107:1019, 1973

Harris RL, Riley HD: Reactions to aerosol medication in infants and children. *JAMA* 201:953–955, 1967

Hay R, Miller WC: Efficacy of a new hygroscopic condenser humidifier. *Crit Care Med* 16:277–279, 1982

Hayes B, Robinson, JS: An assessment of methods of humidification of inspired gas. *Br J Anaesth* 42:94–104, 1970

Hedstrand U, Liw M, Rooth G, Ogren CH: Effect of respiratory physiotherapy on arterial oxygen tension. *Acta Anaesthesiol Scand* 22:349–352, 1978

Heisterberg L, Staehr Johansen T, Werner Larsen H, Holm M, Anderson B: Postoperative pulmonary complications in upper abdominal surgery. *Acta Chir Scand* 145:505–507, 1979

Hilding AC: Ciliary streaming in the lower respiratory tract. *Am J Physiol* 191:404–410, 1957

Hirsh JA, Tokayer JL, Robinson MJ, Sackner MA: Effects of dry air and subsequent humidification on tracheal mucous velocity in dogs. *J Appl Physiol* 39:242–246, 1975

Hofmeyr JL, Webber BA, Hodson ME: Evaluation of positive expiratory pressure as an adjunct to chest physiotherapy in the treatment of cystic fibrosis. *Thorax* 41:951–954, 1986

Huber GL, Finley TN: Effect of isotonic saline on alveolar architecture (abstract). *Anesthesiology* 26:252–253, 1965

Hughes RL: Do no harm—cheaply (editorial). Chest 77:582–584, 1980

Ikeda S: Flexible bronchofiberscope. Ann Otol Rhinol Laryngol 79:916–923, 1970

Indihar FJ, Forsberg DP, Adams AB: A prospective comparison of these procedures used in attempts to prevent postoperative pulmonary complications. Respir Care 27:564–568, 1982

Intermittent Positive Pressure Breathing Trial Group: Intermittent positive pressure breathing therapy of chronic pulmonary disease. Ann Intern Med 99:612–620, 1983

Iverson LI, Ecker RR, Fox HE, May IA: A comparative study of IPPB, the incentive spirometer, and blowbottles: The prevention of atelectasis following cardiac surgery. Ann Thorac Surg 25:197–200, 1978

Jaworski A, Goldberg SK, Walkenstein MD, Wilson B, Lippmann ML: Utility of immediate postlobectomy fiberoptic bronchoscopy in preventing atelectasis. Chest 94:38–43, 1988

Jenkins SC, Soutar SA: A survey into the use of incentive spirometry following coronary artery bypass graft surgery. Physiotherapy 72:492–493, 1986

Jenne JW: Theophylline as a bronchodilator in COPD and its combination with inhaled Beta-adrenergic drugs. Chest 92:75–145, 1987a

Jenne JW: Introduction. Chest 92:1S, 1987b

Jones FL: Increasing postoperative ventilation: A comparison of five methods. Anesthesiology 29:1212–1215, 1968

Jones JG, Clarke SW, Oliver DR: Two-phase gas-liquid flow in airways (abstract). Br J Anaesth 41:192–193, 1969

Jones RH, MacNamara J, Gaensler EA: The effects of intermittent positive pressure breathing in simulated pulmonary obstruction. Am Rev Respir Dis 82:164–185, 1960

Jorgensen JR, Falliers CJ, Bukantz SC: Pneumothorax and mediastinal and subcutaneous emphysema in children with bronchial asthma. Pediatrics 31:824–832, 1963

Jung R, Wight J, Nusser R, Rosott L: Comparison of three methods of respiratory care following upper abdominal surgery. Chest 78:31–35, 1980

Kahn RC: Humidification of the airways. Adequate for function and integrity (editorial)? Chest 84:510–511, 1983

Kamat SR, Dulfano MJ, Segal MS: The effects of intermittent positive pressure breathing (IPPB/I) with compressed air in patients with severe chronic nonspecific obstructive pulmonary disease. Am Rev Respir Dis 86:360–380, 1962

Karetzky MS, Garvey JW, Brandstetter RD: Effect of fiberoptic bronchoscopy or arterial oxygen tension. NY State J Med 1:62–63, 1974

Karetzky MS, Asthma mortality associated with pneumothorax and intermittent positive-pressure breathing. Lancet 1:828–829, 1975

Kasik JE, Schilling JP: Good news! Bad news? The status of respiratory therapy in the 1980s (editorial) JAMA 245:2059, 1981

Khan MA: Fiberoptic bronchoscopy revisited (editorial). Chest 74:119–120, 1978

Khan MA, Whitcomb ME, Snider GL: Flexible fiberoptic bronchoscopy. Am J Med 61:151–155, 1976

Kilburn KH: Mucociliary clearance from bullfrog (Rana cantesbiana) lung J Appl Physiol 23:804–810, 1967

Kittredge P: IPPB—the pressure is building (editorial). Respir Care 18:644–648, 1973

Klain M, Nordin U, Keszler H: Musociliary transport with and without humidification in high frequency ventilation (abstract). Anesthesiology 57:86, 1982

Klein EF, Shah DA, Shah NJ, Modell JH, Desautels D: Performance characteristics of conventional and prototype humidifiers and nebulizers. Chest 64:690–696, 1973

Kleinholz EJ, Fussell J, McBrayer R: Arterial blood gas studies during fiberoptic bronchoscopy. Am Rev Respir Dis 108:1014, 1973

Kovnat DM, Rath GS, Anderson WM, Snider GL: Maximal extent of visualization of bronchial tree by flexible fiberoptic bronchoscopy. Am Rev Respir Dis 110:88–90, 1974

Krastins IRB, Corey ML, McLeod A, Edmonds J, Levison H, Moes F: An evaluation of incentive spirometry in the management of pulmonary complications after cardiac surgery in a pediatric population. Crit Care Med 10:525–528, 1982

Landa JF: Indications for bronchoscopy. Chest [Suppl] 73:686–690, 1978

Lederer DH, Van de Water JM, Indech RB: Which deep breathing device should the postoperative patient use? Chest 77:610–613, 1980

Leith DE: Review of comments concerning presentations and discussions of intermittent positive pressure breathing session. Am Rev Respir Dis 110:200–201, 1974

Lindholm C-E, Ollman B, Snyder J, Millen E, Grenvik A: Flexible fiberoptic bronchoscopy in critical care medicine—diagnosis, therapy and complications. Crit Care Med 2:250–261, 1974

Loren M, Chai H, Miklich D, Barwise G: Comparison between simple nebulization and intermittent positive-pressure in asthmatic children with severe bronchospasm. Chest 72:145–147, 1977

Luck JC, Messeder OH, Rubenstein MJ, Morrissey WL, Engel TR: Arrhythmias from fiberoptic bronchoscopy. Chest 74:139–143, 1978

Lundgren R, Haggmark S, Reiz S: Hemodynamic effects of flexible fiberoptic bronchoscopy performed under topical anesthesia. Chest 82:295–299, 1982

Lyager S, Wernberg M, Rajani N, Bøggild-Madsen B, Nielsen L, Nielsen HC, Andersen M, Møller J, Silberschmid M: Can postoperative pulmonary complications be improved by treatment with the Bartlett-Edwards incentive spirometer after upper abdominal surgery? Acta Anaesthesiol Scand 23:312–319, 1979

Mackenzie CF, Shin B, McAslan TC: Chest physiotherapy: The effect on arterial oxygenation. Anesth Analg (Cleve) 57:28–30, 1978

Mackenzie CF, Shin B: Chest physiotherapy vs. bronchoscopy (letter). Crit Care Med 14:79, 1986

MacIntyre NR, Anderson HR, Silver RM, Schuler FR, Coleman RE: Pulmonary function in mechanically-ventilated patients during 24-hour use of a hygroscopic condenser humidifier. Chest 84:560–564, 1983

Macklin MT, Macklin CC: Malignant interstitial emphysema of the lungs and mediastinum as an important occult complication in many respiratory diseases and other conditions: an interpretation of the clinical literature in light of laboratory experiment. *Medicine* 23:281–358, 1944

Mahajan VK, Catron PW, Huber GL: The value of fiberoptic bronchoscopy in the management of pulmonary collapse. *Chest* 73:817–820, 1978

Malik SK, Jenkins DE: Alterations in airway dynamics following inhalation of ultrasonic mist. *Chest* 62:660–664, 1972

Mapleson WW, Morgan JG, Hillard EK: Assessment of condenser-humidifiers with special reference to a multiple-gauze model. *Br Med J* 1:300–305, 1963

Marini JJ, Pierson DJ, Hudson LD: Acute lobar atelectasis: A prospective comparison of fiberoptic bronchoscopy and respiratory therapy. *Am Rev Respir Dir* 119:971–978, 1979

Marini JJ, Pierson DJ, Hudson LD: Comparison of fiberoptic bronchoscopy and respiratory therapy (letter). *Am Rev Respir Dis* 126:368, 1984

McConnell DH, Maloney JV, Buckberg GD: Postoperative intermittent positive pressure breathing treatments. *J Thorac Cardiovasc Surg* 68:944–952, 1974

McCool FD, Mayewski RF, Shayne DS, Gibson CJ, Griggs RC, Hyde RW: Intermittent positive pressure breathing in patients with respiratory muscle weakness. *Chest* 90:546–552, 1986

McGovern JP, Ozkaragoz K, Roett K, Haywood TJ, Hensel AE: Mediastinal and subcutaneous emphysema complicating atopic asthma in infants and children. *Pediatrics* 27:951–960, 1961

Mertz JJ, Scharer L, McClement JH: A hospital outbreak of *Klebsiella* pneumonia from inhalation therapy with contaminated aerosol solutions. *Am Rev Respir Dis* 95:454–460, 1967

Meyers JR, Lembeck L, O'Kane H, Baue AE: Changes in functional residual capacity of the lung after operation. *Arch Surg* 110:576–583, 1975

Milledge JS: Therapeutic fiberoptic bronchoscopy in intensive care. *Br Med J* 2:1427–1429, 1976

Modell JH, Giammona ST, Davis JH: Effect of chronic exposure to ultrasonic aerosols on the lung. *Anesthesiology* 28:680–688, 1967

Moffet HL, Allan D, Williams T: Survival and dissemination of bacteria in nebulizers and incubators. *Am J Dis Child* 114:13–20, 1967

Moore RB, Cotton EK, Pinney MA: The effect of intermittent positive pressure breathing on airway resistance in normal and asthmatic children. *J Allergy Clin Immunol* 49:137–141, 1972

Morris JF, Robertson WE, Glauser FL: Comparative study of two hand-held respirators. *JAMA* 211:802–806, 1970

Motley HL, Lang LP, Gordon B: Use of intermittent positive pressure breathing combined with nebulization in pulmonary disease. *Am J Med* 5:853–856, 1948

Murray JF: Review of the state of the art in intermittent positive pressure breathing therapy. *Am Rev Respir Dis* 110:193–199, 1974

Newhouse MT, Ruffin RE: Deposition and fate of aerosolized drugs. *Chest* 73:936–943, 1978

Noehren TH, Lasry JE, Legters LJ: Intermittent positive pressure breathing (IPPB) for the prevention and the management of postoperative pulmonary complications. *Surgery* 43:658–665, 1958

Nunn JF, Coleman AJ, Sachithanandan T, Bergman NA, Laws JW: Hypoxaemia and atelectasis produced by forced expiration. *Br J Anaesth* 37:3–11, 1965

Nussbaum E: Flexible fiberoptic bronchoscopy and laryngoscopy in children under 2 years of age. *Crit Care Med* 10:770–772, 1982

O'Connor MJ: Comparison of two methods of postoperative pulmonary care. *Surg Gynecol Obstet* 140:615–617, 1975

O'Donnell JE: Fiberoptic endoscopy of the respiratory tract in the intensive care ward. *Anaesth Intensive Care* 3:139–141, 1975

O'Donohue WJ: Maximum volume IPPB for the management of pulmonary atelectasis. *Chest* 76:683–687, 1979

O'Donohue WJ: IPPB past and present. *Respir Care* 27:588–590, 1982

O'Donohue WJ: National survey of the usage of lung expansion modalities for the prevention and treatment of postoperative atelectasis following abdominal and thoracic surgery. *Chest* 87:76–80, 1985

Ophoven JP, Mammel MC, Gordon MJ, Boros SJ: Tracheobronchial histopathology associated with high-frequency jet ventilation. *Crit Care Med* 12:829–832, 1984

Oulton JL, Hobbs GM, Hicken P: Incentive breathing devices and chest physiotherapy: A controlled trail. *Can J Surg* 24:638–640, 1981

Perch SA, Realey AM: Effectiveness of the Servo SH 150 "artificial nose" humidifier: a case report. *Respir Care* 29:1009–1012, 1984

Pereira W, Kovnat D, Iacovino J, Kahn M, Natsios G, Spivack M, Snider GL: Fever and pneumonia following fiberoptic bronchoscopy (abstract). *Am Rev Respir Dis* 109:692, 1974

Pereira W, Kovnat DM, Snider GL: A prospective study of the complications following flexible fiberoptic bronchoscopy. *Chest* 73:813–816, 1978

Perruchoud A, Ehrsam R, Heitz M, Kopp C, Tschan M, Herzog H: Atelectasis of the lung: Bronchoscopic lavage with acetylcysteine. Experience in 51 patients. *Eur J Respir Dis* 61(Suppl):163–168, 1980

Perry LB: Topical anesthesia for bronchoscopy. *Chest [Suppl]* 73:691–693, 1978

Petty TL: A critical look at IPPB (editorial). *Chest* 66:1–3, 1974

Petty TL, Guthrie A: The effects of augmented breathing maneuvers on ventilation in severe chronic airway obstruction. *Respir Care* 16:104–112, 1971

Pflug AE, Cheney FW, Butler J: The effects of an ultrasonic aerosol on pulmonary mechanics and arterial blood gases in patients with chronic bronchitis. *Am Rev Respir Dis* 101:710–714, 1970

Pierson DJ, Iseman MD, Sutton FD, Zwillich CW, Creagh CE: Arterial blood gas changes in fiberoptic bronchoscopy during mechanical ventilation. *Chest* 66:495–497, 1974

Pierson RN, Grieco MH: Isoproterenol aerosol in normal and asthmatic subjects. *Am Rev Respir Dis* 100:533–541, 1969

Ploysongsang Y, Branson R, Rashkin MC, Hurst JM: Pressure flow characteristics of commonly used heat-moisture exchangers. *Am Rev Respir Dis* 138:675–678, 1988

Pontoppidan H: Mechanical aids to lung expansion

in non-intubated surgical patients. *Am Rev Respir Dis* 122(2):109–119, 1980

Powner DJ, Sanders CS, Bailey BJ: Bacteriologic evaluation of the Servo 150 hygroscopic condenser-humidifier. *Crit Care Med* 14:135–137, 1986

Primiano FP, Moranz ME, Montague FW, Miller RB, Sachs DPL: Conditioning of inspired air by a hygroscopic condenser humidifier. *Crit Care Med* 12:675–678, 1984

Rao S, Wilson DB, Brooks RC, Sproule BJ: Acute effects of nebulization of N-acetylcysteine on pulmonary mechanics and gas exchange. *Am Rev Respir Dis* 102:17–22, 1970

Rashad K, Wilson K, Hurt HH, Graff TD, Benson DW: Effect of humidification of anesthetic gases on static compliance. *Anesth Analg (Cleve)* 46:127–132, 1967

Rauscher C: Respiratory failure. Direct visualization of the bronchial tree. *J Kans Med Soc* 73:481–482, 1972

Reinarz JA, Peirce AK, Mays BB, Sanford JP: The potential role of inhalation therapy equipment in nosocomial pulmonary infection. *J Clin Invest* 44:831–839, 1965

Ricksten SE, Bengtsson A, Soderberg C, Thorden M, Kvist H: Effects of periodic positive airway pressure by mask on postoperative pulmonary function. *Chest* 89:774–781, 1986

Riley RL: Effect of lung inflation upon the pulmonary vascular bed. In *Pulmonary Structure and Function (A Ciba Foundation Symposium)*, edited by AVS de Reuck and M O'Connor, pp 261–272. Little, Brown, Boston, 1962

Ringrose RE, McKown B, Felton FG, Barclay BO, Mushmore HG, Rhoades ER: A hospital outbreak of *Serratia marcescens* associated with ultrasonic nebulizers. *Ann Intern Med* 69:719–729, 1968

Robinson JS: Humidification. In *Scientific Foundations of Anaesthesia*, edited by C Scurr and S Feldman, pp 488–496. William Heinemann Medical Books, London, 1974

Ruben H, Knudsen EJ, Carugati G: Gastric insufflation as influenced by the pressure used during intermittent positive pressure ventilation. *Nord Med* 6:957–959, 1961

Sackner MA: State of the art—bronchofiberscopy. *Am Rev Respir Dis* 111:62–88, 1975

Sackner MA: Tracheobronchial toilet. Weekly update. *Pulm Med* 1–8, 1978

Sackner MA, Wanner A, Landa J: Applications of bronchofiberscopy. *Chest [Suppl]* 62:70–78, 1972

Sahn SA, Scoggin C: Fiberoptic bronchoscopy in bronchial asthma, a word of caution. *Chest* 69:39–42, 1976

Salisbury BG, Metzger LF, Altose MD, Stanley NN, Cherniack NS: Effect of fiberoptic bronchoscopy on respiratory performance in patients with chronic airways obstruction. *Thorax* 30:441–446, 1975

Sanders CV, Luby JP, Johanson WG, Barnett JA, Sanford JP: *Serratia marcescens* infections from inhalation therapy medications: Nosocomial outbreak. *Ann Intern Med* 73:15–21, 1970

Sanderson DR, McDougall JC: Transoral bronchofiberscopy. *Chest [Suppl]* 73:725–726, 1978

Sands JH, Cypert C, Armstrong R, Ching S, Trainer D, Quinn W, Stewart D: A controlled study using

routine intermittent positive-pressure breathing in the post-surgical patient. *Dis Chest* 40:128–133, 1961

Sara C: The management of patients with a tracheostomy. *Med J Aust* 1:99–103, 1965

Sara CA, Clifton BS: Techniques and mechanical aids for artificial respiration. *Med J Aust* 2:447–458, 1962

Sara C, Currie T: Humidification by nebulization. *Med J Aust* 1:174–179, 1965

Sawyer WD: Airborne infection. *Milit Med* 128:90–93, 1963

Scheffler RM, Delaney M: *Assessing Respiratory Therapy Modalities: Trends and Relative Costs in Washington DC*, Backround Paper #2, Case Studies of Medical Technology, Office of Technology Assessment of the US Congress. Government Printing Office, Washington DC, 1981

Schulze T, Edmondson EB, Pierce AK, Sanford JP: Studies of a new humidifying device as a potential source of bacterial aerosols. *Am Rev Respir Dis* 96:517–519, 1967

Schuppisser JP, Brandli O, Meili U: Postoperative intermittent positive pressure breathing versus physiotherapy. *Am J Surg* 140:682–686, 1980

Schwieger I, Gamulin Z, Forster A, Meyer P, Gemperle M, Suter PM: Absesnce of benefit of incentive spirometry in low-risk patients undergoing elective cholecystectomy. *Chest* 89:652–656, 1986

Shapiro BA, Peterson J, Cane RD: Complications of mechanical aids to intermittent lung inflation. *Respir Care* 27:467–470, 1982

Shim C, Bajwa S, Williams MH: The effect of inhalation therapy on ventilatory function and expectoration. *Chest* 73:798–801, 1978

Shrader DL, Lakshminarayan S: The effect of fiberoptic bronchoscopy on cardiac rhythm. *Chest* 73:821–824, 1978

Siemens-Elema: *Servo Humidifier 150 and 151 Operating Manual.* Siemens-Elema, Solna, Sweden, 1979

Sinha R, Bergofsky EH: Prolonged alteration of lung mechanics in kyphoscoliosis by positive pressure hyperinflation. *Am Rev Respir Dis* 106:47–57, 1972

Smeltzer TH, Barnett TB: Bronchodilator aerosol, comparison of administration methods. *JAMA* 223:884–889, 1973

Smith RM: Diagnosis and treatment: Nasotracheal intubation as a substitute for tracheostomy. *Pediatrics* 38:652–654, 1966

Stange K. Bygdeman S: Do moisture exchangers prevent patient contamination of ventilators? *Acta Anaesth Scand* 24:487–490, 1980

Stock MC, Downs JB, Gauer PK, Alster JM, Imrey PB: Prevention of postoperative pulmonary complications with CPAP, incentive spirometry, and conservative therapy. *Chest* 87:151–157, 1985

Sukumalchantra Y, Park SS, Williams MH: The effect of intermittent positive pressure breathing (IPPB) in acute ventilatory failure. *Am Rev Respir Dis* 92:885–893, 1965

Suratt PM, Smiddy JF, Gruber B: Deaths and complications associated with fiberoptic bronchoscopy. *Chest* 69:747–751, 1976

Swift DL: Aerosols and humidity therapy, generation and respiratory deposition of therapeutic aerosols. *Am Rev Respir Dis* 122(2):71–77, 1980

Sykes MK, McNicol MW, Campbell EJM: *Respiratory Failure*, pp 187–192. Blackwell Scientific Publications, London, 1976

Thomson ML, Pavia D, Jones CJ, McQuiston TAC: No demonstrable effect of S-carboxymethylcysteine on clearance of secretions from the human lung. *Thorax* 30:669–673, 1975

Thornton JA, Darke CS, Herbert P: Intermittent positive pressure breathing (IPPB) in chronic respiratory disease. *Anaesthesia* 29:44–49, 1974

Timms RM, Harrell JH: Bacteremia related to fiberoptic bronchoscopy. *Am Rev Respir Dis* 111:555–557, 1975

Toremalm NG: Air-flow patterns and ciliary activity in the trachea after tracheotomy. *Acta Otolaryngol* 53:442–454, 1961

Torres G, Lyons HA, Emerson P: The effects of intermittent positive pressure breathing on the intrapulmonary distribution of inspired air. *Am J Med* 29:946–954, 1960

Van de Water JM, Watring WG, Linton LA, Murphy M, Byron RL: Prevention of postoperative pulmonary complications. *Surg Gynecol Obstet* 135:229–233, 1972

Van de Water JM: Preoperative and postoperative techniques in the prevention of pulmonary complications. *Surg Clin N Am* 60:1339–1348, 1980

Vraciu JK, Vraciu RA: Effectiveness of breathing exercises in preventing pulmonary complications following open heart surgery. *Phys Ther* 57:1367–1371, 1977

Walley RV: Humidifier for use with tracheotomy and positive-pressure respiration. *Lancet* 1:781–783, 1956

Waltemath CL, Bergman NA: Increased respiratory resistance provoked by endotracheal administration of aerosols. *Am Rev Respir Dis* 108:520–528, 1973

Wanner A, Rao A: Clinical indications for and effect of bland, mucolytic, and antimicrobial aerosols. *Am Rev Respir Dis* 122(2):79–87, 1980

Wanner A, Landa JF, Neiman RE, Vevaina J, Delgado I: Bedside bronchofiberscopy for atelectasis and lung abscess. *JAMA* 224:1281–1283, 1973

Weeks DB: Evaluation of a disposable humidifier for use during anesthesia. *Anesthiology* 54:337–340, 1981

Weeks DB, Ramsey FM: Laboratory investigation of six artificial noses for use during endotracheal anesthesia. *Anesth Analg* 62:758–763, 1983

Weibel ER: *Morphometry of the Human Lung*, p 139. Academic Press, New York, 1963

Wells RE, Perera RD, Kinney JM: Humidification of oxygen during inhalation therapy. *N Engl J Med* 268:644–647, 1963

Winning TJ, Brock-Utne JG, Goodwin NM: A simple clinical method of quantitating the effects of chest physiotherapy in mechanically ventilated patients. *Anaesth Intensive Care* 3:237–238, 1975

Wohl MEB: Atelectasis. *Phys Ther* 48:472–477, 1968

Wood RE, Fink RJ: Complications of flexible fiberoptic bronchoscopes in infants and children. *Chest [Suppl]* 73:737–740, 1978

Wu N, Miller WF, Cade R, Richburg P: Intermittent positive pressure breathing in patients with chronic bronchopulmonary disease. *Am Rev Tuberc Pulm Dis* 71:693–703, 1955

Zavala DC: Complications following fiberoptic bronchoscopy (editorial). *Chest* 73:783–786, 1978

Zibrak JD, Rossetti P, Wood E: Effect of reductions in respiratory therapy on patient outcome. *N Engl J Med* 315:292–295, 1986

Ziment I: Why are they saying bad things about IPPB? *Respir Care* 18:677–689, 1973

Ziment I: Letter. *Respir Care* 19:586–587, 1974

Ziment I: Theophylline and mucociliary clearance. *Chest* 92:38S–43S, 1987

CHAPTER 10

Undesirable Effects, Precautions, and Contraindications of Chest Physiotherapy

Colin F. Mackenzie, M.B., Ch.B., F.F.A.R.C.S.

Undesirable Effects
Contraindications and Precautions
  Respiratory System
  Cardiovascular
  Central Nervous System
  Gastrointestinal
  Genitourinary
  Musculoskeletal System
  Hemopoietic System
  Burns and Skin Grafts or Flaps
  Pain

Any therapy is associated with disadvantages, side effects, and contraindications. This chapter attempts to cover the undesirable effects, precautions during administration, and contraindications of chest physiotherapy. During the years 1974–1987 chest physiotherapy was used at our institution to treat over 7,000 critically ill trauma patients who had multiple ailments besides trauma. The additional problems included sepsis, coagulopathy, chronic and acute respiratory failure, and neurological, renal, hepatic, and cardiac diseases. Some undesirable effects were seen, and many potential problems were considered during this 13-year experience. When standard therapy was not carried out, the compromises and alternatives that were used are described. This chapter is intended to illustrate the contraindications, precautions, and side effects that were routinely observed.

UNDESIRABLE EFFECTS

The undesirable effects that may potentially occur with chest physiotherapy for the critically ill patient are tabulated in Table 10.1. This table identifies the problem and when in the course of chest physiotherapy it may occur. Effects and appropriate remedies or alternatives to prevent recurrence are suggested.

CONTRAINDICATIONS AND PRECAUTIONS

In order to simplify reading, comprehension, and information retrieval, contraindications and precautions are covered in a systematic manner.

Table 10.1
Potential Undesirable Effects of Chest Physiotherapy (CPT) in the Critically Ill Patient

Problem	Effects	Treatment/Prevention
During Turning		
Displacement of intravenous or intraarterial lines, hemofiltration devices, or shunts	Exsanguination, air embolus Lack of venous access Trauma of reinsertion	Suture and tape lines and shunts Secure
Tracheal extubation	Hypoxia	Tape tracheal tube well, restrain patient if necessary
Tracheal trauma from tube movement	Tracheal stenosis after extubation	Move ventilator tubing with patient or disconnect during turning
Displacement of fractures or joint injury	Hematoma, malalignment, pain	Use mobile traction or an external fixator; turn patient with extremity in neutral alignment
Open abdominal wounds or dehiscence	Evisceration	Use abdominal binder, synthetic mesh; remove or treat source of infection; therapist should be aware of problem
Chest tube dislodgement	Pneumothorax, infection	Suture and tape tube adequately; position drainage bottle to prevent tension on chest tube
Cardiovascular and respiratory dysfunction	Dysrhythmia, dyspnea or hypoxia	Monitor carefully during and following turning; increase FIO_2, change ventilator settings, call a physician; return to supine if problem
Pain	Patient distress causes raised heart rate, blood and intracranial pressures	Use analgesics, barbiturates, lidocaine, regional block, extradural or intrathecal narcotics, inhaled N_2O, TENS, or patient controlled analgesia (PCA); careful handling of the patient; turn in stages
During Segmental Drainage		
Head-down position	In spontaneously breathing patient, this may cause respiratory distress if there is already compromised respiratory function, distended abdomen, or obesity	Assume head-down position gradually; if there is distress, reduce head-down tilt and notify physician
	In mechanically ventilated patient, tracheal tube may become kinked when the patient is turned or positioned prone; ventilator pressures may rise	Tracheal tube position to prevent kinking is shown in Figure 3.7; larger tracheal tube will reduce peak airway pressures, or the ventilator pressure limit may be set higher
	Cardiovascular disturbance including dysrhythmia, pulmonary edema and hypertension	Put flat or sit up; reevaluate after therapeutic intervention
	Elevation of intracranial pressure	Give barbiturate, short acting narcotic, or lidocaine intravenously, vent CSF through intraventricular catheter, give diuretics, and elevate the head on a pillow (in reference to the body)
	Loss of cervical spine traction	Secure feet to foot of turning frame

Table 10.1 *continued*
Potential Undesirable Effects of Chest Physiotherapy (CPT) in the Critically Ill Patient

Problem	Effects	Treatment/Prevention
Head-up position	Hypotension, shock, dysrhythmia	Place flat, give fluids to increase cardiac filling pressures, then intropic agents; slowly sit the patient up
	Respiratory function in the quadriplegic is best with a slight head-down tilt	Use abdominal binder if sitting up a quadriplegic because respiratory function is compromised
Side position	If patient is in a halo vest, this may dig into shoulder	Turn the patient more prone or place rolls under the vest
	With pelvic injury there may be displacement of bony fractures	Use pelvic external fixators; fracture brace provides stability and allows turning
	Fractured clavicle, scapula or humerus may be displaced, and a previously dislocated shoulder may be redislocated	More prone position may relieve pressure on fractured scapula, clavicle, or humerus; internal or external fixation or fracture brace on humerus may prevent displacement
	Rib fracture may puncture lung, causing pneumothorax	Chest monitoring is advisable; if pneumothorax develops a chest tube is required
	Pain when turning onto flail chest	Pain relieved with systemic local or inhaled analgesics or TENS
	Major plastic surgery or neurosurgery on the head and face may be traumatized	Protect all operative sites; place intravenous bag around craniotomy or operative site; protect eyes, especially in unconscious patients; monitor increasing facial edema following facial surgery frequently
	Secretions may pass into dependent lung	Treat dependent lung last
	In mechanically ventilated patients, side-lying with the affected lung uppermost increases leakage through bronchopleural fistula	Limit duration of position with bronchopleural fistula uppermost
Prone position	Airway obstruction; reduced respiratory excursion, occlusion of vascular lines, and disruption of monitoring devices; injury to eyes or operative site	Turn head to the side or position with a roll under forehead where possible; rolls under chest or across pelvis (roll may help chest excursion and allow function of vascular lines and monitoring devices); protect eyes and operative sites, especially in unconscious patients
During Chest Physiotherapy Percussion	Petechiae, pain and fractured rib displacement if incorrectly performed; pathological rib fractures may occur independent of chest percussion	Use systemic, local, or inhaled analgesics, regional, PCA, or TENS for pain

Table 10.1 *continued*
Potential Undesirable Effects of Chest Physiotherapy (CPT) in the Critically Ill Patient

Problem	Effects	Treatment/Prevention
Vibration	Pain, fractured ribs, and rib or thoracic spine fracture displacement; tracheal cuff pressure rises	The therapy should cease, and the therapist should receive instruction in correct procedure techniques; only trained therapists should treat critically ill patients; patient should be investigated for cause of rib fractures; avoid vibration over rib fractures and in patients with thoracic spine fractures
Bagging	Patient distress, pneumothorax, cardiac output changes; increased intracranial pressure	Sedate patient or omit procedure entirely; use chest tube for pneumothorax
Suctioning	May produce hypoxemia (see Chapter 5)	Give additional O_2; suction through a port adaptor; limit duration and choose appropriate suction catheter size
	Reduction in PEEP or CPAP[a]	Many devices advocated; port adaptors can minimize loss of PEEP; ventilator flow rates must exceed suctioning flow rates; high-frequency positive pressure ventilation may be the most effective prevention
Cough	May cause airway closure, dizziness and syncope if repetitive; raises airway, blood and intracranial pressure (see Chapter 5)	Usually considered an advantage in aiding the clearance of secretions but should be used discriminately; repetitive cough may be disadvantageous; forced expiratory technique is an alternative (see Chapter 3); if cough is undesirable, prevent with lidocaine, sedation, or muscle paralysis
Transbronchial aspiration of pus, blood, or secretions	Lung abscess may cause infection in opposite lung; pulmonary hemorrhage may occur with lung contusion, infection, or carcinoma of bronchus eroding into pulmonary vessels; secretions loosened with CPT may pass into anatomically opposite and dependent lung	Lung abscess rupture, fatal pulmonary hemorrhage, and transbronchial aspiration of secretions may occur independently of CPT; clinical examination showing deterioration of respiratory function and impairment of oxygenation (fall in SaO_2) should strongly suggest transbronchial aspiration; a chest x-ray and treatment to the newly affected areas of suspected aspiration should be carried out

[a]CPAP, continuous positive airway pressure.

Respiratory System

Hypoxemia

Chest physiotherapy may cause a fall in partial pressure of arterial oxygen (PaO_2) in neonates (Holloway et al., 1969; Fox et al., 1978), in mechanically ventilated patients with cardiovascular instability (Gormenzano and Branthwaite, 1972), and in acutely ill patients who do not produce much sputum (Connors et al., 1980). The use of higher inspired oxygen concentrations (FIO_2) may overcome these falls in arterial oxygenation (Kigin, 1981). Increased FIO_2 should be used, before and during chest physiotherapy, for patients in whom a drop in PaO_2 of 20 mm Hg or less would be considered hazardous. Monitoring of arterial saturation (SaO_2) by pulse oximetry enables rapid bedside indication of hypoxemia. When during chest physiotherapy, SaO_2 falls below 90% (equivalent to a PaO_2 of about 60 mm Hg) FIO_2 should be increased.

Chest physiotherapy is used to clear secretions from the airways of children with acute bronchiolitis. There is no clinical evidence of benefit (Webb et al., 1985). Furthermore there is an anecdotal report that babies with bronchiolitis may deteriorate rapidly during handling and vigorous chest physiotherapy. Tracheal intubation and mechanical ventilation may be required (Milner and Murray, 1989).

If a patient is hypoxemic ($PaO_2 < 60$ mm Hg), positive end-expiratory pressure (PEEP) may be used to improve intrapulmonary shunt. This may subsequently allow chest physiotherapy to be performed. There is a relative contraindication to chest physiotherapy for patients with persistent hypoxemia that occurs despite the use of high levels of PEEP and FIO_2. Restriction of chest physiotherapy in these circumstances should be considered in comparison to the advantages that may be gained if chest physiotherapy is able to reverse a process that standard therapy (i.e., PEEP) has failed to improve.

Removal of PEEP during suctioning may cause hypoxemia. Several techniques that maintain or increase inspired gas flow during passage of a suction catheter through a side arm adapter are available. In order for any of these techniques to minimize the loss of PEEP and not induce atelectasis, the ventilator flow rates must greatly exceed the vacuum produced by suctioning, because suction is applied in a closed system.

In the hypoxemic patient, suctioning must be limited in duration and performed by using an appropriately sized catheter, only when secretions are audible in the larger airways. Mechanical ventilatory support may be necessary before a hypoxemic spontaneously breathing patient can tolerate chest physiotherapy.

Blind nasotracheal suctioning is not advocated (see pp. 179–180) and may result in cardiac arrest (Fineberg et al., 1960). Suctioning may cause cardiac dysrhythmias, hypotension, and hypoxemia. Recent evidence identifies a significant fall in mixed venous O_2 saturation with suctioning. O_2 consumption increases while cardiac output rises or even falls with the suctioning procedure. Fall in cardiac output occurred when suctioning was not accompanied by coughing. The fall was thought to occur due to a decrease in intrathoracic pressure diminishing left ventricular preload (Walsh et al., 1989). If this is the mechanism then closed sheath suction catheters that prevent entrainment of air during suctioning may potentiate this effect.

The effects of ventilation/perfusion changes occurring with postural drainage may be reduced by shortening postural drainage time or by administration of supplemental oxygen. The prone position is associated with improved oxygenation (Douglas et al., 1977; Albert et al., 1987). When there is unilateral lung disease due to atelectasis or pneumonia, oxygenation is optimized when the patient is placed with the good lung dependent (Zack et al., 1974; Seaton, 1979; Remolina et al., 1981). However positioning the good lung down is likely to be less efficacious for other types of localized pulmonary disease such as bullae (Fishman, 1981). These techniques are used during treatment of the hypoxemic patient. Lastly, unless there is a specific indication other than prophylaxis and unless some sputum is produced, the patient should not receive any therapy.

Lung Contusion

If pulmonary contusion is the indication for chest physiotherapy, treatment should begin as soon as the patient is stabilized. In a 22-month period, 179 patients with rib fractures were treated with chest physiotherapy. One hundred and fifty of these patients (83.7%) had multiple rib fractures and, therefore, most probably had some degree of underlying lung contusion. Over a 7-year period 1,141 patients with chest injury received chest physiotherapy (see Appendix I). Chest physiotherapy was usually uneventful and appeared beneficial. In this patient population the advantages outweighed the problems.

The most frequent problem occurred in patients with copious bloody tracheal secretions and severe lung contusion who required multiple blood transfusions and developed a coagulopathy. It may be inadvisable in these patients to posturally drain the lung contusion until hemorrhage is reduced or the coagulopathy is controlled. If postural drainage is used, the anatomically dependent, noninjured lung may become filled with blood. Therefore, the "good lung," not the contused lung, should be treated, keeping the contused bleeding lung dependent with the patient supine or turned to the contused side. This may reduce the effectiveness of oxygenation of the good lung. In our experience nondependent placement of the good lung preserves gas exchange. If the good lung is placed down blood drains transbronchially and gas exchange is compromised in both lungs. A double-lumen tracheal tube with an endobronchial cuff may be helpful in these circumstances to prevent spillage and allow postural drainage. However, in our practice, this was only used for greater than 24 hr with independent lung ventilation. The potential complications of airway obstruction with dislodgment of the double-lumen tube and damage to the bronchi from the endobronchial cuff should be considered. The apparently "good lung" may also have suffered an injury similar to the contused lung; this "contre coup" effect may become apparently only later.

Pulmonary Hemorrhage

There are two case reports of fatal pulmonary hemorrhage associated with chest physiotherapy (Hammond and Martin, 1979; Rasanen et al., 1988) and a letter (Campbell, 1980) describing a fatal pulmonary hemorrhage temporally associated with chest physiotherapy. All three patients had carcinoma of the lung and had received radiation therapy. Whether chest physiotherapy was related to the hemoptysis is not certain, since hemoptysis as a cause of death with bronchial carcinoma and radiation is well documented. In none of the patients was chest vibration given and only one received chest percussion. All patients had hemoptysis independent of chest physiotherapy. It remains uncertain whether fatal pulmonary hemorrhage would have occurred irrespective of chest physiotherapy. In our opinion these reports do not justify withholding chest physiotherapy in all patients with hemoptysis.

Major Airway Rupture

Major airway rupture may occur due to blunt or penetrating trauma. This is considered by some following surgical repair to be a contraindication to suctioning, coughing or positive airway pressure. It is thought that these maneuvers may cause breakdown of the tracheobronchial anastomosis. In penetrating lung injury not associated with blunt chest trauma (Fig. 10.1A and B), early extubation, patient mobilization, breathing exercises, and assisted coughing are the rule. However, the patient who sustains a tracheobronchial tear as the result of a high-speed automobile accident may have an associated lung contusion and other extrathoracic injuries (Fig. 10.2A and B). Management of these injuries requires mechanical ventilation, PEEP, and vigorous chest physiotherapy. Chest physiotherapy, if indicated, should not be withheld because of the possibility of dehiscence of the anastomosis. Restriction of turning, coughing and suctioning, and

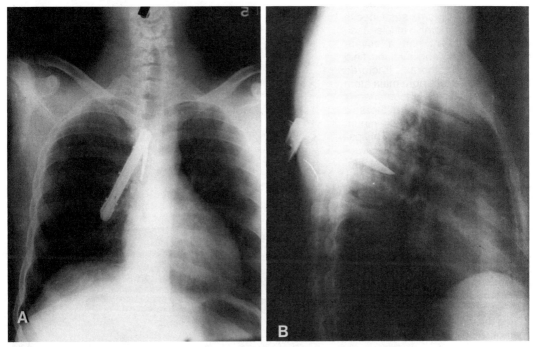

Figure 10.1. **(A)** Anteroposterior (AP) chest x-ray shows midline penetrating trauma. **(B)** Lateral chest x-ray shows extent of penetration into lung. This patient was extubated immediately after aortography and surgical removal of the knife. No vascular, neurological, or respiratory sequelae persisted, and the patient was discharged from the hospital 2 days after surgery.

early extubation in the patient with major blunt chest injury and a tracheobronchial tear increase the likelihood of anastomosis infection. Infection is the most common reason for dehiscence.

Pneumothorax and Hemothorax

Any maneuver, such as coughing, suctioning, or frequent turning, that could result in significant increases of airway pressure is a contraindication to chest physiotherapy for a mechanically ventilated patient with an unrelieved pneumothorax. Such patients should have a chest tube placed to prevent the development of a tension pneumothorax. If, however, the pneumothorax is loculated or minimal, conservative observation may be used instead of a chest tube. In this case, frequent clinical examination, observation of ventilator airway pressures, and monitoring with serial chest x-rays and pulse oximetry are indicated. If the pneumothorax remains stable on this regimen, chest physiotherapy is not contraindicated.

A hemopneumothorax or large fluid collection may make maneuvers such as percussion and vibration ineffective. Drainage of the fluid would seem worthwhile before percussion and vibration are attempted. However, following a single treatment with chest physiotherapy after reexpansion of an atelectasis, small effusions may reabsorb completely (Fig. 10.3A and B). Therefore, a treatment may be tried; if it is unsuccessful, the effusion should be tapped, and if this is bloody or recurrent, it should be drained. Hemothorax and pneumothorax may occur in association with other chest injuries. A common denominator may be a fractured rib that punctured the lung and caused the pneumothorax or that tore an intercostal or pulmonary vessel.

Flail Chest

Should physical maneuvers be performed on the patient with a flail chest? Displacement of fractured ribs occurs during inspiration, expiration, and turning. The rib displacement that occurs

Figure 10.2. (A) Admission supine portable AP chest x-ray after insertion of a right-sided chest tube for tension pneumothorax sustained in a high-speed motor vehicle accident. This patient had a severe right upper lung and midlung field contusion, hemothorax, fractured ribs 2–6, and a torn right main stem bronchus. Massive subcutaneous emphysema outlines the thoracic musculature and the mediastinum and ascends into the neck. This patient also had multiple facial fractures, dislocation of the right hip, and fractures of the left tibia and fibula and right ankle. He required mechanical ventilation for 5 days after repair of the torn bronchus. (B) Twelve days after injury the chest x-ray showed resolution. During this time the patient received chest physiotherapy. One therapeutic bronchoscopy was necessary to remove a blood clot after suctioning was restricted. Following this episode, standard chest physiotherapy techniques were reinstituted.

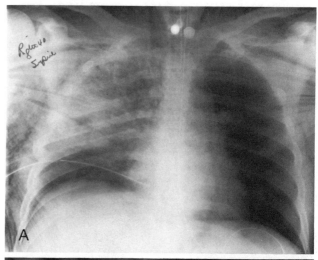

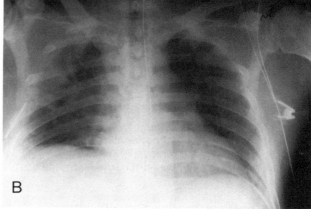

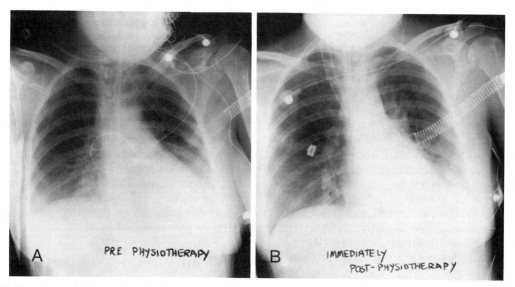

Figure 10.3. (A) AP erect portable chest x-ray shows atelectasis of the basal segments of the left lower lobe. There is loss of the left hemidiaphragm shadow and a pleural effusion at the left base. (B) After chest physiotherapy and reexpansion of all but the posterior basal segment atelectasis, the lateral two-thirds of the left hemidiaphragm and the left costophrenic angle become visible. The pleural effusion has reabsorbed.

during coughing, defecation, sitting up, and lying down may be considerably more than can be achieved with appropriate percussion and vibration. Controlled positive pressure mechanical ventilation was introduced for internal pneumatic stabilization of the flail chest (Avery et al., 1956). However, there are now many advocates of intermittent mandatory ventilation (IMV) who suggest that this is more physiological because of the substmospheric intrathoracic pressure associated with the spontaneous breath. Although the spontaneous breath may have advantages in aiding cardiac filling, for the patient with flail chest it results in considerable rib displacement (Shin et al., 1979a). This is impressively demonstrated in Figure 10.4A–C. Ventilation with pressure support is a means of preventing the subatmospheric intrathoracic pressures that caused such inward rib displacement as shown in Figure 10.4.

There are numerous other maneuvers that the patient carries out, or that are part of the daily routine of nursing procedure, that cause some, if not more, rib displacement than does chest physiotherapy. No one would dispute that the jagged edge of a fractured rib sticking into the lung is hazardous, but the additional hazard associated with correctly performed percussion is grossly overrated. When correctly performed by a trained therapist, percussion is not forceful, because of the air trapped in the cupped hand. However, novice therapists and nontherapists may perform percussion incorrectly; this should be avoided, especially in patients with flail chest. Therefore, percussion should be carried out by a trained therapist. When lung contusion accompanies flail chest, percussion may be most beneficial, since it is frequently the lung under the rib fractures that requires the therapy (Fig. 10.5A–C). Vibration is a more forceful maneuver; since the chest wall is manually compressed, it should not be performed over rib fractures. For the spontaneously breathing patient who has rib fractures with little underlying lung injury, pain relief and breathing exercises with supportive coughing and ambulation may be all that is required to main-

tain a clear chest. Does chest physiotherapy cause rib fractures? One report in a neonate with hyaline membrane disease suggests that percussion of the chest was a probable additive or singular cause of rib fractures (Purohit et al., 1975). However, rib fractures are known to occur with hyaline membrane disease independent of chest physiotherapy (Burnard et al., 1965). Pathological rib fractures in adults are associated with secondary carcinoma, myeloma, and chronic cough.

Chest Tubes and Subcutaneous Emphysema

Chest tubes are not a contraindication to chest therapy; in fact, they usually indicate that the patient has a respiratory problem and may benefit from chest therapy. Care should be taken when turning such patients to prevent the tube from becoming dislodged or kinked. Chest tubes should be sutured in place and taped to the chest wall and the drainage bottle should be positioned to prevent tension on chest tubes. If the tube slips out, subcutaneous emphysema or a pneumothorax may result. A pneumothorax may also occur if a chest tube becomes disconnected from its underwater seal. All connections should be made with plastic adaptors and should be wired and taped in place. Subcutaneous air may occur following rupture of a small airway. This may be a relatively common finding during mechanical ventilation, especially if the patient is out of phase with, or "fighting," the ventilator. Subcutaneous air may be a precursor of pneumothorax and may appear in the mediastinum, in the neck, or beneath the diaphragm (Macklin and Macklin, 1944). It is not, however, a contraindication to chest physiotherapy, provided that there is no pneumothorax present. Chest physiotherapy may be effectively carried out despite subcutaneous emphysema, with no apparent increase in crepitus or radiological evidence of air (Ciesla et al., 1981).

Empyema

Empyema may result from an inadequately drained pleural cavity, an under-

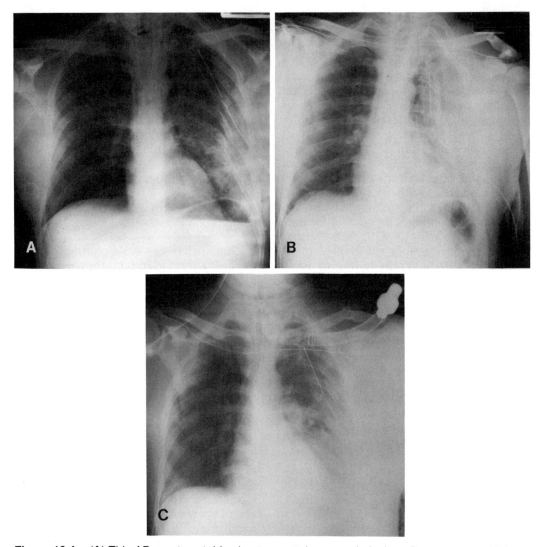

Figure 10.4. (**A**) This AP erect portable chest x-ray taken on admission after a motor vehicle accident shows multiple left rib fractures, a left lung contusion, and a left clavicular fracture. The patient is intubated and receiving controlled mechanical ventilation. (**B**) The patient was placed on IMV 24 hr after admission. This AP erect portable chest x-ray was taken after 4 hr of IMV, when the mandatory rate was 6 breaths/min. During the 4 hr, the patient showed paradoxical movement of the left chest wall but maintained adequate arterial blood gases. (**C**) The patient had a tracheostomy performed and was placed on controlled mechanical ventilation. This chest x-ray shows chest wall reexpansion which took place within 4 hr of reinstitution of controlled mechanical ventilation. [Figure 10.4**A–C** is from a presentation by B. Shin et al. (1979a) at the Eighth Annual Meeting of the Society of Critical Care Medicine, May 1979.]

lying pneumonia or a bronchopleural fistula. For treatment of this condition, a chest tube, or empyema tube (as it is frequently called), may stay in position for weeks rather than days and is often not connected to an underwater seal. Adequate drainage is imperative; therefore, loculations should be searched for and drained. If adequate drainage cannot be obtained or if pleural thickening prevents adequate lung reexpansion, decortication may be indicated. Chest physiotherapy is not effective if the pleura is grossly fibrotic and thickened.

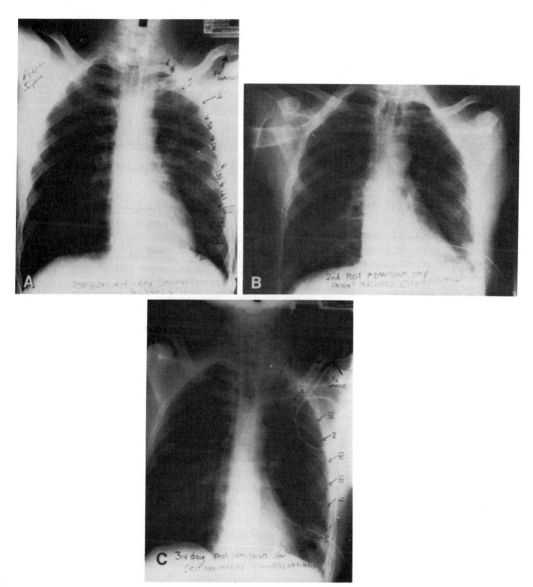

Figure 10.5. (**A**) Admission AP supine portable chest x-ray shows fractured left clavicle and ribs 2–11. There is also a left pneumomediastinum, most visible around the aortic knob. A left lung contusion is apparent underlying fractured ribs 5–7. (**B**) A left lower lobe basal segment atelectasis developed the day after admission, and the patient became hypoxemic despite controlled mechanical ventilation and routine turning and suctioning. A left chest tube was placed, but the pneumomediastinum persisted. A pulmonary artery catheter was placed to exclude cardiac causes for deteriorating pulmonary function (see **C**). (**C**) Chest physiotherapy, including postural drainage, percussion, coughing, and tracheal suctioning, was carried out despite the clavicular fracture, multiple rib fractures, pneumomediastinum, and detriorating pulmonary function. This chest x-ray was taken within 12 hr of a single treatment with chest physiotherapy and shows clearance of the left lower lobe atelectasis and radiological improvement of the left lung contusion. Respiratory function improved, and the patient was extubated 5 days after admission.

Lung Abscess

A loculated empyema may rupture into the airway or a traumatic cyst at the center of a lung contusion may become infected. Lung abscess is also associated with pneumonia, pulmonary malignancy, and tuberculosis. Rupture of a localized abscess is preceded by blood staining of the sputum. Abscesses may rupture spontaneously and result in coughing with expectoration of large quantities of pus. If rupture occurs in association with chest physiotherapy spillage may occur into the opposite lung resulting in a spread of infection (Rasanen et al., 1988). If transbronchial aspiration of infected material occurs the dependent lung opposite the abscess should be managed with chest physiotherapy including postural drainage.

Bronchopleural Fistula

Chest physiotherapy may be carried out despite a bronchopleural fistula. By reexpansion of atelectatic lung around a fistula, closing of the fistula may be hastened. If the fistula is acute, drainage of lung secretions may abort infection. However, in mechanically ventilated patients, prolonged periods of postural drainage with the fistula uppermost increase the leakage through the fistula and may result in a sudden rise in $PaCO_2$. This occurs when the patient is lying on the normal lung, because the upper lung is preferentially ventilated with positive pressure ventilation, as it has a higher compliance. In patients ventilated with PEEP, the reduction in alveolar ventilation and increased fistula leak may be particularly troublesome. Chest therapy, while the fistula is uppermost, should be carried out provided secretions are obtained. Since the patient is usually nursed supine or with the unaffected lung uppermost, it is essential that the lungs be kept clear of secretions. The newer methods of mechanical support, such as pressure support, airway pressure release (Stock et al., 1981), and inverse ratio ventilation (Willats, 1985), high frequency oscillation (Butler et al., 1980) or ventilation (Carlon et al., 1979a; Sjostrand and Eriksson, 1980), may turn

out to be the approach of choice to reduce bronchopleural pressure differences and allow rapid healing. Several authors have suggested reducing the leak from the fistula by applying positive pressure equally through the tracheobronchial tree and a chest tube. (Downs and Chapman, 1976; Gallagher et al., 1976; Powner and Grenvik, 1981).

Extrapleural Hematoma

Extrapleural hematomas associated with rib fractures or chest wall injury commonly may overlie damaged lung. Restriction of therapy to other areas of the chest prevents treatment of the lung most likely to benefit. Chest physiotherapy is often cited as a cause for extrapleural hematoma associated with rib fractures. In our experience chest physiotherapy does not increase the incidence of extrapleural hematomas and need not be withheld. Twenty-four of 252 patients with rib fractures had extrapleural pathology diagnosed by chest x-ray. In 10 this was noted before chest physiotherapy and in 14 after 313 chest physiotherapy treatments. There was no statistical difference in the incidence of extrapleural bleeding, pneumo- or hemothorax, or displacement of rib fractures before and after chest physiotherapy. There was also no difference in the changes occurring with chest physiotherapy whether the patients had single or multiple rib fractures. (Ciesla et al., 1988, personal communication). Therefore, unless the extrapleural hematoma is expanding (when percussion or vibration may stimulate further bleeding) or the patient has a coagulopathy, chest physiotherapy need not be restricted. Novice therapists and nontherapists should not treat these patients, as incorrect application of manual external chest pressure must be avoided.

Cardiovascular

Cardiac Failure

For patients in whom there is doubt about the diagnosis of cardiac failure, assessment of reserve cardiac function may be made before chest physiotherapy is performed. This can be achieved by leg raising, inflation of MASTrousers, or rapid fluid infusion sufficient to raise cardiac filling pressures greater than 2 mm Hg above baseline. If "flat" ventricular function curves are obtained, cardiac contractility may be improved by inotropic agents or reduction of systemic vascular resistance, before placing the patient in the head-down position for postural drainage and chest physiotherapy.

Patients in borderline cardiac failure should be observed very carefully during chest physiotherapy. They are frequently monitored with intravascular catheters, as well as electrocardiogram (ECG) and pulse oximetry when in the intensive care unit (ICU). In our institution in the past 13 years over 1,300 patients with some degree of heart failure were monitored with pulmonary artery and arterial indwelling catheters and also received chest physiotherapy. Although dysrhythmias rarely occurred during percussion or vibration, some of these patients became tachycardic or bradycardic or noticeably cyanotic in the head-down position. The detrimental effects of the head-down position on cardiorespiratory function for patients with impaired cardiac function may be diminished by inotropic drugs, reducing the duration of postural drainage, or by support with controlled mechanical ventilation and PEEP. In this sort of patient, others believe that the desired effect of chest physiotherapy may be obtained with the patient flat (B. A. Webber, personal communication). Bradycardia is seen with suctioning in patients with borderline cardiac failure. The hazards of suctioning are fully described in Chapter 5. In the last 5 years use of pulse oximetry has enabled direct feedback of detrimental effects on SaO_2 of maneuvers such as head-down positioning and suctioning. If saturation falls below 90% the intervention should cease. Inspired O_2 is increased to allow therapy to continue.

During physiotherapy treatment of patients with impaired cardiac function, the therapist should continually observe the ECG, intravascular pressures, and SaO_2. Development of a dysrhythmia is visible on the ECG and frequently diminishes cardiac output; this may readily be observed immediately on occurrence, as a diminution in the wave form of an arterial pressure tracing. Provided mechanical damping is excluded, the decrease in pulse pressure should be treated by ceasing the stimulus, placing the bed horizontal, placing the patient supine, and taking appropriate pharmacological action. Pharmacology may include increased inspired oxygen concentrations as the initial step before antiarrhythmic drugs. Sitting the patient up decreases cardiac filling pressures and may assist the return to sinus rhythm for the patient in cardiac failure.

With a 3 μg/kg continuous infusion of fentanyl, cardiac output rose 20–25% above baseline values during chest physiotherapy. Without analgesic infusion cardiac output rose 50%. O_2 consumption and CO_2 production increase during chest physiotherapy. The rise in blood pressure and heart rate that occurs when no analgesic is given is attenuated by fentanyl infusion (Klein et al., 1988). In our opinion these changes are not an indication to withhold chest physiotherapy in patients with cardiac dysfunction because these are often the very patients who can least tolerate respiratory compromise. Baseline values of cardiac function return within 15 min of ceasing chest physiotherapy (Mackenzie and Shin, 1985; Klein et al., 1988). The appropriate management includes use of analgesia and sedation to reduce the adverse cardiovascular and metabolic affects of chest physiotherapy.

Pulmonary Edema

The patient with borderline cardiac failure or impaired cardiac function can usually tolerate chest physiotherapy in the head-down position if the above precautions are taken. If, however, the patient cannot tolerate the head-down position because of severe cardiac failure and pulmonary edema, this should be avoided. There should be a definite restriction of tracheal suctioning. The more suctioning that is performed, the more surfactant and protein are lost in the edema fluid. It is a vicious circle. Surfactant loss allows small airways to close, increasing secretion retention and the indication for chest physiotherapy. Acute cardiac failure needs treatment directed at decreasing cardiac preload or afterload or increasing cardiac contractility. Because of loss of sympathetic innervation to the heart and peripheral vasculature, patients with acute cervical spinal cord injury may be unable to increase cardiac contractility in response to elevation of cardiac filling pressures (Mackenzie et al., 1985). Pulmonary edema is a common cause of death during spinal shock and may be precipitated by head-down positioning that may elevate central venous pressures. Patients with acute spinal cord injury who are positioned head down should be monitored for signs of pulmonary edema.

Pulmonary edema may occur secondary to noncardiac as well as cardiac causes. Therefore, not all pink frothiness seen on suctioning is caused by fluid overload or inadequate cardiac function. The most frequent cause of noncardiogenic pulmonary edema seen in the trauma patient is lung contusion. Chest physiotherapy is indicated to treat lung contusion, and suctioning need not usually be restricted because the edema is localized, not generalized. Massive bleeding from an associated lung laceration or a major coagulopathy may, however, contraindicate chest therapy and suctioning. The lung laceration may require bronchoscopy (although frequently nothing can be visualized because of all the blood) and operation. The coagulopathy requires correction with blood products. Other noncardiogenic causes of pulmonary edema include nitrogen dioxide inhalation, high inspired oxygen concentration, heroin overdosage, and high-altitude pulmonary edema. These and other causes are fully described elsewhere (Fishman, 1980).

If cardiac failure and pulmonary edema develop during therapy, sitting the patient up and PEEP (in the already tracheally intubated patient) are the immediate bedside therapies of choice.

Myocardial Ischemia

Myocardial ischemia or infarction commonly reduces cardiac output and is associated with dysrhythmia. Since myocardial perfusion occurs mostly during diastole, maneuvers that cause tachycardia reduce coronary perfusion and should be avoided, where possible, in the patient with coronary artery disease. If, for example, the patient becomes tachycardic after 15 min in the head-down position, rather than persisting in order to complete the treatment, the therapist should elevate the head of the bed. The therapy may be finished later when heart rate has slowed or the patient has received sedation, such as morphine.

Myocardial Contusion

Myocardial contusion is a commonly touted but rarely proved diagnosis in the living, traumatized patient. In 173 consecutive patients who died following direct helicopter admission from road accidents to a trauma unit 17 had some degree of myocardial contusion (Mackenzie et al., 1979). The significance of myocardial contusion remains unknown. Despite ECG and cardiac enzyme changes suggestive of myocardial contusion, Technetium-99m scans in 12 trauma patients did not demonstrate any abnormality (A. Rodriguez, personal communication). Sutherland and colleagues (1981) report that radionuclide angiography is the diagnostic tool of choice. During chest physiotherapy these patients are not treated any differently from those patients with impaired cardiac function.

Ruptured Aorta

Traumatic rupture of the aorta may occur secondary to rapid deceleration in automobile accidents. At our institution an average of 5 patients/year have been diagnosed, with a reported survival rate of 75% (27/36) (Ayella et al., 1977). There is again no contraindication to chest physiotherapy following repair, provided monitoring equipment is appropriately observed during maneuvers that may cause cardiovascular disturbance, such as acute position change and tracheal suctioning.

Pulmonary Embolus

Pulmonary embolus is reported to occur frequently following long-bone or pelvic fractures. It may present as either the results of fat embolization or as acute cardiovascular collapse from embolization of a massive thrombus. Clinically, significant embolization may not always occur. In our experience it was extremely rare. Considering the patient population studied, it was not a frequent cause of death. Only 1 pulmonary embolus was identified in 124 consecutive full autopsies of patients who died following motor vehicle accidents (Mackenzie et al.) Conventional autopsy studies in intensive care unit patients report an incidence of 9–27% of pulmonary emboli (Pingelton, 1988). Pulmonary thrombi also occur and confuse the diagnosis. Despite the availability of lung scans and pulmonary angiograms the diagnosis of pulmonary embolus is difficult. In 5 years (1975–1980) only 2 patients of 3,210 consecutive trauma admissions were seen showing the classic signs of fat embolus.

The possibility of precipitating thrombus or fat embolization by chest physiotherapy and turning seems, in our experience, remote. In fact, this low incidence suggests that the aggressive approach with early mobilization may be a possible mechanism preventing pulmonary embolus.

Central Nervous System

Cerebral Contusion

The most common pathology of the central nervous system found in trauma patients is cerebral contusion. Forty-seven percent of 173 deaths from road accidents occurring in a 2-year period were due to head injury (Mackenzie et al.). The distressing factor associated with cerebral trauma is that the damage is frequently irreversible despite appropriate therapy. Use of predictors of outcome, such as the Glasgow Coma Scale (Jennett et al., 1976) and the Maryland Coma Scale (Salcman et al., 1981), are important in order to determine those patients in whom aggressive treatment is likely to improve the prognosis. Prevention of chest complications in this group of patients is of great importance. Despite all the intracranial pressure monitoring, hyperventilation, intracranial pressure reducing drugs, and maneuvers, unless adequate lung function is maintained, cerebral outcome may be jeopardized in the important group of patients with head injury who survive.

The great recent advance in the treatment of the patient with cerebral contusion was the use of intracranial pressure monitoring. Previously, therapy was withheld that might, in some circumstances, be thought to affect cerebral perfusion adversely. Now, with the intelligent use of the intracranial pressure monitor, therapy can be tailored to its effect on cerebral perfusion. The patient may no longer need to be dehydrated, to the detriment of the kidney and ciliary activity of airway mucosa. Barbiturates may be given more discriminately to only those patients with persistently high intracranial pressure. Chest physiotherapy with the head-down position may be used allowing clearance of retained secretions. During 1979–88 1,684 patients with head injury received chest physiotherapy. Of these 720 (42.7%) patients required intracranial pressure monitors. Over 90% of these patients had lower lobe problems that required a head-down position for postural drainage and therapy. Intracranial pressure monitoring enabled this to be carried out while allowing any resultant compromise in cerebral perfusion to be observed and, therefore, rectified (see Figs. 8.4 and 8.5).

Sixteen patients with pulmonary complications and severe head injury (average Glasgow Coma Scale = 5) had resting ICP sitting up of 15 mm Hg and were randomly assigned to head-down (HD) or flat (HF) positioning for CPT (Imle et al., 1988). Although ICP rose during 15 min of CPT while both HD and HF, cerebral perfusion pressure (CPP) was not different. There were no differences in heart rate, mean arterial pressure, or end-tidal CO_2 after CPT. CPT while HD does not result in decreased CPP despite the increased ICP because of cerebrovascular autoregulation. CPP (mean arterial BP-

ICP) is a more clinically relevant monitor of the cerebral effects of CPT than simple measurement of ICP. Perfusion and chest vibration were not found to adversely affect ICP or CPP in this study.

Cerebrospinal Fluid (CSF) Leak

A CSF leak due to a dural tear may be a relative contraindication to the head-down position for chest therapy. Leakage implies decompression of any intracranial pressure elevation, but if the leakage increases during the head-down position and persists at a higher rate despite head elevation, the dural tear was most probably reopened. CSF leaks may be associated with facial injury and skull fracture. Leakage may occur through the ear, the nose or an open fracture. If leakage continues, operative closure of the dural tear may be required.

Spinal Cord Injury

Cervical spinal cord transection causes interruption of the autonomic nervous system and loss of motor function below the level of the spinal cord injury. This disturbs the normal compensatory cardiovascular reflexes because of loss of sympathetic nervous system control over the heart and peripheral circulation. Quadriplegia also results in impairment of respiratory function. Chest physiotherapy in a quadriplegic patient must, therefore, be performed with caution, since acute postural changes may precipitate cardiac decompensation and cause acute pulmonary edema or profound hypotension. Acute pulmonary edema is a commonly reported cause of death in acute quadriplegia (Meyer et al., 1971). Suctioning is also reported to be a hazardous procedure in the acute quadriplegic (Welply et al., 1975). In our experience of treating 51 patients with cervical spine injury during 15 months, there were two deaths that occurred during suctioning of quadriplegic patients when they were in the prone position on a Stryker frame. Both instances occurred at night in the step-down unit when the patients were in their recovery phase. Tolerance of the prone position in spontaneously breathing quadriplegic patients

can be improved by placing pillows or rolls across the anterior iliac crests and enlarging the hole in the canvas of the Stryker frame to allow free movement of the diaphragm and dependent abdomen. Suctioning should be carried out with monitoring of ECG and SaO_2 (by pulse oximetry). Tracheal suctioning in a patient in the prone position on a Stryker frame is an acrobatic achievement performed kneeling; this may not allow the monitors to be seen by the person suctioning.

Despite all these precautions, attention to respiratory therapy on a prophylactic basis is of the utmost importance in reducing early mortality in quadriplegic patients (Fugl-Meyer, 1976; McMichan et al., 1980) (see Chapter 8). For the paraplegic patient in whom prognosis is more likely to be favorable and chest complications less common, chest physiotherapy is usually applied only when specifically indicated. With functional arm movement, the abdomen can be compressed by the high paraplegic, greatly enhancing the effectiveness of coughing. If treated on a Stryker frame initially, patients with cervical spine injury and no neurological deficit can often be mobilized by means of a halo vest or other type of orthopedic stabilization. Because of the early mobilization allowed by surgical fusion or external stabilization, respiratory problems may be prevented. However, if the orthotic device restricts chest excursion it may lead to secretion retention. Some patients with thoracic spine injury may require prolonged bed rest. Nonetheless, these patients may be instructed in breathing exercises and can be log-rolled to allow appropriate chest therapy when required. Most thoracic spine injuries are inherently stable and allow the performance of chest physiotherapy. However, an unstable thoracic spine injury is considered to be a contraindication to vigorous chest vibration.

Surgical Procedures about the Head

Patients with a craniotomy and removal of bone flap should be carefully positioned during turning and head-down tilt. The edges of the surgical area should be supported. A 500- or 1,000-ml plastic infusion bag may be used (see Fig. 3.13). Ear injuries or major plastic surgical repairs around the head and neck should be supported similarly if the area might be traumatized during positioning; this protection is especially important when treating the unconscious patient and should include measures to prevent damage to the eyes when the patient is turned from the supine position. Similarly, care should be taken when turning and positioning patients with skin grafts or flaps or those with extensive burns. Chest percussion and vibration are contraindicated over recent plastic or skin graft procedures. A sterile drape should cover chest burns to prevent contamination during chest physiotherapy.

Gastrointestinal

Dehiscence

Dehiscence of an abdominal wound occurs as a complication after surgery. The precipitating factors causing dehiscence include diminished healing due to malnutrition, age, use of corticosteroids, inadequate surgical technique, obesity, diabetes, infection, or hemorrhage in the wound (Schwartz, 1979). Coughing is a possible mechanical cause of early dehiscence. However, chest physiotherapy should not be restricted, nor is it withheld even when dehiscence has occurred. Mechanical means, such as binders and synthetic mesh, can be used to prevent evisceration if the abdomen is open or the dehiscence is infected and draining. Turning and posturing for chest physiotherapy can then be achieved (Fig. 10.6).

Tracheoesophageal Fistula

In order to prevent leakage and allow adequate alveolar ventilation, overinflation of the tracheal tube cuff may be unavoidable in mechanically ventilated patients with increased dead space, carbon dioxide production, intrapulmonary shunt, and PEEP. Carbon dioxide excretion capabilities of the lung may be considerably compromised in the critically ill patient by hyperalimentation (Kinney et al., 1980). Because of tracheal cuff overinflation, causing compression of the esophagus, tracheoesophageal fistula may occur during prolonged intubation. This should not restrict chest physiotherapy even in the critically ill patient; rather, attention to optimizing respiratory function should be mandatory. It is our experience that bronchoscopy is extremely hazardous in patients who require PEEP greater than 15 cm H_2O and have low lung compliance (Mackenzie and Shin, 1988). This is not, therefore, a reasonable alternative to chest physiotherapy for such patients with a tracheoesophageal fistula.

In order to prevent continued aspiration of secretions, palliative occlusion of the lower and upper esophagus and a gas-

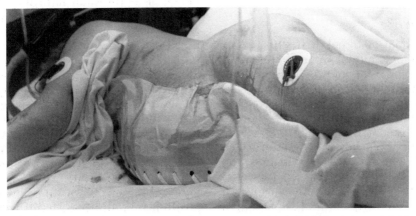

Figure 10.6.   This obese diabetic patient developed peritonitis, abdominal wound dehiscence, and left lower lobe atelectasis. Evisceration was prevented by the abdominal binder. The patient is shown positioned for chest physiotherapy treatment.

trostomy may overcome the immediate problem until respiratory dysfunction can be rectified and any precipitating factors treated. In the critically ill patient a definitive repair must be delayed.

Abdominal Distension

Major abdominal distension or gross obesity may compromise respiratory function in the spontaneously breathing patient. Respiratory dysfunction may be further aggravated in the head-down position. Because of unfavorable changes in diaphragmatic and chest wall function due to abdominal distension and gross obesity, tracheal intubation and mechanical ventilation are often required to assist lung expansion and prevent development of atelectasis.

Generalized edema secondary to alterations in capillary permeability may produce edema of the abdominal wall and bowel. It may also cause peritoneal effusion. Mechanical ventilation would be the treatment of choice for these patients, and the obese patient with Pickwickian syndrome rather than assisted respiration. This would be instituted before chest physiotherapy in the head-down position. Similarly, quadriplegic patients who develop abdominal distension should be decompressed by an endogastric tube and receive mechanical ventilatory support before postural drainage of the lower lobes.

Genitourinary

Pelvic Fracture

The association of pelvic fracture and a bladder injury may in some centers contraindicate turning of the patient. The use of external fixation (Hoffmann, 1954) to the displaced pelvis allows turning but may hinder prone positioning. Alternatively, patients with pelvic fractures may be log-rolled, placed in MASTrousers, a fracture brace, or transferred to a turning frame. In a 7-year period 417 patients received chest physiotherapy despite a fractured pelvis (Appendix I). In less than 5% of patients were any turning restrictions ordered. Pelvic traction was not used at our institution prior to 1979. This did not deter turning when required for a specific respiratory problem. Turning without external stabilization was not knowingly associated with increased hematoma, stimulation of bleeding, or any urethral damage. There were no instances of hematuria after turning for chest physiotherapy, and no patients had marked changes in vital signs, or hematocrit, or went into shock during or after therapy. Most pelvic fractures are relatively stable and self-supported. This clinical impression of stability is confirmed by the considerable amount of traction that is often required to alter the displacement of a fracture, during application of the external pelvic fixators, despite a highly favorable mechanical advantage from an intramedullary pin into the ileum.

Renal Dialysis

Renal dialysis can cause considerable shifts in intravascular volume. Reports of hypoxemia during dialysis have appeared. Explanations include loss of carbon dioxide through the dialysate membrane, which significantly decreases the respiratory quotient (Aurigemma et al., 1977), ventilation/perfusion changes, and diffusion abnormalities related to leukoagglutination (Carlon et al., 1979b). The experience in our institution is frequently the reverse. PaO_2 is noted to increase during dialysis. Aggressive fluid therapy, which has reduced the incidence of acute renal failure and has increased nonoliguric renal failure (Shin et al., 1979b), results in fluid overload in those patients who require dialysis. The improved respiratory function, during and following dialysis can be explained by fluid removal from the lungs. Chest physiotherapy is indicated when respiratory function warrants treatment and may be given during dialysis when the dialysate is draining from the abdominal cavity. It should not be performed in the head-down position, when severe abdominal distension occurs. The head-up position is contraindicated if volume depletion results from hemodialysis. In the unstable patient, chest physiotherapy can be carried out after dialysis is completed and coagulation and intravascular volume have returned to normal.

Musculoskeletal System

Multiple Trauma

Conflicting therapeutic aims inevitably occur in a patient with multisystem trauma. What is the ideal treatment for one system may compromise another; this is the case with musculoskeletal injury. While immobilization is the ideal way to obtain good bony union after satisfactory reduction is achieved, it impairs respiratory function (see Chapter 6). As in any situation when multisystem disease occurs, priorities must be established to determine which problem is potentially the most life-threatening to the critically ill patient. It is not considered good therapeutics for the patient with fractures maintained in perfect alignment to die of pulmonary complications following immobilization; rather, a compromise must be reached.

In instances in which a patient has an isolated bony injury and atelectasis, therapy includes postural drainage and positioning. This may be limited by the restraints of traction and casts. Percussion, vibration, and breathing exercises may be carried out with patient cooperation. However, when the patient is unconscious, has multiple bony injuries, and is suffering from severe acute lung problems requiring high FIO_2 and PEEP, improved positioning must be obtained to allow effective chest physiotherapy. If this is not possible, alternative methods must be employed.

Better positioning may be achieved by altering the means of joint immobilization. Immobilization by means of external fixators (see Fig. 3.15) enables a patient to be turned into all postural drainage positions despite bilateral long-bone fractures. These positions would be impossible to achieve with orthodox splints and traction. If traction needs to be used, a more mobile device allows more complete turning; therefore, more ideal postural drainage positions can be achieved. Neufeld traction has many of

these desirable assets and allows more complete mobilization by altering the point of suspension of the cast during turning. The use of a halo vest, in a patient with cervical spine injury without neurological deficit, also allows turning to both sides for postural drainage and mobilization, neither of which can be achieved with a turning frame.

These alternatives enable more satisfactory treatment to be given to patients immobilized because of bony fractures. This is a major advance in respiratory care for the trauma patient, since bony fractures are a common problem. In a 7-year period 2,029 (30%) of 6,697 trauma patients had peripheral bony fractures (excluding skull, rib and facial bones) and were treated with chest physiotherapy in the critical care recovery unit. Of these patients 70% had more than one system injured (e.g., in addition to peripheral bony injury, there was head, chest, or abdominal injury). Injury severity scores of trauma patients receiving chest physiotherapy are shown in Appendix I. Because of the successful use of alternative techniques, less than 2% had any turning restrictions imposed. Turning restrictions were ordered only if the orthopedist felt bony alignment was unacceptably displaced during turning and the patient's respiratory condition was not life-threatening. Similarly, although osteoporosis of the spine or ribs requires that percussion and vibration be performed with caution, this compromise must be weighed against the necessity for chest physiotherapy.

In 7 years, 1981–88, 380 patients had external fixators used instead of casts; the majority were applied to tibial fractures. In the same period, 736 patients with other orthopedic fixation devices required chest physiotherapy. The other devices included Neufeld traction (5%), internal fixation (41%), spinal rods (7%), and skeletal traction (13%), including traction through a Steinmann pin and Bucks traction or a combination of external fixators and skeletal traction. These alternative traction techniques enabled more complete mobilization of the patient and allowed turning into appropriate postural drainage positions for chest physiotherapy.

The alternative compromise to not using chest physiotherapy was to use some other treatment to clear retained secretions from the lungs. The most often considered alternative was bronchoscopy. Some of the advantages and disadvantages of bronchoscopy are considered in Chapter 9. Other alternatives, such as incentive spirometry, paper coils, and blow bottles, have no application in the unconscious or mechanically ventilated patient and are of unproven value in comparison to deep breaths in spontaneously breathing patients. Circulomatic and kinetic beds were occasionally used as a preventative means but remain unproven in effectiveness and value in clearing pulmonary secretions (see pp. 109 to 117).

Hemopoietic System

Precautions observed during chest physiotherapy for patients with hemopoietic disease relate to the care with which the patient must be handled so that bleeding is not precipitated. Coagulopathy is the most common hemopoietic problem seen in a trauma unit (perhaps also in the average surgical ICU). In the trauma patient this is frequently due to thrombocytopenia. When the platelet count falls below 30,000, problems are likely to be encountered. However, if platelet malfunction is present, even higher levels may give rise to abnormal bleeding. In the surgical patient, anticoagulation may be used to prevent or treat pulmonary embolus, or it may occur as a secondary response to another pathological factor, such as disseminated intravascular coagulation precipitated by shock.

Patients with bleeding disorders should be suctioned very carefully to avoid undue trauma to the airway. Blind nasotracheal suctioning is absolutely contraindicated because of the likelihood of precipitating bleeding from the nasal mucous membranes; it is also contraindicated for its other undesirable effects (see p. 179). If secretions suctioned through a tracheal tube are profusely bloody, therapy should cease until coag-

ulation correction can be achieved. This, however, frequently becomes a vicious circle, since bleeding within the tracheobronchial tree may lead to acute atelectasis and result in a need, and a specific indication, for chest physiotherapy. In this case, postural drainage, percussion, vibration, and assisted coughing with limited tracheal suction are used. When precipitation of bleeding during turning is considered a possibility, turning for chest therapy may coincide with some other necessity, such as changing bed linens or relief of pressure areas. Vigorous percussion, in the presence of an expanding extrapleural hematoma and rib fractures, is contraindicated in patients with a coagulopathy.

Transbronchial aspiration of blood from unilateral lung pathology into an otherwise normal lung during chest physiotherapy should be managed by giving chest physiotherapy to the normal lung at the end of therapy. Varying degrees of pulmonary hemorrhage may occur from hemoptysis to copious frank blood. At all times a cause for hemoptysis should be determined. If frank hemorrhage occurs, bronchoscopy or surgery may be required.

Burns and Skin Grafts or Flaps

Chest physiotherapy may be indicated in patients with chest burns. Care should be taken to avoid contamination of the burned area. During the acute stage the chest should be covered with a thin sterile drape, and the physical therapist should wear a cap, mask, and sterile gown and gloves. Chest percussion and vibration are carried out within the patient's tolerance and depending on the type of burn. For third-degree burns, chest physiotherapy is not painful.

Skin grafts over the chest or other areas of the body should not have any prolonged pressure or shearing forces applied. The patient must be positioned carefully for chest physiotherapy and the graft area supported in the position least likely to cause pressure or dislodgment. Similarly, any pedicle flap grafts should be positioned so that tension is minimized and trauma during chest physiotherapy reduced. Breathing exercises and assisted coughing may be used in place of percussion and vibration for the spontaneously breathing patient with fresh skin grafts.

Pain

Pain associated with chest physiotherapy is a commonly claimed contraindication. There is no doubt that following major surgery or trauma, deep breathing and coughing are painful! Whether chest physiotherapy is contraindicated depends on the consequences of withholding therapy and the initial indication. If it is thought that as a result of not receiving the treatment the patient would suffer respiratory dysfunction and require even more painful and stressful therapy, such as intubation and mechanical ventilation, effective methods of pain relief must be found. If treatment is prophylactic or if breathing exercises and assisted coughing would suffice in place of percussion, vibration, and expectoration, these should be used.

There are several means of pain relief following surgery including systemic analgesic medications, intravenous local anesthetics, nerve blocks with local anesthetics, or narcotics and stimulation-produced analgesia such as transcutaneous electrical nerve stimulation (TENS) and acupuncture. Systemic narcotics bind to specific opiate receptors in the CNS and inhibit conduction of nociceptive stimuli. More recently narcotic agonist–antagonists such as nalbuphine and butorphanol and partial agonists such as buprenorphrine are used for acute pain (Raj, 1988).

Intravenous anesthetics, particularly 2-chloroprocaine, may be safe and efficacious in managing musculoskeletal pain. The mechanism of action is unclear but may involve antagonism of chemical mediators such as substance P or modulations of nociceptive stimuli in afferent nerves within the spinal cord. Monitoring for local anesthetic toxicity is essential during infusion.

Epidural or spinal anesthesia may be given as a single bolus or by continuous infusion. Morphine is the only narcotic approved for epidural or spinal use. A single bolus provides analgesia of 12–24 hr duration. Fentanyl and meperidine are also used epidurally. The continuous infusion techniques avoid the peak and trough concentrations associated with repeated injections. Both intravenous and intraspinal narcotics can be patient controlled within predetermined limits of maximum and minimum infusion rates by using bedside or portable infusion pumps. Techniques such as instillation of local anesthetics through intrapleural catheters are also useful to improve chest movement following upper abdominal surgery. Control of pain can improve respiratory function (Fairley, 1980).

Some patients are more tolerant of pain than others. The relationship with the physical therapist, augmented by the medical and nursing staff, is an important factor in pain tolerance. If patients understand that the treatment is important and beneficial, they are almost always cooperative. The therapist should give the patient a brief, clear description of what is going to happen and why the therapy is required. Rapport is best established before surgery, so that the need for therapy is understood. This is not always possible.

Pain relief should be given when required before the start of chest physiotherapy; time should be allowed for the analgesic effect to occur. Since pain may be a major cause of the initial respiratory difficulty, effective pain relief should greatly assist clearance of retained secretions and prevent their reaccumulation (Fairley, 1980). Reports suggest that pain relief may reduce (Trinkle et al., 1975) or avoid (Shackford et al., 1981) the need for mechanical ventilation. These techniques require a physician's skills and are time-consuming; risks must be weighed against the other available methods of pain control. Continuous intravenous infusion techniques may be useful for providing successful analgesia and allowing chest physiotherapy to be carried out in the ICU (M. A. Branthwaite, personal communication, 1980). Klein (1988) found that 3 μg/kg fentanyl infusion but not 1.9 μg/kg fentanyl attenuated increases in blood pressure and heart rate occurring with chest physiotherapy. Neither dose of analgesic prevented rises in cardiac output averaging

20–25% above baseline or rises in CO_2 production and O_2 consumption during chest physiotherapy.

It is quite apparent that intravenous or intramuscular analgesics are not the panacea for all patients. Local anesthetic techniques have the advantage of little systemic effect, but they require skillful administration and must be frequently repeated. Inhaled 50% nitrous oxide may be useful to enable some patients to breathe and cough more deeply during chest physiotherapy but may cause bone marrow depression and neuropathy (Layzer, 1978). As an alternative to these methods stimulation-produced analgesia such as acupuncture or TENS may be used to relieve pain (Abram et al., 1981); the physical therapist may have considerable expertise in TENS application. The reports of its use in the ICU are favorable (Ali et al., 1981). Encouragement, intravenous or intramuscular analgesics, intravenous local anesthetics, spinal or epidural blocks, or stimulation-produced analgesia, heat, or cold may be used to reduce the patient's appreciation of pain, allowing chest physiotherapy to be performed. The appropriate patient(s) benefiting most from each of these methods of pain relief needs to be established. If a patient finds one aspect of treatment, such as vigorous chest vibration, particularly unpleasant, the therapist can, perhaps, emphasize other aspects, such as postural drainage and assisted coughing. The therapist should be as gentle as possible while treating the patient in pain, yet still be vigorous enough to perform the therapy effectively.

SUMMARY

The complications, precautions, and contraindications presented in this chapter represent the results of an aggressive approach to chest physiotherapy for the trauma patient. In our experience the potential benefits of chest physiotherapy must be weighed against the risk for the patient of continuing the same approach which resulted in deterioration of pulmonary function. Often the risks claimed to be associated with chest physiotherapy are unsubstantiated in practice or

may be minimized by the compromises and precautions outlined in this chapter.

The therapist's role involves coordination of information about the patient from the radiologist and from the physicians and nurses in charge of the patient. A therapist trained in ICU work is best able to integrate this information. Awareness of potential problems that may occur during chest physiotherapy is the therapist's part of the multidisciplinary approach to treatment of the critically ill patient with respiratory complications. It is the physician's responsibility to be similarly aware of the complications and to give considered thought to the hazards of chest physiotherapy in relation to the likelihood of improvement occurring with existing or alternative treatment.

References

Abram SE, Reynolds AC, Cusick JF: Failure of naloxone to reverse analgesia from transcutaneous electrical stimulation in patients with chronic pain. Anesth Analg (Cleve) 60:81–84, 1981

Albert RK, Leasa D, Sanderson M, Robertson HT, Hlastala MP: The prone position improves arterial oxygenation and reduces shunt in oleic acid-induced acute lung injury. Am Rev Respir Dis 135:628–633, 1987

Ali J, Yaffe CS, Serrette C: The effect of transcutaneous electric nerve stimulation on postoperative pain and pulmonary function. Surgery 89:507–512, 1981

Aurigemma NM, Feldman NT, Gottlieb M, Ingram RH, Lazarus JM, Lowrie EG: Arterial oxygenation during hemodialysis. N Engl J Med 297:871–873, 1977

Avery EE, Morch ET, Benson DW: Critically crushed chests. A new method of treatment with continuous mechanical hyperventilation to produce alkalotic apnea and internal pneumatic stabilization. J Thorac Cardiovasc Surg 32:291–311, 1956

Ayella RA, Hankins JR, Turney SZ, Cowley RA: Ruptured thoracic aorta due to blunt trauma. J Trauma 17:199–205, 1977

Burnard ED, Gratton-Smith P, Docton-Warlow CG: Pulmonary insufficiency in prematurity. Aust Paediatr J 1:12–38, 1965

Butler WJ, Bohn DJ, Bryan AC, Froese AB: Ventilation by high frequency oscillation in humans. Anesth Analg (Cleve) 59:577–584, 1980

Campbell C: Appreciation for advice (letter). Phys Ther 60:809–810, 1980

Carlon GC, Howland WS, Klain M, Goldiner PL, Ray C: High frequency positive pressure ventilation for ventilatory support in patients with bronchopleural fistulas. Crit Care Med 7:128, 1979a

Carlon GC, Campfield PB, Goldiner PL, Turnbull AD: Hypoxemia during hemodialysis. Crit Care Med 7:497–499, 1979b

Ciesla ND, Klemic N, Imle PC: Chest physical therapy to the patient with multiple trauma: Two case studies. *Phys Ther* 61:202–205, 1981

Ciesla N, Rodriguez A, Anderson P, Norton B: The incidence of extrapleural hematomas in patients with rib fractures receiving chest physiotherapy. Personal communication, 1988

Connors AF, Hammon WE, Martin RJ, Rogers RM: Chest physical therapy. The immediate effect on oxygenation in acutely ill patients. *Chest* 78:559–564, 1980

Douglas WW, Rehder K, Beynen FM, Sessler AD, Marsh HM: Improved oxygenation in patients with acute respiratory failure; the prone position. *Am Rev Respir Dis* 115:559–566, 1977

Downs JB, Chapman RL: Treatment of bronchopleural fistula during continuous positive pressure ventilation. *Chest* 69:363–366, 1976

Fairley HB: Oxygen therapy for surgical patients. *Am Rev Respir Dis* 122(2):37–44, 1980

Fishman AP: Pulmonary Edema. In *Pulmonary Diseases and Disorders*, edited by AP Fishman, pp 733–753. McGraw-Hill, New York, 1980

Fishman AP: Down with the good lung. (Editorial). *N Engl J Med* 304:537–538, 1981

Fineberg C, Cohn HE, Gibbon JH: Cardiac arrest during nasotracheal aspiration. *JAMA* 174:148–150, 1960

Fox WW, Schwartz JG, Schaffer TH: Pulmonary physiotherapy in neonates: Physiologic changes and respiratory management. *J Pediatr* 92:977–981, 1978

Fugl-Meyer AR: *Handbook of Clinical Neurology, Injuries of the Spine and Spinal Cord*, chap. 19, The Respiratory System, pp 335–349. American Elsevier Publishing, New York, 1976

Gallagher TJ, Smith RA, Kirby RR: Intermittent inspiratory chest tube occlusion to limit bronchopleural cutaneous air leaks. *Crit Care Med* 4:328, 1976

Gormenzano J, Branthwaite MA: Effects of physiotherapy during intermittent positive pressure ventilation. *Anaesthesia* 27:258–263, 1972

Hammon WE, Martin RJ: Fatal pulmonary hemorrhage associated with chest physical therapy. *Phys Ther* 59:1247–1248, 1979

Hoffmann R: Osteotaxis, osteosythese externe par fiches et rotules. *Acta Chir Scand* 107:72–81, 1954

Holloway R, Adams EB, Desai SD, Thambiran AK: Effect of chest physiotherapy on blood gases of neonates treated by intermittent positive pressure respiration. *Thorax* 24:421–426, 1969

Imle PC, Mars MP, Eppinghaus CE, Anderson P, Ciesla ND: Effect of chest physiotherapy (CPT) positioning on intracranial (ICP) and cerebral perfusion pressure. *Crit Care Med* 16:382, 1988

Jennett B, Teasdale G, Braakinar R, Minderhound J, Knill-Jones R: Predicting outcome in individual patients after severe head injury. *Lancet* 1:1031–1034, 1976

Kigin CM: Chest physical therapy for the postoperative or traumatic injury patient. *Phys Ther* 61:1724–1736, 1981

Kinney JM, Askanazi J, Gump FE, Foster RJ, Hyman AI: Use of ventilatory equivalent to separate hypermetabolism from increased dead space ventilation in the injured or septic patient. *J Trauma* 20:111–119, 1980

Klein P, Kemper M, Weissman G, Rosenbaum SH, Askanazi J, Hyman AJ: Attenuation of the hemodynamic responses to chest physical therapy. *Chest* 93:38–42, 1988

Layzer RB: Myeloneuropathy after prolonged exposure to nitrous oxide. *Lancet* 2:1227–1230, 1978

Mackenzie CF, Shin B, Fisher R, Cowley RA: Two year mortality in 760 patients transported by helicopter direct from the road accident scene. *Am Surg* 45:101–108, 1979

Mackenzie CF, Shin B, Krishnaprasad D, McCormack F, Illingworth W: Assessment of cardiac and respiratory function during surgery on patients with acute quadriplegia. *J Neurosurg* 62:843–849, 1985

Mackenzie CF, Shin B: Chest physiotherapy vs bronchoscopy. *Crit Care Med* 14:78–79, 1986

Macklin MT, Macklin CC: Malignant interstitial emphysema of the lungs and mediastinum as an important occult complication in many respiratory diseases and other conditions: An interpretation of the clinical literature in the light of laboratory experiment. *Medicine* 23:281–538, 1944

McMichan JC, Michel L, Westbrook PR: Pulmonary dysfunction following traumatic quadriplegia. *JAMA* 243:528–531, 1980

Meyer GA, Berman IR, Doty DB, Moseley RV, Gutierrez VS: Hemodynamic responses to acute quadriplegia with or without chest trauma. *J Neurosurg* 34:168–177, 1971

Milner AD, Murray M: Acute bronchiolitis in infancy: Treatment and prognosis. Editorial. *Thorax* 94:1–5, 1989

Pingelton SK: Complications of acute respiratory failure: State of the art. *Am Rev Respir Dis* 137:1463–1493, 1988

Powner DJ, Grenvik A: Ventilator management of life threatening bronchopleural fistulae. *Crit Care Med* 9:54–58, 1981

Purohit DM, Caldwell C, Lerkoff AH: Multiple rib fractures due to physiotherapy in a neonate with hyaline membrane disease. *Am J Dis Child* 129:1103–1104, 1975

Raj P: Drug administration techniques for chronic pain. In *Current Practice in Anesthesiology*, edited by M Rogers, B. C. Decker Inc., Toronto, pp 243–248, 1988

Rasanen J, Bools JC, Downs JB: Endobronchial drainage of undiagnosed lung abscess during chest physical therapy. *Phys Ther* 68:371–373, 1988

Remolina C, Khan AV, Santiago TV, Edelman NH: Positional hypoxemia in unilateral lung disease. *N Engl J Med* 304:523–525, 1981

Salcman M, Schepps RS, Ducker TB: Calculated recovery rates in severe head trauma. *Neurosurgery* 8:301–308, 1981

Schwartz SI: *Principles of Surgery*, p 496. McGraw-Hill, New York, 1979

Seaton D: Effect of body position on gas exchange after thoracotomy. *Thorax* 34:518–522, 1979

Shackford SR, Virgilio RW, Peters RM: Early extubation versus prophylactic ventilation in the high risk patient: A comparison of postoperative management in the prevention of respiratory complications. *Anesth Analg (Cleve)* 60:76–80, 1981

Shin B, Mackenzie CF, Chodoff P: Is IMV superior

to controlled ventilation in the management of flail chest? *Crit Care Med* 7:138, 1979a

Shin B, Mackenzie CF, McAslan TC, Helrich M, Cowley R: Postoperative renal failure in trauma patients. *Anesthesiology* 51:218–221, 1979b

Sjostrand UH, Eriksson IA: High rates and low volumes in mechanical ventilation—not just a matter of ventilatory frequency. *Anesth Analg (Cleve)* 59:567–576, 1980

Sutherland GR, Calvin JE, Driedger AA, Holliday RL, Sibbald WJ: Anatomic and cardiopulmonary responses to trauma with associated blunt chest injury. *J Trauma* 21:1–12, 1981

Trinkle JK, Richardson JD, Franz JL, Grover FL, Aro KV, Holmstrom FMG: Management of flail chest without mechanical ventilation. *Ann Thorac Surg* 19:355–363, 1975

Tyler ML: Complications of positioning and chest physiotherapy. *Resp Care* 27:458–466, 1982

Walsh JH, Vanderntarf C, Hoscheit D, Fahey NPJ: Unsuspected hemodynamic alterations during endotracheal suctioning. *Chest* 95:163–165, 1989

Webb MSC, Martin JA, Cartlidge PHT, Ng YK, Wright NA: Chest physiotherapy in acute bronchiolitis. *Arch Dis Child* 60:1078–1079, 1985

Welply NC, Mathias CJ, Frankel HL: Circulatory reflexes in tetraplegics during artificial ventilation and general anaesthesia. *Paraplegia* 13:172–182, 1975

Willats SM: Alternative modes of ventilation. Part II. High and low frequency positive pressure ventilation, PEEP, CPAP, reverse ratio ventilation. *Intensive Care Med* 11:51–55, 1985

Zack MB, Pontoppidan H, Kazemi H: The effect of lateral positions on gas exchange in pulmonary disease. *Am Rev Respir Dis* 110:49–55, 1974

APPENDIX I

Chest Physiotherapy Statistics Showing Type and Number of Patients Treated

Table AI.1
Number of Patients Treated with Chest Physiotherapy 1974–87[a]

Fiscal Year	Number of Admissions	Number of Patients Treated	Total Admissions (%)
1974	872	372	0.43
1975	920	330	0.36
1976	1105	418	0.38
1977	1023	580	0.57
1978	1053	590	0.56
1979	1249	681	0.55
1980	1240	322[b]	0.27
1981	1324	396	0.30
1982	1505	342	0.23
1983	1692	532	0.31
1984	1953[c]	778	0.40
1985	2104	676	0.32
1986	2445	705	0.29
1987[d]	2534	401	0.16
Total	20994	7123	0.36

[a]Data collected by Department of Physical Therapy MIEMSS.
[b]Calculated from 6 months of available data.
[c]MIEMSS available beds increased from 32 to 107 in this time frame. Acute beds increased from 26 to 42. Note that although available beds increased by 64% there is only a 38% increase in acute beds.
[d]Fiscal year 1987 three staff physical therapy positions were vacant.

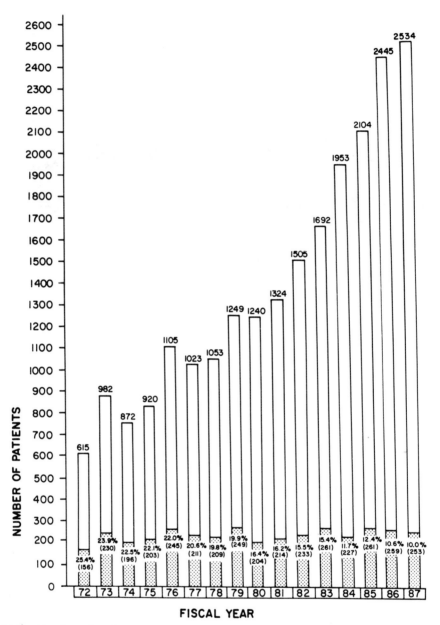

Figure AI.1. Number of patients admitted for fiscal years 1972–87. Mortality is shown as the dotted portion of the histogram. The percentage mortality varies from 25.4% to 10.0%. The number of patients this mortality represents is shown in parentheses. Data from C.F. Mackenzie and from Annual Report of MIEMSS.

Figure AI.2. Information included in this profile shows that 768/1221 (62.9%) of patients arrived directly from the scene of injury and 453/1221 indirectly after management at another medical institution. Only 520/1221 (42.6%) required surgery in the operating room and 29/1221 (2.4%) were inappropriate admissions and were discharged home directly from the admitting area. Data from M. Moody.

Distribution of 1,221 admissions* to OR,† CCRU, ICU and ward together with duration of stay and placement for 1979.

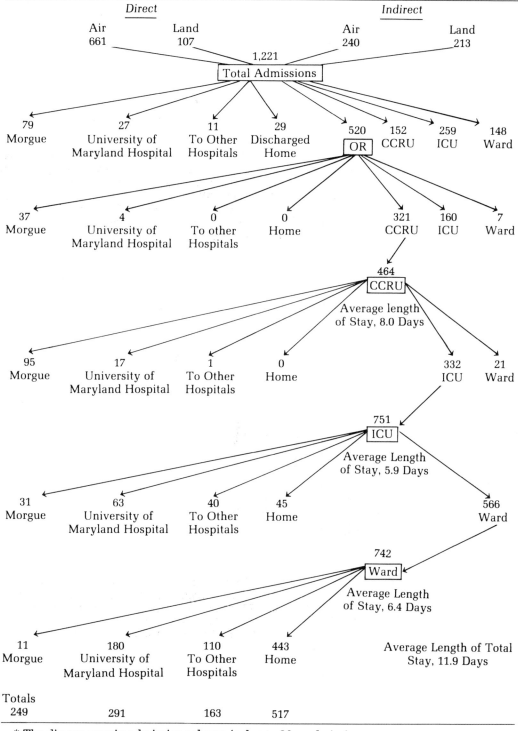

Direct   *Indirect*

| Air | Land | | Air | Land |
| 661 | 107 | | 240 | 213 |

1,221
Total Admissions

| 79 | 27 | 11 | 29 | 520 | 152 | 259 | 148 |
| Morgue | University of Maryland Hospital | To Other Hospitals | Discharged Home | OR | CCRU | ICU | Ward |

| 37 | 4 | 0 | 0 | 321 | 160 | 7 |
| Morgue | University of Maryland Hospital | To other Hospitals | Home | CCRU | ICU | Ward |

464
CCRU
Average length of Stay, 8.0 Days

| 95 | 17 | 1 | 0 | 332 | 21 |
| Morgue | University of Maryland Hospital | To Other Hospitals | Home | ICU | Ward |

751
ICU
Average Length of Stay, 5.9 Days

| 31 | 63 | 40 | 45 | 566 |
| Morgue | University of Maryland Hospital | To Other Hospitals | Home | Ward |

742
Ward
Average Length of Stay, 6.4 Days

| 11 | 180 | 110 | 443 | Average Length of Total Stay, 11.9 Days |
| Morgue | University of Maryland Hospital | To Other Hospitals | Home | |

Totals
| 249 | 291 | 163 | 517 |

* The discrepancy in admissions shown is due to 28 readmissions.
† OR, operating room.

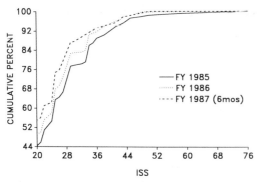

Figure AI.3. Injury severity score (ISS) above 20 is plotted against cumulative percentage of patients with that ISS admitted for years 1985–1987. There is a remarkable similarity in ISS score over the 3 years with a trend for higher scores, indicating more severe injury, with each successive year. Data from Annual Report of MIEMSS.

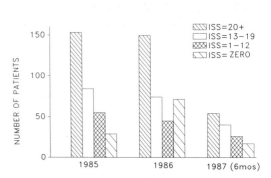

Figure AI.4. ISS for patients receiving chest physiotherapy during 1985, 1986, and 6 months of 1987. The number of patients in each category of ISS is shown on the vertical axis. Data from Trauma Registry Database and data collected by Department of Physical Therapy MIEMSS.

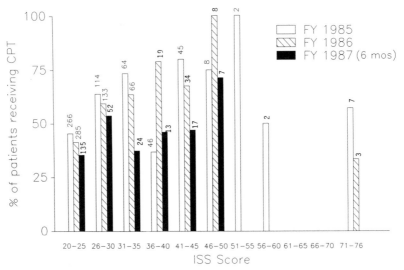

Figure AI.5. The annual number of patients (1985–87) with a specific ISS above 20 (the most severely injured patients) treated with CPT is shown as a number at the top of each bar histogram. This number of patients who were treated with CPT is plotted as a percentage of the total number of patients who had the same ISS (on the vertical axis). For example, in 1986 100% (8 of 8) patients with ISS score 46–50 received CPT. Data from Annual Report of MIEMSS and data collected by Department of Physical Therapy MIEMSS.

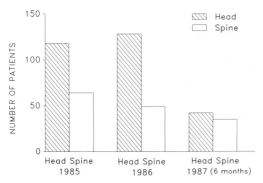

Figure AI.6. Number of severe head injured and spine injured patients who received chest physiotherapy during 1985, 1986, and 1987 (6 months). Data collected by Department of Physical Therapy MIEMSS.

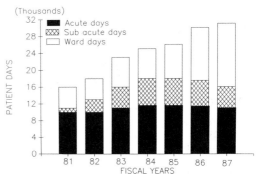

Figure AI.7. MIEMSS patient days 1981 to 1987. Note consistency of acute days and significant increase in subacute and ward days over 7 years. The increase in subacute and ward days accounts for the decrease in percentage of admissions receiving chest physiotherapy since most patients were managed with chest physiotherapy while in acute beds. Data from Annual Report of MIEMSS.

Table AI.2
Patients in Acute Beds Treated with Chest Physiotherapy, Fiscal Years 1981–1987 (July–Dec)[a]

Critical care recovery unit	1588
Intensive care unit	1229
Neurotrama unit	682
Total	3499

[a]Note: 3639 patients received chest physiotherapy in this time period; 96% of patients treated were in acute beds.

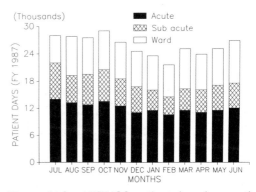

Figure AI.8. MIEMSS patient days by month in 1987. Note consistent proportions of acute, subacute, and ward days and also seasonal changes. Patient days were under 2,400 in January, February, and April. Data from Annual Report of MIEMSS.

Table AI.3
Chest Physiotherapy Treatments to Specific Lung Lobes, Fiscal Years 1981–1987[a,b]

	Percentage of Total Treatments						
	1981 (3,510)[c]	1982 (2,675)	1983 (3,915)	1984 (6,211)	1985 (5,230)	1986 (5,396)	1987 (3,888)
Lung Lobe							
Right upper lobe	3	2	4	3	4	3	5
Left upper lobe(excluding lingula)	1	1	1	1	1	1	1
Right middle lobe	3	2	3	3	2	3	4
Lingula	1	1	1	1	2	3	2
Right lower lobe	40	41	39	41	38	38	36
Left lower lobe	52	53	52	51	53	52	52
Additional coughing and deep breathing exercise sessions	249	226	348	886	530	348	313

[a]Data collected by Department of Physical Therapy MIEMSS.
[b]Note consistency of chest physiotherapy treatments to specific lung lobes. Ninety-one percent were directed to the lower lobes, 52% left lower lobe, 39% right lower lobe. Patients mobilized as part of chest physiotherapy treatment are not represented in this table.
[c]Total number of treatments.

Table AI.4
Average Chest Physiotherapy Treatment Time (Minutes), Fiscal Years 1981–1987[a,b]

Year	Time (min)
1981	29
1982	29
1983	30
1984	27
1985	29
1986	33
1987	34

[a]Data collected by Department of Physical Therapy MIEMSS.
[b]Seven-year average, 30 min per treatment.

Table AI.5
Number of Trauma and Nontrauma Patients Treated with Chest Physiotherapy, Fiscal Years 1981–1987[a]

Year	Trauma (%)	Nontrauma (%)
1981	91	9
1982	91	9
1983	95	5
1984	85	15
1985	95	5
1986	96	4
1987	96	4
7-year average	93	7

[a]Data collected by Department of Physical Therapy MIEMSS.

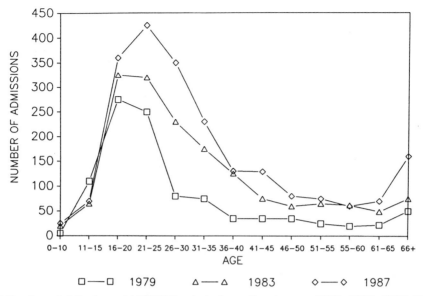

Figure AI.9. Age distribution of MIEMSS admissions, fiscal years 1979, 1983, 1987. The 16–35 year age group accounts for the majority of admissions. There is an increase in the over 65 year age group in 1987. Data from Annual Report of MIEMSS.

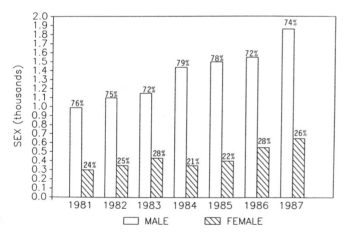

Figure AI.10. Sex distribution for MIEMSS primary admissions (excludes readmissions) for fiscal years 1981–1987. The percentage of annual admissions is shown above each histogram. Admissions increased 48% over the 7 years, although the greatest variance is only 7%. Data from Annual Report of MIEMSS.

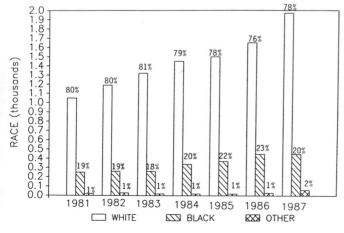

Figure AI.11. Race distribution of MIEMSS primary admissions, fiscal years 1981–1987. The annual percentage is shown above each histogram. Note consistency within 5% for black or white patients. Data from Annual Report of MIEMSS.

Table AI.6
Monitored Status of Patients Treated with Chest Physiotherapy, Fiscal Years 1981–1988 (July–December 1987)[a]

Type of Catheter	Number of Patients
Arterial	2245
Central venous (not PA)	1224
Pulmonary artery (PA)	916
Intraventricular	720

[a]Data collected by Department of Physical Therapy MIEMSS.

Table AI.7
Body Systems Injured Among Patients Receiving Chest Physiotherapy, Fiscal Years 1981–1988 (July–December 1987)[a]

Injury	Number of Patients
Head	1684 (3 CVAs)
Chest	1141
Abdomen	651
Spine	775[b]
Pelvis	417
Limbs injured	2029

[a]Data collected by Department of Physical Therapy MIEMSS.
[b]Fiscal years 1981–1987; 370 spinal injury patients had neurological deficit.

Table AI.8
Patients with Bony Injuries Who Were Treated with Chest Physiotherapy in a 34-Month Period[a]

Injury	Number of Patients
Rib fracture	226 (39 single)
Scapular fracture	16
Clavicular fracture	60
Limb fracture	379
Pelvic fracture	136
Total	817
Total number of limbs fractured	671

[a]Data collected by Department of Physical Therapy MIEMSS.

Table AI.9
Spinal Injury Level of Injury Among Patients Treated with Chest Physiotherapy, Fiscal Years 1981–1988 (July–December 1987)[a,b]

Injury	Number of Patients Treated
Cervical	446 (1 cancer)
Thoracic	153
Lumbar	84

[a]Data collected by Department of Physical Therapy MIEMSS.
[b]Data available on 683 of 775 patients; 297 of the 775 spinal injury patients received chest physiotherapy on a turning frame.

Table AI.10
Orthopedic Fixation Devices in Use on Patients Treated with Chest Physiotherapy, Fiscal Years 1981–1988 (July–December 1987)[a,b]

Device	Number of Patients
Internal fixation	452
External fixator	380
Skeletal traction	148
Spinal rods	83
Neufeld traction	53

[a]Data collected by Department of Physical Therapy MIEMSS.
[b]In the first 6 months of fiscal year 1988 20 patients were also treated with continuous passive motion of the hip and knee.

APPENDIX II

Abbreviations and Symbols

AP	anteroposterior
ARDS	adult respiratory distress syndrome
a-ADCO$_2$	arterial alveolar carbon dioxide difference
A-aDO$_2$	alveolar arterial oxygen difference
AV	assisted ventilation
A-$\bar{v}$DO$_2$	arterial venous oxygen difference
C	cervical or centigrade
CCRU	critical care recovery unit
cm	centimeter
CO$_2$	carbon dioxide
COPD	chronic obstructive pulmonary disease
CPAP	continuous positive airway pressure
CPM	continuous passive motion
CPP	cerebral perfusion pressure
CPT	chest physiotherapy
CNS	central nervous system
CSF	cerebrospinal fluid
C$_T$	total lung/thorax compliance
cv	closing volume
CXR	chest x-ray
DNA	deoxyribonucleic acid
ECG	electrocardiogram
EEG	electroencephalogram
EMG	electromyography
ERV	expiratory reserve volume
F	fahrenheit
FET	forced expiratory technique
FEV$_1$	forced expiratory volume in one second
FIO$_2$	fraction of inspired oxygen
FLS	flow limiting segment
FRC	functional residual capacity
FVC	forced vital capacity
gm	gram
GPB	glossophrayngeal breathing
HD	head down
HF	head flat
HFCWC	high-frequency chest wall compression
HFV	high frequency ventilation
Hg	mercury
H/L ratio	high/flow amplitude electromyogram ratio
HMD	hyaline membrane disease
H$_2$O	water
Hz	Hertz or cycles per second
ICP	intracranial pressure
ICU	intensive care unit
ID	internal diameter
I/E	inspiratory to expiratory ratio
IMT	inspiratory muscle training
IMV	intermittent mandatory ventilation
IPNV	intermittent positive negative ventilation
IPPB	intermittent positive pressure breathing
IPPV	intermittent positive pressure ventilation
IS	incentive spirometry
ISS	injury severity score
I.V.	intravenous
kg	kilogram
L	lumbar
LLL	left lower lobe
LUL	left upper lobe
MASTrousers	military antishock trousers

MIEMSS	Maryland Institute for Emergency Medical Services Systems	$\dot{Q}_t$	cardiac output per mintue
mg	milligram	R_{aw}	airway resistance
ml	milliliter	R_{pul}	pulmonary vascular resistance
mm	millimeter	R_{syst}	systemic vascular resistance
MSVC	maximum sustained ventilatory capacity	**RDS**	respiratory distress syndrome
N	normal	**RH**	relative humidity
N_2O	nitrous oxide	**RLL**	right lower lobe
NHLI	National Heart and Lung Institute	**RML**	right middle lobe
NHLBI	National Heart, Lung and Blood Institute	**RNA**	ribonucleic acid
		RUL	right upper lobe
O_2	oxygen	SaO_2	arterial oxygen saturation
P	pressure		
p	probability	**SD**	standard deviation
$PaCO_2$	partial pressure of arterial carbon dioxide	**SE**	standard error
		T	thoracic
$\bar{P}_{art}$	mean arterial pressure	$TcPO_2$	transcutaneous oxygen tension
PaO_2	partial pressure of arterial oxygen	$TcPCO_2$	transcutaneous carbon dioxide tension
PCA	patient controlled analgesia	**TENS**	transcutaneous electrical nerve stimulation
P_{CWP}	pulmonary capillary wedge pressure		
P_{EE}	end-expiratory pressure	**TLC**	total lung capacity
PEEP	positive end-expiratory pressure	T_{max}	maximum daily temperature
PEF	peak expiratory flow	**TMC**	tracheal mucus clearance
PEP	positive expiratory pressure	**torr**	the pressure supporting 1 mm Hg at 0°C and standard gravity
Pe_{Max}	maximum expiratory mouth pressure		
$P_{ET}CO_2$	partial pressure of end-tidal carbon dioxide	**V**	volume
		VC	vital capacity
$P_{ET}O_2$	partial pressure of end-tidal oxygen	V_d	dead space volume
		$\dot{V}_E$	expired minute ventilation
PFT	pulmonary function test		
pH	$-\log_{10}[H^+]$	$\dot{V}O_2$	oxygen consumption per minute
P_{IE}	end-inspiratory pressure		
PI_{max}	maximum inspiratory mouth pressure	$\dot{V}/\dot{Q}$	ventilation/perfusion per minute
PmCrit	critical mouth pressure	V_t	tidal volume
P_{max}	maximum airway pressure	**WBC**	white blood cell count
		x-ray	roentgenogram
PNIP	peak negative inspiratory pressure	μ	micron (micrometer)
		$\downarrow$	decrease
PsO_2	skin oxygen tension	$\uparrow$	increase
PT	physical therapist	$\nearrow\searrow$	slightly increased or decreased
$P_{tc}O_2$	transcutaneous oxygen tension		
		%	percent
$P\bar{V}O_2$	partial pressure of mixed venous oxygen	$<$	less than
		$>$	greater than
$\dot{Q}_s/\dot{Q}_t$	intrapulmonary shunt	Δ	change

Summary of Chest Physiotherapy Treatment and Evaluation

FREQUENCY OF TREATMENT

As Symptoms and Signs Indicate

1. Ideal frequency.
2. Therapist must be well trained in clinical evaluation.
3. Close communication with the physician is essential.
4. Works well with experienced therapists assigned to a specific unit.

Four Hourly

1. Usual frequency that is necessary for critically ill patients.
2. Treatment is continued throughout a 24-hr period for mechanically ventilated patients.
3. Spontaneously breathing patients in no acute distress usually benefit from sleep at night; cooperation is then improved with daytime treatments.

More Frequently than Four Hourly

1. Indicated for patients with copious secretions that are not removed by four hourly chest physiotherapy treatments.
2. Patients with closed head injuries and secretion retention who are limited in the amount of time they may remain in the head-down position.
3. The need for treatment more frequently than four hourly should be reevaluated after 12–24 hr of treatment.
4. Increased frequency of treatment often makes optimal treatments impossible because of multiple other therapeutic interventions.

Less Frequently than Four Hourly

1. Mobilized patients.
2. Patients who clear their secretions spontaneously with deep breathing and coughing.
3. Patients with minimal secretions with or without radiological evidence of atelectasis or pneumonia.

4. Acute lobar collapse usually responds to 1–2 vigorous chest physiotherapy treatments and may then be replaced by patient mobilization.

ROUTINE EVALUATION OF CHEST PHYSIOTHERAPY

During Mechanical Ventilation

1. Examine the patient as previously described (pp. 73–80). Particularly auscultate the chest over the area to be treated and compare with the opposite side. A sigh or mandatory breath may be useful in evaluation of breath sounds.
2. Note the mode of ventilation. Identify tidal volume, minute ventilation, inspired oxygen concentration, and respiratory rate. Measure airway pressures with the bed flat and the patient supine, calm, and in phase during a tidal volume ventilated breath.
3. Obtain the most recent values for arterial blood gas analysis.
4. Obtain information about the most recent chest x-ray.
5. Position the patient appropriately. Make a note of any change in vital signs, auscultatory findings, ventilator airway pressures, and volumes when the patient is correctly positioned.
6. Apply therapy as described in the section "Essentials of Chest Physiotherapy Treatment."
7. Note changes in airway pressures. A fall in peak airway pressure (fall in R_{aw}) usually indicates secretion removal from the central larger airways. A fall in plateau or end-expiratory pressure (increase in C_T) usually indicates secretion removal from more peripheral smaller airways.
8. Note changes in auscultation of the chest. Changes in the character of the breath sounds from bronchial to vesicular or in the clearance of adventitial sounds or in improvement of air entry are favorable findings.
9. Note sputum volume removed. This may be measured.
10. Clinical examination of the chest and measurement of airway pressure (in the postural drainage position) are repeated throughout therapy. Clearance of the chest to auscultation, increased C_T, and termination of sputum production are all suitable end points for therapy.
11. The patient is returned to the supine flat position, the chest is reexamined, airway pressures and volumes are remeasured, and vital signs noted. Arterial blood gases are analyzed if PaO_2/FIO_2 was less than 250 before therapy.
12. If a complete lobar atelectasis was present before therapy, a chest x-ray is repeated.

During Spontaneous Respiration

1. Examine the patient. Particularly observe the rate and pattern of respirations and use of accessory muscles. Auscultate the chest over the area to be treated and compare with the opposite side.
2. Obtain the most recent values for arterial blood gas analysis.
3. Obtain information about the most recent chest x-ray.
4. Position the patient appropriately. Make note of any complaints of discomfort, dyspnea, or wheezing. Observe the patient for appearance of cyanosis or change in respiratory rate. Reexamine the patient in the postural drainage position. Observe ECG or other monitoring devices.
5. Apply therapy as described in the section "Essentials of Chest Physiotherapy Treatment."
6. Note changes in auscultation of the chest. Changes in the character of the breath sounds from bronchial to vesicular or in the clearance of adventitial sounds or in improvement of air entry are favorable findings.
7. Note sputum volume removed. This may be measured.

8. Clinical examination of the chest is repeated throughout therapy. Clearance of the chest to auscultation and termination of sputum production are suitable end points for therapy.
9. The patient is returned to the supine position, the chest is reexamined, and vital signs noted. Arterial blood gases are analyzed if PaO_2/FIO_2 was less than 250 before therapy.
10. If a complete lobar atelectasis was present before therapy, a chest x-ray is repeated.

POSITIONING THE PATIENT FOR CHEST PHYSIOTHERAPY TREATMENT

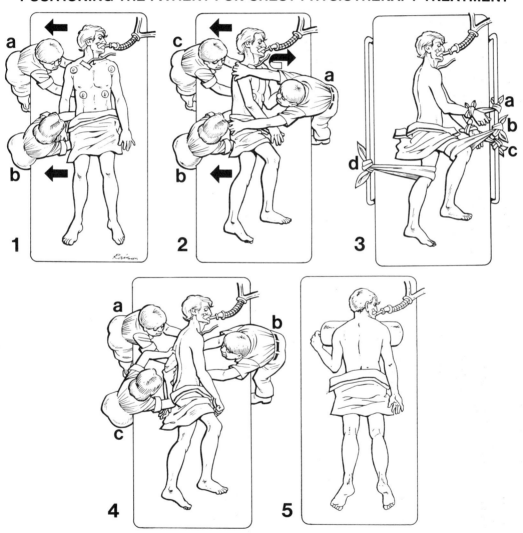

Figure AIII.1. **(1)** Both hands are placed under the trunk (**a**) while a second person places both hands under the hips (**b**). The patient is lifted to the side of the bed. **(2)** (**a**) With one hand over the uppermost shoulder and the other over the uppermost hip, the patient is pulled onto the side. (Crossing the patient's legs prior to turning facilitates rolling the patient.) (**b**) A second person lifts the hips back. (**c**) For obese or difficult patients, a third person may simultaneously lift the shoulders back. **(3)** To keep an agitated patient side-lying, the wrists are restrained (**a** and **b**), and sheets are tied around the thighs to the bed rail. The upper hip is flexed (**c**) and the lower hip is extended (**d**). **(4)** To turn the patient from the side to prone, two people (**a** and **b**) lift the trunk while a third person (**c**) pulls the dependent arm under the patient. **(5)** If a tracheal tube is present, while two people hold up the patient's trunk, the third places a roll under the upper thorax. The patient remains positioned as in Part 5.

Essentials of Chest Physiotherapy Treatment

Treatment Components	Purpose	How to Perform	When to Use	Things to Avoid	Important Details to Remember
Postural drainage	Mobilize retained secretions through assistance of gravity	Patient positioned so that involved segmental bronchus is uppermost (see pp. 97–99 for postural drainage positions)	When coughing or suctioning, breathing exercises, forced expiratory technique, and patient mobilization are not adequate to clear retained secretions	Avoid significant changes in patient's vital signs, increase in intracranial pressure, and stress to intravascular lines and indwelling tubes	Patient must be properly positioned for bronchial drainage of the involved lung segment; this can be attained despite the presence of multiple injuries, monitoring equipment, and lines (p. 101)
Percussion	As an adjunct to postural drainage for mobilization of secretions	Rhythmical clapping of cupped hands over bare skin or thin material covering area of lung involvement; performed during inspiration and expiration	Same as above	Avoid skin redness or petechiae (indicates improper hand positioning by therapist, or patient coagulopathy)	May be performed in the presence of rib fractures, chest tubes, and subcutaneous emphysema; should produce a hollow sound; should not cause undue pain; does not need to be forceful to be effective if performed properly
Vibration	As an adjunct to postural drainage for mobilization of secretions	Intermittent chest wall compression over area of lung involvement; performed during expiration only	Same as above	Avoid excessive pressure, pinching, or shearing of soft tissue	Not recommended for use over rib fractures or unstable thoracic spine injuries; be sure to vibrate chest wall, not just shake soft tissue; forcefulness should vary according to patient's needs and tolerance
Breathing exercises	Assists in removing secretions, relaxation, and to increase thoracic cage mobility and tidal volume; inspiratory resistive devices or weights to improve ventilatory muscle strength/endurance	Patient taught to produce a full inspiration followed by a controlled expiration; use hand placement for sensory feedback; leaning forward posture used with COPD; increased resistance applied during inspiration using resistors or abdominal weights (see p. 119)	For use with spontaneously breathing patients	Avoid use of undesired respiratory muscles and fatigue	May be used independently or in conjunction with other chest physiotherapy techniques; patient must be cooperative; breathing exercises aimed at relaxation should not increase the work of breathing; strength versus endurance should be considered with respiratory muscle training
Coughing	Removal of secretions from the larger airways	Steps: 1. Inspiratory gasp 2. Closing of the glottis 3. Contraction of expiration muscles 4. Opening of the glottis (see p. 155)	For use with spontaneously breathing patients	Avoid bronchospasm induced by repetitive coughing	Coughing is less effective in tracheally intubated patients; coughing ability can be improved by manual support of the patient's incision and tracheal stoma, following tube removal; an effective cough is preceded by a large inspiration; methods of cough stimulation, including "huffing," vibration, summed breathing, external tracheal compression, and oral pharyngeal stimulation, are used (see p. 162)

Technique	Purpose	Procedure	Indication	Precautions	Comments
Forced expiratory technique	As an adjunct to clear excess secretions	Patient performs a controlled diaphragmatic inspiration, followed by huffing, or forced expirations from mid to low lung volume	Same as above; used as an alternative to other breathing exercises and coughing	Avoid excessive fatigue	May be used independently or with other chest physiotherapy techniques; requires patient cooperation; use not reported in patients with tracheal tubes; described for patients with cystic fibrosis and other chronic lung diseases; may be as effective as postural drainage or manual techniques for these patients
Suctioning	Removal of secretions from the larger airways	Use aseptic technique 1. Provide supplemental oxygen, if indicated 2. Fully insert suction catheter without applying suction; be gentle 3. Apply suction while withdrawing catheter 4. Reexpand lung with mechanical ventilator or resuscitator bag 5. PEEP, tidal volume, and FIO_2, are better maintained using a port adapter (see p. 177)	Tracheal suctioning for use only with patients who have an artificial airway in place	Avoid hypoxemia (cyanosis and significant changes in vital signs) and cardiac dysrhythmias, mechanical trauma and bacterial contamination of tracheobronchial tree, and increase in intracranial pressure	In intubated patients, suctioning is performed routinely and is an integral part of chest physiotherapy; frequency is determined by the quantity of secretions; the suctioning procedure should be limited to a total of 15 sec; the suction catheter can reach only to the level of the main stem bronchus; it is more difficult to cannulate the left main stem bronchus than the right; nasotracheal suctioning should be avoided (see p. 179)
Bagging	Provide artificial ventilation; restore oxygen and reexpand the lungs after suctioning	Attach the manual resuscitator bag to an oxygen source, then carefully connect it to the patient's tracheal tube; squeeze bag rhythmically in coordination with the patient's own breathing pattern; expiration is passive (see p. 181)	Before and after suctioning patients who are not mechanically ventilated and who cannot spontaneously take a deep breath	Avoid barotrauma and tracheal irritation	Bagging can be used to improve clinical assessment of breath sounds; it is also used in conjunction with vibration when treating patients not breathing deeply; hyperinflation can produce alterations in cardiac output and intracranial pressure; know the limitations of manual resuscitator bags at your facility
Patient mobilization	To prevent the detrimental sequelae of bedrest and immobilization; to decrease rehabilitation time	Turning and passively positioning the patient; appropriate splint usage; passive and active range of motion; active and resistive exercises; sitting, standing, and ambulating the patient	Used to some degree with every patient according to patient's diagnosis and tolerance	Avoid patient fatigue, stress to intravascular lines, and indwelling tubes, orthostatic hypotension, significant changes in vital signs, and dyspnea	Mobilization is possible to some degree for every patient; minimal supplies are needed for mobilization; emphasis should be placed on functional activities; proper positioning may decrease contracture formation and spasticity; ECG leads and arterial and central monitoring lines should be temporarily disconnected from the recording module during ambulation; at the physician's discretion, chest tubes and abdominal sumps may be disconnected from wall suction to allow ambulation

Duration, Type, and Frequency of Interventions in Four Critically Ill Patients

To document the interventions likely to cause cardiac or respiratory changes, four critically ill patients were observed in the CCRU at MIEMSS between 8 A.M. and 4 P.M. All interventions were recorded and timed. The weekday of observation was randomly chosen, but the patients observed were four of the most ill patients in the CCRU.

PATIENT #1

Problem: Gunshot wound to abdomen with lacerations of liver, right renal vein, gallbladder, and inferior vena cava, renal failure
Admission: 12 days previously
Monitors: ECG, temperature, Foley catheter, central venous and radial arterial lines, orogastric tube, abdominal sump

Medications:

Amphojel	Gentamycin	Parenteral nutrition
Ticarcillin	Morphine sulfate	Dopamine infusion
Afrin spray	Blood and fresh frozen	
Tylenol	plasma	

State: Sedated, mechanically ventilated through translaryngeal tracheal tube

Time:	8:00	9:00	10:00	11:00	12:00	13:00	14:00	15:00
Temperature (°C):	39.2		39.4	39.4	39.3	39.2	39.3	39.4

8:10–11	Ventilator adjusted
8:11–20	Physicians' rounds
8:22	Bed adjusted
8:23–25	Vital signs taken
8:25–50	Physicians discussing patient
8:50–00	Vital signs and blood taken; respiratory function testing
9:20–25	Examined by chest physical therapist
9:27–57	Chest physiotherapy
9:41	Dopamine infusion rate decreased
10:01	Nurse applied cream to perineum
10:00–10	Physician altering ventilator
10:15	Mouth suctioned

10:25–55	Clean abdominal sump and wound
10:47	New intravenous line started
10:53	Dialysis started
10:55–00	Suture of abdominal wound that had minimally dehisced
11:00–12	Nurse dressed wound
11:08	Physician working on mass spectrometer attachment to ventilator
11:18	Dopamine infusion readjusted
11:21	Fluid infusion increased
11:21	Bed position readjusted
11:25–30	Vital signs taken
11:30–35	Ventilator adjusted
11:34	Plasma given and infusion rate of other fluids increased
11:43	Arterial and central venous lines flushed
11:45	Trachea suctioned
11:47–02	Physician irrigating abdominal sump tube; dressing of internal jugular central venous insertion site
12:03	Intravenous infusion rate adjusted
1:40	Morphine given intravenously
1:45–55	Ankles bandaged
2:00–07	Manual ventilation by resuscitator; mouth suctioned and mouth care performed
2:40–50	ECG trace taken
3:30	Vital signs taken
3:47–49	Eyes checked; eye drops added
3:51	Nurse auscultated chest and abdomen
3:54	Tube feeding
3:58	Tracheal tube suctioned
3:59	Nose suctioned
4:00	Patient still on dialysis (started 10:53)

PATIENT #2

Problems: Ruptured left diaphragm
Right hip fracture
Left femur fracture with Neufeld traction
Facial fracture and lacerations
Hematuria from ruptured bladder

Admission: 20 days previously

Monitors: ECG, temperature, indwelling arterial line, Foley catheter, chest tube on left, nasogastric tube

Medications:

Maalox	Valium	Tobramycin
Amphojel	Tylenol	Parenteral nutrition

State: Patient is conscious and mechanically ventilated through a tracheostomy tube and was on a Roto-Rest bed

Time:	8:00	9:00	10:00	11:00	12:00	13:00	14:00	15:00	16:00
Temperature (°F)	99.8		100.2		100		100		100.2

8:20–23	Ventilator adjusted
8:23	Vital signs taken
8:25–28	Physicians' examination and rounds
8:30–31	Nurse filled water in Pleurivac
8:33–36	Mouth care
8:37–45	Tracheostomy area cleaned
8:46–48	Physicians' examination of patient
8:48–51	Nurse placed intravenous line in arm

8:45–01	Nurse cleaned intravenous site
9:02	Urine volume measured and recorded
9:03–04	Tracheal suctioning and manual ventilation while tracheal stoma is suctioned
9:05–10	Nurse shaving patient
9:10–15	Cleaned other intravenous sites
9:26–27	Tracheal suctioning and manual ventilation with resuscitator
9:29–30	Steinmann pin in left femur cleaned
9:30–35	Teeth brushed
9:32	Nails cut
9:36–42	Trachea suctioned; patient lifted further up the bed
9:42–47	Roto-Rest bed fixtures rearranged
9:47	Bed turned on to right side
9:55	Bed turned further on same side
9:56–10	Chest physical therapist examined patient and chart
10:10	Bed starts rotating
10:24	Bed stopped rotating (15 min); trachea suctioned
10:27	Dextrose started intravenously
10:32–35	Manual resuscitator bag ventilation while patient is suctioned by nurse
10:40	Bed starts rotating
11:30–35	Vital signs and blood taken; neck cleaned
11:45	Trachea suctioned
12:05	Blood taken
12:07	Urine volume measured and charted
12:09	Trachea suctioned
12:13–15	Bed turned supine; rotation stopped (93 min); bed fixtures taken off
12:15–18	Patient pulled further up the bed; fixtures put back in place on bed; bed turned to the left side
12:18–25	Cleaned perineum; repositioned bed in horizontal position
12:25–50	Bed began rotating; eye drops given; bed rotation stopped (25 min)
12:50–1:30	Chest physiotherapy given; bed rotation stopped
1:30	Nasogastric feeding
1:30	Bed rotation begun; stopped at 2:06 (36 min)
2:06–10	Cleaned perineum
2:19–25	Removed bed fixtures after rotation was stopped; patient moved further up the bed; replaced bed fixtures
2:30	Bed turned to right side
2:35	Urine volume measured and recorded; bed turned to right tilt side
2:43–50	Manual ventilation with resuscitator while the ventilator tubing was changed
2:50	Rotating bed started; stopped 10 min later
3:00–10	Chest physical therapist examined the patient; patient position readjusted on the Roto-Rest bed
3:10	Chest physiotherapy given for 20 min (no bed rotation)
3:35	Bed repositioned: rotation started for 10 min
3:45	Vital signs taken; fixtures taken off; patient adjusted on bed
3:48	Urine volume measured and recorded
3:50	Bed fixtures replaced
3:50–53	Patient given range of motion exercises in bed
3:53–4:00	Bed rotation restarted (8 min)

PATIENT #3

Problem: Extensive gangrenous cellulitis of the left thigh
Admission: 16 days previously
Monitors: ECG; temperature; triple-lumen, thermistor-tipped, pulmonary artery catheter; radial arterial line; Foley catheter; nasogastric tube
Medications:

Cortisporin	Amphojel	Insulin
Silvadene	Morphine sulfate	Hyperalimentation
Ticarcillin	Plasma	Blood
Tobramycin	Lasix	

State: Conscious and mechanically ventilated through a translaryngeal tracheal tube

Time:	8:00	9:00	10:00	11:00	12:00	13:00	14:00	15:00
Temperature (°F)	99.8						98.9	

8:00–10	Dressing wound
8:15–18	Blood intravenous line started
8:22–26	Vital signs taken
8:25–27	Intravenous infusion rate increased
8:28–32	Nasogastric feeding
8:28–33	Physicians' examination and rounds
8:33–43	Nurse cleaned wound area and changed dressing
8:47	Given intravenous antibiotics
8:50–00	Vital signs and blood taken
9:00–06	Physicians' examination
9:07–30	Wound area cleaned and dressing changed
9:34	Fluid infusion rate changed
9:41	Foley catheter taped into place on leg
9:42–49	New intravenous line started
10:17–22	Patient moved to a stretcher
10:37	Fluid infusion rate adjusted
10:53	Patient taken to hyperbaric chamber and for whirlpool and debridement
2:35	Patient returned
2:30	Patient reattached to monitors
2:30–55	Dressing of gangrenous wound
3:00	Arterial blood drawn; line flushed
3:15–25	Nurse removed bandage
3:25–42	Suture procedure on wound
3:42–50	Wound bandaged
3:53	Patient lifted to put sheet underneath

PATIENT #4

Problem: 19-year-old female ejected from automobile; bilateral temporal contusions, subarachnoid hematoma, multiple facial and mouth lacerations, left pneumothorax

Admission: 15 days earlier

Monitors: ECG, Foley catheter, central venous and arterial lines, Richmond screw, orogastric tube

Medications:

Pentobarbital	Tylenol	Nafcillin
Nystatin	Sublimaze	Lipids
KCL	Lidocaine	Alupent

State: In Pentobarbital coma, mechanically ventilated through a tracheostomy tube

Time:	8:00	9:00	10:00	11:00	12:00	13:00	14:00
Temperature:					101.8		102

Time	Intervention	HR	MABP	PA	ICP	CPP
8:35	Change ventilator tubing					
8:40	Resting on right side					
	Head of bed 45°	97	96	17	8	88
8:43	Calibrating respiratory monitoring system	97	95	17	9	86

Time	Intervention	HR	MABP	PA	ICP	CPP
8:43–8:57	Resting (same position)	100	95	17	8	87
8:58–9:02	Physicians examining patient	99	106	19	7	99
9:06–9:25	Resting (same position)	105	106	21	11	95
9:25	Lower head of bed (0° incline)	112	97	19	26	71
9:26	Nurse administers sublimase	117	101	19	27	74
9:27	Nurse rolls patient to side	106	98	26	38	60
9:28	Roll patient back supine	100	94	20	34	60
9:29	Uncross legs, preparation for pull up in bed	103	93	17	29	64
9:30	Pull straight up in bed	106	91	17	30	61
9:31	Raise head of bed 45°	96	97	22	15	82
9:31	Readjust ventilator tubing	100	100	21	10	90
9:32	Retape catheter tubing	94	96	20	04	92
9:34	Retape arterial and intravenous line	85	98	19	03	95
9:37	Resting	86	95	19	01	94
9:39	x-ray	102	118	25	02	116
9:40	After x-ray and lift	93	99	23	08	91
9:41–9:43	Lower head of bed 0°	112	94	21	20	74
9:44	Turn onto left side	116	92	26	30	62
9:44	Raise head of bed 45° (still on side)	109	103	26	19	84
9:45–9:47	Reposition head and arms	119	146	26	24	122
9:48	Lower head slightly	101	124	23	18	106
9:49	Resting	98	110	22	16	94
9:51	Raise head back to 45°	94	102	22	15	87
9:52–9:54	Physical therapy (ankle exercises)	116	106	24	15	91
9:55	Readjust neck collar	120	102	26	17	85
9:56	Readjust legs	117	150	25	21	129
9:57	Bagging	127	138	42	35	103
9:58	Reposition (uncross legs)	124	101	26	18	83
10:00–10:02	Suctioning	121	114	35	33	81
	Suctioning	123	120	43	48	72
	Bagging	123	116	37	56	60
	Suctioning	120	111	49	52	59
	Bagging	126	117	31	30	87
	Mouth care	126	115	31	20	95
10:02	Lidocaine instillation through tracheostomy	116	116	27	30	86
10:03	Readjust arterial line	114	122	28	37	85
10:05	Resting	101	107	24	25	82
10:07	Pentothal	109	98	23	07	91
10:10	Resting on left side	91	103	19	04	99
10:15–10:20	Shivering	115	109	21	8	101
10:21	Adjustments to lower arterial line	121	124	24	13	111
10:23	Resting	121	107	23	14	156
10:24	Physical therapy (goniometry)	116	121	21	10	111
10:26	Resting	109	104	21	7	97
11:24	Checking pupils—nurse talking	118	108	21	9	99
11:30–11:40	Resting	125	117	24	13	104
11:41	Gagging	117	107	33	22	85
11:42	Suction of mouth	120	110	23	14	96
11:43	Nurse talking to patient	123	112	25	16	96
11:49	Resting	119	112	24	15	97
11:51	Sublimase given	124	117	23	11	106
11:52	Head of bed lowered (0°)	106	92	16	19	73
11:53	Pulled up in bed	113	85	17	20	65
11:54	Rolled to right side	114	96	19	27	69
11:55	Head up 45°	104	102	22	16	86
11:56	Alupent inhaler	104	101	21	11	90
12:00	Nursing care	97	103	19	9	94
12:03	Wedging PA line	87	104	19	8	96
12:08	Application of lacrilube ointment around eyes	108	127	22	11	116

Time	Intervention	HR	MABP	PA	ICP	CPP
12:09	Karaphate down N/G tube	110	112	25	13	99
12:10	Application of lotion on buttocks/thigh	110	107	24	15	92
12:12	Thermometer inserted	118	107	25	18	89
12:12	Rolled head flat	109	95	21	25	70
12:14–12:16	Chest P.T. by nurse	110	91	22	23	68
12:16	Na pentothal given i.v.	104	105	23	19	86
12:17	Thermometer (101.8) taken out	95	97	19	18	79
12:17	Resume chest P.T.	102	98	18	18	80
12:20	Stop chest P.T.	94	98	18	19	79
12:22	Suctioning	118	123	60	67	56
	Bagging	128	104	57	50	54
	Suctioning	128	112	24	34	78
	Bagging	120	108	35	58	50
	Suctioning	130	112	57	75	37
	Bagging	114	126	45	55	71
12:25	End suctioning	125	120	31	40	80
12:26	Head of bed up	119	123	31	41	82
12:27–12:28	Suction out mouth	128	125	42	45	80
12:30–12:35	Resting—45° of back up—on right side	104	119	23	10	109
1:00–1:14	Resting—same position	108	109	22–25	8	111
1:15	Gagging	121	112	33	16	96
1:20–1:30	Resting	119	113	23	9	104
1:34–1:38	Dressing change (left chest tube)—start	120	108	25	14	94
1:39	Suction—mouth	126	115	35	26	89
1:43–1:44	Discontinue pentobarbital	117	110	22	12	98
1:45	Auscultation	114	108	22	10	98
1:48	Resting	111	107	21	11	96
1:50	Insertion of thermometer	102	104	20	11	93
1:51	Nurse speaking to patient for response	115	105	22	10	95
1:55	Hanging intralipid infusion	117	109	22	10	99
1:58	Resting	125	123	38	27	96
1:58	Suctioning	119	147	60	56	91
	Bagging	121	138	49	25	113
	Suctioning	118	135	51	46	89
2:00	Bagging	119	130	35	40	90
	Suctioning	118	125	28	31	94
	Bagging	118	126	32	35	91
2:01	Suction by mouth	121	123	29	21	102
2:02	Head down	114	113	23	28	85
2:03	Rolled on right side—remove thermometer	116	113	23	28	85
2:04	Cleaned up and lotioned	114	108	25	28	80
2:05	Turn back	116	109	22	26	83
2:05	Rolled to left side	105	105	21	30	75
2:06–2:12	Head of bed raised	107	157	26	18	139
2:13	Resting (left side—head of bed at 45°)	111	108	21	6	102
2:14–2:49	Visitors	103	104	20	6	98
2:50	Na pentothal given i.v.	112	108	24	9	99
2:50	Suctioning	111	149	56	30	119
2:51	Bagging	118	124	37	22	102
2:52	Suction mouth	120	122	26	14	108
2:56–3:04	Arterial line, reposition patient	112	136	23	11	125
3:30	Resting—wedging PA catheter	108	109	27	11	98
3:32	Pupils checked	112	111	28	11	100
3:37	Resting	106	109	26	11	98
3:45	Resting	111	116	29	10	106
3:46–47	Gagging	116	114	36	14	100
3:48	Cough/gagging	123	116	50	27	89
3:50	Resting	115	120	29	12	108
3:55	Occupational therapy	119	113	28	13	100
4:00	Resting	105	110	26	11	99

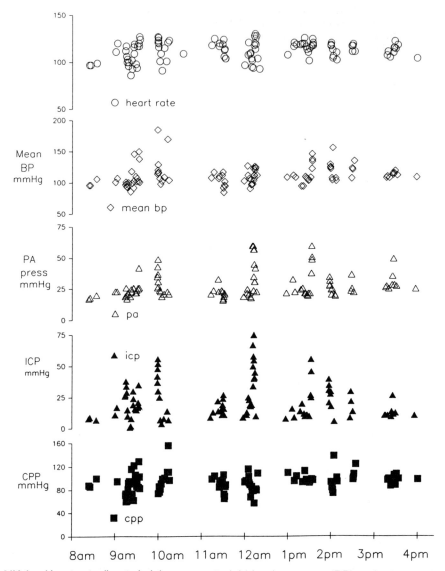

Figure AIV.1.   Heart rate (beats/min), mean arterial blood pressure (BP), pulmonary artery (PA), intracranial (ICP), and cerebral perfusion pressure (CPP) are plotted against time from 8 A.M. to 4 P.M. for Patient 4. The raw data are tabulated. The plotted data in this figure illustrate the great variability in all these measured parameters. Because of therapeutic interventions or general nursing care it is extremely difficult, if not impossible, for these vital signs to reflect only the effects of a single intervention such as chest physiotherapy.

Index